Acquired Immune Deficiency Syndrome

ACQUIRED IMMUNE DEFICIENCY SYNDROME

Biological, Medical, Social, and Legal Issues

Second Edition

GERALD J. STINE

University of North Florida, Jacksonville

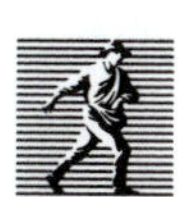

PRENTICE HALL, *Englewood Cliffs, New Jersey 07632*

Library of Congress Cataloging–in–Publication Data

Stine, Gerald James.
Acquired immune deficiency syndrome: biological, medical, social, and legal issues/Gerald J. Stine. –2nd ed.
p. cm
Includes bibliographical references and Index.
ISBN 0-13-356890-3
1. AIDS (Disease) I. Title.
RC607.A26S75 1996
362.1'969792—dc20 95-2430
CIP

Editorial/production supervision
and interior design: ***Carol Bollati-Barbara***
Acquisitions editor: ***David Kendric Brake***
Cover design: ***Bruce Kenselaar***
Manufacturing buyer: ***Trudy Pisciotti***

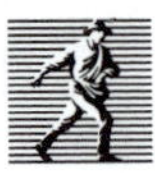

A Simon & Schuster Company
Englewood Cliffs, New Jersey 07632

Printed in the United States of America

10 9 8 7 6 5 4 3 2

ISBN 0-13-356890-3

PRENTICE-HALL INTERNATIONAL (UK) LIMITED, LONDON
PRENTICE-HALL OF AUSTRALIA PTY. LIMITED, SYDNEY
PRENTICE-HALL CANADA INC., TORONTO
PRENTICE-HALL HISPANOAMERICANA, S.A., MEXICO
PRENTICE-HALL OF INDIA PRIVATE LIMITED, NEW DELHI
PRENTICE-HALL OF JAPAN, INC., TOKYO
SIMON & SCHUSTER ASIA PTE. LTD., SINGAPORE
EDITORA PRENTICE-HALL DO BRASIL, LTDA., RIO DE JANEIRO

This book is dedicated to those who have died of AIDS,
those who have HIV disease,
and to those who must prevent the spread of this plague—

EVERYONE, EVERYWHERE.

Contents in Brief

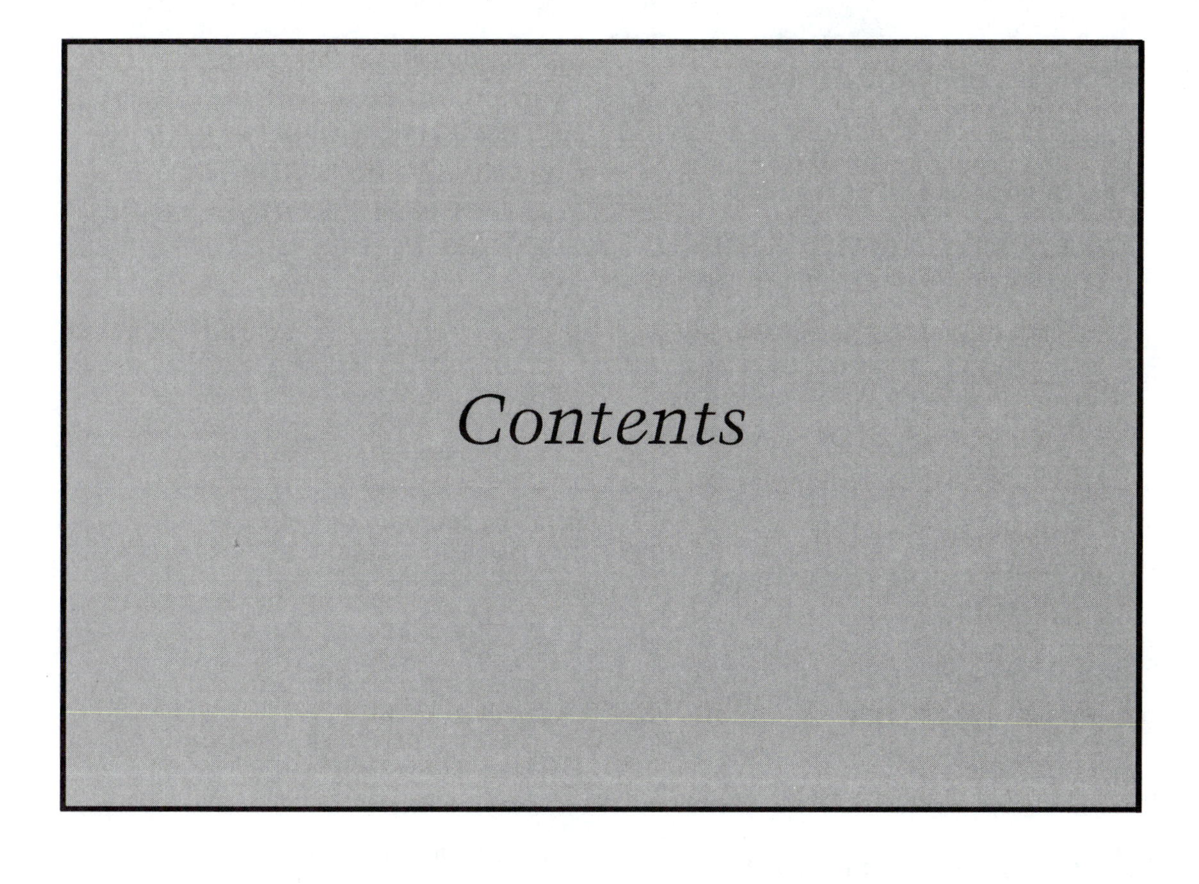
Contents

12 Testing for Human Immunodeficiency Virus 327

13 Counseling for HIV Testing, HIV Disease, and AIDS 355

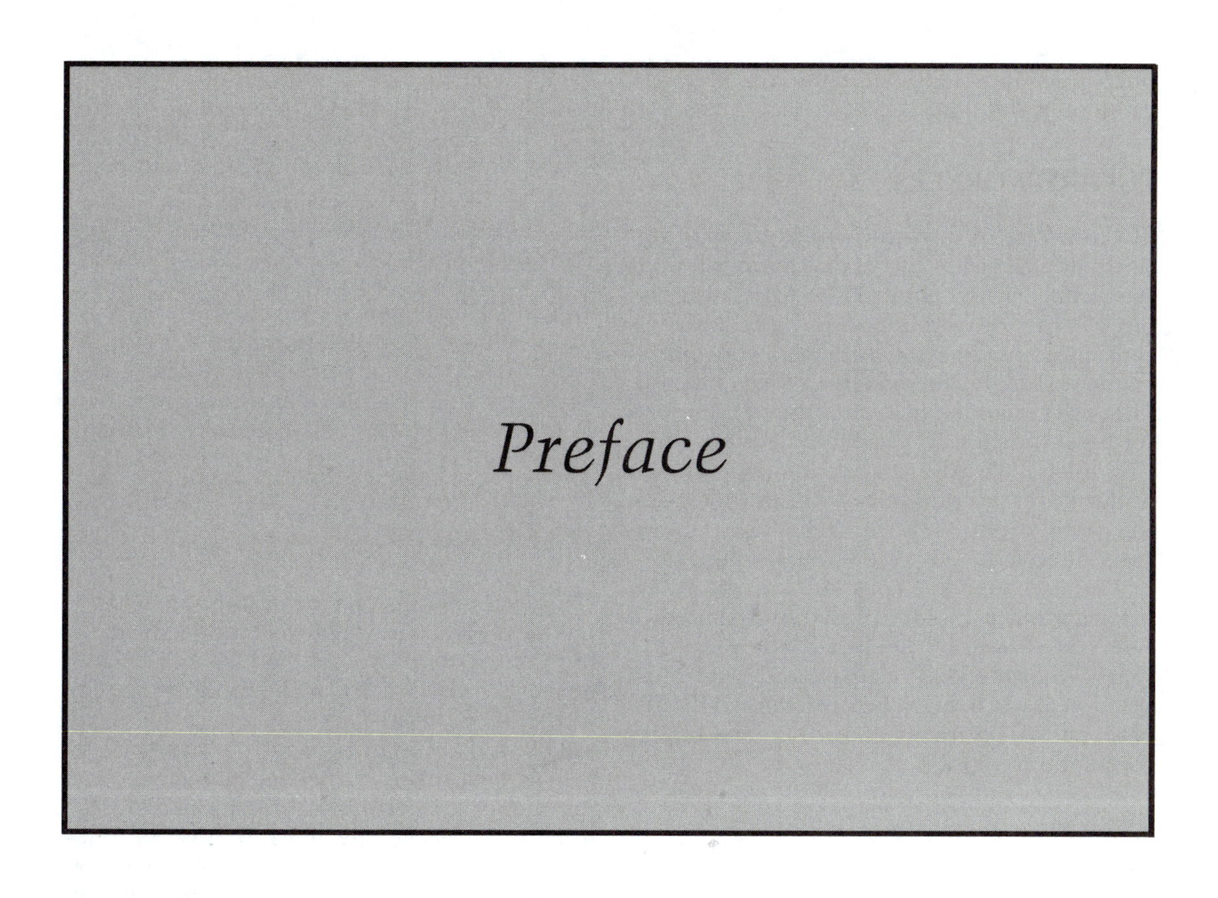

Preface

To place the HIV/AIDS pandemic in perspective, consider Michael Creighton's *The Andromeda Strain.* The essence of this story revolves around the release of an unidentified and untreatable lethal strain of bacteria into the human population. With a few changes—substituting HIV for bacterium, adjusting the time of death after infection, and describing how one dies from the disease—Creighton could have been writing about HIV/AIDS. But with HIV/AIDS, the onset of a real human tragedy, we are learning about our social contradictions, our strengths and our weaknesses, and we are questioning whether this is a morally acceptable disease. How long will it take for this to become a socially acceptable disease?

This text reviews important aspects of HIV infection, HIV disease, and the acquired immune deficiency syndrome. It presents a balanced review of factual information about the biological, medical, social, economic, and legal aspects of this modern-day pandemic.

The intricacy of the HIV/AIDS pandemic has unfolded over the last 15 years. Many of the details of basic research, applied biology, medicine, and social unrest are presented in an attempt to convey the few victories and many setbacks within this ongoing saga. Medical and social anecdotes help to convey a sense of the HIV/AIDS tragedy worldwide. The history of the disease describes how the virus is and is not transmitted. Throughout the text there is a special focus on risk behaviors and risk situations involved in HIV transmission and the means to prevent its transmission. The number of social issues raised by this disease are mind-boggling. Many of these issues are presented—some as open-ended questions for class discussions.

Such questions help the student reflect on what he or she has read.

PURPOSE

The purpose of this text is to present an understandable scientific explanation of what has been learned about HIV/AIDS over the last 15 years. In addition, it is particularly important to provide students with a conceptual framework of the issues raised by the HIV/AIDS pandemic so that they will be better able to deal with the challenges posed by this disease. Clearly, this pandemic poses new and unforeseen problems with no quick biological solutions. Only through reason can we respond in a socially acceptable fashion.

Because there is a constant stream of new information to be interpreted and shared, a new edition will be published about every 2 years. What has been learned and what must still be learned to bring HIV infection, HIV disease, and AIDS under control is valuable information to most, if not all, of us.

Text Use

This text is intended for use in college-level courses on AIDS and as a supplemental HIV/AIDS resource in medical and nursing schools, in colleges of allied health sciences, in psychology department courses on human sexuality and human behavior, in courses on sexually transmitted diseases, in summer teachers programs, in the training of AIDS counselors, in state-mandated AIDS education courses for health care workers, and for physicians who need a ready source of information on how to prevent HIV infection, HIV disease and its progression to AIDS, and types of therapy available. This text is suitable in those cases where information and education about the various aspects of HIV infection, disease, and AIDS are either wanted or required.

During the 15 years since HIV/AIDS was defined as a new disease, more manpower and money has been poured into HIV/AIDS research than into any other disease in history. Information on the AIDS virus has accumulated at an unprecedented pace. Since the discovery of the AIDS virus in 1982–1983, scientists have learned much about how it functions and how it affects the immune system. More was learned about the AIDS virus in the first 6 years after its discovery than had been learned about the polio virus in the first 40 years of the polio epidemic. During the first 6 years of AIDS research, the virus's genetic material was cloned, its structure ascertained, and individual viral genes identified. In fact, so many billions of dollars have been spent on HIV/AIDS that many now believe that HIV/AIDS research has taken away much-needed resources from other diseases that kill many times more people per year than does AIDS.

TEXT OVERVIEW

This text offers answers to questions many people have about the AIDS virus and how their immune systems are affected by it. Covered herein are the activity of the immune system with respect to HIV disease, where the virus might have come from, how it is transmitted, who is most likely to become infected, viral prevalence (geographical distribution of the number of people infected and those expressing HIV disease and AIDS), possible means of preventing infection, signs and symptoms of HIV disease and AIDS, chronological definitions of AIDS, the opportunistic infections most often associated with AIDS, FDA-approved and nonapproved drugs and their effectiveness, the potential for a vaccine to the AIDS virus, the tests available to detect HIV infection, the accuracy of these tests, their cost, availability, and confidentiality. The last three text chapters present the social, economic, and legal issues associated with HIV disease and AIDS. These chapters deal with the fear of HIV infection, the social reaction of the uninfected toward the HIV-infected, AIDS as an economic industry, and acts of discrimination and the laws in place to protect HIV/AIDS persons.

The majority of references herein are dated between 1987 and 1995. Every state in the United States has reported HIV-infected people and people diagnosed with AIDS. The World Health Organization (WHO) reports that of 178 nations reporting to it, 160 have reported diagnosed cases of AIDS. The virus is truly pandemic and now threatens most of the human population. Yet it is a preventable disorder, and the steps to prevention are presented in Chapter 9.

Organization of the Text

Chapter 1 presents information on the discovery of the disease and naming of the illness. Chapter 2 discusses the cause of AIDS and the possible origin of the AIDS virus. Chapter 3 presents the biological characteristics of the virus. Chapter 4 discusses the human immune system as it relates to HIV disease and the loss of the immune system's function. Chapter 5 presents the various opportunistic diseases and forms of cancer associated with HIV disease and AIDS. Chapter 6 discusses the clinical profile of biological indicators of HIV disease and AIDS. Chapter 7 deals with currently available FDA-approved drugs, drugs in experimental trials, and the use of non-FDA-approved drugs purchased through HIV/AIDS buying clubs. Chapter 8 presents the means by which HIV is most efficiently transmitted among humans. Chapter 9 details the most effective means to date of preventing HIV infection. Chapter 10 gives the incidence of HIV infections, HIV disease, and AIDS cases among high and low behavioral at-risk persons for HIV infection in the United States. Chapter 11 provides the incidence of HIV infections, HIV disease, and AIDS in countries outside the United States. Chapter 12 presents those tests most often used to detect the presence of HIV, biological shortcomings of the tests, the confidentiality or lack of confidentiality before and after test results, and costs. Chapter 13 offers pre- and posttest counseling procedures and communication problems between counselor and client. Chapter 14 offers insight to the many social ramifications of having HIV disease or AIDS, human attitudes, and behaviors. Chapter 15 presents the economic costs of this disease, the AIDS industry. Chapter 16 presents the legal aspects of AIDS as a handicap and laws to prevent discrimination. There is also a glossary of terms and a list of telephone numbers to federal, state, and other groups that offer information and help with all aspects of the HIV/AIDS pandemic.

Special Features

Each chapter contains chapter concepts, a summary, review questions, and references. Answers to these questions appear at the back of the book. Chapters also contain definitions for new terms as they are introduced, illustrations, photographs, and tables. All 16 chapters contain boxed information. Some of the chapters contain points of view, points of information, cases in point, and pro and con discussions. They illustrate and highlight important information about HIV infection, HIV disease, and AIDS. At certain places in the text, discussion statements are provided. Instructors may wish to entertain class discussions in these areas.

As science educators, it is our job to expose our students to the new concepts in biology that are shaping humanity's future. To do that, we must expose them to new vocabulary, new methodologies, and new ideas. It is my hope that this text will help in this endeavor.

IN APPRECIATION

The help of the following organizations or people is most deeply appreciated: The Centers for Disease Control and Prevention (CDC), Atlanta, Georgia, for use of slides and literature produced in their *National Surveillance Report* and the *Morbidity and Mortality Weekly Report*; Mara Lavitt and *The New Haven Register* for information on William Bluette; Robert N. Kermescher, Chief of Education and Training at the CDC for his valuable references on AIDS information; E. E. Buff, Biological Administrator, and Barry Bennett, head of Retroviral Testing Services, for their permission and guidance on photographing HIV testing procedures at the Florida Health and Rehabilitation Office of Laboratories Services, Jacksonville, Florida; to Karen Rodriguez and Roni Sanlo, AIDS Unit, Public Health Service, Jacksonville, Florida; Russ Havlak of the Infectious Disease Unit, CDC, Atlanta, Georgia; personnel of the National Institute for Allergy and Infectious Diseases, the

National Center for Health Statistics, Brookwood Center for Children with AIDS in New York, the George Washington AIDS Policy Center in Washington, D.C., the National Institutes for Health, Hoffman-LaRoche Co., Abbott Laboratories, the Pharmaceutical Mfg. Association, the National Cancer Institute, Pan American Health Organization, and the Office of Technological Assessment; Teresa M. St. John, University of North Florida for illustrations; the individuals who have contributed photographs; the text reviewers whose work has been greatly appreciated; Larry Monette, who spent countless hours word processing this manuscript; Guy Selander, M.D., who, over the years, has shared his medical journals with me; James Alderman, Eileen Brady, Mary Davis, Signe Evans, Paul Mosley, Ricky Moyer, Sarah Philips, and Barbara Tuck—reference/research librarians at the University of North Florida; Marie Cimmino for out-of-state library research; and to my special family, wife Delores and children Sherri and Garrett, who helped with proofreading and demonstrated a great deal of patience and understanding and gave up family weekends so the text could be completed on time.

This book has benefited from the critical evaluation of the following reviewers:

- Dr. Paul R. Elliott, Florida State University
- Dr. Robert Fulton, University of Minnesota
- Dr. Robert M. Kitchin, University of Wyoming
- Dr. Richard J. McCloskey, Boise State University
- Dr. Wayne B. Merkley, Drake University
- Dr. Linda L. Williford Pifer, University of Tennessee
- Dr. Bernard P. Sagik, Drexel University
- Professor James D. Slack, Cleveland State University
- Dr. Carl F. Ware, University of California, Riverside
- Dr. Phyllis K. Williams, Sinclair Community College
- Dr. Charles Wood, University of Kansas

Gerald J. Stine, Ph.D.

My son has AIDS. He lives in Miami, and he's not ready to come and stay with us; he wants to remain independent. Eventually he will come home to die. I must be prepared to care for him and to deal with all the issues our family will face. We are active in our community and in our church. I am also a high school teacher, but I've never told anyone about our son. When he comes home it will be impossible to hide the fact that he has AIDS. I am not sure how the community and our friends are going to respond. But we love him regardless.

Mom
(Anonymous)

Acquired
Immune
Deficiency
Syndrome

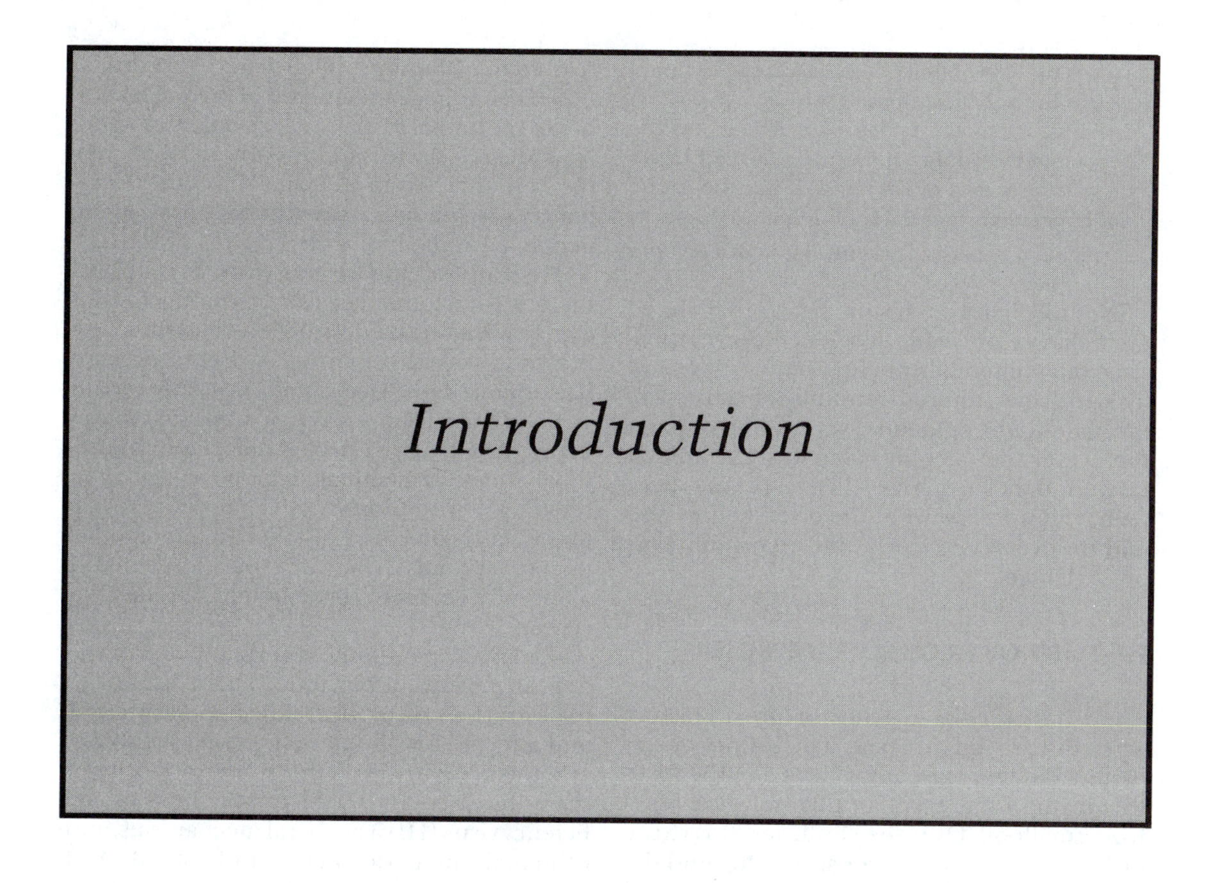

Introduction

TEST OF YOUR CURRENT KNOWLEDGE

Before reading this book, review and answer the following statements about HIV infection and AIDS and answer either True or False to test your current knowledge:

- The first retrospective recorded case of AIDS occurred in the United States in 1952.
- Infection by the AIDS virus, HIV, can be prevented.
- Worldwide, the virus is primarily spread through sexual contact.
- Asymptomatic infected persons can infect others.
- High infection risk is associated with having many sexual partners.
- HIV is fragile and easily destroyed by environmental agents when outside the human body.
- Casual contact does not spread HIV.
- HIV is not transmitted to humans via insects.
- The current risk of acquiring HIV via blood transfusions in the United States is low.
- Children can safely attend school with a classmate who is HIV-infected or has AIDS.
- Even without using precautions, health care workers are at a low risk for acquiring HIV infection.
- There is no cure for HIV infection or AIDS.
- About 60% of those persons expressing AIDS have died.
- AIDS may be close to 100% lethal—sooner or later a person who expresses AIDS dies.
- It is believed that 95% of those infected with HIV will eventually progress to AIDS.

All of the preceding statements are true. Information concerning these statistics and answers to other questions that you may have can be found within.

It was the best of times, it was the worst of times, it was the age of wisdom, it was the age of foolishness, it was the epoch of belief, it was the epoch of incredulity, it was the season of Light, it was the season of Darkness, it was the spring of hope, it was the winter of despair. . .

Charles Dickens, *A Tale of Two Cities*

Nothing in recent history has so challenged our reliance on modern science nor emphasized our vulnerability before nature. We have lived with the acquired immune deficiency syndrome (AIDS) epidemic, witnessing its paradoxes every day. People living with the human immunodeficiency virus live with the fear, pain, and uncertainty of the disease; they also endure prejudice, scorn, and rejection. **This must change!**

HISTORY OF GLOBAL EPIDEMICS

There has never been a time in human history when disease did not exist. The history of epidemics dates at least as far back as 1157 BC to the death of the Egyptian pharaoh Ramses V from smallpox. Over the centuries, this extraordinarily contagious virus spread around the world, changing the course of history time and again. It killed 2,000 Romans a day in the 2nd century AD, more than 2 million Aztecs during the 1520 conquest by Cortez, and some 400,000 Europeans a year during the late 1700s. Three out of four people who survived the high fever, convulsions, and painful rash were left deeply scarred and sometimes blind. Because victims' skin looked as if it had been scalded, smallpox was known as the "invisible fire." Even now, malaria in underdeveloped countries afflicts 300 million people, killing about 1.5 million each year. The problem is compounded by development of drug-resistant malarial strains of protozoa. Thus epidemics are not new to humankind, but the fear they impose on each generation is.

Major recorded pandemics (global) and epidemics (regional) that have devastated large populations are described in Table I-1.

The 1970s witnessed the emergence of Lyme disease (1975), Legionnaires disease (1976), and toxic shock syndrome (1978). In 1981, the Acquired Immune Deficiency Syndrome (AIDS) emerged, and in 1993, there was an outbreak of the hantavirus in Arizona, Colorado, New Mexico, and Utah. By early 1995, 98 people were infected in 21 states with the rodent-borne (deermouse) virus and half of these people have died of acute respiratory distress. There is no vaccine for this virus. In mid-1994 there was an outbreak of necrotizing fasciitis (fash-e-i-tis)—tissue destruction caused by a tissue-invasive strain of Group A streptococcus, a bacterium. This bacterium is a deadly variant strain of the Group A streptococcus that causes "strep throat". The infected may die from bacterial shock, disseminated blood coagulation (clotting), or respiratory or renal (kidney) failure. Clearly some new diseases are more lethal than others and AIDS may be the most lethal of all "new" diseases to strike humans in the 20th century.

The AIDS pandemic is certainly one of the defining events of our time. There are stories to be told from it, stories of the people infected and affected by it—the well, the ill, the dying, and the survivors. And there are the stories of scientific discovery, of the human immunodeficiency virus (HIV) and viral mechanisms, and of genetic mysteries being understood. And then there are stories of scientific politics, claims and counterclaims, and the manipulating that goes on in the stratosphere of high-level science.

"A third of the world died," wrote Jean Froissart at the end of the 14th century, when medieval medicine had little to offer against the Black Death. Now, at the end of the 20th century, we see modern science registering its progress about a plague of our own time.

AIDS is the most dramatic, pervasive, and tragic pandemic in recent history. So deep an impression has the AIDS epidemic made on public perceptions that according to a Louis Harris poll in 1994, almost 30% of the population now believes that the "greatest threat to human life" is AIDS or some other kind of plague. The HIV/AIDS pandemic consists of two parts: one medical, the other social. HIV/AIDS infection has provoked a reassessment of society's approaches to public health strategy, health care resource allocation, medical research, and sexual behavior. Fear and

TABLE I-1 Plague in History

Disease	Dates	Place	Number Killed	Causative Organism	Time to Prevention/Cure (in years)
Measles	from 430 BC	Greece /Rome/World	Millions	Paramyxovirus	1,712
Bubonic Plague	1347–1351	Europe/Asia/Africa	75 million	Pasteurella pestis	580
Cholera	1826–1837	New Jersey	900,000	Vibrio cholerae	75
	1849	United Kingdom	53,293		
	1947	Egypt	11,755		
Tuberculosis	1930–1949	United States	1,000,000	Mycobacterium tuberculosis	85
	1954–1970		150,000		
Malaria	1847–1875	Africa/India	20 million +	Plasmodia	100
Scarlet Fever	1861–1870	United Kingdom	972 per million people	Beta-Hemolytic streptococci	45–44
Polio	1921–1970	North America	37,000	Polio viruses Types I, II, III	30–50
Typhus	1917–1921	Russia	2,500,000	Rickettsias	25
Influenza	1918–1919	U.S./Europe	21,640,000	Influenza virus	57
Small Pox	from 1157 BC	Europe (middle ages)	Many millions	Smallpox virus	2,390
	1926–1930	India	423,000		
	from 590 BC				
Gonorrhea	1921–1992	United States	57,477	Neisseria gonorrhoeae	1,832
	from AD				
Yellow Fever	1986–1988	Nigeria	10,000	Arbovirus	488
AIDS			*Deaths* / *Cases*	Human	Treatments
	1981–95	United States (estimated)	280,000 / 509,000	Immunodeficiency Virus	but no
	1981–95	World (estimated)	4,400,000 / 7,000,000		cure

discrimination have affected virtually every aspect of our culture. Both the medical challenge and, in particular, the social challenge will continue in the foreseeable future. Arthur Ashe, a world-class tennis player, so feared discrimination against himself and family that he lived with AIDS for 3½ years before he was forced to reveal he had AIDS (Figure I-1).

The fear of HIV infection and the ignorance about its causes have created bizarre behavior and at times barbaric practices, strange rituals, and the attempt to isolate those afflicted.

The Black Plague during its most destructive time killed over 500 people a day. Instead of being concerned about providing care to the victims, people spent their time deciding how deep to dig the graves so that none of the horrid fumes would come up and infect others. It was determined that a grave should be six feet deep; and that is exactly how deep it is today. Plague victims were herded together into cathedrals to die or to pray for faith healing to save them. In 14th century Germany and Switzerland, the Christians blamed the Jews for the outbreak of bubonic plague, believing that the Jews were poisoning the water—the very same water that the Jews were drinking. As a result, whole communities of Jews were slaughtered. And in the 1400s and 1500s, when syphilis was spreading across the world killing thousands, the Italians called it the French disease. Of course, the French called it the Italian disease. In the 1930s, cholera was considered a punishment for people unwilling to change their lives—the poor and the immoral. In New York the Irish were blamed. In the early 20th century, polio in America was believed to be caused by Italian immigrants.

Three agents of disease, the smallpox virus, measles virus, and the bubonic plague bacterium are responsible for hundreds of millions of human deaths throughout history. The most recent outbreak of bubonic plague occurred in India in August of 1994.

Worldwide, smallpox killed over 100 million people by 1725. Smallpox is the only disease ever eradicated. The smallpox death of Egyptian pharaoh Ramses V in 1157 b.c. is the first known. Invading armies then spread smallpox through Africa and Europe. The Spanish brought it to Mexico. Edward Jenner

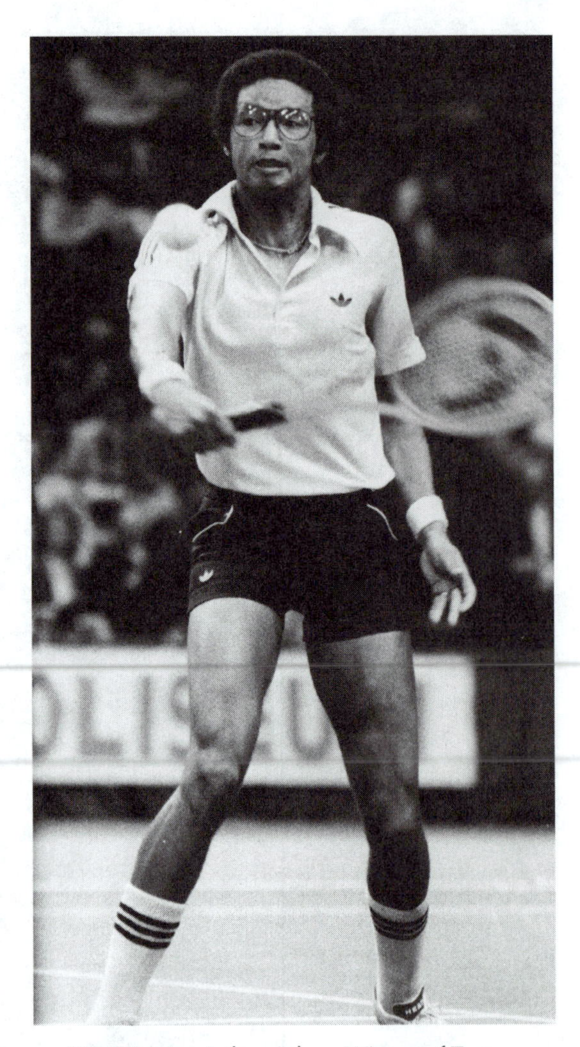

FGURE I-1 Arthur Ashe—Winner of Two United States Tennis Championships. On April 8, 1992 Ashe announced that he had AIDS. He died on February 6, 1993 at age 49. He became infected with HIV from a blood transfusion during heart bypass surgery in 1983. In 1988 his right hand suddenly became numb. Brain surgery revealed a brain abscess caused by toxoplasmosis. He asked two questions, "Why do bad things happen to good people?" and "Is the world a friendly place?" Ashe was the United States Davis Cup Captain for 5 years and supported the NCAA Proposition 42 academic requirements for athletes. In 1975 he became the first black to win a Wimbledon men's title. After learning that he had AIDS, Ashe completed his third book, *A Road to Glory*, a three-volume history of black athletes in the United States. (*Photograph courtesy of AP/Wide World Photos*)

discovered a virus related to smallpox and created a vaccine in the 1870s. Only humans got smallpox. It disappeared after a global vaccination campaign in the 1960s. The last known natural case was in Somalia in 1977. Each year as winter approaches, millions of shots of influenza (flu) vaccine are given, mainly to people who are especially susceptible to the virus (the very young, the elderly, asthmatics, and diabetics). The vaccine is a cocktail of recent influenza A and B strains and affords some protection against genetic changes in these vaccine strains. Nevertheless, in recent history thousands have died from influenza infection; in the 1957–1958 epidemic, for instance, 1 in 300 over age 65 died. There is evidence that the flu virus has been with us since 430 b.c. But in 1890 in China, the duck-borne virus crossed over into swine, then into humans, causing thousands of deaths. This epidemic was followed by severe flu epidemics in 1900, 1918 (the Spanish flu), 1957 (the Asian flu), and 1968 (the Hong Kong flu). The flu epidemic of 1918 and 1919 caused between 20 and 50 million deaths worldwide in people between the ages of 20 and 40. It could happen again, even though there is a vaccine. During the epidemic of 1918, in San Francisco, all citizens were required to wear masks. One form of therapy was "cabbage baths." People did not jump into a tub with some cooked cabbage; they ate the cabbage and urinated into the tub. The flu victims then got into the tub. There may have been a positive side to the bath because once you got out, a distance was created between you and other people. In this way, the baths may have helped stop person-to-person transmission.

The incidence of influenza-related deaths in the United States currently ranges from about 10,000 in years with low influenza activity to more than 40,000 in more severe influenza epidemics (Influenza 1994–1995: Now's The Time To Prepare. (1994) J. Resp. Dis., 15:675).

In 1937, 112,000 Americans contracted tuberculosis and 70,000 died. And even now, in 1995, over 2 million adults worldwide will die of hepatitis B and of the 44 million children who will contract measles, 1.5 million will die. Four thousand people die every day from malaria. Parents and children quietly cope; the ill were and are served, not shunned—that is, until the HIV/AIDS epidemic. The nine leading causes of death due to bacterial, protozoal or viral infections are given in Table I-2.

OVERVIEW ON HIV/AIDS

Acquired Immune Deficiency Syndrome (AIDS), first identified in 1981, is the final stage of a viral infection caused by the Human Immunodeficiency Virus (HIV). Medical experts recognize two strains: HIV-1, discovered in 1983, which is generally accepted as the cause of most AIDS cases throughout the world; and HIV-2, discovered in West Africa in 1986 and later found in some former Portuguese colonies elsewhere and in Europe. HIV is a retrovirus: a virus that inserts—probably for life—its genetic material into the cells of the host at the time of the infection. Inasmuch as the ability to remove genetic material from cells is beyond the capability of current medical science, the infection may be said to be incurable. AIDS is characterized by a profound loss of cell-mediated immune function and the depletion of a special kind of white blood cell called a CD4 or T4 lymphocyte.

Course of HIV Infection

Following infection with HIV, only the most sophisticated tests can detect its presence for the first weeks or months. After this period, the in-

TABLE I-2 Microbes Causing Most Deaths Worldwide

Infectious disease	Cause	Annual Deaths
Acute respiratory infections (mostly pneumonia)	Bacterial or viral	4,300,000
Diarrheal diseases	Bacterial or viral	3,200,000
Tuberculosis	Bacterial	3,000,000
Hepatitis B	Viral	1,000,000–2,000,000
Malaria	Protozoan	1,000,000
Measles	Viral	880,000
Neonatal tetanus	Bacterial	600,000
AIDS	Viral	550,000
Pertussis (whooping cough)	Bacterial	360,000

Sources: World Health Organization; Harvard School of Public Health, 1990 figures.

fected person's system begins producing antibodies to HIV, which blood testing can reveal. Such tests were first available in 1985 and vary as to their ability to detect HIV. About half the infected people will have developed AIDS symptoms in 10 years, some within 5 years. Once diagnosed, death from AIDS usually occurs in 1 to 2 years; infants and persons over age 60 generally proceed more rapidly to AIDS than do others. Almost everyone infected with HIV will progress to AIDS, and, to date, AIDS appears to be always fatal.

Transmission

Three main routes of transmission exist:

1. Contact with infected blood or blood products via transfusions, transplants, or shared needles
2. Sexual contact with an infected person (exposure to body fluids).
3. Infection of infants born to an infected mother.

Prevention

A contaminated blood supply is relatively easy to control. Donated blood is tested for HIV; infected blood is destroyed.

When the virus infects an injection drug user (IDU), it spreads rapidly through the sharing of needles. Free needle exchanges in the United States and in some foreign countries are one way of combating HIV transmission, although there are differing claims as to the success and social desirability of such an approach.

The spread of HIV in the general population has been slow, yet potentially it is the source of far greater numbers of AIDS cases than in the smaller group of IDUs and male homosexuals. Once the infection is established in the general population, it spreads mainly by sexual contact and thus may be impossible to eradicate. Reducing the prevalence of other sexually transmitted diseases can slow the transmission but would require worldwide public health expenditures far greater than any to date.

In addition to these steps, behavioral changes—less promiscuity and more frequent condom use—by large numbers of people are essential for effective control. The major programs to stop the transmission of HIV to date involve educating the public and distribution of condoms. Many public health scientists are pessimistic about the prospect that the necessary behavioral changes will occur.

AIDS—A RECENT CAUSE OF DEATH

AIDS is now the seventh leading cause of death among 1- to 4-year-olds, sixth among 15- to 24-year-olds, and third among 25- to 44-year-olds in the United States. In New York and New Jersey, it is the leading cause of death among men and women 20 to 49 years old.

There is the expectation that parents will die before their children. Because of the HIV/AIDS epidemic, it is not working out that way for many thousands of parents. They are watching their children die in the prime of life.

The facts on HIV infection, disease, and AIDS that are presented in the following chapters, when understood, clearly place the responsibility for avoiding HIV infection on *YOU*. You must assess your lifestyle; if you choose not to be abstinent, you must know about your sexual partner and you must practice safer sex. Never think that you are immune to HIV infection.

FIRST REPORTS ON AIDS CASES IN THE UNITED STATES

On June 5, 1981, the first cases of the illness now known as acquired immunodeficiency syndrome were reported from Los Angeles in five young homosexual men diagnosed with *Pneumocystis carinii* pneumonia and other opportunistic infections.

Initially, AIDS appeared among homosexual males; most frequently those who had many sex partners. Further study of the gay population led to the conclusion that the agent responsible for AIDS was being transmitted through sexual activities. In 1982, cases of AIDS were reported among hemophiliacs, people who had received blood transfusions, and injection drug users. These reports all had one thing in common—an exchange of body fluids, in particular blood or semen, was involved. In January 1983, the first cases of AIDS in heterosexuals were documented. Two females, both sexual partners of IDUs, became AIDS patients. This was clear evidence that the infectious agent could be transmitted from male to female as well as from male to male. Later in 1983, cases of AIDS were reported in Central Africa, but with a difference. The vast majority of African AIDS cases were among heterosexuals who did *not* use injection drugs. These data supported the earlier findings from the American homosexual population: that AIDS is primarily a sexually transmitted disease. And the risk for contracting AIDS increased with the number of sex partners one had and the sexual behaviors of those partners. Thus early empirical observations on which kinds of social behavior placed one at greatest risk of acquiring AIDS were later supported by surveillance surveys, testing, and analysis.

AIDS is now a major cause of morbidity and mortality in children and young adults in the United States, ranking seventh among estimated years of potential life lost before age 65 in 1987 and 15th among leading causes of death in 1988. In 1981, 248 adults and 15 children were reported to have AIDS. By mid-1995 (15 years later), 442,000 people have been reported to have AIDS and over 261,000 have died from the disease.

The first 50,000 cases of AIDS were reported to the Centers for Disease Control and Prevention (CDC) from June 1981 to December 1987 (7 years); the second 50,000 were reported between January 1988 and July 1989 (17 months). The third 50,000 cases were reported between August 1989 and the end of October 1990 (13 months). The fourth and fifth 50,000 were reported over the next 10 month intervals. The sixth 50,000 reports took 8 months and the seventh and eighth 50,000 took 6 months each. The ninth and tenth 50,000 will take about 10 months each (1995 and 1996). It took 8 years and 5 months to record the first 100,000 AIDS cases, 23 months for the second 100,000, 18 months for the third 100,000, about 12 to 14 months for the fourth 100,000, about 20 months to August of 1995, for the fifth 100,000. The sixth 100,000 should be reported by the end of 1997.

Epidemiological data collected worldwide clearly indicate that HIV is transmitted during sexual activities that involve the exchange of HIV-infected semen or vaginal fluids, by receipt of HIV-infected blood or blood products, and from HIV-infected mothers to their fetuses or to their newborns during breast feeding.

Although homosexual/bisexual men still account for most reported AIDS cases, IDUs, their sex partners, and their children represent an increasing proportion of cases. Of AIDS cases reported before 1985, 63% were homosexual/bisexual men with no history of IDU, 18% were female or heterosexual male IDUs, and 2% were the sex partners or children of IDUs. In contrast, of the AIDS cases reported in 1993, 46.6% were homosexual/ bisexual men with no history of injection drug use, 27.7% were female or heterosexual male IDUs, and 4% were the sex partners or children of IDUs. The proportion of AIDS cases among women has also increased from 7% before 1985 to almost 12% through 1994. Blacks and Hispanics continue to be disproportionately represented, particularly among IDUs with AIDS.

Accuracy

The 476,000 AIDS cases reported in the United States by mid-1995 does not represent the true number of people with AIDS. Because of underreporting of AIDS cases and manifestations of HIV infection that do not meet the CDC AIDS surveillance case definition, the number of people with AIDS is still underestimated. If all of the estimated 1,500,000 HIV-infected persons in the United States were diagnosed (found) and their T lymphocyte counts were determined, it is estimated that between 180,000 and 285,000 people, who are asymptomatic or at least do not have AIDS-indicator diseases, would have T4 lymphocyte counts of less than 200 cells/microliter (200 cells/μL). As such individuals are found, each will be diagnosed with AIDS. The number of estimated AIDS cases for 1993 increased 111% over 1992 figures due to the use of the new "1993" definition of what constitutes a person with AIDS. Accuracy in diagnosing and reporting AIDS cases varies by geographic region and patient population; however, mortality studies suggest that 70% to 90% of HIV-related deaths are identified through national surveillance.

The number of AIDS cases is one indication of the larger pandemic of HIV infection. An estimated 1 to 2 million people are infected with HIV in the United States. Probably only 20% to 30% of HIV-infected people know they are infected. Based on there being 1.5 million HIV-infected people in the United States, about 700,000 to 800,000 do not know they are HIV-infected!

Health Care

By the end of 1994, research and health care costs for HIV-infected people and those with the AIDS reached 28 billion dollars. The large number of newly HIV-infected and those progressing to AIDS each year has already placed a strain on the United States health care system, and the situation promises to get worse.

THE EDUCATIONAL COMMUNITY

Like most complex problems, the AIDS epidemic poses special problems for educators. One of the most disturbing is discrimination against HIV-infected children. Guidelines from the U.S. Surgeon General, federal and state health officials, and the medical community have not calmed the fears of misinformed parents. Many stories have made headlines and television news concerning children who have been barred from attending school. While the courts can order admission, they cannot assure acceptance. Persuasion must come through a better understanding of the disease. Parents can be reassured through reminders that HIV/AIDS is not transmitted by casual contact. Students must also be educated about HIV/AIDS. The following Gallup Poll results (Table I-3), although taken in 1988, are about what one would still find true in 1995.

Since the latter half of the 1980s, schools throughout the United States have been offering education programs to teach adolescents about human immunodeficiency virus (HIV) infection. By 1994, 34 states required HIV/AIDS education for adolescents. (10 states required HIV/AIDS education in their elementary schools). However, the effect of such programs on HIV-related knowledge and behavior among adolescents is largely unknown.

WORLD INTERNATIONAL AIDS CONFERENCES

In 1983, there were relatively so few groups involved with HIV/AIDS research that they could stay in contact by telephone. As the virus spread many countries became involved in HIV/AIDS research and clinical care. International, national and state meetings were formed as a way to exchange new information. The international meetings continue to receive the most press coverage. Since the first international AIDS conference in 1985, the conferences have grown in size to the point that scientists are questioning their usefulness. Some idea of the size increase can be gained by comparing the first and fifth meetings:

THE First International Conference on AIDS, Atlanta, 1985:

- Number of AIDS cases 9,608, USA
- Number of deaths 4,712, USA
- Number of delegates 2,000

TABLE I-3 1988 Gallup Poll Results on Age Related HIV/AIDS School Education

	National Totals %	Public School Parents %	Non-Public School Parents %
The Gallup Poll asked those who favored having public schools developed an HIV education program (90% of all respondents) the following questions:			
At what age should students begin participating in an HIV education program?			
Under 5 years	6	5	11
5–9 years	40	43	42
10–12 years	40	39	32
13–15 years	10	11	13
16 years or older	1	1	1
Don't know	3	1	1
Should public schools teach what is called "safer sex" for HIV prevention? (This was understood to mean teaching about the use of condoms.)			
Should	78	81	72
Should not	16	16	25
Don't know	6	3	3

Source: 20th Annual Gallup Poll on the Public's Attitudes Toward the Public Schools.

BOX I.1

MARY D. FISHER SPEAKS ABOUT AIDS AT THE 1992 REPUBLICATION NATIONAL CONVENTION

I bear a message of challenge, not self-congratulation. I want your attention, not your applause. I would never have asked to be HIV-positive. But I believe that in all things there is a good purpose, and so I stand before you, and before the nation, gladly.

The reality of AIDS is brutally clear. Two hundred thousand Americans are dead or dying; a million more are infected. Worldwide, 40 million, or 60 million, or 100 million infections will be counted in the coming few years. But despite science and research, White House meetings and congressional hearings, despite good intentions and bold initiatives, campaign slogans, and hopeful promises—despite it all, it's the epidemic which is winning tonight.

In the context of an election year, I ask you—here, in this great hall, or listening in the quiet of your home—to recognize that the AIDS virus is not a political creature. It does not care whether you are Democrat or Republican. It does not ask whether you are black or white, male or female, gay or straight, young or old.

Tonight, I represent an AIDS community whose members have been reluctantly drafted from every segment of American society. Though I am white, and a mother, I am one with a black infant struggling with tubes in a Philadelphia hospital. Though I am female, and contracted this disease in marriage, and enjoy the warm support of my family, I am one with the lonely gay man sheltering a flickering candle from the cold wind of his family's rejection.

This is not a distant threat; it is a present danger. The rate of infection is increasing fastest among women and children. Largely unknown a decade ago, AIDS is the third leading killer of young adult Americans today—but it won't be third for long. Because, unlike other diseases, this one travels. Adolescents don't give each other cancer or heart disease because they believe they are in love. But HIV is different. And we have helped it along—we have killed each other—with our ignorance, our prejudice, and our silence.

We may take refuge in our stereotypes, but we cannot hide there for long. Because HIV asks only one thing of those it attacks: Are you human? And in this is the right question: Are you human? Because people with HIV have not entered some alien state of being. They are human. They have not earned cruelty and they do not deserve meanness. They don't benefit from being isolated or treated as outcasts. Every one of them is exactly what God made: a person. Not evil, deserving our judgment; not victims, longing for our pity. People. Ready for support and worthy of our compassion.

My call to the nation is a plea for awareness. If you believe you are safe, you are in danger. Because I was not hemophiliac, I was not at risk. Because I did not inject drugs, I was not at risk. My father has devoted much of his lifetime to guarding against another holocaust. He is part of the generation who heard Pastor Neimoller come out of the Nazi death camps to say, "They came after the Jews and I was not a Jew, so I did not protest. They came after the Trade Unionists, and I was not a Trade Unionist, so I did not protest. They came after the Roman Catholics, and I was not a Roman Catholic, so I did not protest. Then they came after me, and there was no one left to protest."

The lesson history teaches is this: If you believe you are safe, you are at risk. If you do not see this killer stalking your children, look again. There is no family or community, no race or religion, no place left in America that is safe. Until we genuinely embrace this message, we are a nation at risk.

Tonight, HIV marches resolutely towards AIDS in more than a million American homes, littering its pathway with the bodies of the young. Young men. Young women. Young parents. Young children. One of the families is mine. If it is true that HIV inevitably turns to AIDS, then my children will inevitably turn to orphans.

My family has been a rock of support. My 84-year-old father, who has pursued the healing of the nations, will not accept the premise that he cannot heal his daughter. My mother has refused to be broken; she still calls at midnight to tell wonderful jokes that make us laugh. Sisters and friends, and my brother Philip (whose birthday is today)—all have helped carry me over the hardest places. I am blessed, rich and deeply blessed, to have such a family.

But not all of you have been so blessed. You are HIV seropositive but dare not say it. You have lost loved ones, but you dare not whisper the word AIDS. You weep silently, you grieve alone.

I have a message for you: It is not you who should feel shame. It is we. We who tolerate ignorance and practice prejudice, we who have taught you to fear. We must lift our shroud of silence, making it safe for you to reaczh out for compassion. It is our task to seek safety for our children, not in quiet denial, but in effective action.

Some day our children will be grown. My son Max, now four, will take the measure of his mother; my son Zachary, now two, will sort through his memories. I may not be here to hear their judgments, but I know already what I hope they are.

I want my children to know that their mother was not a victim. She was a messenger. I do not want them to think, as I once did, that courage is the absence of fear; I want them to know that courage is the strength to act wisely when most we are afraid. I want them to have the courage to step forward when called by their nation, or their Party, and give leadership, no matter what the personal cost. I ask no more of you than I ask of myself, or my children.

To the millions of you who are grieving, who are frightened, who have suffered the ravages of AIDS firsthand: Have courage and you will find comfort.

To the millions who are strong, I issue the plea: Set aside prejudice and politics to make room for compassion and sound policy.

To my children, I make this pledge:

I will not give in, Zachary, because I draw my courage from you. Your silly giggle gives me hope. Your gentle prayers give me strength. And you, my child, give me reason to say to America, "You are at risk."

And I will not rest, Max, until I have done all I can to make your world safe. I will seek a place where intimacy is not the prelude to suffering.

I will not hurry to leave you, my children. But when I go, pray that you will not suffer shame on my account.

To all within the sound of my voice, I appeal: Learn with me the lessons of history and grace, so my children will not be afraid to say the word AIDS when I am gone. Then their children, and yours, may not need to whisper it at all.

God bless the children, and bless us all—and good night.

The Fifth International Conference on AIDS, Montreal, 1989:

- Number of AIDS cases 97,193, USA
- Number of deaths 56,468, USA
- Number of delegates 12,000

The Seventh International Conference on AIDS, 1991:

- Number of AIDS cases 222,000, USA
- Number of deaths 131,000, USA
- Number of delegates 9,000

The Seventh International Conference on AIDS took place in Florence, Italy. The slogan for this conference was "Science Challenging AIDS." Perhaps it should have been the reverse: "AIDS Challenging Science." Few advances in HIV/AIDS therapy or vaccine development were presented. Perhaps the most notable event was the squabble about where the 1992 conference would be held. Organizers of the 1992 conference, which was scheduled for Boston, decided that because of the United States government's restriction on HIV-positive immigrants, it would be held in Amsterdam.

The Eighth International Conference on AIDS, Amsterdam, 1992:

- Number of AIDS cases 263,000, USA
- Number of deaths 166,000, USA
- Number of delegates 11,000

The Promise of Victory— Wars are usually launched with the promise of a quick victory; the campaign against AIDS was no exception. Soon after researchers announced that they had discovered the virus that causes AIDS, U.S. health officials confidently stated that a vaccine would be ready in 2 years. The most frightening scourge of the late 20th century would succumb to a swift counterattack of human ingenuity and high technology. But no one made victory speeches in Amsterdam. The atmosphere was tense yet somber, reflecting the 11 years of failure, frustration, and a mounting death toll. Participants learned that there will not be a vaccine ready for years, nor will there be a drug cure—that our best defense is still education. Perhaps the most interesting moment of the meeting occurred with the announcement that some 30 people are known to have AIDS but are not HIV-infected. The news media rushed in with reports of a new and different AIDS virus. They failed to realize that severe immunodeficiency long predates the discovery of HIV. And that there was no apparent clustering of such cases. If the 1992 conference is to be remembered, it is because of the straightforward admission by the representatives of rich, industrialized nations that the HIV/AIDS pandemic is everyone's responsibility. That no magic bullet or quick fix will emerge to save us and that we are in this together for the long haul.

The Ninth International Conference on AIDS, Berlin, Germany, June 7–11, 1993:

- Number of AIDS cases: 339,000 USA
- Number of deaths: 203,000 USA
- Number of delegates: 14,000

The same pessimism of the Eighth International Conference held stage during the Ninth Conference. People from 166 nations attended the conference. They were exposed to over 800 oral presentations, 4,500 posters, and two guides the size of telephone directories filled with abstracts. The general theme in Berlin has become a familiar one: Although a cure for AIDS has not yet been found, medical science has made more progress in a shorter period of time toward understanding acquired immune deficiency syndrome and the viruses that cause it than it has for any other disease. Although true, this observation is no longer comforting to AIDS patients.

In fact, an undercurrent in many of that year's presentations, especially those by top AIDS researchers and public health officials, was a seemingly conscious effort to diminish expectations. A drug to cure AIDS is not just around the corner; a safe, effective AIDS vaccine remains problematic; and incremental advances in AIDS prevention should be counted as successes. The hopes to finding agents to cure an HIV infection or, at lest, significantly delay the progress of HIV disease to AIDS and death have dimmed. The agents that have been approved for use in treating AIDS—nucleoside analogs that inhibit the HIV enzyme reverse transcriptase—are not very good drugs. They are toxic, HIV develops resistance to them, and they are only moderately successful in maintaining patients' health. In addition, a large, controversial French and British study of zidovudine (commonly referred to as AZT), The Concorde Trials, indicates that early use of the drug in HIV infected individuals provides no survival benefits.

The Tenth International Conference on AIDS, Yokohama, Japan, August 7–12, 1994:

- Number of AIDS cases: 420,000 USA
- Number of Deaths: 231,000 USA
- Number of Delegates: 12,000

The 10th International Conference on AIDS ended with no major breakthroughs reported and with the world's researchers still far from defeating AIDS.

In the five days it took to conduct the conference, an estimated 41,000 people around the world became infected by the virus that causes the disease.

The grim statistic underscored the gap that became more evident between the rapidly spreading epidemic and the slow pace of progress in fighting the disease. Neither cure nor vaccine is expected by the end of the decade.

But as the conference ended participants said they could take some solace in the belief that painstaking advances are being made in basic science. Eventually this may set the stage for a new assault on the disease.

This Conference set itself apart from its nine predecessors not so much by what happened, but by what did not. In contrast to past years, no clinical trials of anti-HIV drugs stirred the delegates. No AIDS vaccine tests in monkeys or chimps had the conference halls abuzz, as they have in the past. Even the AIDS activistis who have traditionally disrupted the conference sessions with provocative signs and blaring bulhorns were absent. The conference ended with pledges of renewed efforts in basic research and because of the lack of progress, to meet every two years. The next meeting will occur in 1996. In short, the 10th International AIDS conference was more of a symbol of the AIDS pandemic then it was for the demonstration of progress against the disease.

THE AIDS MEMORIAL QUILT

The purpose of the quilt is to educate. The "AIDS Quilt" is made up of individual fabric panels, each the size of a grave, measuring three feet by six feet, stitched together. In October 1987, the AIDS quilt was first put on display on the mall in Washington, D.C. At that time it contained 1,920 panels and covered an area larger than two football fields and it took less than 2 hours to read all the names. In 1992 it took 60 hours. By mid-1994, the quilt contained over 28,000 panels bearing over 40,000 names, required over 30 acres to lay out and weighed 28 tons. There are about 50 miles of seams and 26 miles of canvas edging. There are panels from each of the 50 states. Each day new panels arrive from across the United States and 29 foreign countries to be added to the quilt (Figure I-2). For those left behind, the panels represent an expression of love and a sign of grief—a part of the healing process (Figure I-3).

Many of the names listed below can be found on the quilt: Michael Bennett, director/choreographer; Mel Boozer, Leonard Matlovich, Michael Callen, and Pedro Zamora gay rights activists; Sonia Singleton, AIDS activist; Arthur Bressan, Jr. and Colin Higgins, film makers; Roy Cohn, attorney; Perry Ellis, fashion designer; Dan Eicholtz, cartoonist; Wayland Flowers, comedian; Michel Foucault, philosopher; Philip-Dimitri Galas, playwright; Keith Haring, artist; Brad Davis (Figure I-4), Rock Hudson (Figure I-5), Ray Sharkey, Court Miller, Christopher Stryker, and Stephen Stucker, actors; Liberace, performer (Figure I-6); Charles Ludlum, actor/director/playwright; Robert Mapplethorpe, photographer; Stewart McKinney, U.S. Congressman, RCT; Ed Mock and Michael Peters choreographers; Klaus Nomi, performance artist; Rudolf Nureyev, renowned dancer and choreographer; Max Robinson, ABC news anchor; Tom Cassidy, Cable News Network business anchorman; Jerry Smith, Washington Redskins football player; Willi Smith, fashion designer; Sylvester, singer; Dan Turner, AIDS activist; Dr. Tom Waddell, Olympic athlete; Stephen Kolzak, casting

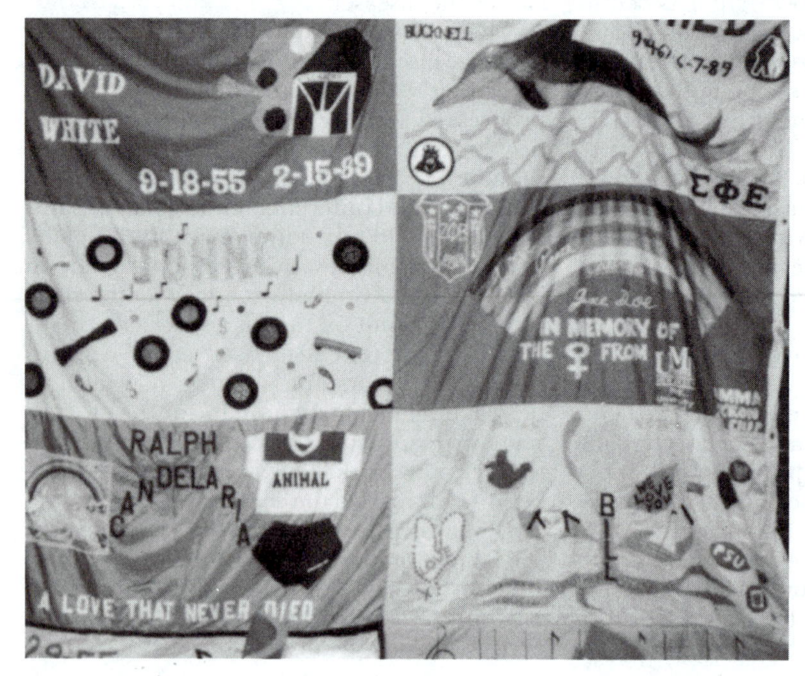

FIGURE I-2 Photograph taken of a section of the quilt in July of 1991.

Connie
one year
one week
one day
12·23·86—12·30·87
one eternity

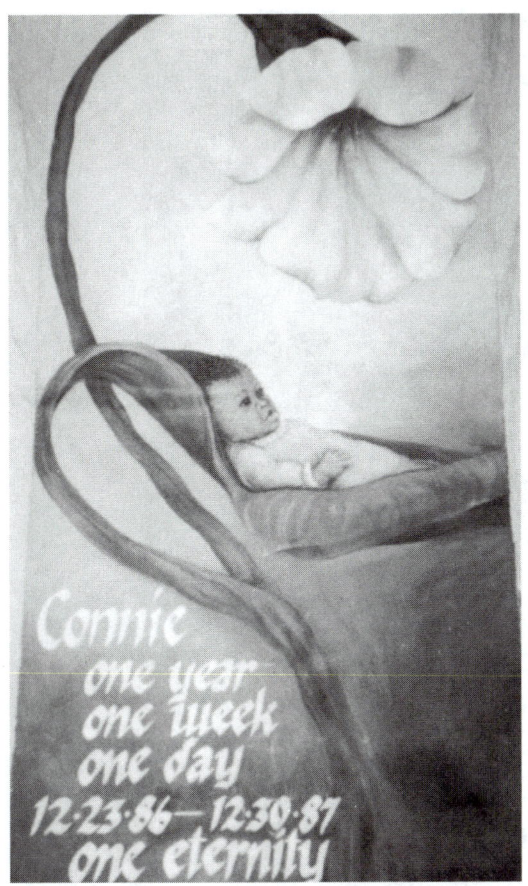

FIGURE I-3 A photograph of a single panel of the quilt taken in July of 1991.

director for *Cheers*; Ryan White, teenager; Rickey Wilson, guitarist with the B-52s; Freddie Mercury, rock singer of Queen; Peter Allen, songwriter and pianist; Dan Bradley, funded a legal agency for the poor; Esteban DeJesus, lightweight boxing champion; Belinda Mason, only member with AIDS on President Bush's National Commission on AIDS; Kimberly Bergalis, first case of HIV infection from a health care provider—her dentist; Rob McCall, winner of the Olympic bronze medal for ice skating/dancing; Howard Ashman, Oscar winner for Best Original Score and Best Song for the 1991 film, *Beauty and the Beast;* Anthony Perkins, best known for his work as Norman Bates in the movie *Psycho;* Alison Gertz, ice skating champions Brian Pocker, Dennis Coi, Rob McCall, Shaun McGill, Ondrej Nepela, John Carrell, Tim Brown, and James Hulick; and Arthur Ashe, tennis champion; Stephen Kritsick, veterinarian who presented pet care on ABC's *Good Morning America*; Randy Shilts, journalist/author—*And the Band Played on*; and authors Paul Sergios, and John Preston.

Portions of the quilt are on tour in major cities. Donations made for viewing the quilt are being used to support local Names Project chapters and their staffs.

Each panel has its own story. The stories are told by those who make the panels for their lost friends, lovers, parents, and children. The complete quilt was displayed in Washington, D.C., October 9–11, 1992 for the last time—it is too large to view again as a whole.

For more information about the Names Project's AIDS Memorial Quilt, call (415) 863-5511.

For information about your state chapter, contact the Names Project coordinator at (201) 888-1790.

WORLD AIDS DAY

December 1, 1988 was the first acclaimed *World AIDS Day* (WAD). World AIDS Day is a day set aside to pay tribute to those who have AIDS and to those who have died of AIDS. Its purpose is to increase our awareness of AIDS. The first WAD did not attract much attention outside the gay community. But in 1989, artists got together and held the first annual *Day Without Art* to coincide with World AIDS Day. For the second annual Day Without Art/World AIDS Day on December 1, 1990, at least 3,000 art organizations in the United States were involved. They included the Smithsonian Institution as well as small American art galleries and art galleries in Canada, England, France, and the Netherlands.

The second annual Day Without Art/ World AIDS Day was commemorated by shrouded sculptures, darkened marquees, and exhibits depicting the loss of life to HIV infection and AIDS. At 8 PM on December 1, 1990, the Manhattan and San Francisco skylines were dimmed for 15 minutes. On Broadway, the marquees were darkened for 1 minute and 23 cable TV stations as well as broadcasts in England,

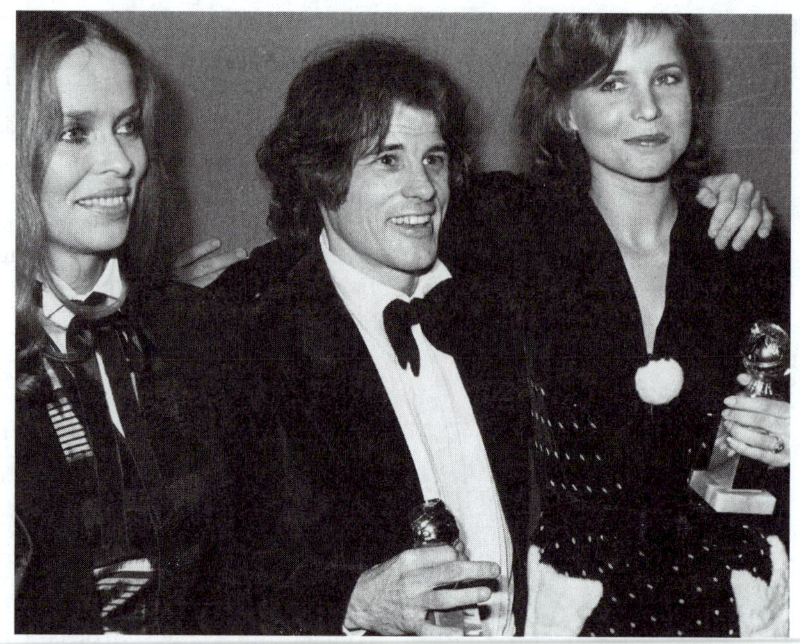

FIGURE I-4 Brad Davis, Film Star. Voted best actor by the Foreign Press Associations Golden Globes Awards (1979) for his work in *Midnight Express.* The film was the story of an American imprisoned in Turkey. Brad became HIV-infected through drug use and died at age 41 in 1991. (*Photograph Courtesy of AP/Wide World Photos*)

Canada, and Australia were interrupted with a 1-minute announcement about AIDS.

The third annual Day Without Art/World AIDS Day was the largest AIDS event ever. The theme was "Sharing the Challenge." It was intended to underline the global nature of the pandemic and to foster awareness that only by pooling efforts, resources, and imagination can hope prevail against the common threat. Many more people, businesses, and industries became involved for the first time. World AIDS Day 1992 adopted the theme "A Community Commitment." The theme for World AIDS Day 1993 was "A Time to Act." Topics covered were: fighting denial, discrimination, and complacency; bridging the resource gap; reducing women's vulnerability to infection; prevention; and providing humane care. The theme for 1994 was "The Global Challenge; AIDS and the Family." For information on World AIDS Day 1995/1996, write 108 Leonard Street, 13th Floor, New York, NY 10013 or call (212) 513-0303, or world AIDS Day Public Information Office, WHO-GPA, 1211 Geneva 27, Switzerland.

THE WORLD HEALTH ORGANIZATION

The World Health Organization (WHO) has established a global program on HIV infection and AIDS. The program has three objectives: to prevent new HIV infections, to provide support and care to those already infected, and to link international efforts in the fight against HIV infection and AIDS. By mid 1995, the WHO estimated that there were about 6 million AIDS cases and some 20 million cases of HIV infection worldwide. By the end of 1995, there will be 22 million HIV infections and over 7 millon AIDS cases. Michael Merson, current director of the WHO's Global Program on AIDS, said in a recent interview, "It is very unlikely that the global prevalence of HIV infection will stabilize or level off for at least several decades." The WHO estimates that 10 million children and 30 million adults will be HIV-infected by the year 2000. This is a minimum estimate. Merson added, "The global balance of HIV infection is rapidly tipping toward the developing countries. In 1985, some-

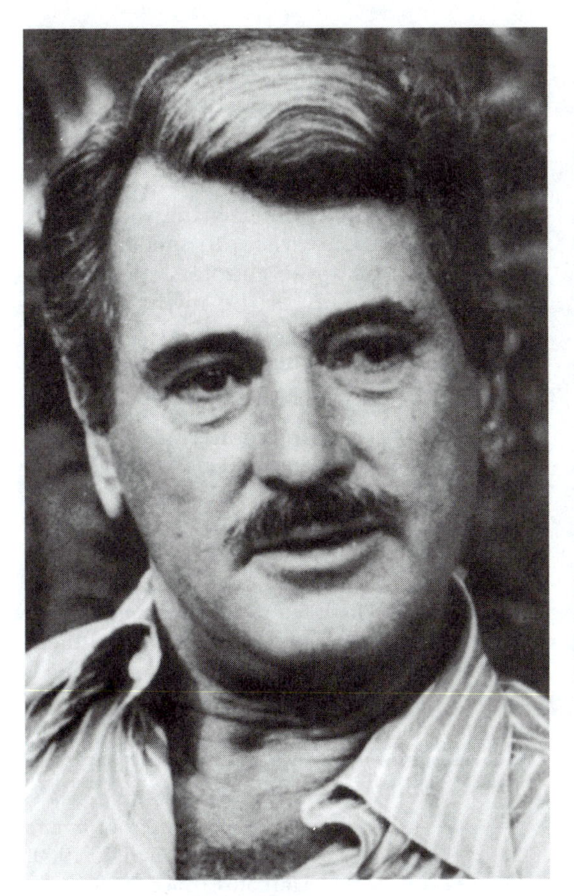
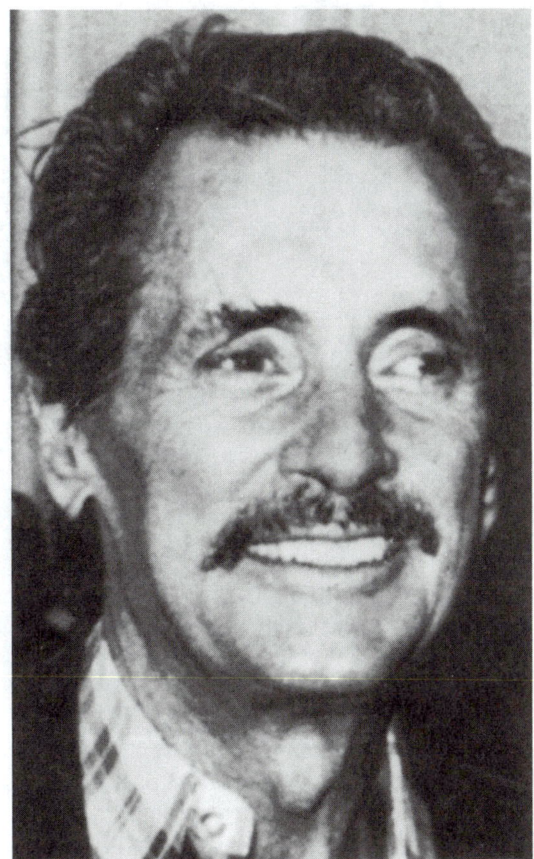

FIGURE I-5 Rock Hudson, Movie and Television Star. A Hollywood legend and undisclosed homosexual. He was the first major public figure to reveal he had AIDS. Hudson died in 1985 at age 59. (*Photograph courtesy of AP/Wide World Photos*)

where around 50% of the world's total infections, we estimated, were in developing countries. But now we estimate that by the year 2000, 75 to 80% will be in developing countries and by the year 2010, as many as 90%."

In addition, if HIV infection increases as rapidly in Asia and Latin America as it did in Africa, then the current projection of 40 million will need to be significantly revised upward. A recent study by Harvard scientists and a team of 40 HIV/AIDS experts states that by the year 2000 there will be 38 million to 110 million HIV-infected adults. Twenty-four million adults will have AIDS. There are some estimates that if an effective vaccine is not produced, the number of HIV-infected may reach 1 billion by the year 2025. This would mean about 1 in 10 people worldwide would be HIV-infected!

THE FUTURE

The history of HIV/AIDS is one of remarkable scientific achievement. Never in the history of man has so much been learned about so complex an illness in so short a time. We moved into the 1990s with hope and the determination to find better therapies and a vaccine. The task is formidable but it has to be done and it will be accomplished. The evolving story of the HIV/AIDS epidemic has been one of the

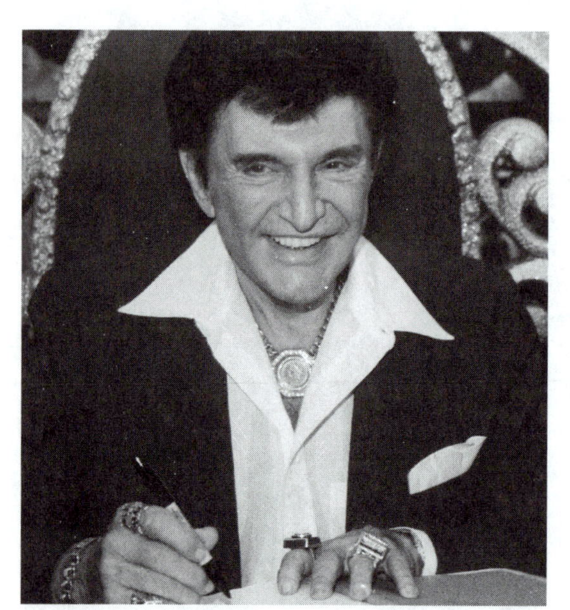

FIGURE I-6 Wladziu Valentino (Lee) Liberace, Internationally Known Pianist and Entertainer. Died of AIDS February 4, 1987 at the age of 67. (*Photograph courtesy of AP/Wide World Photos*)

major medical news events of the past 15 years. It is getting hard to imagine medicine without HIV/AIDS. But we must be careful not to blame this disease on our already failing health care system. As the National Commission on AIDS said:

> The AIDS epidemic did not leave 37 million or more Americans without ways to finance medical care, but it did dramatize their plight. This epidemic did not cause the problems of homelessness—but it has expanded it and made it more visible. The epidemic did not cause the collapse of the health care system—but it has accelerated the disintegration of our public hospitals and intensified their financing problems. The AIDS epidemic did not directly augment problems of substance abuse—but it has made the need for drug treatment for all who request it a matter of urgent national priority.

HIV/AIDS is a truly persistent global epidemic and will require a proportionate response to bring it to heel. It will be the plague of our lifetimes—and probably that of our children's lives as well. We already have children age 14 and younger who don't know what an HIV-free world is. They were born into this epidemic. To survive this epidemic, we must prevent the faces from becoming faceless. The chapters on HIV infection, HIV disease, and AIDS in this book will help bring widespread information on the virus into focus. The information within these chapters should also help eliminate many of the myths and irrational fears, or FRAID (fear of AIDS), generated by this disease. There is much work to be done by both scientists and society.

> Perhaps a borrowed anecdote says it best:
>
> As the old man walked the beach at dawn, he noticed a young woman ahead of him picking up starfish and flinging them into the sea. Finally catching up with the youth, he asked her why she was doing this. The answer was that the stranded starfish would die if left to the morning sun.
>
> "But the beach goes on for miles and there are millions of starfish," countered the old man. "How can your effort make any difference?"
>
> The young woman looked at the starfish in her hand and threw it to safety in the waves. "It makes a difference to this one," she said.
>
> (Adapted from *The Unexpected Universe* by Loren Eiseley. Copyright 1969, Harcourt Brace, New York)

Too easily can we become overwhelmed by the enormity of the AIDS pandemic. The numbers of patients and their constant needs have caused many to become paralyzed into inactivity and lulled into indifference. Like the old man, many ask "Why bother?"

For the sake of every individual living with HIV, we must focus on what each one of us can do. Each person can make a difference. Believing this, we are empowered to cope with the larger whole. **WE MUST NOT LET AIDS DICTATE THAT 49 IS OLD AGE AND AGE 39 OUR LIFE EXPECTANCY.**

Toll-Free National AIDS Hotline

- For the English-language service (open 24 hours a day, 7 days a week), call 1-800-342-AIDS (2437).
- The Spanish service (open from 8 AM to 2 AM, 7 days a week) can be reached at 1-800-344-SIDA (7432).

- A TTY service for the hearing impaired is available from 10 AM to 10 PM Monday through Friday at 1-800-243-7889.

For additional help you may wish to consult with your college or community library. They may have access to the following AIDS-related data bases:

- Aidsline—90,000 references to journals, books, and audiovisuals
- Aidstrials—information on 500 clinic trials of drugs and vaccines
- Aidsdrugs—a dictionary of drugs and experimental chemicals and biological agents against the virus
- Dirline—lists over 2,300 organizations and services that provide public information on HIV disease and AIDS

Toll-Free State AIDS Hotlines

For information about HIV-specific resources and counseling and testing services, call your state AIDS hotline:

State	Hotline	State	Hotline
Alabama	800-228-0469	Montana	800-233-6668
Alaska	800-478-2437	Nebraska	800-782-2437
Arizona	800-548-4695	Nevada	800-842-2437
Arkansas	501-661-2133	New Hampshire	800-324-2437
California (No.)	800-367-2437	New Jersey	800-624-2377
California (So.)	800-922-2437	New Mexico	800-545-2437
Colorado	800-252-2437	New York	800-541-2437
Connecticut	800-342-2437	North Carolina	800-733-7301
Delaware	800-422-0429	North Dakota	800-472-2180
District of Columbia	202-332-2437	Ohio	800-332-2437
Florida	800-352-2437	Oklahoma	800-535-2437
Georgia	800-551-2728	Oregon	800-777-2437
Hawaii	800-922-1313	Pennsylvania	800-662-6080
Idaho	208-345-2277	Puerto Rico	800-765-1010
Illinois	800-243-2437	Rhode Island	800-726-3010
Indiana	800-848-2437	South Carolina	800-322-2437
Iowa	800-445-2437	South Dakota	800-592-1861
Kansas	800-232-0040	Tennessee	800-525-2437
Kentucky	800-654-2437	Texas	800-299-2437
Louisiana	800-922-4379	Utah	800-366-2437
Maine	800-851-2437	Vermont	800-882-2437
Maryland	800-638-6252	Virginia	800-533-4148
Massachusetts	800-235-2331	Virgin Islands	800-773-2437
Michigan	800-827-2437	Washington	800-272-2437
Minnesota	800-248-2437	West Virginia	800-642-8244
Mississippi	800-537-0851	Wisconsin	800-334-2437
Missouri	800-533-2437	Wyoming	800-327-3577

Acquired Immune Deficiency Syndrome
AIDS

What do we know about AIDS? The next 16 chapters will present the many faces of the AIDS pandemic in the United States and other countries. Unlike people, the AIDS virus (HIV) does not discriminate; and it appears that most humans are susceptible to HIV infection, its suppression of the human immune system, and the consequences that follow. The viral infection that leads to AIDS is the most lethal, the most feared, and the most socially isolating of all the sexually transmitted diseases. *We must, as a people, fight against AIDS, not against each other* (Figure P-1).

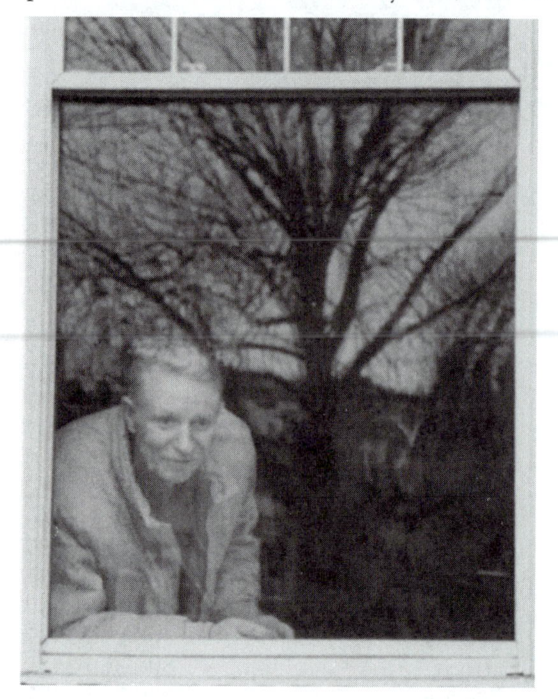

FIGURE P-1 The Loneliness of AIDS. Skip Bluette, diagnosed with AIDS July 1986, died July 1988. He suffered the indignity of having to lie to a dentist to get treatment. He suffered the ignorance of nurses afraid to touch him. He suffered the loss of his greatest pleasures—discos, gourmet meals, movies, and sex with men. Family was vital to Skip. So vital that on July 17, the day he died, their presence was his final wish.

Skip Bluette wanted his story told. Photographer Mara Lavitt interviewed and photographed him during the last 8 months of his life. Portions of Lavitt's article, which appeared in *The New Haven Register*, are presented in the following chapters. (*By permission of Mara Lavitt and* The New Haven Register)

CHAPTER

1

Discovering the Disease, Naming the Illness

Chapter Concepts

- AIDS is a syndrome, not a single disease.
- The first cases of AIDS-related *Pneumocystis carinii* pneumonia (PCP) were reported by the Centers for Disease Control and Prevention (CDC) in June of 1981; the first case of Kaposi's sarcoma in July 1981.
- Luc Montagnier discovered the AIDS virus in 1983.
- The first CDC definition of AIDS was presented in 1982 and expanded in 1983, 1985, and 1987, and again on January 1, 1993.

The letters A, I, D, S (AIDS) are an acronym for Acquired Immune Deficiency Syndrome.

A =	acquired	=	a virus received from someone else
I =	immune	=	a protection against disease-causing microorganisms
D =	deficiency	=	a loss of this protection
S =	syndrome	=	a group of signs and symptoms that together define AIDS as a human pathology

AIDS: A DISEASE OR A SYNDROME?

AIDS has been presented in journals, nonscience magazines, newspaper articles, and on television as a disease. But a disease is a pathological condition with a single identifiable cause. As we learned from the days of Louis Pasteur and Robert Koch, there is a single identifiable organism for each infectious disease.

AIDS patients may have many diseases. Most AIDS patients have more than one disease. Each produces its own signs and symptoms. Collectively, the diseases that are expressed in an AIDS patient are referred to as a **syndrome.** The number of different diseases an AIDS patient has and the severity of their expression reflects the functioning of that person's immune system.

In 1982–1983, the agent that destroys an essential portion of the human immune system was identified by French scientists as a virus. From that point on there was a specific infectious agent associated with the cause of AIDS. The symptoms of viral-induced AIDS can begin *only* after one has been infected with a specific virus. This virus is now called the *H*uman *I*mmunodeficiency *V*irus (HIV). The specific viral induced disease is referred to specifically as HIV/AIDS because there are other reasons for a suppressed immune system, like cancer chemotherapy, that also produce AIDS-like symptoms. ***Because individuals can express AIDS for reasons other than becoming HIV-infected, unless stated otherwise all information herein will refer only to AIDS caused by HIV and referred to as HIV/AIDS.***

Over time the AIDS virus depletes a subset of T cells, the T4 helper cells, that are essential in the proliferation of cells necessary to cell-mediated immunity and in the production of antibodies (Figure 1-1). Thus, cell-mediated immunity and antibodies are critical components of the human immune system. Without the ability to produce a sufficient number of immune specific cells and immune specific antibodies, the body is vulnerable to a large variety of infections caused by organisms that normally do not cause human disease. It is these infections that create the symptoms and progression of illnesses that eventually kill AIDS patients. Thus AIDS begins with HIV infection. Technically it can be called **HIV disease** or **HIV T4 helper cell disease,** but the popular press, scientists, and others still refer to HIV disease as AIDS. But, AIDS is the end stage of chronic HIV infection. AIDS is not transmitted, the virus is.

It is believed that eventually everyone who is correctly diagnosed with HIV/AIDS will die. But all who become HIV-infected may not progress to AIDS. Estimates are that some 5% of the HIV-infected population will not progress to AIDS (*Medical World News*, 1988). This implies that there is a percentage of the population that is resistant to HIV-associated immune system suppression.

Naming the Disease

In June of 1981, the Centers for Disease Control and Prevention (CDC) first reported on diseases occurring in gay men that previously had only been found to occur in people whose immune systems were suppressed by drugs or disease (*Morbidity and Mortality Weekly Report (MMWR)*, 1981).

The report stated that five young men in Los Angeles had been diagnosed with *Pneumocystis carinii* pneumonia (PCP) in three different hospitals. Because cases of PCP occurred almost exclusively in immune suppressed patients, five new cases in one city at one time were termed by the report as "unusual." The report also suggested "an association between some aspects of homosexual life-style or disease acquired through sexual contact and PCP in this population. Based on clinical examination of each of these cases,the possibility of a cellular immune dysfunc-

POINT OF INFORMATION 1.1

ANNOUNCEMENT OF CDC NAME CHANGE

The U.S. Congress, as part of the Preventive Health Amendments of 1992, has recognized CDC's leadership role in prevention by formally changing its name to the Centers for Disease Control and Prevention. The President signed the bill on October 27. In making this change, and acknowledging CDC's responsibility for "addressing illness and disability before they occur," the congress also specified that the agency should continue to be recognized by the acronym "CDC."

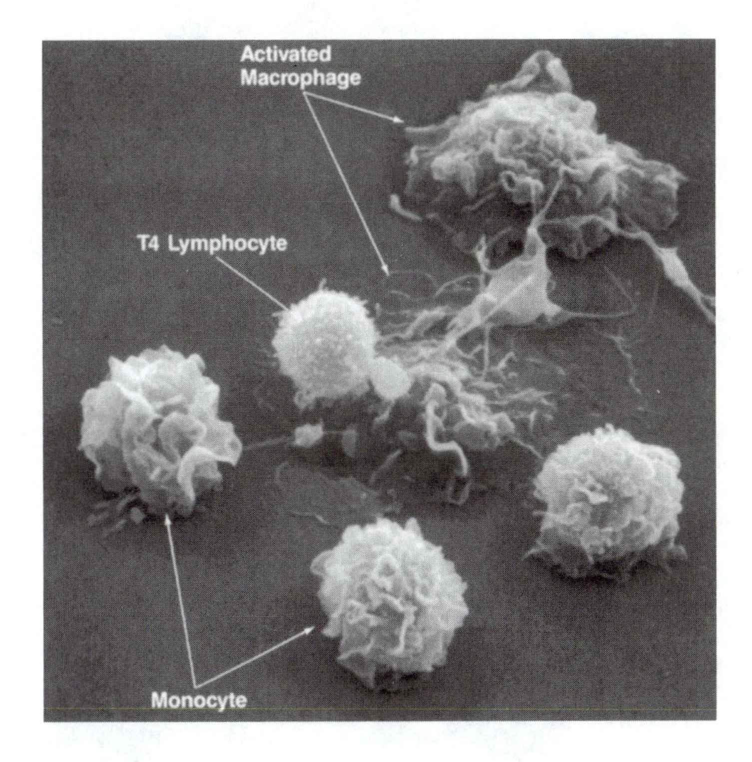

FIGURE 1-1 Normal Human T Lymphocytes, Monocytes, and Macrophages. Scanning electron micrograph of monocytes, macrophages, and a T4 lymphocyte, magnified 9,000 times. These white blood cells are the targets of HIV infection. Note that the T4 lymphocyte (round cell, at the center) is adhered to a flattened macrophage. (*Photograph courtesy of Dr. M. A. Gonda, Program Resources, Inc., NCI-Frederick Cancer Research Facility. Reprinted from Gonda,* Natural History, *95:78-81, 1986, with permission from* Natural History.)

tion related to a common exposure might also be involved."

In July 1981, the CDC (*MMWR*, 1981) reported that an uncommon cancer, *Kaposi's sarcoma* (KS), had been diagnosed in 26 gay men who lived in New York City and California. This was also an unusual finding because KS, when it occurred, was usually found in *older* men of Hebrew or Italian ancestry. The sudden and dramatic increase in pneumonia cases, all of which were caused by a widespread but generally harmless fungus, *P. carinii*, indicated that an infectious form of immune deficiency was on the increase. This immune deficiency disease, initially called GRID for Gay-Related Immune Deficiency, was noted to be quickly spreading in the homosexual community, among users of injection drugs, and among blood transfusion recipients. This new mysterious and lethal illness appeared to be associated with one's lifestyle. These early cases of immune deficiency heralded the beginning of an epidemic of a previously unknown illness. But before long, the disease was reported in heterosexuals and was subsequently called AIDS.

DISCOVERY OF THE AIDS VIRUS

There was no shortage of ideas on what caused AIDS. It was believed by some to be an act of God, a religious curse or penalty against the homosexual for practicing a biblically unacceptable lifestyle that included drugs, alcohol, and sexual promiscuity. Some believed it was due to sperm exposure to amyl nitrate, a stimulant used by some homosexuals to heighten sexual pleasure (Gallo, 1987). Others believed there was no specific infectious agent. They believed that certain people who *excessively stressed their immune systems* experienced immune system failure, and before it could recover, other infections killed them. But many scientists who had expertise in analyzing the sudden onset of "new" human diseases felt the cause of this form of human immune deficiency was an infectious agent. They believed that the agent was transmitted through sexual intercourse, blood, or blood products and from mother to fetus. They also believed that this agent which led to the loss of T cells was smaller than a bacterium or fungus because it passed through a filter normally used to remove those microorganisms. It turned out after further studies that this agent fit the profile of a virus.

In January of 1983, Luc Montagnier (Mont-tan-ya) and colleagues at the Pasteur Institute in Paris isolated the AIDS virus (Hobson et al., 1991). In May of that year, he published the first report on a T cell retrovirus found in a patient with **lymphadenopathy** (lim-fad-eh-nop-ah-thee), or swollen lymph glands. Lymphadenopathy is one of the early signs in patients progressing toward AIDS. The French scientist (Figure 1-2) named this virus **lymphadenopathy**-associated virus (LAV) (Barre-Sinoussi et al., 1983).

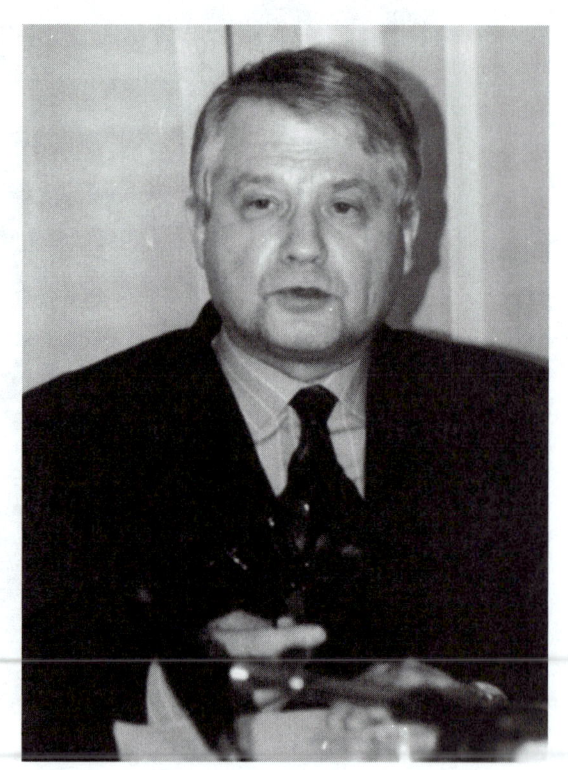

FIGURE 1-2 Luc Montagnier, from the Pasteur Institute in Paris. He discovered the human immunodeficiency virus (HIV), the cause of AIDS. *(Photograph courtesy of AP/Wide World Photos)*

Naming the AIDS Viruses: HIV-1, HIV-2

During the search for the AIDS virus, several investigators isolated the virus but gave it different names. For example, Robert Gallo (Figure 1-3) named the virus HTLV III (Human T Cell Lymphotropic Virus). Because the collection of names given this virus created some confusion, the Human Retrovirus Subcommittee of the Committee on the Taxonomy of Viruses reduced all of the names to one: **human immunodeficiency virus** or **HIV**. This term has now been accepted for use worldwide.

In 1985, a second type of HIV was discovered in West African prostitutes. It was named HIV type 2 or **HIV-2**. The first confirmed case of HIV-2 infection in the United States was reported in late 1987 in a West African woman with AIDS. By December 1990, 16 additional cases of HIV-2 infection were reported to the CDC (*MMWR*, 1990). Since then, a few new HIV-2 infections have been identified. Cases of HIV-2 infection have been found in Massachusetts, Connecticut, Rhode Island, Florida, and New York. Case histories of all of the HIV-2 infected patients revealed that they had recently immigrated to the United States from West Africa, had sexual contact with West Africans, or had traveled to West Africa. Clinically, what has been learned about HIV-1 appears to apply to HIV-2, except that HIV-2 appears to be less harmful (cytopathic) to the cells of the immune system, and it reproduces more slowly than HIV-1.

Unless stated otherwise, all references to HIV in this book refer to HIV-1.

DEFINING THE ILLNESS: AIDS SURVEILLANCE

Data gathered from AIDS patients in 1981 indicated that all demonstrated a loss of T4 lym-

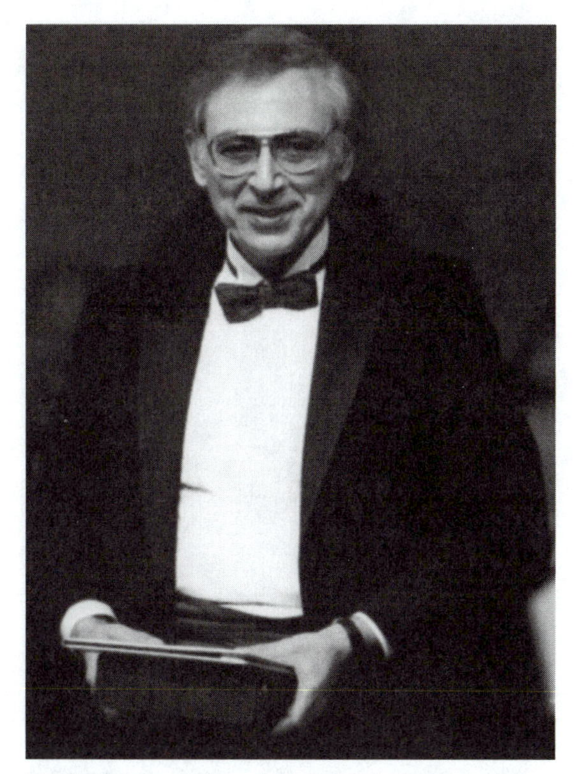

FIGURE 1-3 Robert Gallo, Chief of Tumor Cell Biology, National Cancer Institute. *(Photograph courtesy of AP/Wide World Photos)*

phocytes, and that 42% of AIDS patients had already died as a result of severe opportunistic infections. Opportunistic infections are caused by organisms and viruses that are normally present but do *not* cause disease unless the immune system is damaged. Clearly there was an immediate need for a name and definition for this disease so that a rational surveillance program could begin.

Definitions of AIDS for Surveillance Purposes

The initial objective of AIDS surveillance was to describe the epidemic in terms of time, place, and individual; and to recognize immediately changes in rate and pattern in the spread of AIDS. Early surveillance was done to gather data in order to generate information of value in planning control programs. Because a *cellular deficiency of the human immune system* was found in every AIDS patient, along with an assortment of other signs and symptoms of disease, and because the infection was *acquired* from the action of some environmental agent, it was named **AIDS** for **Acquired Immune Deficiency Syndrome.**

In order to establish surveillance, a system for monitoring where and when AIDS cases occurred and a workable definition had to be developed. The definition had to be *sensitive* enough to detect every possible AIDS patient while at the same time *specific* enough to exclude those who may have AIDS-like symptoms, but were not infected by the AIDS virus.

In 1982, there was no *single characteristic* of AIDS that would allow for a useful definition for surveillance purposes. Because immunological testing was essentially unavailable, the first AIDS surveillance definition was based on the clinical description of symptoms. The *first* of many criteria for the diagnosis of AIDS were: (1) the presence of a reliably diagnosed disease at least moderately predictive of cellular immune deficiency; and (2) the absence of an underlying cause for the immune deficiency or for reduced resistance to the disease (*MMWR*, 1982).

The definition of AIDS was thus an arbitrary one, reflecting the partial knowledge of the consequences that prevailed at the time. Various systems for classifying HIV-related illnesses have been devised since 1982 to take into account increasing knowledge about the spectrum of those illnesses. But the definition of AIDS has remained largely unchanged, partly for epidemiological reasons: a standard definition of AIDS makes it easier to monitor the incidence of the disease over time. Had the whole picture of HIV infection and its consequences been known in 1982, the term "AIDS" would never have been coined. Instead, we would refer to the various stages of "HIV disease" (or perhaps, following an older tradition, "Gottlieb's disease," after Dr. Mike Gottlieb, who first described it).

The 1982 definition was modified in 1983 to include new diseases then found in AIDS patients. With this modification, AIDS became reportable to the CDC in every state. In 1985, additional diseases were included in the AIDS case definition. Those diseases were disseminated histoplasmosis, chronic isosporiasis, and some of the non-Hodgkin's lymphomas (a form of cancer).

Part of the 1982 through 1985 AIDS case definitions was the description of patients with AIDS-related complex (ARC). The symptoms of ARC included swollen lymph nodes (lymphadenopathy), weight loss, loss of appetite, fever, rashes, night sweats, and fatigue. But ARC patients did not have opportunistic infections, and because HIV testing was not widely available, their antibody status was unknown. By 1987, the need for a mid-AIDS classification was unnecessary. Antibody tests were available and much more was known about the onset of opportunistic infections. Thus the CDC dropped ARC from their 1987 AIDS definition. Extrapulmonary tuberculosis, HIV encephalopathy (brain disease), HIV wasting syndrome, presumptive *Pneumocystis carinii* pneumonia (PCP), and esophageal candidiasis (both fungal infections) were added to the definition (Table 1-1). For AIDS diagnoses in children, multiple or recurrent bacterial infections were added.

Broadly speaking, the term *AIDS* may be understood as referring to the onset of life-threatening illnesses as a result of HIV disease that results from an HIV infection. AIDS is the end stage of a disease process which may have been developing for 5, 10, or 15 years, for most of which time the infected person will have been perfectly well and quite possibly unaware that he or she has been infected.

Thus the number of AIDS cases reported from 1987 through 1992 reflects the revisions of the initial surveillance case definition. One major drawback to all of the CDC AIDS definitions is the fact that through 1992, the Social Security Administration (SSA) used the CDC AIDS definition to determine disability. But all the definitions were primarily based on symptoms and opportunistic infections in men. Therefore, about 65% of women with HIV/AIDS were excluded from SSA benefits. They were excluded because of failure to be diagnosed with AIDS by the CDC AIDS definition (Sprecher, 1991).

TABLE 1-1 1987 CDC Definition of AIDS

ADULT

A. Without laboratory evidence for HIV infection:
- Lymphoma of brain (<60 years of age)
- Lymphoid interstitial pneumonitis (<13 years of age)

B. With laboratory evidence for HIV infection:
- Disseminated coccidioidomycosis
- HIV encephalopathy
- Isosporiasis (persisting > 1 month)
- Lymphoma of brain (any age)
- Non-Hodgkin's lymphoma (B cell or undifferentiated)
- Recurrent Salmonella septicemia
- Extrapulmonary tuberculosis
- HIV-wasting syndrome
- Recurrent bacterial infections (<13 years of age)
- Disseminated histoplasmosis

PEDIATRIC

Children with AIDS may have infectious diseases that are not covered by the adult CDC AIDS definitions. Thus children under 15 months are classified separately from older children because passive maternal antibodies may be present.

To Be HIV-Infected, Children Under 15 Months Must:

1. Show HIV in blood and tissues.
2. Show evidence of humoral and acquired immune deficiency and have one or more opportunistic infections associated with AIDS.
3. Show other symptoms meeting the CDC definition of AIDS.

TO BE HIV-INFECTED, CHILDREN BETWEEN 16 MONTHS AND 12 YEARS MUST:

1. Show 1 and 3 above.
2. Show HIV antibodies.

This definition was updated on January 1, 1993 to include all persons with a T4 cell count of less than 200/μL. See text for additional details.

(Adapted from Roger J. Pomerantz, M.D., "The Chameleon Called AIDS," Harvard Medical School, 1988.)

Impact of the 1993 Expanded AIDS Case Definition— On January 1, 1993, the newest definition of AIDS was put into the surveillance network. The reason for the new CDC definition was that epidemiologists felt the 1987 definition failed to reflect the true magnitude of the pandemic. In particular, it failed to address AIDS in women. In addition, those with T4 counts under 200/µL are most likely to be severely ill or disabled and in greatest need of medical and social services. With the new AIDS definition, these people are eligible earlier in their illness for federal and state medical and social assistance programs.

CDC revised the classification system for HIV infection to emphasize the clinical importance of the T4 lymphocyte count in the categorization of HIV-related clinical conditions. Consistent with this revised classification system, CDC has expanded the AIDS surveillance case definition to include all HIV-infected persons who have less than 200 T4 lymphocytes/µL, or a T4 lymphocyte percent less than 14% of total lymphocytes (Table 1-2). In addition to retaining the 23 clinical conditions in the 1987 AIDS surveillance case definition, the expanded definition includes (1) pulmonary tuberculosis, (2) invasive cervical cancer, and (3) recurrent pneumonia in persons with documented HIV infection (Table 1-3). This expanded definition requires laboratory evidence for HIV infection in persons with less than 200 T4 lymphocytes/µL or with one of the added clinical conditions. The objectives of these changes are to simplify the classification of HIV infection and the AIDS case reporting process, to be consistent with standards of medical care for HIV-infected persons, to better categorize HIV- related morbidity, and to reflect more accurately the number of persons with severe HIV-related immunosuppression who are at highest risk for severe HIV-related morbidity and most in need of close medical follow-up. The addition of the three clinical conditions reflects their documented or potential importance in the HIV epidemic. Invasive cervical cancer is included on the basis of an epidemiological link between HIV infection and cervical dysplasia, and reports that HIV speeds the

TABLE 1-2 T4 Lymphocyte Counts Related to Percentages of Total Lymphocytes

T4 Cell Category	T4 Cells/µL	Percent T4 Cells of Total Lymphocytes
(1)	≥ 500	≥ 29
(2)	200–499	14–28
(3)	<200	<14

1. Normal T4 cell count ranges from 900 to 1,200 T4 cells/µL of blood.

2. The equivalences of T4 cells to percent of total lymphocytes were derived from analyses of more than 15,500 lymphocyte subset determinations from seven different sources: one multistate study of diseases in HIV-infected adolescents and adults, and six laboratories (two commercial, one research, and three university-based). The six laboratories are involved in proficiency testing programs for lymphocyte subset determinations.

(Adapted from *MMWR*, 1993.)

TABLE 1-3 List of 26 Conditions in the 1993 AIDS Surveillance Case Definition

- Candidiasis of bronchi, trachea, or lungs
- Candidiasis, esophageal
- Cervical cancer, invasive[a]
- Coccidioidomycosis, Disseminated or extrapulmonary
- Cryptococcosis, extrapulmonary
- Cryptosporidiosis, chronic intestinal (>1 month duration)
- Cytomegalovirus disease (other than liver, spleen, or nodes)
- Cytomegalovirus retinitis (with loss of vision)
- HIV encephalopathy
- Herpes simplex: chronic ulcer(s) (>1 month duration); or bronchitis, pneumonitis, or esophagitis
- Histoplasmosis, disseminated or extrapulmonary
- Isosporiasis, chronic intestinal (>1 month duration)
- Kaposi's sarcoma
- Lymphoma, Burkitt's (or equivalent term)
- Lymphoma, immunoblastic (or equivalent term)
- Lymphoma, primary in brain
- *Mycobacterium avium complex* or *M. kansasii,* disseminated or extrapulmonary
- *Mycobacterium tuberculosis,* disseminated or extrapulmonary
- *Mycobacterium tuberculosis,* any site (pulmonary[a] or extrapulmonary)
- *Mycobacterium,* other species or unidentified species, disseminated or extrapulmonary
- *Pneumocystis carinii* pneumonia
- Pneumonia, recurrent[a]
- Progressive multifocal leukoencephalopathy
- Salmonella septicemia, recurrent
- Toxoplasmosis of brain
- Wasting syndrome due to HIV

[a]Added in the 1993 expansion of the AIDS surveillance case definition.

(Adapted from the CDC, Atlanta, Georgia.)

progression of both cervical dysplasia and cancer. From January 1, 1993 through December 1993, 5,729 new AIDS cases were reported based on the presence of one of the three clinical conditions.

The expanded AIDS surveillance case definition has had a substantial impact on the number of reported cases in 1993.

Of the 105,990 Adult/Adolescent AIDS cases reported in 1993, 57,235 (54%) were reported based on conditions added to the definition in 1993; and 48,755 (46%) were reported based on pre-1993 defined conditions (Table 1-4). Of the 57,235 cases reported based on 1993-added conditions, 51,511 persons (91%) had severe HIV-related immunosuppression only; 4,006 (7%), pulmonary tuberculosis (TB); 1,445 (2%), recurrent pneumonia; and 273 (1%), invasive cervical cancer (19 persons were reported with more than one of these opportunistic illnesses). A substantial increase in the number of reported AIDS cases occurred in all regions of the United States. Of areas reporting more than 250 cases, the proportion of cases based on the 1993-added criteria ranged from 35% in North Carolina (n = 1,353) to 71% in Colorado (n = 1,323).

The increase in reported cases in 1993 was greater among females (151%) than among males (105%). Proportionate increases were greater among blacks and Hispanics than among whites. The largest increases in case reporting occurred among persons aged 13–19 years and 20–24 years; in these age groups, a greater proportion of cases were reported among women (35% and 29%, respectively) and were attributed to heterosexual transmission (22% and 18%, respectively).

TABLE 1-4 AIDS Cases by Race/Ethnicity Reported for 1994, United States

Race/Ethnic Group	AIDS Cases	Percentage of Cases
White	36,628	45.5
Black	28,819	35.8
Hispanic	14,248	17.7
Asian/Pacific Islander	536	0.7
American Indian	242	0.3
Total	80,473[a]	100

[a]Pediatric AIDS cases for 1994, 990.

Compared with homosexual/bisexual men, proportionate increases in case reporting were greater among heterosexual injecting-drug users (IDUs) and among persons reportedly infected through heterosexual contact.

Women, blacks, heterosexual IDUs, and persons with hemophilia were more likely than others to be reported with 1993-added conditions. Most of these differences were attributable to reports of the three opportunistic illnesses added in 1993; of 5,729 persons reported with a 1993-added opportunistic illness, 26% were women, 48% were heterosexual IDUs, and 63% were black. The number of Hispanics reported under the 1993-added criteria reflected reports from Puerto Rico: 38% of the 3,173 reports from Puerto Rico were based on the 1993-added criteria, compared with 54% of the 15,145 cases among Hispanics from other areas.

The pediatric AIDS surveillance case definition was not changed in 1993. During 1993, 990 children aged <13 years were reported with AIDS, an increase of 21% compared with the 783 cases reported in 1992. Of those 990 children, 50% were female, and most were either black (55%) or Hispanic (27%) and were infected through perinatal HIV transmission (93%). New York, Puerto Rico, and Florida reported 489 (51%) of the pediatric AIDS cases (MMWR, 1994).

If all of the approximately 1 million plus persons in the United States with HIV infection were diagnosed and their immune status known, it is estimated that 120,000–190,000 persons who do not have AIDS-indicator diseases would be found to have T4 lymphocyte counts < 200/μL. However, since all of these persons are not aware of their HIV infection status, and of those who are, not all have had an immunological evaluation, the immediate impact on the number of AIDS cases will be considerably less. Under the 1987 AIDS surveillance criteria, approximately 49,106 AIDS cases were reported in 1992, but 105,990 were reported for 1993. In 1994, there were 80,473 new AIDS cases. For 1995, the number of new cases should be about 60,000 with 53,000 new cases occurring in 1996 and in 1997.

The effects of the expanded surveillance definition was greatest in 1993 because of the backlog in number of persons who fit the new AIDS definition. Once most of these cases are reported, the yearly incidence should fall off to between 50,000 and 60,000 cases a year through the rest of the 1990s. Finally, the expanded HIV classification system and the AIDS surveillance case definition have been developed for use in conducting public health surveillance. They were not developed to determine whether any statutory or other legal requirements for entitlement to federal disability or other benefits are met.

The revised surveillance case definition does not alter the criteria used by the Social Security Administration in evaluating claims based on HIV infection under the Social Security disability insurance and Supple-mental Security Income programs. The Social Security Administration has recently proposed a new method for the evaluation of HIV infection and criteria to determine eligibility for disability. Other organizations and agencies providing medical and social services should develop eligibility criteria appropriate with the services provided and local needs (*MMWR*, 1993).

Problems Stemming from Changing the AIDS Definition for Surveillance Purposes

Each time the definition of AIDS has been altered by the CDC, it has led to an increase in the number of AIDS cases. In 1985, the change in definition led to a 2% increase over what would have been diagnosed prior to the change. The 1987 change led to a 35% increase in new AIDS cases per year over that expected using the 1985 definition. The 1993 change resulted in a 52% increase in AIDS cases over that expected for 1993. Such rapid changes alters the baseline from which future predictions are made and makes the interpretations of trends in incidence and characteristic of cases difficult to process.

SUMMARY

Much continues to be written about HIV/AIDS. Some of it, especially in lay articles, has been less than accurate and has led to public confusion and fear. **HIV infection is not AIDS.** HIV infection is now referred to as HIV disease. AIDS is a syndrome of many diseases, each resulting from an opportunistic agent or cancer cell that multiplies in humans who are immunosuppressed. The new 1993 CDC AIDS definition will allow, over the long term, earlier access to federal and state medical and social services for HIV-infected individuals.

REVIEW QUESTIONS

(Answers to the Review Questions are on page 478.)

1. The letters A, I, D, and S are an acronym for?
2. Is AIDS a single disease? Explain.
3. When was the AIDS virus discovered and by whom?
4. In what year did CDC first report on a strange new disease which later was named AIDS?
5. Name one acronym for HIV.
6. How many times has CDC changed and expanded the definition of AIDS? In what years?
7. Why did the CDC do away with the ARC definition?
8. What is one major advantage of the new CDC AIDS definition for the HIV-infected?

REFERENCES

BARRE-SINOUSSI, FRANCOISE, et al. (1983). Isolation of a T-lymphocyte retrovirus from a patient at risk for acquired immune deficiency syndrome (AIDS). *Science,* 220:868–871.

GALLO, ROBERT C. (1987). The AIDS virus. *Sci. Am.,* 256:47–56.

HOBSON, SIMON WAIN, et al. (1991). LAV revisited: Origins of the early HIV-1 isolates from Institut Pasteur. Science, 252:961–965.

Medical World News. (1988). Researchers blast CDC projections of AIDS deaths—AIDS update, 29:73.

Morbidity and Mortality Weekly Report. (1981). Pneumocystis pneumonia—Los Angeles, 30:250–252.

Morbidity and Mortality Weekly Report. (1982). Update on acquired immune deficiency syndrome (AIDS)—United States, 31:507–508, 513–514.

Morbidity and Mortality Weekly Report. (1990). Surveillance for HIV-2 infection in blood donors—United States, 1987–1989, 39:829–831.

Morbidity and Mortality Weekly Report. (1993). 1993 Revised classification system for HIV infection and expanded surveillance case definition for AIDS among adolescents and adults, 41:1–19.

Morbidity and Mortality Weekly Report. (1994). Update: Impact of the expanded AIDS surveillance case definition for adolescents and adults on case reporting—United States, 1993, 43:160–170.

SPRECHER, LORRIE. (1991). Women with AIDS: Dead but not disabled. *The Positive Woman,* 1:4.

CHAPTER

2

What Causes AIDS: Origin of the AIDS Virus

CHAPTER CONCEPTS

- HIV does not cause AIDS?
- AIDS is caused by the Human Immunodeficiency Virus (HIV).
- An unbroken chain of HIV transmission has been established between those infected and the newly infected.

THE CAUSE OF AIDS: THE HUMAN IMMUNODEFICIENCY VIRUS

The unexpected appearance and accelerated spread of an unknown lethal disease soon raised several important questions: *What* is causing the disease? Where did it come from? *How* does the causative agent function? *What* are the characteristics of the agent? These four questions will be answered.

This section has a subtitle which implies that AIDS is the result of HIV infection. There are a relatively small number of scientists and nonscientists as of this writing who claim that HIV does **not** cause AIDS. For a balanced HIV/AIDS presentation, this claim will be presented first.

HIV Does Not Cause AIDS: A Minority Point of View

Peter Duesberg is perhaps the most vocal in his concern that the scientific community is investigating the wrong causative agent. Duesberg is a molecular biologist at the University of California at Berkeley and a member of the National Academy of Sciences. Duesberg has advanced his anti-HIV/AIDS hypothesis at great expense to himself. He states that "I have been excommunicated by the retrovirus-AIDS community

BOX 2.1

SEX AND HIV DO NOT CAUSE AIDS!

Medical Doctor puts his life on the Line to Prove It.

On 28 October, Robert Willner held a press conference at a North Carolina hotel, during which he jabbed his finger with a bloody needle he had just stuck into a man who said he was infected with HIV. Willner is a physician who recently had his medical license revoked in Florida for, among other infractions, claiming to have cured an AIDS patient with ozone infusions. He is also the author of a new book, *Deadly Deception: The Proof that SEX and HIV Absolutely DO NOT CAUSE AIDS.* He insists that jabbing himself with the bloody needle, which he describes as "an act of intelligence," was not meant to sell books. "I'm interested in proving to people that there isn't one shred of scientific evidence that HIV causes any disease".

USA Today, October 3, 1994, carried a full-page advertisement to promote the selling of Willner's book. A full-page ad in this newspaper, regardless of location, if carried nationally costs $57,500. **Question for class discussion:** Did *USA Today* management provide socially responsible advertisement or did money talk and responsibility walk? What is the potential medical downside of this advertisement?

The scientific journal *Science* (1994; 226:1642–1649) presented a series of six articles by Jon Cohen concerning the *question* of whether HIV causes AIDS. The articles are a balanced review of the scientific facts as they relate to the question.

with noninvitations to meetings, noncitations in the literature and nonrenewals of my research grants, which is the highest price an experimental scientist can pay for his convictions."

In 1971, he co-discovered cancer-causing genes in viruses. In the March 1987 issue of *Cancer Research,* Duesberg published "Retroviruses as Carcinogens and Pathogens: Expectations and Reality." The article provoked wide-based scientific discussion and received a lot of popular press coverage. Duesberg argued that there is no evidence that HIV causes AIDS. He has published additional articles in *Science* (1988) and in the *Proceedings of the National Academy of Sciences* (1989) stating that HIV is not the cause of AIDS. In May of 1992, Duesberg was the featured speaker at an alternative AIDS conference, "AIDS: A Different View," promoted by homeopathic physician Martien Brands. The week of meetings was spent giving new interpretations to some of the data used to establish HIV as the causative agent of AIDS. In short, Duesberg suggests that there is no single causative agent, that the disease is due to one's "lifestyle." He marshals arguments to support his theory that, in the United States and probably in Europe, AIDS is a collection of noninfectious deficiencies predominantly associated with drug use, malnutrition, parasitic infections, and other specific risks.

Duesberg believes that the tests which detect HIV antibodies are useless. In the June 1988 issue of *Discovery* he said, "If somebody told me today that I was antibody positive, I wouldn't worry one second. I wouldn't take Valium. I wouldn't write my will. All I would say is that my immune system seems to work. I have antibodies to a virus. I am protected."

In June 1990, Weiss and Jaffe wrote a critical refutation of Duesberg's theory that HIV cannot be the cause of AIDS. Duesberg's response suggested that he was unaware of published data that clearly answer the questions he raises concerning HIV involvement in AIDS. For example, one of Duesberg's major points is that no one has yet shown that hemophiliacs infected with HIV progress to AIDS. The data on matched groups of homosexual males and hemophiliacs which show that *only* those infected with HIV develop AIDS have been available for a number of years. Summary data on matched pairs from these two groups were presented by Weiss and Jaffe in *Nature* (1990). These data clearly show that only HIV-infected gay males and hemophiliacs progress to AIDS.

Duesberg's arguments and disagreements with the vast majority of prominent scientists who have researched the causal agent of AIDS are many. But they pale when placed next to the overwhelming evidence which leaves no doubt in the opinion of most scientists that HIV causes AIDS (see Cohen, 1995; Andrews, 1995).

Based on an August 1992 report in *Newsweek*, a father discussed his decision, based on Duesberg's claims, to counsel his infected hemophiliac son to avoid zidovudine (ZDV) treatment. This situation is similar to what happened when desperate cancer patients followed the advice of a credentialed academician who recommended vitamin therapy as the cure for cancer. Based on this advice, some people failed to undergo truly effective therapy. **Questions**: Is Duesberg's opinion on this issue inadvertently harmful to humans? To the scientific process? Will the use of his idea, that HIV does not cause AIDS, provide a course of action that will stop the Acquired Immune Deficiency Syndrome? As of mid-1995, Duesberg still insisted that HIV does not cause AIDS. He believes that HIV is just another opportunistic agent like those that cause other opportunistic diseases (Duesberg, 1993, 1995). Robert Root-Bernstein authored "Rethinking AIDS" in 1993. This book attempts to support Duesberg's hypothesis that there is no link between HIV and AIDS. His main thesis is that scientists do not have the necessary information to conclude that HIV causes AIDS. He believes, first, that the right studies on the cause of immunosuppression have not been done and, second, that there need not be a common thread (such as the virus) associated with this new disease, no common denominator such as a causative transmissible agent, but on the other hand he does not rule out the case for a single infectious organism that has yet to be identified.

In 1993, Britain's *Sunday Times* took the Duesberg claim that HIV does not cause AIDS to a new level by runing a series of articles disclaiming HIV as the cause of AIDS. The *Sunday Times* continued to run these articles throughout 1994 (Dickson, 1994; Karpas, 1994). In mid-1994, Kary Mullis (reciepent of the Nobel prize in chemistry for his invention of the polymerose chain reaction—see Chapter 12 for explanation) joined Duesberg and the *Sunday Times* by saying, "the idea that HIV was the 'probable cause of AIDS' was not a scientifically proven fact, nor, indeed, was there any clear evidence that AIDS was spread through sexual contact. I think we [spread] retroviruses by our lungs, not by our genitals." Mullis continued by saying, "it is not a scientitic fact, or even a supposed fact, that HIV is the probable cause of AIDS." Mullis is unrepentant in the face of those who complained his ideas were undermining the activities of AIDS health-workers around the world. Critics of Mullis state that he has limited knowledge of HIV/AIDS and no scientific authority to speak on the cause of AIDS (Dickson, 1994). Robin Weiss, director of research at the Institute of Cancer Research, wrote that Mullis "has about as much knowledge and authority to speak on the cause of AIDS as William Shockley, the Nobel Laureate who invented the transistor, had when he used to speak on the intellectual superiority of whites compared to blacks."

Mullis himself appeared unfazed by such criticisms. His main concern was that the efforts of "a lot of talented people in the medical profession had been diverted" by misconceptions about HIV.

In April 1989, Shyh-Ching Lo of the Armed Forces Institute of Pathology started a second round of controversy. In an article, he claimed to have discovered a non-HIV "virus-like infectious agent" in 7 of 10 AIDS patients. Lo and colleagues stated that either this was a new opportunistic infection or "an agent which plays a more fundamental role as a cofactor in the process associated with infection by HIV." Later they discovered that the mysterious agent was a mycoplasma (a bacterium without cell walls). It appears to serve as a cofactor for HIV infection but is not necessary for HIV infection to occur. According to Montagnier, the person who discovered HIV, the virus is essential but may need a cofactor to establish HIV disease and AIDS.

Evidence That HIV Causes AIDS

It has been firmly established that there is a high correlation between HIV infection and the development of AIDS. With respect to establishing HIV as the causative agent of AIDS, let's look at the evidence:

1. The virus has now been identified in virtually all AIDS patients tested; in over 90% of those with pre-AIDS symptoms (formerly called AIDS related complex or ARC), that is, individuals who are HIV-positive and have symptoms of HIV disease; and in individuals who are HIV-positive but appear to be healthy.
2. The virus has been identified by electron microscopy inside and on the surface of T4 cells in HIV-positive and AIDS patients (Figure 2-1A,B).
3. Recent work of Bruce Patterson and Steven Wolinsky has shown that the genetic material of HIV (HIV-DNA) can be found in as many as 1 in 10 blood lymphocytes of persons with HIV disease (Cohen, 1993).
4. Antibodies against the virus, viral antigens, and HIV RNA have been found in HIV-positive and AIDS patients.
5. There is an absolute chronological association between the emergence of AIDS and the appearance of HIV in humans worldwide. For example, among homosexual males treated in a San Francisco STD clinic, the proportion of HIV-positive men increased from 1% in 1978 to 25% in 1980 to 65% in 1984.
6. There is a chronological association of HIV-positive individuals who progress to AIDS. People who are truly HIV-negative, and without the need for chemotherapy or radiation treatments, do not demonstrate HIV antibodies and never demonstrate AIDS. For example, prior to 1985, 75% to 90% of hemophiliacs in the United States tested HIV-positive. They became HIV-infected because the virus was present in blood factor VIII concentrates self-administered by hemophiliacs to clot their blood. In addition, the use of blood donor prepared blood factor VIII concentrates prior to 1985 has been linked to HIV infections wherever the blood

FIGURE 2-1 Viral Replication in Human Lymphocytes. Scanning electron micrograph of HIV-infected human T4 lymphocyte. **A**, A single cell infected with HIV showing virus particles and microvilli on the cell surface (magnified 7,000 times). **B**, Enlargement of a portion of the cell surface in (**A**) showing multiple virus particles budding or attached to the cell surface (magnified 20,000 times). (*Photograph courtesy of K. Nagashima, Program Resources, Inc., NCI-Frederick Cancer Research Facility*)

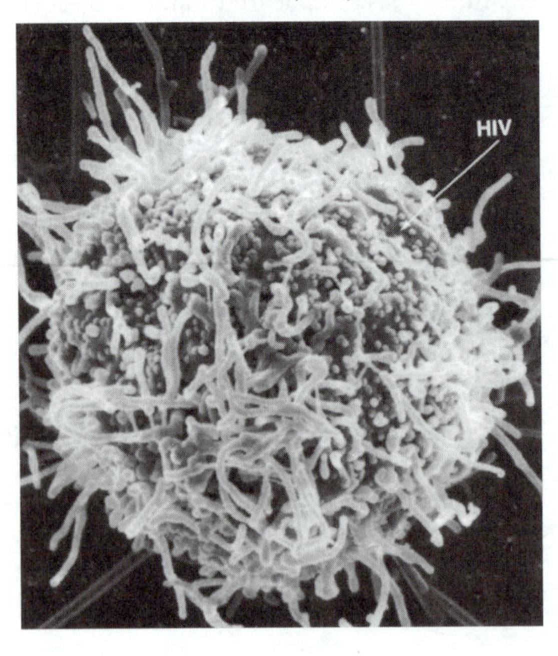

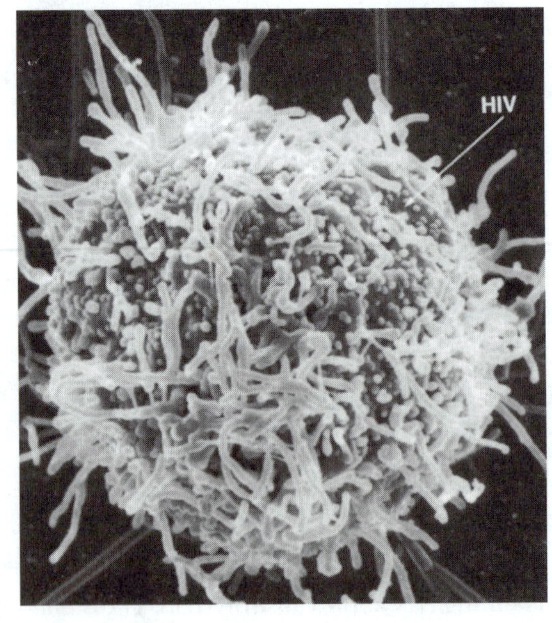

concentrate was used. Over half of these HIV-infected individuals have developed AIDS and 56% have died from it.

7. Hemophiliacs from low- and high-risk behavior groups were equally infected from HIV-contaminated blood factor VIII concentratee.
8. The virus is found in HIV-positive and AIDS patients but not in healthy low behavioral risk individuals.
9. With the exception of persons who had their immune systems suppressed due to genetic causes or by drug therapy, prior to the appearance of the virus, there were no known AIDS-like cases. The virus has been isolated worldwide—but only where there are HIV-positive people and AIDS patients.
10. An HIV-positive identical twin born to an HIV-positive mother developed AIDS, but the HIV-negative twin did not.
11. Finally, there have been numerous reports in the literature on HIV-infected individuals (homosexual, bisexual, and heterosexual) transmitting the virus to their sexual partners, both eventually dying of AIDS. *The unbroken chain of HIV transmission between prostitutes and their customers, between injection drug users sharing the same syringe, from infected mothers to their unborn fetuses, and so on all lead to the inescapable conclusion that HIV does cause AIDS.* Thus the identification of HIV as the causative agent of AIDS is now firmly accepted by scientists worldwide.

ORIGIN OF THE AIDS VIRUS

The object of determining the origin of the AIDS virus is to gain insight into how the virus may have evolved the unique set of characteristics that enable it to destroy the human immune system. Such information will offer valuable clues as to how rapidly the virus is evolving.

If, for example, HIV is a new virus, say less than 30 years old, the many different varieties of HIV now infecting people worldwide probably evolved from a common ancestor sometime after World War II. And new varieties can be expected to continue evolving at what would be a frightening pace for several more decades, possibly producing new strains of the virus that are even more dangerous than those now infecting people. This could mean that vaccines now being developed based on current virus strains may not be useful in 20 or 30 years. But, should the known strains of the virus prove to be hundreds or thousands of years old, it might be possible that the current types of HIVs are in a state of global balance and they would not be expected to offer scientists any shocking evolutionary surprises in the future. Such information is useful for the development of treatments or vaccine against HIV and to predict future emergence of other diseases.

UFOs, Biological Warfare, and Cats

Fear stimulates the imagination. Out of human fear have come some rather strange explanations for the cause of AIDS. Early reports had unidentified flying objects (UFOs) crashing to Earth and releasing a "new organism" that would wipe out humanity.

There have been frequent reports in the Soviet press linking AIDS with American biological warfare research. The Soviets agreed in August 1987 to stop these reports (Holder, 1988). There are also reports of extremism, as in the case of Illinois State Representative Douglas Huff of Chicago who told the *Los Angeles Times* that he gave over $500 from his office allowance fund to a local official of the Black Hebrew sect to help the group investigate its claim that Israel and South Africa created the AIDS virus in a laboratory in South Africa. Huff said AIDS is "clearly an ethnic weapon, a biological weapon" designed specifically to attack nonwhites (*CDC Weekly*, 1988).

Still another myth to surface is that the AIDS virus came from domestic cats. Because of its similarities to human AIDS, feline immunodeficiency virus has been called "feline AIDS." The cat retrovirus may damage cats' immune systems leaving the animals vulnerable to opportunistic infections *or* it may cause feline leukemia. However, the cat virus has never been shown to be passed to humans.

The origin of HIV has been attributed to HIV-contaminated polio, smallpox, hepatitis and tetanus vaccines, the African green monkey, African people, their cattle, pigs, and sheep—and the CIA. With respect to the use of HIV-contaminated vaccines, a number of recent articles suggest that early monkey kidney cultures used to produce the polio vaccine carried HIV. Review of the literature offers *no* evidence that this occurred. And the argument for the safety of the polio vaccine lies in the absence of any AIDS-related diseases among the hundreds of millions of persons vaccinated worldwide (Koprowski, 1992).

Now over 15 years (1980–1995) into the AIDS epidemic, researchers are still baffled by the question: Where did the AIDS virus come from? AIDS is now known to be caused by two human immunodeficiency viruses, HIV-1 and HIV-2. The former, the cause of most AIDS cases worldwide, *appears to have spread from Central Africa; while the latter has so far been confined mainly to West Africa and the islands off its coast.* Several theories have been proposed to explain the origins of the AIDS epidemic. Most have been speculative rather than verifiable; and several have caused offense, particularly those which refer to sexual practices with monkey blood (Gilks, 1991). Charles Gilks (1992) states that HIV may have entered the human population by the direct inoculation of malaria-HIV-infected blood into human prisoner-volunteers. The problem with this theory is that it is not testable so it, like others, will remain an unproven theory proposed to explain the origin of HIV/AIDS.

At the Fifth International Conference on AIDS in Montreal (1989), Vanessa Hirsch and colleagues presented evidence that a virus isolated from a species of West African monkey, the sooty mangabey (an ash-colored monkey), may have infected humans 20 to 30 years ago. They believe this virus subsequently *evolved into HIV-2.* Hirsch et al. studied a virus known as the simian immunodeficiency virus (SIVsm) that infects both wild and captive sooty mangabey monkeys. They molecularly cloned and sequenced the DNA of the virus and constructed an evolutionary tree of the several known primate immuno-deficiency viruses. This tree showed SIVsm to be more closely related to HIV-2 than to HIV-1.

Gerald Meyers of Los Alamos National Laboratory states that SIVsm and HIV are so closely related that when HIV-2 is found in a human, it may be the sooty mangabey virus. However, HIV-1, that causes AIDS, does not sufficiently resemble HIV-2 or SIVsm, thus HIV-1 probably did not evolve from SIVsm/HIV-2. Still, the prevailing theory is that humans were first infected through direct contact with HIV-infected primates. The pri- mate to human scenario is easier to accept than humans infecting primates. Humans have hunted, handled, and even eaten primates for thousands of years. Recent laboratory accidents have shown that SIV can infect humans. Even though at the moment, no identifiable disease has been associated with the SIV/human infections, such accidents have demonstrated the potential for cross-species transmission of HIV-related viruses. Why not believe the same for the origin of HIV-1?

There also remains the possibility that HIV has been present but remained an obscure virus in the human population for a long time before it was recognized as a lethal agent, similar perhaps to the polio virus which surely existed in the human population for years prior to its being discovered as the cause of the polio epidemic of 1894. After all, there is ample evidence that primates, historically, have harbored lentiviruses (the class that includes SIV and HIV). Why should humans be any exception?

Adam Carr (*AIDS in Australia,* 1992) writes that the most widely accepted view on the origin of HIV is that the virus is endemic to a remote part of central Africa, possibly in the mountains of eastern Zaire, and that it began to spread to other parts of Africa only after the area had been penetrated by Europeans in the twentieth century.

In colonial Africa, it is quite possible that a low but persistent level of AIDS cases could have gone unnoticed by the poorly developed health services of the time. In the 1970s, when rapid urbanization and its attendant social changes began in Zaire and neighboring countries, the epidemic began to accelerate and come to the attention of health authorities. By this time it would have begun to spread to other countries. Tourists, soldiers (there were thousands of Cuban troops in neighboring Angola in the mid-1970s), guest workers, and other travelers would have taken the virus to Europe, the Caribbean, and North America.

The first documented case of AIDS in Europe was seen in a Danish surgeon who had worked in Zaire. She died in 1976.

Discussion of the African origins of HIV has caused controversy. Some African governments protested at suggestions that Africa was "responsible" for the AIDS epidemic, and even denied that AIDS was a problem in their countries. For most of the 1980s, the military government of Zaire would not allow outsiders to investigate the spread of AIDS and did not report AIDS cases to the World Health Organization. Some Africans denounced "racist" Western media for reporting AIDS as an African plague. Carr states that "by 1990, when it was obvious to all that HIV infection was tragically widespread in central, southern, and eastern Africa, this controversy had largely ended. HIV infection is far too widespread in Africa to be the result of recent importation from outside; the African epidemic clearly precedes the Western one." Regardless, where HIV/AIDS arose is irrelevant to medical science—when and how HIV entered the human population is relevant.

In summary, there are at least three possible origins of the AIDS virus: (1) it is a human-made virus, perhaps from a germ warfare laboratory; (2) it originated in the animal world and crossed over into humans; and (3) HIV has existed in small isolated human populations for a long time and, given the right set of conditions, it escaped into the larger population. Computer modeling of DNA sequence in HIV and SIVsm suggests that HIV evolved within the last 100 years. So, for now, the question remains: Is AIDS a new disease or an old disease which was late being recognized—so late that we will never know its true source of origin, the origin of HIV?

Perhaps the real question is not where HIV-1 came from but whether it has always caused disease. From the study of human history, as it relates to human disease, scientists have numerous examples that show that as human habits change, new diseases emerge. Regardless of whether HIV is old or new, history will show that social changes, however small or sudden, have most likely hastened the increase in virulence and the spread of HIV. In the 1960s, war, tourism, and commercial trucking forced the outside world on Africa's once isolated villages. At the same time, drought and industrialization prompted mass migrations from the countryside into newly teeming cities. Western monogamy had never been common in Africa, but as the French medical historian Mirko Grmek notes in his book, *History of AIDS* (1990), urbanization shattered social structures that had long contained sexual behavior. Prostitution exploded, and venereal disease flourished. Hypodermic needles came into wide use during the same period, creating yet another mode of infection. Did these trends actually turn a chronic but relatively benign infection into a killer? The evidence is circumstantial, but it's hard to discount.

Whatever the forces are that brought us AIDS, they can surely bring other diseases. By encroaching on rain forests and wilderness areas, humans are placing themselves in ever-closer contact with animal species and their deadly parasites. Activities, from irrigation to the construction of dams and cities, can expose humans to new diseases by expanding the range of the rodents or insects that carry them. Stephen Morse, a Rockefeller virologist, studies the movement of microbes among populations and species. He worries that human activities are speeding the flow of viral traffic. More than a dozen new diseases have shown up in humans since the 1960s, nearly all of them the result of once exotic parasites exploiting new opportunities.

The Ebola virus is often cited as an example of the pathogens in our future. The virus first struck in August 1976, when a trader arrived at a mission hospital in northern Zaire with a raging fever and blood oozing from every orifice. Within days the man died, and nearly half of the nurses at the hospital were stricken. Thirty-nine died, and as hospital patients contracted the virus, it spread to 58 neighboring villages. Ebola fever ended up striking 1,000 people in Zaire and nearby Sudan, killing 500. Epidemiologists feared it would spread more widely, but the outbreaks subsided as quickly as they had begun. From an evolutionary perspective, that's no great surprise. A parasite that kills that rapidly has little chance of sustaining a chain of infection unless it can survive independently of its host. HIV may take 10 to 20 years to kill its host. Surely, by that time it can be passed on.

IS IT AIDS OR IDIOPATHIC CD4 LYMPHOPENIA (ICL)?

The July 1992 issue of *Newsweek* broke a story about persons with "AIDS-like symptoms" who are HIV-negative. The social and scientific impact was immediate. Occurrences of non-HIV AIDS cases became the unscheduled focus of the following 8th International Conference on AIDS. Scientists Jeffrey Lawrence reported on patients with low CD4 counts and Sidhir Gupta and David Ho stated that they had evidence of a new virus in such persons (Culliton, 1992). Ho said he found high levels of the reverse transcriptase, an enzyme present in HIV. But finding reverse transcriptase is not enough to prove the existence of a virus. Scientists turned out to be wrong when they earlier reported finding reverse transcriptase in Kawasaki's disease, a childhood illness; in hepatitis C, a liver infection, and in Graves's disease, a cause of hyperthyroidism.

It should be mentioned that ICL by definition is not AIDS because AIDS stands for acquired immune deficiency syndrome which is caused by HIV. To diagnose ICL the CDC lists three criteria: Two CD4 tests that show counts of less than 300 of the T4 immune cells per microliter of blood, **no HIV infection**, and no other illness or therapy associated with T4 cell depletion. Severe immunosuppression **not** associated with HIV can result from a congenital immunodeficiency or a variety of other causes, for example, cancer, genetic defects, chemo-therapy, radiation, or large amounts of corticosteroids.

Collectively, by mid-1995, *worldwide,* less than 100 cases of HIV-negative AIDS-like persons had been reported. A small number of persons when compared to an estimated 20 million HIV-infected persons and 6 million AIDS cases. Persons with unexplained T4 lymphocyte depletion but without detectable HIV infection have been described since 1985. The 40 cases reported in the United States constitute a remarkably varied collection of people. They live in 15 states, range from 18 to 70 years old, and the majority (54%) have no known risk factors for HIV. This heterogeneity has led epidemiologists to conclude that, whatever is going on, there probably is not a single cause for all the cases. And the notion that a single transmissible agent does not account for all these cases was bolstered by the fact that although most of the patients' sexual and household contacts have yet to be studied, the few that have been examined appear to have normal T4 counts (Cohen, 1992).

In summary, the cause or causes of immunodeficiency and persistently low T4 cell counts in the patients described with ICL are unknown. They may represent a condition that was not detected until T4 cell counting became widely available. Alternatively, they may represent a different syndrome of immunodeficiency associated with T4 cell depletion. Of 26 cases described by the CDC, there has been speculation that some of these cases result from infection by a "new virus," but the existence of such a virus has not been proven. To date, the number of cases is small, and there is no report of transmission to close contacts. Of the 26 cases reported on by the CDC, five had received transfusions before onset of illness, five were men who had sex with men, and the remaining 16 had no known risk factors for HIV infection. Follow-up investigation of the blood donors for one patient found that they were HIV-negative, in good health, and had no evidence of immune deficiency. For an update on this scientific mystery, information is available from HRS (904) 487-2478 and CDC (404) 639-2981.

SUMMARY

The AIDS virus was discovered and reported on by Luc Montagnier of France in 1983. Identifying the virus that caused the immunosuppression that caused AIDS allowed for AIDS surveillance definitions that began in 1982. The recent recognition of non-HIV AIDS cases is not unexpected and can be explained. There is no new threat of another AIDS causing biological agent.

REVIEW QUESTIONS

(Answers to the Review Questions are on page 478.)

1. What may be the strongest nonlaboratory evidence for saying that AIDS is caused by an environmental agent?
2. Where might HIV have originated and where did the first HIV infections appear?

REFERENCES

ANDREWS, CHARLA. (1995). "The Duesberg Phenomenon." What does it mean? *Science,* 267:157.

CDC Weekly. (1988). Extremists seek to blame AIDS on Jews. July: 11.

COHEN, JON. (1992). Mystery virus meets the skeptics. *Science,* 257:1032–1034.

COHEN, JON. (1993). Keystone's blunt message: 'It's the Virus, Stupid'. *Science,* 260:292–293.

CULLITON, BARBARA J. (1992). The mysterious virus called "Isn't." *Nature,* 358:619.

DICKSON, DAVID. (1994). Critic still lays blame for AIDS on lifestyle, not HIV. *Nature,* 369:434.

DUESBERG, PETER H. (1990). Duesberg replies [to the charges of Weiss and Jaffe]. *Nature,* 346:788.

DUESBERG, PETER H. (1993). HIV and AIDS. *Science,* 260:1705–1708.

DUESBERG, PETER H. (1995). The Duesberg Phenomenon: Duesberg and other voices. *Science,* 267:313.

GILKS, CHARLES. (1991). AIDS, monkeys and malaria. *Nature,* 354:262.

GILKS, CHARLES. (1992). AIDS and malaria experiments. *Nature,* 355:305.

GRMEK, MIRKO. (1990). History of AIDS: Emergence and orgin of a modern pandomic. Princeton, NJ: Princeton University Press.

HOLDER, CONSTANCE. (1988). Curbing Soviet disinformation. *Science,* 242:665.

KARPAS, ABRAHAM. (1994). AIDS plagued by journalists. *Nature,* 368:387.

KOPROWSKI, HILARY. (1992). AIDS and the polio vaccine. *Science,* 257:1024–1026.

ROOT-BERNSTEIN, ROBERT. (1993). *Rethinking AIDS.* New York: Free Press, 512 pp.

WEISS, ROBIN A., et al. (1990). Duesberg, HIV and AIDS. *Nature,* 345:659–660.

CHAPTER

3

Characteristics of the AIDS Virus

CHAPTER CONCEPTS

- Retroviruses are grouped into three families: oncoviruses, lentiviruses, and foamy viruses.
- HIV is a lentivirus.
- HIV RNA produces HIV DNA which integrates into host cell to become a proviral DNA.
- HIV contains nine genes; its three major structural genes are GAG-POL-ENV.
- Six HIV genes regulate HIV reproduction and at least one gene influences infection.
- HIV undergoes rapid genetic changes within infected people.
- The reverse transcriptase enzyme is highly error prone.
- HIV causes immunological suppression by destroying T4 helper cells.

Viruses are microscopic particles of biological material, so small that they can be seen only with electron microscopes. A virus consists solely of a strip of genetic material (nucleic acid) within a protein or fatty (lipid) coat.

Viruses are parasitic organisms; they live inside the cells of their host animal or plant, and can perpetuate themselves only by forcing the host cell to make viral copies. The new virus leaves the host cell and goes on to infect more cells. By damaging or killing these cells, some viruses cause diseases in the host animal or plant. Genetically, viruses are the simplest forms of "life" ; the genetic blueprint for the structure of the **human immunodeficiency virus (HIV)** is 100,000 times smaller than that contained in a human cell, and the complete sequence of 9,749 molecules (nucleotides) which form the code for this information has been identified and their arrangement sequenced (mapped).

Scientists have produced a great deal of information about the human immunodeficiency virus over a relatively short time. The immediate involvement of so many scientists followed by the rapid identification of the causative agent of AIDS is unequaled in the history of medical science. More is known about HIV than about the viruses that cause such long-standing human diseases as polio, measles, yellow fever, hepatitis, flu, and the common cold. Now let us review some of the characteristics of the AIDS virus.

HUMAN IMMUNODEFICIENCY VIRUS (HIV)

HIV is a retrovirus (Figure 3-1). Retroviruses are so named because they reverse the usual flow of genetic information within the host cell. In all living cells, normal gene expression results from the genetic information of DNA being copied into RNA (Figure 3-2). The RNA is translated into a specific cellular protein. In all living cell types, the directions for protein synthesis come from the species' genetic information contained in its DNA:

DNA $\rightarrow$ RNA $\rightarrow$ Protein Synthesis

In brief, retrovirus RNA is copied, using its reverse transcriptase enzyme, into a complementary single strand of DNA (Figure 3-3). The single-strand retroviral DNA is then copied into double-stranded retroviral DNA (this replication occurs in the cell's cytoplasm). At this point the viral DNA has been made according to the instructions in the retroviral RNA. This retroviral DNA migrates into the host cell nucleus and becomes integrated (inserted) into the host cell DNA. It is now a **provirus** (Figure 3-4). The provirus is like the "mole" in a John LeCarre spy novel, it may hide for years before doing its specific job.

Before the provirus's genes can be expressed, RNA copies of them that can be read by the host cell's protein-making machinery must be produced. This is done by transcription. Transcription is accomplished by the cell's own enzymes. But the process cannot start until the cell's RNA polymerase is activated by various molecular switches located in two stretches near the ends of the provirus: the long terminal repeats. This requirement is reminiscent of the need of many genes in multicellular organisms to be "turned on" or "off" by proteins that bind specifically to controlling sequences.

Some of the cellular signaling proteins that bind to HIV's long terminal repeats are members of an important family of proteins known as NF-kB/Rel. Present in virtually all human cells, these regulatory proteins increase the transcriptional activity of many genes. Significantly, cells increase production of some protein members of this family when they are stimulated by foreign proteins or by hormones that control the immune system. It appears that HIV utilizes the NF-kB/Rel proteins resulting from activation of immune cells to boost its own transcription!

Production of Viral RNA Strands or RNA Transcripts

Within the host cell nucleus, proviral DNA, when activated, produces new strands of RNA. Some of the RNA strands behave like messenger RNA, producing proteins essential for the production of HIV. Other RNA strands become encased within the viral core proteins to become the new viruses (Figure 3-4). Whether the transcribed RNA strands become mRNA or RNA strands for new viruses depends on whether or not the newly synthesized RNA strands undergo complex processing. RNA processing means that after the RNA is produced, some of it is cut into segments by cellular emzymes and then reassociated or **spliced** into a length of RNA suitable for protein synthesis. The RNA strands that are spliced become the mRNA used in protein synthesis. The unspliced RNA strands serve as new viral strands that are encased in their protein coats (capsids) to become new viruses that bud out of the cell (Figure 3-5).

Two distinct phases of transcription follow the infection of an individual cell by HIV. In the first or early phase, which lasts roughly 24 hours, RNA strands or transcripts produced in the cell's nucleus are snipped into multiple copies of shorter sequences by cellular splicing enzymes. When they reach the cytoplasm,

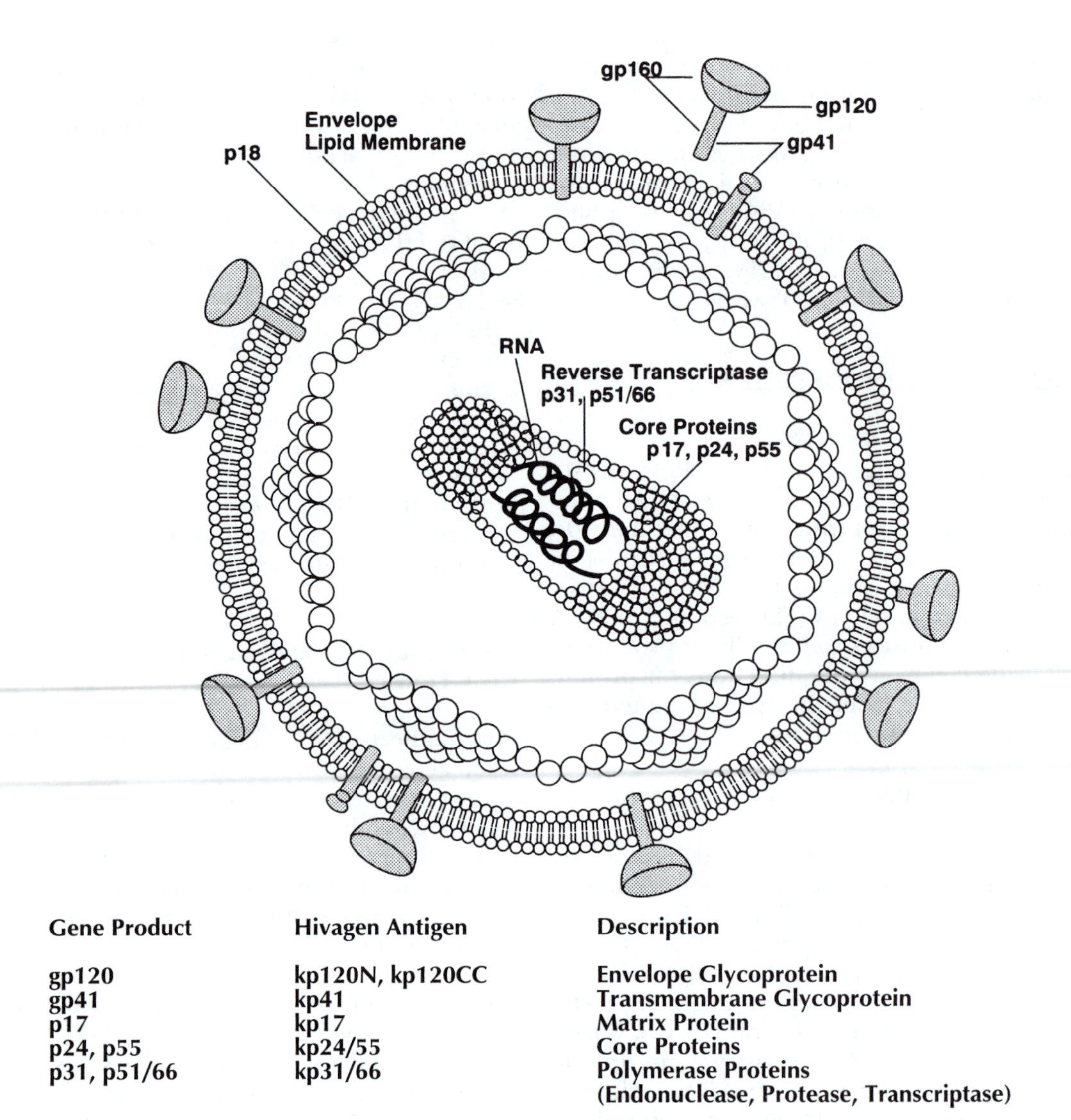

Gene Product	Hivagen Antigen	Description
gp120	**kp120N, kp120CC**	**Envelope Glycoprotein**
gp41	**kp41**	**Transmembrane Glycoprotein**
p17	**kp17**	**Matrix Protein**
p24, p55	**kp24/55**	**Core Proteins**
p31, p51/66	**kp31/66**	**Polymerase Proteins (Endonuclease, Protease, Transcriptase)**

FIGURE 3-1 Human Immunodeficiency Virus. The virus is a sphere measuring 1,000 A or 1/10,000 mm in diameter. The truncated cone-shaped core in a spherical envelope is the dominant feature. In this diagram the virus has been cut through its diameter. Surrounding it is a membrane derived from the host cell. The virus gains the membrane while "budding" out or exiting the cell. The membrane consists of two lipid (fat) layers impregnated with some human proteins, for example Class I and Class II human lymphocyte antigen complexes important for controlling the immune response. The external viral membrane also contains molecules of viral glycoproteins **(gp)**— a sugar chain attached to protein. Each glycoprotein appears as a spike in the membrane. Each spike consists of two parts: **gp41** which extends through the membrane; and **gp120** which extends from the end of gp41 to the outside and beyond the membrane (the numbers 41 and 120

(continued on next page)

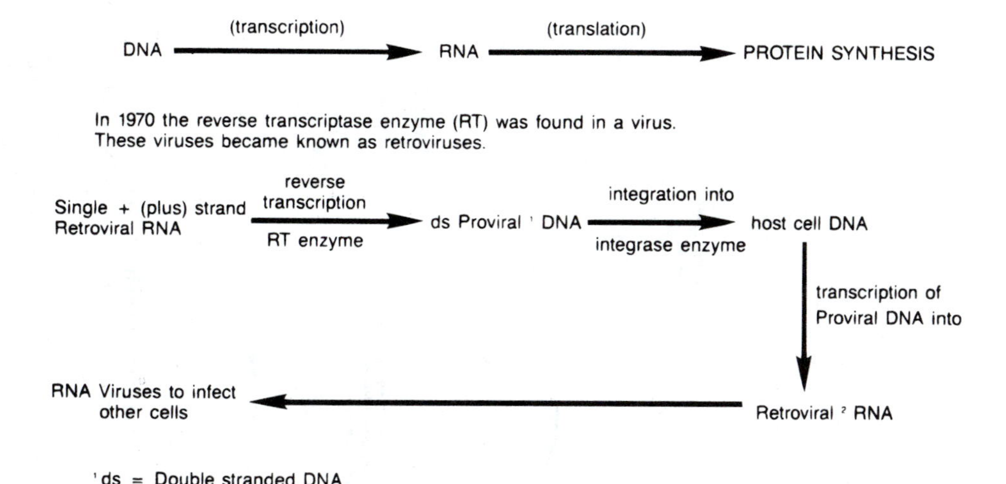

FIGURE 3-2 Human and Retroviral Flow of Genetic Information. The general directional flow of genetic information in all living species is from DNA, where the information is stored, into RNA, which serves as a messenger for the construction of proteins which are the cells' functional molecules. This unidirectional flow of genetic information has been referred to as the "central dogma' of molecular biology. In the 1960s, Howard Temin and colleagues discovered an enzyme that copied RNA into DNA, a reverse of what was normally expected, thus the name *reverse transcriptase.*

(continued)

represent the mass of the individual gps in thousands of daltons). As a complete unit, gp41 plus gp120 is called gp160. These two membrane or **envelope** proteins play a crucial role in binding HIV to CD4 protein molecules found in the membranes of several types of immune system cells. The gp160 precursor is cleaved into envelope (gp120) and transmembrane (gp41) proteins in the cell's Golgi compartment. The HIV envelope complex is transported via vesicles to patches in the outer cell membrane. Full-length HIV RNA is complexed with capsid proteins and the nucleocapsid is transferred to the cell surface membrane at envelope-containing sites. The binding of gp to CD4 makes such immune system cells vulnerable to infection. Other HIV proteins are located and described in this figure.

Within the cone-shaped core there are two strands of viral genomic RNA 9,749 nucleotide bases long. They are attached to molecules of an enzyme, reverse transcriptase, which transcribes the viral RNA into DNA once the virus has entered a cell. Also present with the RNA are an integrase, a protease, and a ribonuclease enzyme. The released virus is processed internally by HIV protease to form the characteristic dense lentivirus core. Most HIV appear to have initiated DNA synthesis prior to completion of budding and maturation.

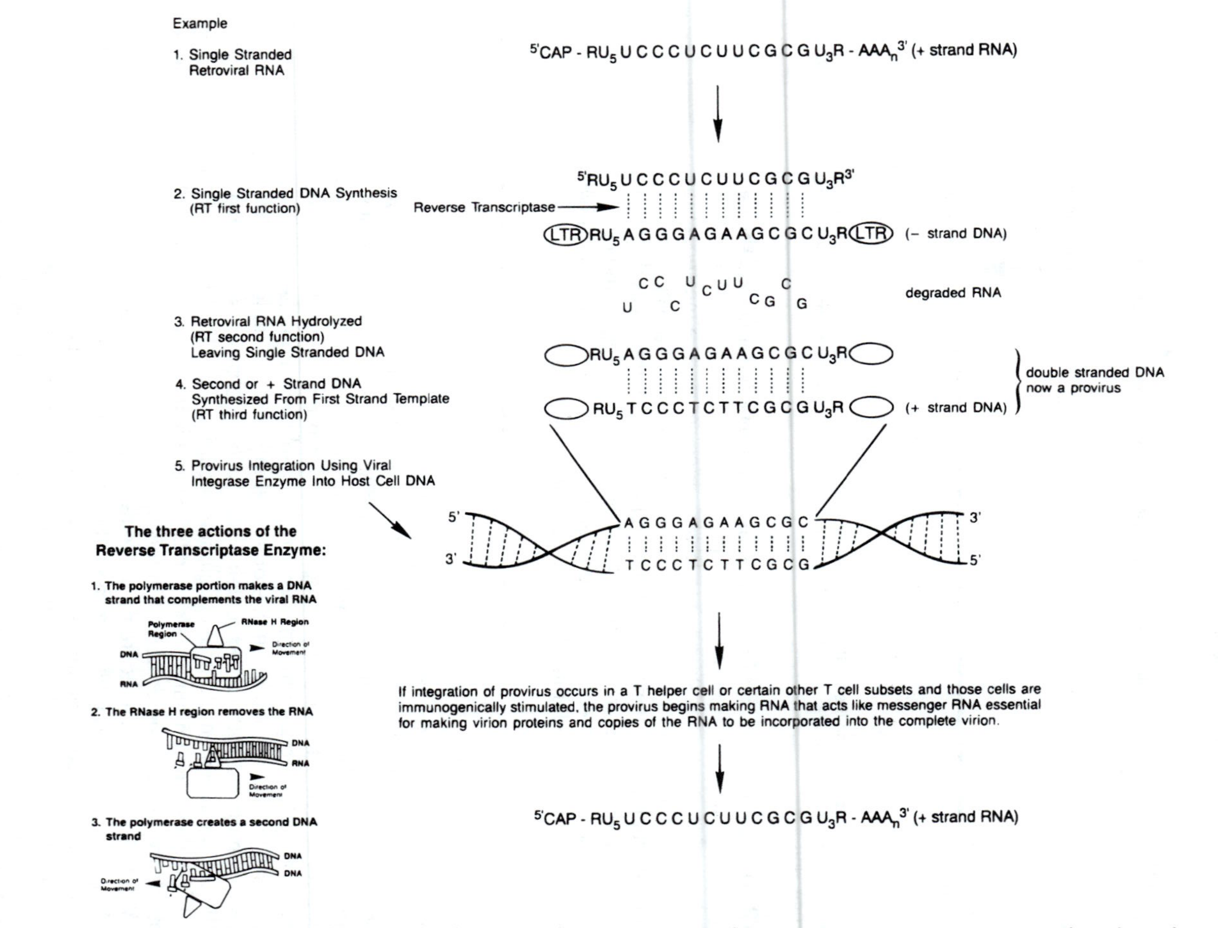

FIGURE 3-3 Proposed Production and Function of Retroviral Provirus. Note the reverse transcriptase enzyme has three functions: (1) to act as an RNA-dependent DNA polymerase transcribing single-strand DNA from viral RNA; (2) to demonstrate RNase H activity (RNase H is a subunit of the RT enzyme) by hydrolyzing the retroviral RNA off the RNA–DNA complex; and (3) to act as a DNA- dependent polymerase and transcribe the second DNA strand complementary to the first DNA strand. The process of viral RNA transcription is complex. When completed, the viral RNA gives rise to the formation of either linear or circular molecules of proviral DNA. Each end of the provirus contains an identical long series of terminal-repeating nucleotides or LTRs. LTRs are not a part of the viral genome. Although retroviral DNA integration is considered to be the normal route for RNA virus reproduction, retroviral reproduction may occur without proviral integration (see Figure 3-4).

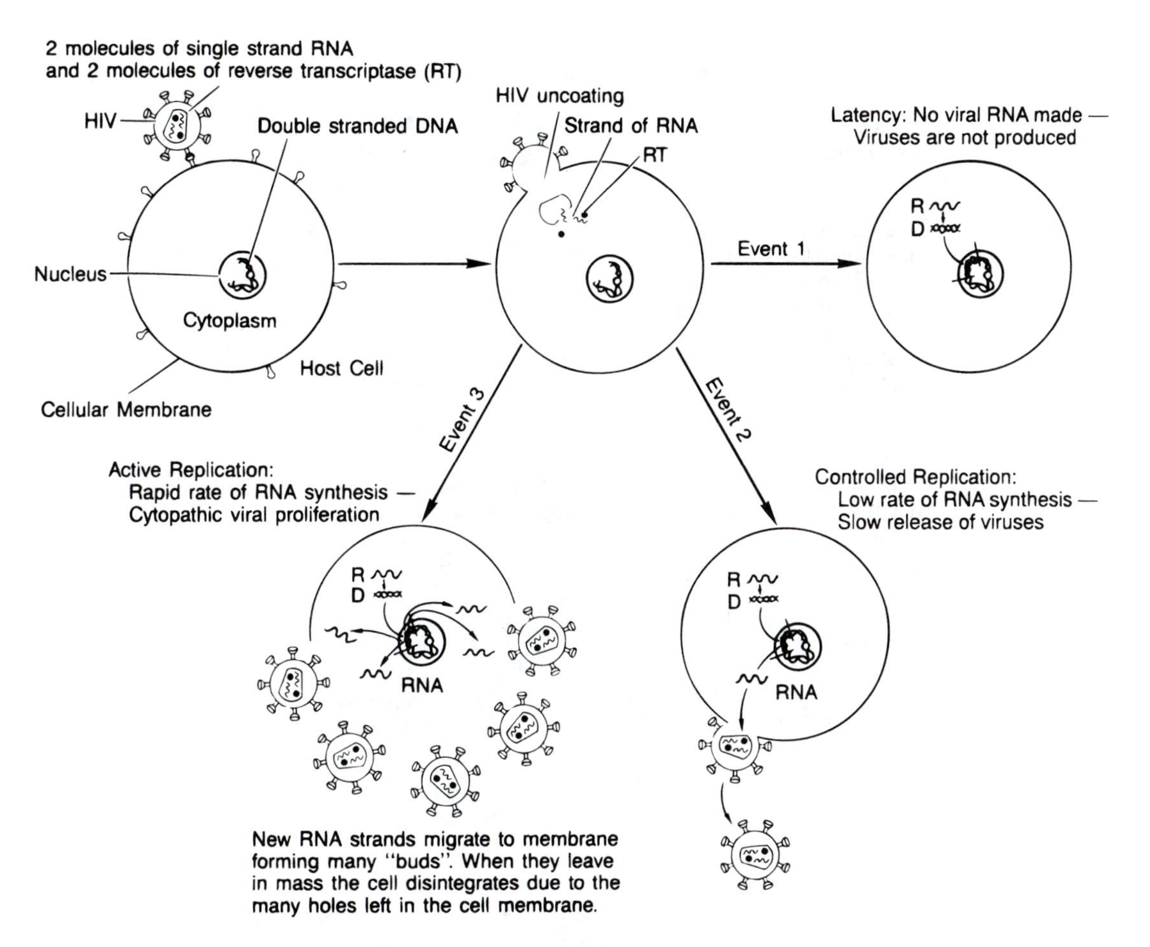

FIGURE 3-4 Proposed Reproductive Cycle for HIV. After cellular infection, HIV may have three choices with regard to its reproduction. The choice for reproduction occurs after the virus enters the cell's cytoplasm and its RNA is exposed to the cell's environment. *In all three choices, single-stranded HIV retroviral RNA is first transcribed into single-stranded retroviral DNA*. This ss DNA is then transcribed into a double stranded molecule that may begin producing HIV RNA, some used for production of virus proteins and others to be incorporated into the mature virus. As the virus accumulate, they move to the cell membrane, become imbedded, and when the cell ruptures it releases the membrane- enveloped viruses. The most common route for retroviruses, the ds DNA migrates to the host cell nucleus, circularizes, and becomes integrated (inserted) into the cellular DNA. Occasionally the retroviral DNA is transcribed and new viruses exit through the membrane. Choice 3 is similar to Choice 2 except it takes immunogenetic stimulation to activate the steady production of virions which exit through the cell membrane. Evidence for the use of all three choices has been found in vivo for HIV. (See text for further details on retroviral reproduction.)

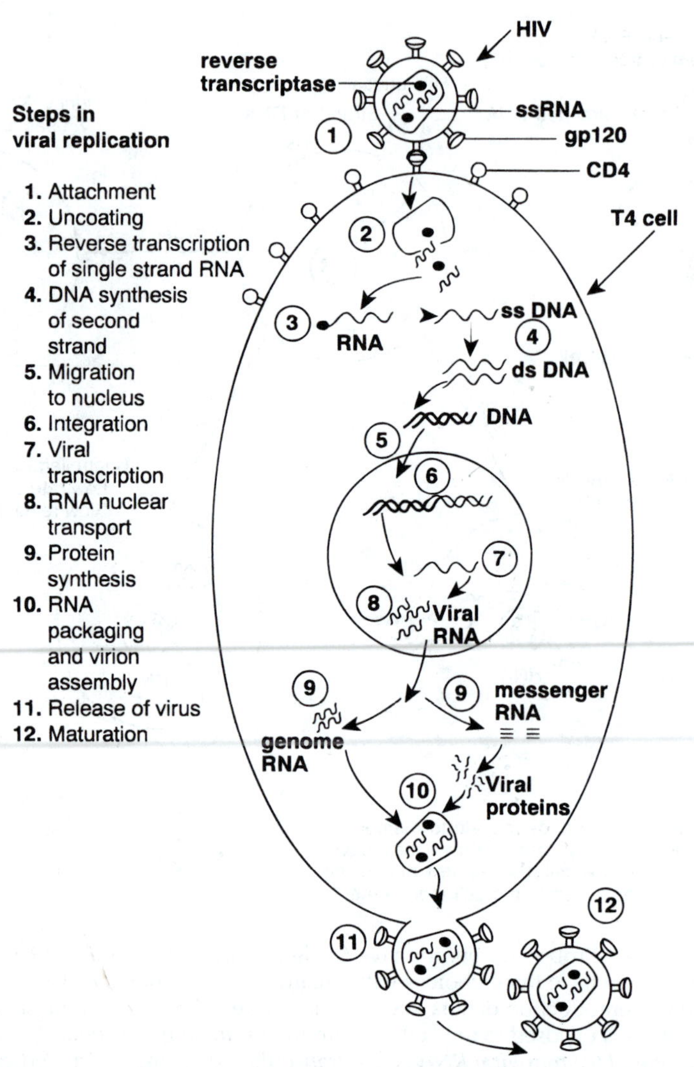

FIGURE 3-5 Life Cycle of HIV. There is still some confusion as to whether HIV becomes a latent infection once HIV-DNA becomes inserted or integrated into the host DNA. The most recent evidence (1993, 1994) is that HIV is never truly latent; it is constantly being reproduced at a very low rate in lymphocytes within the lymph nodes. However, there is some evidence of HIV latency in blood circulating T4 cells. Therefore, a latent period following DNA integration has not been shown in this diagram.

they are only about 2,000 nucleotides in length. These early-phase short transcripts encode only the virus's **regulatory proteins**; the structural genes that constitute the rest of the genome are among the parts that are left behind. In the second or late phase, two new size classes of RNA—long (unspliced) transcripts of 9,749 bases making up the new viral genome and medium-length (singly spliced) transcripts of some 4,500 bases—move out of the nucleus and into the cytoplasm. The 4,500 base transcripts encode HIV's structural and enzymatic proteins (Greene, 1993).

Experimental results reported by Somasundaran et al. (1988) showed that when lymphoid cell lines or peripheral blood lymphocytes were infected with a laboratory strain of HIV, up to 2.5 million copies of the viral RNA were produced by cells; and within 3 days of infection, up to 40% of the total protein synthesized by the cells was viral protein. This is an unprecedented takeover for a retrovirus which typically makes only modest amounts of RNA and protein.

Much of what HIV does after entering the host cell or while integrated as a retroprovirus depends on the activity of the retroviral genes.

BASIC GENETIC STRUCTURE OF RETROVIRAL GENOMES

The first retrovirus was isolated from a sarcoma in chickens by Peyton Rous in 1911 and named the Rous sarcoma virus. The basic genetic structure of the Rous sarcoma virus and all animal retroviruses is the same. They all contain retroviral RNA sequences that code for the *same three genes* abbreviated GAG, POL, and ENV. Flanking each end of the retroviral genome is a sequence of similar nucleotides called long terminal repeats or redundancies (LTRs).

$$5' \underset{\text{LTR}}{=} \overline{\text{GAG POL ENV}} \underset{\text{LTR}}{=} 3'$$

Some of the animal retroviruses such as the Rous sarcoma virus contain an additional *onc* or *oncogene* that, along with its LTRs, causes a rapid form of cancer in chickens which kills them in 1 to 2 weeks after infection. Without the *onc* gene the virus causes a *slow progressive cancer.*

Retroviral Genome of HIV

What sets the HIV genome apart from all other known retroviruses is the number of genes in HIV and the apparent complexity of their interactions in regulating the expression of the GAG-POL-ENV genes (Figure 3-6).

The Nine Genes of HIV— The HIV genome contains at least nine recognizable genes. As can be seen in Table 3-1, five of the nine genes are involved in regulating the expression of the GAG-POL-ENV genes.

The letters **GAG** stand for group-specific antigens (proteins) that make up the viral nucleocapsid. The GAG gene codes for the production of the dense cylindrical core proteins (p**24**, a nucleoid shell protein with a molecular weight of 24,000; and several internal proteins, p7, p15, p17, and p55) which have been visualized by electron microscopy. The GAG protein has the ability to direct the formation of virus-like particles when all other major genes (POL and ENV) are absent. It is only when the GAG gene is nonfunctional that retroviruses (HIV) lose their capacity to bud out of a host cell. Because of these observations, the GAG protein has been designated the virus particle-making machine (Wills et al., 1991).

The **POL** gene codes for protease (p10), the virus-associated polymerase that is active in two forms, p51 or p66, and endonuclease (integrase, p31) enzymes. The integrase enzyme cuts the cell's DNA and inserts the HIV DNA. Evidence from retroviral deletion studies shows that the loss of LTRs and the 3' side of the POL gene stops viral DNA integration into the host genome. However, nonintegrated DNA, without its LTRs and integrase enzyme, can still produce new viruses. This clearly demonstrates that viral DNA integration is not essential for viral multiplication even though integration is the normal course of events (Dimmrock et al., 1987).

The regulation of HIV transcription appears to be intimately related to the onset of HIV disease and AIDS. Thus interruption or inactivation of the POL gene would appear to have therapeutic effects (Kato et al., 1991).

The ENV gene codes for two major envelope glycoproteins (gp120, located on the external "spikes" of HIV and gp41, the transmembrane protein that attaches gp120 to the surface of HIV) that become embedded throughout the host cell membrane, which ultimately becomes the **envelope** that surrounds the virus as it "buds" out (Figure 3-7). Studies on how HIV kills cells have revealed at least one way that the envelope glycoproteins enhance T helper cell death. The envelope glycoproteins cause the formation of **syncytia**; that is, healthy T cells fuse to each other forming a group around a single HIV-in-

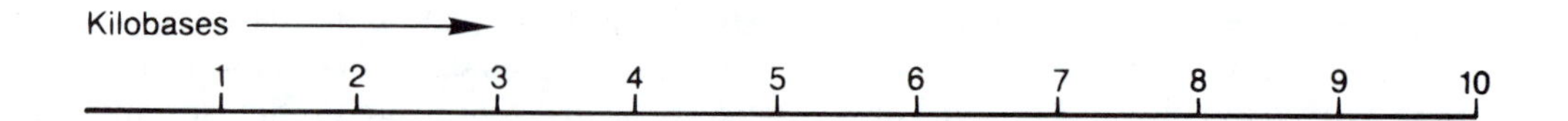

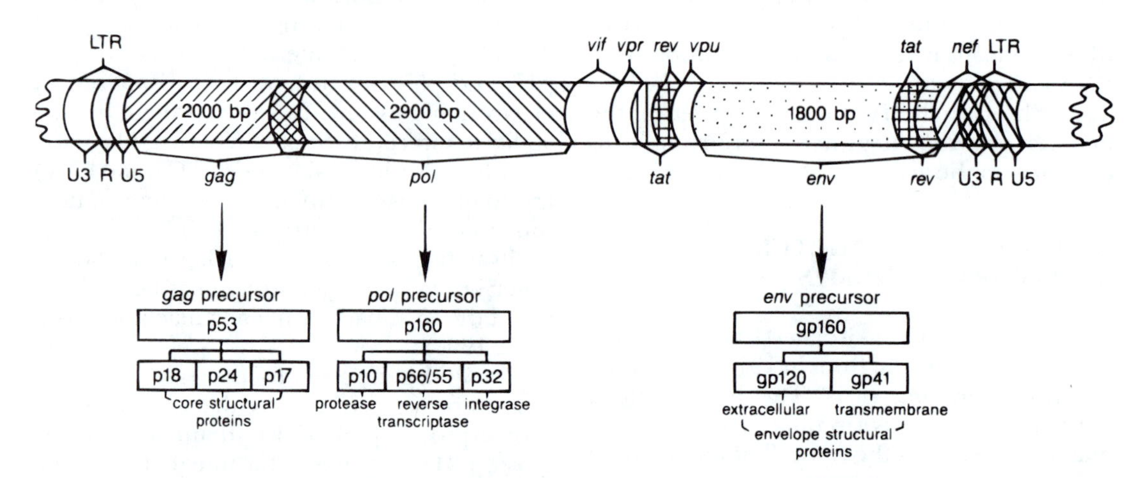

FIGURE 3-6 Genome of HIV. Nine of the genes making up the HIV genome have been identified. They are positioned as shown. Six of these genes are involved in a complex set of interactions that modify the regulation of the GAG-POL-ENV genes. Five are essential for HIV replication and six control reproduction (see text for details). The maxtrix protein, p17, forms the outer shell of the core of HIV, lining the inner surface of the viral membrane. Key functions of p17 protein are: orchestrates HIV assembly, directs gag p55 protein to host cell membrane, interacts with transmembrane protein, gp41, to retain envelope coded proteins within HIV and contains, a nuclear localization signal that directs HIV-RNA integration complex to the nucleus of infected cells. This feature permits HIV to infect *nondividing cells,* a distinguishing feature of HIV (Matthews et al., 1994).

fected T4 cell. Individual T cells within these syncytia lose their immune function (Figure 3-8). Starting with a single HIV-infected T4 helper cell, as many as 500 *uninfected* T4 helper cells can fuse into a single syncytium. Continued creation of these syncytia could deplete a T4 cell population.

It should be noted that the T4 lymphocyte level in an 18-month-old child is approximately 2,500/µL (a very small number of cells when compared to the 4.5 to 5.5 million red blood cells [RBCs]/µL or the 5,000 to 7,000 white blood cells [WBCs]/µL) and T4 numbers decrease from this age on with average numbers in 15- to 50-year-olds at 900 to 1,500/µL. This may help clarify why the loss of the long-lived T4 cells from HIV is so critical. That is, in adults there is a lower level of T4 cells to begin with.

The Six Genes of HIV That Control HIV Reproduction— Collectively, the six additional HIV genes tat, rev, nef (regulatory genes) and vif, vpu, vpr (auxiliary genes) working together with the host cell's machinery actually control the reproductive retroviral cycle: adhesion of HIV to a cell, penetration of the cell, uncoating of HIV genome, reverse transcription of the RNA genome producing proviral DNA and immediate production of new viral RNA, or the integration of the provirus and later viral multiplication. The six genes allow for the entire reproductive scenario to occur in 12 to 24 hours in growing cells.

Gene Sequence— The HIV proviral genome has been well characterized with regard to gene location and sequence (Figure 3-

TABLE 3-1 Genes of the HIV-1 and HIV-2 Genomes

Old Name(s)	New Name	Molecular Mass (kDa)	Function
GAG (group antigen)	MA	p17	Matrix (protection)
	CA	p24	Capsid (protection)
	NC	p7	Nucleocapsid (protection)
POL (polymerase)	PR	p10	Protease (enzyme)
	IN	p32	Endonuclease (enzyme)
	RT	p66, p51	Reverse transcriptase (enzyme)
ENV (envelope)	SU	gp120	Surface envelope
	TM	gp41	Transmembrane envelope
tat III, ta	tat (transactivator protein)[a]	p14	Transactivation of all HIV proteins
art, trs	rev (differential regulator of expression of virus protein)	p19	Regulation of expression of virus proteins
sor, A, P, Q	vif (virus infectivity factor)	p23	Required for ineffectivity as cell-free virus
3' ORF, B, E', F	nef (negative regulator) factor)	p27	Retards HIV replication
R	vpr (virus protein R)	?	Undetermined
U	vpu (virus protein U)[b]	p16	Required for efficient viral replication and release
X	vpx (virus protein X)[c]	p14	Undetermined

[a] Transactivator gene—the product of their genes influences the function of genes some distance away.

[b] Found only in HIV-1.

[c] Found only in HIV-2 and SIV (Simian Immunodeficiency Virus).

6), but the function of each gene is not completely understood. The genes for producing regulatory proteins can be grouped into two classes: genes that produce proteins essential for HIV replication (*tat* and *rev*), and genes that produce proteins that perform accessory functions that enhance replication and/or infectivity (vif, nef, vpr, and vpu) (Rosen, 1991).

The entire genome is 9,749 bases in length. Each end of the proviral genome contains an identical long sequence of bases, the long terminal repeats. Although these LTRs are not considered to be genes of the HIV genome, they do contain regulatory base sequences that help the five regulatory genes control GAG-POL-ENV gene expression (Figure 3-6). For example, it is known that the **vif** gene is associated with the infectious activity of the virus. Vif may also be involved in viral replication, but it does not appear to influence the production of GAG-POL-ENV proteins.

The **tat** gene is one of the first vital genes to be transcripted. The tat gene produces a transactivator protein, meaning that the gene produces a protein that exerts its effect on viral replication from a distance rather than interacting with genes adjacent to *tat* or their gene product. *Tat* contains two coding regions or exons—areas that contain genetic information for producing a diffusible protein—which, through the help of the LTR sequences, increases the expression of HIV genes thereby increasing the production of new virus particles. Tat protein consists of 86 amino acids and binds to cadmium or zinc. The tat protein interacts with a short nucleotide sequence called TAR located within the 5' LTR region of HIV messenger RNA (mRNA) transcripts (Matsuya et al., 1990). Once that tat protein binds to the TAR sequence, transcription of the provirus by cellular RNA polymerase II accelerates at least 1,000-fold. Margaret Fischl (1994) reported that although the *tat* gene can increase the number of HIV produced, *tat* may not be essential for viral replication. Because of this finding the development of drugs to inhibit tat expression has been discontinued.

The **rev** gene (regulator of expression of viral protein) also contains two exons that together code for a 116-amino acid protein.

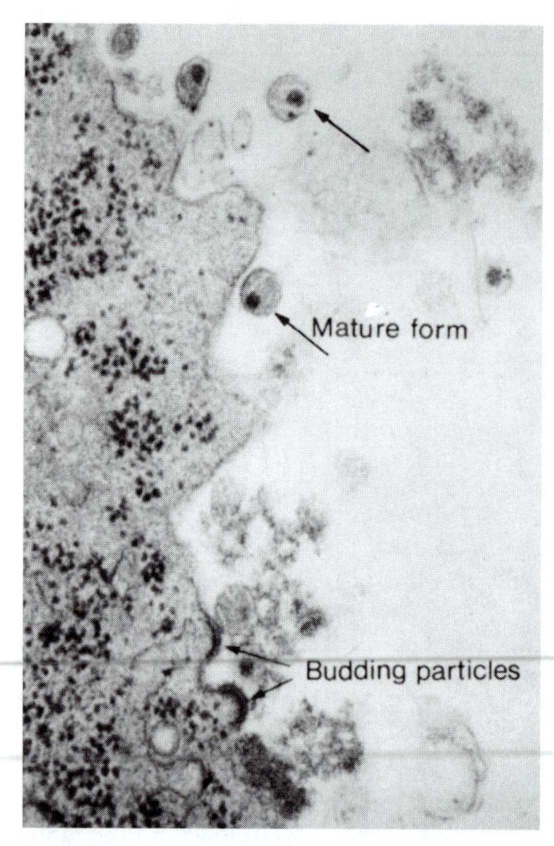

FIGURE 3-7 Budding and Mature Retroviruses. This is a photograph of HIV taken by electron microscopy. Note the difference between the free or mature HIV and those that are just budding out through the membrane of a T4 helper cell. This cell came from an HIV-infected hemophiliac. Closely observing the mature HIV, one can make out the core protein area surrounded by the cell's membrane (virus envelope). (*Courtesy CDC, Atlanta*)

What the *rev* gene does is selectively increase the synthesis of HIV structural proteins in the latter stages of HIV disease, thereby maximizing the production of new viruses. It does this by regulating splicing of the HIV-RNA transcript (cutting out nucleotide sequences that exist between exons and bringing the exons together) and transporting spliced and unspliced RNAs from the nucleus to the cytoplasm (Patrusky, 1992).

The **nef** gene (negative regulator protein) produces a protein that is maintained in the cell cytoplasm next to the nuclear membrane. It is believed **nef** functions by making the cell more capable of producing HIV. Several antigenic forms of nef protein have been found which suggest multiple activities of nef within HIV-infected cells (Kohleisen et al., 1992).

The functions of the **vpr** gene, which codes for viral protein R, and the **vpu** gene, which codes for viral protein U, are not completely understood. Recently, it has been learned that the vpu protein is required for the efficient assembly or release of new HIV viruses. All three genes, vif, vpr, and vpu appear to be necessary for HIV to cause disease.

Genetic Stability of Species— The individual or collective characteristics (phenotypes) of any virus, cell, or multicelled organism depend on the expression of their genes and the interaction of gene products within a given environment. From a biological point of view, changes in phenotype (observable characteristics) that are inheritable are by definition genetic changes. Such changes occur due to changes in the hereditary material. Changes in hereditary material may occur by nucleotide addition, substitution, and deletion. These changes are referred to as **genetic mutations**. Genetic mutations provide biological heterogeneity and genetic diversity (similarity as a species but dissimilarity with regard to certain characteristics). Genetic diversity results from slow but ever-present mutations that alter the phenotype. Investigations on the rate at which genetic mutations occur in living species indicate that DNA is a stable molecule with relatively low mutation rates for any given gene. Because of low mutation rates within the DNA of a species's gene pool (all of the genes that can be found in the DNA of a species) and selection pressures by a slowly changing environment, species evolution is constant but very slow.

Genetic mutations in the strain of an organism or virus produce genetic and phenotype **variants** (different members) of that strain. Regardless of the rate at which mutations occur, they are genetic mistakes—they are not intentional, they just happen by chance. Most mutations or genetic mistakes ei-

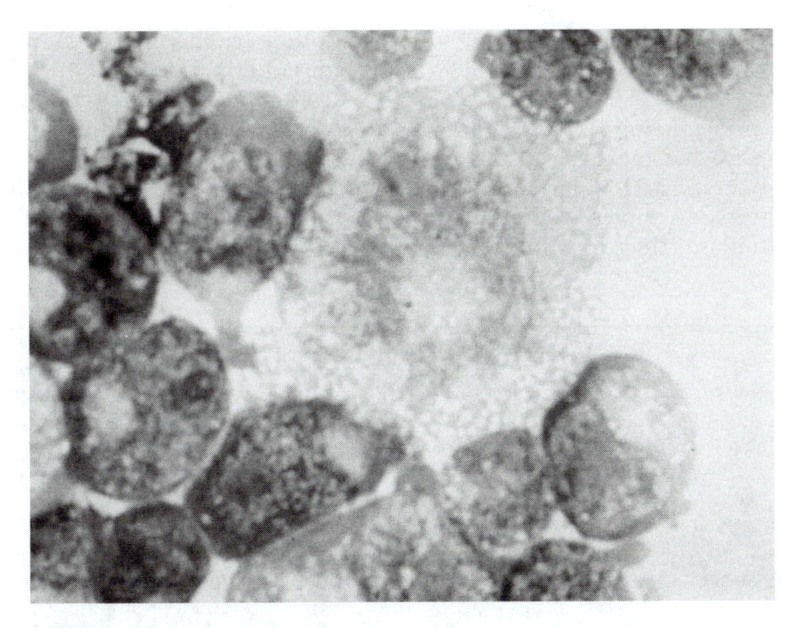

FIGURE 3-8 Formation of T4 Helper Cell Syncytia. A single infected T4 helper cell can fuse with as many as 500 uninfected T4 helper cells. The formation of syncytia lead to a loss or depletion of T4 helper cells from the immune system. *(Courtesy of Dr. Tom Folks, National Institute of Allergy and Infectious Diseases)*

ther make no difference to an organism or virus (silent mutations) or they cause a change. Few genetic mistakes within a stable environment improve the species. After all, the species arrived at this point in time via genetic and environmental selection pressures—those with the best constellation of genes survived to reproduce those genes. In species that produce large numbers of offspring, genetic mistakes that are lethal or lead to an early death are of little consequence to the species. A genetic mistake that improves the chance of survival and reproduction is retained.

Genetic Stability of HIV— A virus like HIV can produce thousands of replicas within a single cell. Genetic mistakes during viral replication produce variant HIVs. In economic terms, HIV replicas are inexpensive to make. Even if most of these mutant HIV replicas are inactive or throwaway copies, it makes little if any difference to the HIV per se. However, if a few HIV replicas received environmentally advantageous mutant genes, these HIV mutants would survive as well as or better than the parent HIVs. Both parent HIV and mutant HIV would reproduce in the same cell. Over time, if only the mutant or variant HIVs were transmitted to other people and undergo still further genetic changes, these variant HIVs could, with sufficient accumulative genetic changes, become a new subtype of HIV—for example, an HIV-3 strain.

Investigations of some of the *RNA* viruses revealed relatively high mutation rates. Thus some of the RNA viruses are our best examples of evolution in "real" time. Because of their high error rate during replication they show, as expected, both high genetic diversity and biological heterogeneity in their host, and a rate of evolution about a million times faster than DNA-based organisms (Nowak, 1990). The human immunodeficiency virus in particular fits this category. Heterogeneity of HIV is reflected by: (1) the difference in the kinds of cells variant HIV infects; (2) the way different HIV mutants replicate; and (3) the way different variants of HIV harm infected cells.

Mechanisms of Producing HIV Variants—What is puzzling is what mechanisms are responsible for generating HIV variants. One theory is tha as new RNA copies accumulate in the host cell cytoplasm they recombine with each other (exchange parts), producing new varieties of HIV (Levy, 1988).

Another mechanism of producing HIV variants results from a highly error-prone reverse transcriptase (RT) enzyme of HIV. Preston and colleagues (1988) found that HIV transcriptase makes at least on error in each HIV genome per round of replication in a cell!

POINT OF INFORMATION 3.1

BACTERIAL MUTATIONS: A DISASTER IN PROGRESS

Anytime a new antibiotic or antimicrobial against bacteria becomes widely used, the very compound that saves your life, it is at the same time, acting as a selective agent allowing cells resistant to the compound to increase. It does this by killing off those bacterial cells that are sensitive to the compound, while at the same time allowing those cells that carry a genetic mutation for resistance to the compound to multiply (reproduce new cells that are also resistant to the compound). Thus, over time, the more widely a specific antimicrobial compound is used, the more likely it is to become ineffective!

For people, the consequences of resistant infections range from larger medical bills to permanent disability or death. Drug resistant infections lead not only to more hospitalizations, but also to lengthier stays. Treatment is prolonged and may require the use of more costly agents with greater toxicity. One estimate suggests that antibiotic resistance costs more than $30 billion per year in the United States.

Decades ago, gonorrhea responded to low doses of penicillin. Throughout the 1950s and 1960s, the necessary dosage climbed; in the 1970s, in the 1980s some strains of the causative organism, became completely resistant to penicillin. Those infections were treated with tetracycline. Ultimately tetracycline resistance developed. The current treatment of choice is ceftriaxone sodium, a parenteral third-generation cephalosporin.

Another example of changing therapeutic drug use: In the early 1970s, *Haemophilus influenzae* meningitis was treated with ampicillin. But strains of the organism became resistant to the drug, spurring recommendations that serious infections be treated with ampicillin and oral chloramphenicol or intravenous chloramphenicol sodium succinate. When *H. influenzae* became resistant to both drugs, the primary treatment became a third-generation cephalosporin.

Today, scientists are monitoring a number of ominous situations. The most frightening is the emergence of enterococci resistant to vancomycin HCl. An increasingly common cause of nosocomial hospital-associated infections, enterococci have always had powerful intrinsic resistance. Even drug-susceptible strains can stand up to most oral agents. Treatment of endocarditis and other serious infections typically requires combinations of a penicillin or vancomycin along with an aminoglycoside.

Currently, about 14% of all nosocomial enterococcal infections among patients in U.S. intensive care units are resistant to vancomycin (*MMWR*, 1993).

A major fear now is that *Staphylococcus aureus* resistant to methicillin sodium will also develop resistance to vancomycin, currently the treatment of last resort. Methicillin-resistant *S. aureus* is a significant problem in large university teaching institutions and small community hospitals. Reports to the Centers for Disease Control and Prevention indicate that more than 20% of staphylococci are resistant to methicillin. Another major concern is the emergence of penicillin-and cephalosporin-resistant strains of *Streptococcus pneumoniae.* This bacterium causes meningitis, otitis media (middle ear infections), and pneumonia.

FACTORS THAT CONTRIBUTE TO DRUG RESISTANCE

While technological and social changes in recent decades have fostered bacterial drug resistance, doctors and their patients also encourage its emergence. Overuse of antibiotics—particularly broad-spectrum agents—is a major contributor. Other factors are underdosing and inappropriate or extended prophylaxis. Noncompliance with therapy and self-administration of leftover medication worsen the situation. (Cohen etal., 1994).

Other investigators say that reverse transcriptase, on average, introduces a mutation once in every 2,000 nucleotides or about six mutations per round of replication! This unusually high rate of nucleotide misincorporation (substitution, addition, and deletion) as proviral DNA is being made by RT is responsible for generating the genetic diversity and heterogeneity found among the isolates of HIV. In short, the high error rate in producing proviral DNA means that each HIV-infected cell will carry variant HIV, most of which will be genetically unique (Vartanian et al., 1992). This high rate of mutation underlies HIV's remarkable ability to become resistant to drug therapies.

Other means of creating HIV genetic variability can involve one or all of the steps in the retroviral reproductive cycle, beginning with the fact that HIV carries two identical RNA molecules that are joined together in parallel at one end (5' end). This RNA strand relationship makes it possible for genetic (RNA) recombination between the strands which contributes to the remarkable genetic variability of HIV.

Michael Saag and colleagues (1988) examined the generation of molecular variation of HIV by sequential HIV isolates from two chronically infected people. They found 39 distinguishable but highly related genomes (HIV variants). Similar changes in the HIV genome did not occur in vitro (in tissue culture). These results indicate that HIV heterogeneity occurs rapidly in infected individuals; and that a large number of genetically distinguishable but related HIVs rapidly evolve in parallel and coexist during chronic infection. That is, whenever a drug or the immune response successfully attacks one variant, another arises in its place. Pools of related genetic variants are often referred to as quasispecies (Delwart et al., 1993).

Additional evidence indicates that some HIV genetic variants demonstrate a preference as to the cell type they infect. This means that one genetic change may allow the virus to attach to cells that were once immune to the virus. The rapid genetic change which results in altered viral products makes it very difficult to design a vaccine or drug that will be effective against all HIV variants. Zidovudine, dideoxycytosine, and dideoxyinosine-resistant (nucleoside analog drugs used in treating HIV/AIDS patients) HIV mutants have already been found in AIDS patients. HIV mutants have also been found for the new nonnucleoside drugs used for HIV therapy.

Antigenic Variation— This is the product of the mutations that occur in the GAG-POL-ENV genes. Immunological nvestigations on GAG and POL gene proteins show that these two genes are relatively stable. That is, although mutant GAG and POL gene proteins have been found in different viral isolates, the amount of variation for these gene products appears to be minimal. Antibodies are made against the GAG-POL-ENV gene proteins, but it is the antibodies made against the ENV gene protein that appear to be the most important. These antibodies neutralize the envelope glycoproteins that seem to be an essential part of HIV's infecting process. However, it is the ENV gene that is subject to frequent mutations, producing HIV with different envelope glycoproteins within a given individual. Some HIV strains cannot infect certain CD4 cell lines due to a genetic change that has altered the virus-CD4 binding/fusion reaction (Putney et al., 1990). AIDS investigators Mayer-Cheng, E.V. Fenyo, K. Dehurst, and N. Tersmette report that virus isolates obtained from patients with advanced AIDS contain HIV that is more cytopathic than the HIV isolated earlier in the course of the disease and that these more cytopathic strains of HIV have demonstrated host cell tropism. HIV isolated from asymptomatic people normally infects CD4 lymphocytes and monocytes, but the more cytopathic HIV is capable of infecting and replicating in a variety of non-CD4 cell types in the brain, gastrointestinal tract, kidney, and other tissues (Nowak et al., 1991).

It now appears that HIV can constantly change its surface antigenic composition, thereby allowing it to escape antibody neutralization. This immune selection of HIV mutants allows the virus to persist in the presence of an immune response. This immune selection viral phenomenon is not new. It is what the influenza virus does yearly so that last year's vaccine will not protect people from this year's variation.

BOX 3.1

WHY DO SOME HIV-INFECTED PERSONS LIVE SO LONG?

In 1983, at age 71, a man became HIV-positive. He received a contaminated blood transfusion while undergoing colon surgery. Unlike most long-term HIV survivors, he has suffered no symptoms and no loss of immune function. He is celebrating his 81st birthday. He is one of five patients who came to the attention of an AIDS researcher as he was preparing a routine update on transfusion-related HIV infections. All five people were infected by the same donor. And 7 to 10 years later, no one has suffered any effects.

The blood donor was a gay male who had contracted the virus during the late 1970s or early 1980s and gave blood at least 26 times before learning he was infected. After locating the donor it was found that the man was just as healthy as the people who got his blood.

It has been known that relatively few patients remain well for long periods, but it has never been known why. Over 150 long-term HIV-positive people have been identified, about half of them are being studied. Statistically it is estimated that about 5% of HIV-infected people will be long-term survivors. That is, they are HIV-positive without consequences. Is it the environment, say in the vitamins they take, or is it some gene they have in common? These findings suggest that it has more to do with the strain of virus and on individual immune responses. Such findings might imply that HIV has been infecting humans for centuries before it began causing disease. As HIV screening becomes more acceptable, many more such cases may turn up. If the number of such cases increases significantly worldwide, the data may be evidence to support the idea that HIV is an ancient nonlethal virus that, in our lifetime, has undergone the changes necessary to cause a human disease. (For additional information on long-term AIDS survivors, see Box 6.4.)

However, HIV differs from viruses such as influenza. Influenza and other viruses do not have an RNA to DNA replication step so they are not as mutable as the retroviruses. Because of the error-prone reverse transcriptase enzyme used by the retroviruses, the possibility of genetic change far exceeds that for any other known nonretroviral human pathological virus.

DISTINCT GENOTYPES (VARIANTS) OF HIV-1 WORLDWIDE

Because HIV changes so rapidly, it is a moving target, hard to hit with a single drug or single vaccine. Gerald Meyers has been tracking HIV variants for several years. To do this he has sequenced the nucleotides of the GAG gene. From his analysis he has found five major genotypes of HIV-1 variants worldwide. Each genotype differs from the other by about 35%. Other families of variants are likely to appear over time. Meyers believes that all five families arose from a common viral HIV source and the differentiation of one HIV into another began around 1960 (Goldman, 1992). Two of the five families have been found in Thailand. One family, genotype E, infects heterosexuals almost exclusively. Genotype B and E are found in injection drug users (Moore, 1994). Joost Louwagie and colleagues (1993) sequenced the GAG gene from 55 international HIV isolates from people in 12 countries on four continents. Their work resulted in finding seven separate and distinct HIV genotypes (A, B, C, D, E, F, and G). None of these genotypes was contained within the physical boundaries of one country. Genotype B was found globally. Genotypes A and D were found in a broad east to west belt across sub-Saharan Africa from Senegal to Kenya. Genotype C was found in a north-to-south pattern in Africa.

Worldwide, at least six genetic subtypes exist, based on **envelope genetic sequence**, and each subtype differs at the nucleotide level from any other subtype by as much as 35%. Envelope sequences of isolates within a subtype can vary genetically by as much as 30%. Although there are geographic patterns of strain prevalence, multiple strains are found in many countries. A **single sequence envelope subtype** is dominant in the United States, probably related to a strong **founder effect** (the initial subtype to become established in the United States).

In addition to the genotypes listed above, there is a genotype O that contains up to 30 different variants of the virus. Each of the 30 variants is genetically different from the others but, taken as a group, they are so different from the other known HIV genotypes that these 30 variants have been given the designation "O" for "outlier" because these variants lie outside the known genotypes. The O variants have been known since 1987 but have been found mainly in Cameroon and surrounding African countries that, to date, have only been marginally affected by AIDS. To date O variants have not been found in the United States, but then though 1994 they have not been tested for. Currently, the commercial HIV blood tests used in the United States and Europe do *not* detect antibodies to the O variants! Adjustments to detect O antibodies using the current HIV testing kits are underway.

The rapid evolution of HIV families of variants has researchers abandoning hopes of developing a single vaccine effective against all variants. It may be feasible to concoct multiple-strain cocktail vaccines like those used in the flu vaccinations. (There are three major flu virus families.)

POINT OF INFORMATION 3.2

GAPS IN OUR KNOWLEDGE REQUIRE BASIC RESEARCH

The goal of policies for funding HIV/AIDS research should be to continue to search for a solution to this complex scientific, medical, and human problem. If the money allocated to AIDS research is to be spent wisely, finding effective therapeutic and preventive measures must be based on adequate scientific and epidemiological information.

Despite rapid progress in certain areas of HIV/AIDS research, serious limitations in our capacity to study HIV infection have become apparent. The lack of a suitable animal model means that fundamental questions about the pathogenesis of HIV disease can not yet be answered. Understanding the pathogenesis of HIV infection is central to an appreciation of the way in which HIV weakens the immune system and how the virus could be modified to stimulate effective immunity in infected men and women. The lack of an animal model was solved, in part, when infection by the simian immunodeficiency virus (SIV) in monkeys was recognized a natural counterpart to the human infection. Other animal models have appeared, but there is no truly useful small-animal model that faithfully replicates the human disease.

Money allocated to other areas of HIV/AIDS research or from other sources must now be given to revitalizing basic research per se. When searching for the cure for a human disease, both basic and medical engineering are critical. If one understands fully how a disease works, then it is more likely that a cure might be engineered or produced. But if fundamental scientific gaps exist, then broader based scientific research is needed.

Our capacity to move quickly to identify HIV as the cause of AIDS came from a commitment to viral oncology and retrovirus research made in the late 1960s and 1970s. Thus it was a commitment to attack cancer that led to the identification in the 1980s of the nature of the AIDS virus. A treatment or preventive strategy for the disease is as likely to come from fundamental discoveries in fields other than AIDS research as from those targeted for AIDS.

Paradoxically, targeting too narrowly, may slow down progress in combating AIDS. We must not compromise research in other areas of basic science at the expense of these directed programs. This would risk eliminating the research project that holds the ultimate answers to a critical piece of the puzzle.

Much basic research must be done to answer questions such as: How does HIV cross mucosal surfaces such as those lining the mouth, vagina, and anus? What are the cells that support primary HIV replication and what molecular and/or immunological factors determine the outcome of viral infection at the primary site? How does HIV spread from its primary site in a human, and how is its spread regulated? Are some strains of the virus more virulent than others? And how does HIV kill cells?

Intimately related to these questions about HIV are related issues such as the nature of the mucosal immune response to HIV; the ability to generate protective mucosal immunity against HIV; the nature of the systemic immune response that limits acute HIV infection; whether HIV can be eliminated from the body after infection; and the precise role of T cells and their products in attacking HIV. The list of unanswered scientific questions is much longer. Although partial answers exist for several of these questions, firm answers on which to base specific therapeutic strategies or vaccine approaches are needed to provide the foundation of the next steps (Fields, 1994).

SUMMARY

HIV is a retrovirus. It has RNA for its genetic material and carries reverse transcriptase enzyme for making DNA from its RNA. HIV, using its enzyme, copies its genetic information from RNA into DNA which becomes integrated into host cell DNA and may remain silent for years, or until such time as it is activated into producing new HIV. HIV contains at least nine genes; three of them, GAG-POL-ENV, are basic to all animal retroviruses. The six additional genes are involved in the infection process and regulate the production of products from the three genes. HIV, because of its error-prone reverse transcriptase enzyme, mutates at an unusually high rate. With time, many mutant HIV variants can be found within a single HIV-infected person. A vaccine against one mutant HIV may not work against a second—like the vaccines made yearly against different mutant influenza viruses.

REVIEW QUESTIONS

(*Answers to the Review Questions are on page 478.*)

1. Why is HIV called a retrovirus?
2. What are the three major genes common to all retroviruses? How many additional genes does HIV have?
3. Why are retroviruses, and HIV in particular, believed to be genetically unstable? Give two reasons for your answer.
4. What is believed to be the major reason for the high rate of genetic mutations in HIV production?

REFERENCES

COHEN, MITCHELL, et al. (1994). When bugs outsmart drugs. *Patient care,* 28:135–146.

DELWART, ERIC, et al. (1993). Genetic relationships determined by a DNA heteroduplex mobility assay: Analysis of HIV envGenes. *Science* 262:1257–1262.

DIMMROCK, N.J., and PRIMROSE, S.B. (1987). *Introduction to Modern Virology,* 3rd Ed. Oxford: Blackwell Scientific Publications.

FIELDS, BERNARD. (1994). AIDS: Time to turn to basic science. *Nature,* 369:95–96.

FISCHL, MARGARET. (1984). Combination retroviral therapy for HIV infection. *Hosp. Pract.,* 29:43–48.

GOLDMAN, ERIK L. (1992). HIV-1 appears to have at least 5 distinct subtypes. *Fam. Pract. News,* 22:9.

GREENE, WARNER. (1993). AIDS and the immune system. *Sci. Am.,* 269:99–105.

KOHLEISEN, MARKUS, et al. (1992). Cellular localization of Nef expressed in persistently HIV-1 infected low-producer astrocytes. *AIDS,* 6:1427–1436.

LEVY, JAY A. (1988). Mysteries of HIV: Challenges for therapy and prevention. *Nature,* 333:519–522.

LOUWAGIE, JOOST, et al. (1993). Phylogenetic analysis of GAG genes from 70 international HIV-1 isolates provides evidence for multiple genotypes. *AIDS,* 7:769–780.

MATSUYA, HIROAKI, et al. (1990). Molecular targets for AIDS therapy. *Science,* 249:1533–1543.

MATTHEWS, STEPHEN, et al. (1994). Structural similarity between p17 matrix protein of HIV and interferon-2. *Nature,* 370:666–668.

MOORE, JOHN, et al. (1994). The who and why of HIV vaccine trials. *Nature,* 372:313–314.

Morbidity and mortality weekly report. (1993). Nosocomial enterococci resistant to vancomycin—United States, 1989–1993, 42:597:599.

NOWAK, MARTIN A. (1990). HIV mutation rate. *Nature,* 347:522.

NOWAK, MARTIN A., et al. (1991). Antigenic diversity thresholds and the development of AIDS. *Science,* 254:963–969.

PATRUSKY, BEN. (1992). The Intron story. *Mosaic,* 23:20–33.

PRESTON, BRADLEY D., et al. (1988). Fidelity of HIV-1 reverse transcriptase. *Science,* 242:1168–1171.

PUTNEY, SCOTT D., et al. (1990). Antigenic variation in HIV. *AIDS,* 4:S129–S136.

ROSEN, CRAIG A. (1991). Regulation of HIV gene expression by RNA-protein interactions. *Trends genet.s,* 7:9–14.

SAAG, MICHAEL S., et al. (1988). Extensive variation of human immunodeficiency virus Type-1 *in vivo. Nature,* 334:440–444.

SOMASUNDARAN, M., et al. (1988). Unexpectedly high levels of HIV-1 RNA and protein synthesis in a cytocidal infection. *Science,* 242:1554–1557.

VARTANIAN, JEAN-PIERRE, et al. (1992). High-resolution structure of an HIV-1 quasispecies: Identification of novel coding sequences. *AIDS,* 6:1095–1098.

WILLS, JOHN W., et al. (1991). Form, function and use of retroviral Gag protein. *AIDS,* 5:639–654.

CHAPTER 4

The Immunology of HIV Disease/AIDS

CHAPTER CONCEPTS

- HIV is attracted to the CD4 receptor sites on T4 lymphocyte, monocyte, and macrophages cells.
- Monocytes and macrophages serve as HIV reservoirs in the body.
- Cofactors may enhance HIV infection.
- Impact of T4 cell depletion is immune suppression.
- Latency refers to inactive proviral HIV DNA, but true latency may not exist for HIV.
- Clinical latency refers to infection with low-level HIV production over time.
- Polymerase Chain Reaction (PCR) is used to multiply the proviral DNA to a measurable state.

Several cell types in the human body can become infected by HIV. The more important of these cells belong to the body's *immune system.* The immune system filters out foreign substances, removes damaged and dead cells and acts as a security system to destroy mutant and cancer cells. It is composed of a number of specialized cells, several organs, and a group of biologically active chemicals. The human immune system is like a jigsaw puzzle—many parts come together to form an overall defense against disease-causing agents. If parts of the immune system are missing or damaged, illness may occur due to an immune deficiency.

Over most of the body, the skin prevents disease-causing agents from entering the body. But they can enter through body openings, cuts, or wounds. Once they enter the body, they trigger an *immune response.* All body cells have special molecules on their membranes that are like flags with the word "self" on them. The cells of the immune system try to destroy anything present in the body that is not carrying the self molecules, anything that is "nonself." Nonself is any substance or object that triggers the creation of antibodies. Such substances are called *antigens.* Antigens may be whole virus or organisms or parts of virus, organisms, or their products.

BOX 4.1

BASIC IMMUNE SYSTEM TERMINOLOGY

Of the many mysteries of modern science, the mechanism of self versus nonself recognition in the immune system must rank near the top. The immune system is designed to recognize foreign invaders. To do so it generates on the order of 10^{12} or one trillion different kinds of immunological receptors so that no matter what the shape or form of the foreign invader there will be some complementary receptor to recognize it and effect its elimination. Understanding how the immune system responds to any foreign substance is puzzle enough, but the added mystery is that the immune system can distinguish foreign carbohydrates, nucleic acids, and proteins from those that exist within us, often in shapes barely distinguishable from the invaders. When the immune system is working well it never gets activated by self substances, but unerringly responds to the nonself substances. When the system is not working well this distinction gets blurred and diseases of autoimmunity occur—our immune cells attack our own tissue!

To understand the human immune system certain basic terminology is reviewed:

Antibody—an immunoglobulin (a protein) which is produced and secreted by B lymphocytes in response to an antigen. Antibodies are able to bind to and destroy specific antigens. Antibodies contribute to the destruction of antigen by their interaction with other components of the immune system.

Antigen—a substance that is recognized as foreign by the immune system when introduced into the body. An antigen can be a whole microorganism (such as a bacterium or whole virus) or a portion or a product of an organism or virus.

Leukocytes—all white blood cells (WBCs) including neutrophils, lymphocytes, and monocytes (phagocytes).

Lymphocytes—mononuclear WBCs which are critical in immune defense because they provide the specificity and memory needed for immune function and long-term or even life-long immunity. The two major classes of lymphocytes are B cells and T cells; both recognize specific antigens. (For an excellent review of lymphocyte life span and memory, see Sprent et al., 1994.)

Cytokines—soluble factors secreted by T cells, B cells, and monocytes which mediate complex immune interactions by acting as messengers. Subcategories of cytokines include: (1) lymphokines (secreted by lymphocytes), and (2) monokines (secreted by monocytes and macrophages). Specific cytokines include interleukin-1 (IL-1), interleukin-2 (IL-2), gamma interferons (γINF), B cell stimulating factor (BCSF), and B cell differentiating factor (BCDF).

The two branches of the human immune system are: Cellular Immunity and Humoral Immunity. Basic terms for each are provided, but as the terms will show, the two branches overlap to provide our immunity. (Adapted from *Mountain-Plains Regional HIV/AIDS Curriculum*, 1992.)

I. ***Cellular Immunity***—immune protection resulting from direct action of cells of the immune system. Key cell types offering Cellular Immunity are:

A. ***Phagocytes***

1. Phagocytes are leukocytes which are specialized for "eating" particles and molecules.
2. The most active phagocytic cells are monocytes and macrophages. Monocytes circulate in the blood but eventually move into body tissues (brain, muscle, etc.) where they mature into macrophages.
3. Phagocytes initiate the cellular immune response. When an invader (e.g., a virus or bacteria) enters the body, it will be trapped and "eaten" by a phagocyte. This attack against invaders occurs in various places in the body: the lining of the gut, throat, skin, bloodstream, or in organized lymphoid tissue such as the tonsils, other lymph nodes, or the spleen.
4. The phagocyte ingests the foreign invader and partially digests it. Pieces of the invader (antigens) can then be displayed on the phagocyte's surface, making the phagocyte an "**antigen-presenting cell**." This process alerts other cells in the immune system that a foreign substance is present.

B. ***Lymphocytes***

1. Ninety-eight percent of lymphocytes reside in lymphoid tissue (Pantaleo et al., 1993). Lymphocytes are uniquely specialized. Each lymphocyte has receptors on its

surface for one, and only one, of the many millions of possible antigens that can invade the body. When the receptors lock with their matched antigen, the process of neutralizing, inactivating, or destroying the foreign particle begins.

2. This requires that the body have an immense variety of receptors for an immense number of antigens. Humans usually have about 100,000 million (one trillion) lymphocytes.
3. There are several types of lymphocytes that play major roles in the immune response.
   a. ***T Lymphocytes*** mature in the thymus and play a central role in the immune response by destroying infected cells, controlling inflammatory responses, and helping B cells make antibodies. There are several subsets of T lymphocytes

      1) ***Helper T cells*** (**T_H**) alert the immune system to the presence of an antigen and activate other cells in the system. Helper T cells carry the CD4 marker and are most often referred to as **T4** cells.
         a) T4 cells have receptors on their surface which are specialized for the recognition of antigens found on the surface of antigen-presenting cells.
         b) When the T4 cell randomly contacts the surface of a phagocyte, its receptor binds to antigen on the phagocyte and the T4 cell becomes activated.
         c) The T4 cell then begins to secrete a variety of stimulatory factors (*lymphokines) into the space around it.*
         d) The T4 cell will eventually divide into two cells of exactly the same specificity. If the foreign substance persists, the two daughter cells will divide, and so on. Thus, the number of cells specific for that foreign antigen is greatly expanded.
         e) The T4 cell probably does little to repel the intruding substance on its own, but it is vital for activating the other main classes of lymphocytes (e.g., B cells, natural killer cells and phagocytes). It does this by means of the lymphokines it secretes when activated. The most familiar of these are interleukin-2 (IL-2) and gamma interferon (γIFN).
         f) As a result of activation by T4 cells, B lymphocytes multiply and produce specific antibodies. The antibodies attach to the antigens on free organisms and infected cells, leading to inactivation and destruction of organisms and cells.

      2) ***Inducer T cells*** (**T_i**) were previously known as the delayed sensitivity T cells. Inducer T cells also carry the CD4 molecule.

         a) When an inducer T cell recognizes antigen on the surface of a phagocyte and is helped by factors from a T4 cell, it also becomes activated and secretes its own family of lymphokines. IL4, IL5, and IL10. These factors attract many more phagocytes from around the body which accumulate in the area where antigen is being recognized.

         b) Phagocytes are specialized for "eating;" they will ingest and destroy the foreign invader.

      3) ***Cytotoxic T cells*** are lymphocytes also known as killer T cells. Cytotoxic T cells express the CD8 molecule and are most often referred to as **T8** cells. They are crucial for the immune response to viral infections. Although they cannot neutralize free virus, by eliminating virus infected-cells they are largely responsible for recovery from a viral infection.

         a) When a cytotoxic T8 cell recognizes antigen and is assisted by an activated T4 cell, it becomes *activated.* An activated cytotoxic T8 cell has the ability to "look inside" other cells and detect abnormalities with-in and destroy the infected cells.

         b) As the infected cell breaks apart, infectious particles can be released from the cell. The released infectious particles may be phagocytized, neutralized by antibody, or may infect new cells.

c) Cytotoxic T8 cells have antigen specificity; this specificity is determined when the cytotoxic T8 cell is exposed to the antigen.

b. ***B LYMPHOCYTES*** or ***B cells*** arise principally in the bone marrow and are responsible for making antibodies. The B cell response is referred to as humoral immunity.

1) B lymphocytes have receptors for antigen and also require help from T4 cells to become activated.
2) When activated, they release large amounts of immunoglobulins, called *antibodies,* into the bloodstream and mucosal surfaces.
3) Antibodies circulate in body fluids. When they encounter the specific antigen with which they can interact, they bind to it.
4) Antigen–antibody interactions block the antigen's harmful potential in a variety of ways. For example, if the antigen is a toxin it may be neutralized or if it is a virus, it may lose its ability to bind to its target tissue.
5) In addition, the complex of antigen and antibody activates a group of proteins in the blood called *complement,* which then facilitates the removal of the antigen by calling in a large number of phagocytes.

c. ***Memory cells***

1) Two groups of T and B lymphocytes become separate T and B memory cells for when the same antigen invades the body again.
2) Memory cells initiate immune response upon re-exposure to an antigen.
3) Memory cells remember, recognize, and induce a more rapid immune response against the antigen.
4) Memory cells are responsible for disease resistance after immunization and are also responsible for natural immunity.

d. ***Suppressor T cells*** also carry the CD8 molecule.

1) The function of suppressor T8 lymphocytes in the immune system is not well understood.
2) Suppressor T8 cells turn off antibody production and other immune responses after an invader has been destroyed or eliminated from the body. This provides a balance in the immune system and allows it to rest when its functions are not required.

e. ***Natural killer (NK) cells***

1) NK cells are antigen nonspecific lymphocytes which recognize foreign cells of many different antigenic types. That is, one NK cell can recognize many different types of invaders. Therefore, NK cells can attack without first having to recognize specific antigens.
2) NK cells are important in fighting viral infections.

II. *Humoral Immunity*—immune protection by the circulating antibodies which are produced by B cells. (See preceding section on **B Lymphocytes**.)

In general, most organisms that damage cells do so from the outside by producing toxic chemicals or in some way externally interfering with the cell's metabolism. But viruses generally invade different cell types forcing them to produce viral replicas at the expense of their own essential metabolic functions. Gradually, like a machine wearing out, the host cell starts to fade and die. The best thing a virus can do is find a host cell that does not die and that can produce replicas indefinitely. In a biological time frame, new disease-causing viruses are often very deadly to new hosts. If a new virus strain is too deadly, it kills its host before other hosts are infected, and the strain dies out. Over biological time, successful viruses and their new hosts learn to accommodate each other. This will most likely happen with human-HIV associations, but how many people over how many years will have to die before human cells learn to accommodate HIV is unknown. Perhaps it will never happen. Smallpox virus has been infecting humans for thousands of years and has never been accommodated by humans.

HUMAN LYMPHOCYTES: T CELLS AND B CELLS

The hallmark of the human immune system is its ability to mount a highly specific response against virtually any foreign entity, even those never seen before in the course of evolution. It is able to do this because of the number of different kinds of cells called lymphocytes. The human immune system contains about one trillion (1×10^{12}) lymphocytes, a relatively small number when compared to the trillions upon trillions of other types of cells in the body. Lymphocytes travel among most other cells; they circulate in blood and lymph tissue and are present in large numbers in the thymus, bone marrow, lymph nodes, spleen and appendix (Figure 4-1). By 1968, lymphocytes had been divided into two classes: lymphocytes called **B cells** that are derived from and mature in bone marrow, and lymphocytes called **T cells** that are derived from bone marrow but travel to and mature in the thymus gland (Figure 4-2). T cells make up 70% to 80% of the lymphocytes circulating in the body. Circulating T cells are a heterogeneous group of cells with a wide range of different functions. Three major kinds of T cells are cytotoxic (CD8) or killer T cells, helper T cells (also called T4 cells), and suppressor T cells (also called T8 cells). Killer T cells bind to

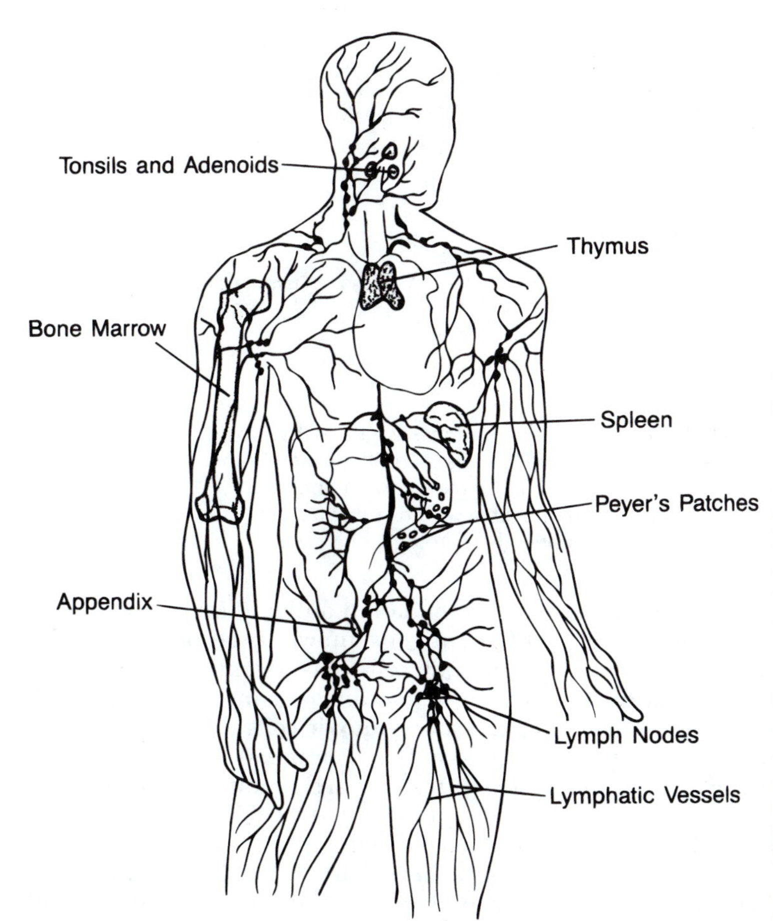

FIGURE 4-1 Organs of the Human Immune System. The organs of the immune system are positioned throughout the body. They are generally referred to as lymphoid organs because they are concerned with the development, growth, and dissemination of lymphocytes, or white cells, that populate the immune system. Lymphoid organs include the bone marrow, thymus, lymph nodes, spleen, tonsils, adenoids, appendix, and the clumps of lymphoid tissue in the small intestine called Peyer's patches. The blood and lymphatic fluids transport lymphocytes to and from all of the immune system organs.

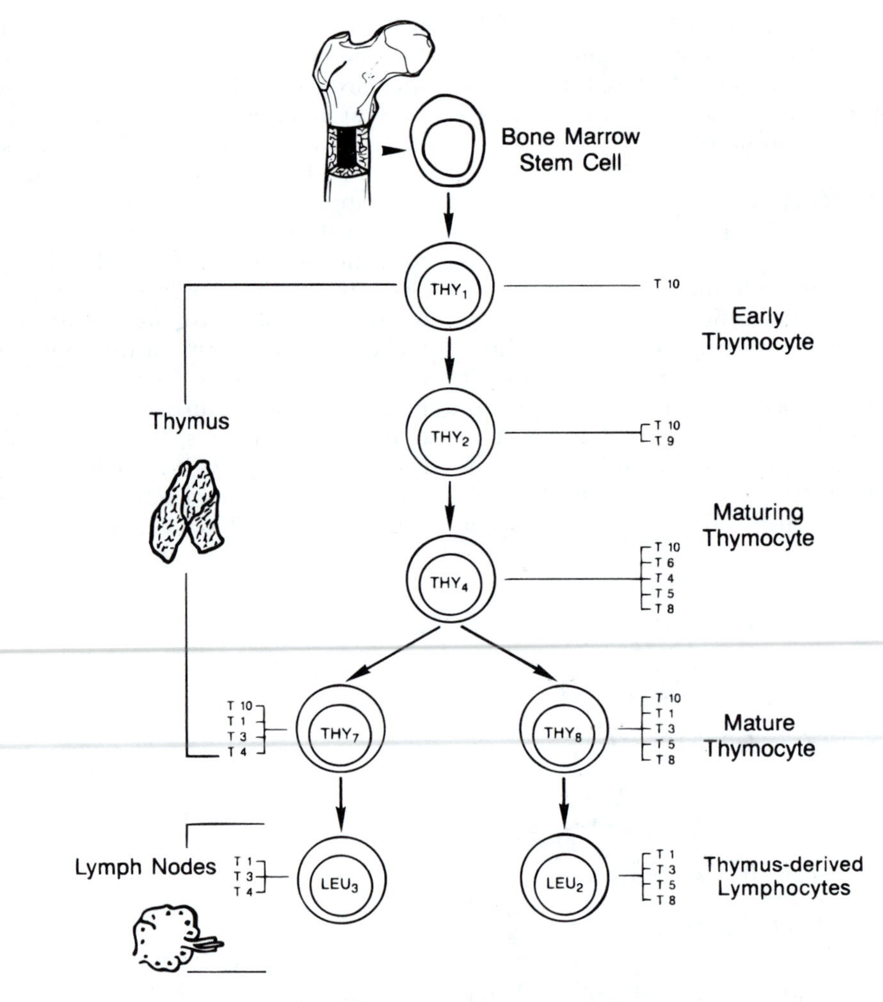

FIGURE 4-2 T lymphocyte Differentiation in Humans. Stages of thymic differentiation (i.e., the presence of the different antigens on their membrane surfaces) are defined on the basis of reactivity to monoclonal antibodies. Schematic pictures of cells represent thymocytes within specific stages of a defined phenotype: T1–T10 and membrane glycoproteins of T cells.

cells carrying a foreign antigen and destroy them. T4 cells do not kill cells; they interact with B cells and killer T cells and help them respond to antigens. All T cells produce proteins called **receptors** that are similar to antibodies in that they recognize specific antigens. The receptor proteins are located on the outer cell membrane.

T cell subsets, called **helper T cells** (whose full name is the CD4+ T lymphocyte or is commonly called the T4 cell; the CD4 means cluster differentiation antigen; there are at least 80 CD antigens known to be present on different body cells), are essential in helping to induce the immune response; while others, **T suppressor/cytotoxic cells** (T8 or CD8 cells), act to regulate (suppress) the immune response after the foreign antigen has been reduced or eliminated (Table 4-1) and to lyse virus-infected cells.

It is believed that T4 cells recognize only those antigens located on viruses, fungi, and

TABLE 4-1 Cells of the Human Immune System

Cell Type	Function
Stem cells	Self perpetuating cells that give rise to lymphocytes, macrophages, and other hematological cells
T helper cells (T_H), also called T4 or CD4 cells	Cells that interact with an antigen before the B cell interacts with the antigen
Cytotoxic cells (Tc)	Recruited by T helper cells to destroy antigens
Suppressor T cells (Ts), also called T8 or CD8 cells	Cells that dampen the activity of T and B cells; they somehow inhibit the immune response
B cells	Bone marrow stem cells that differentiate into plasma cells that secrete antibodies
Plasma cells	Cells devoted to the production of antibody directed against a particular foreign antigen
Monocytes	Precursors of macrophages
Macrophages	Differentiated monocytes that serve as antigen-presenting cells to T cells; they can also engulf a variety of antigens and antibody-covered cells
Killer cells (K)	Lymphocytes that recognize and kill any cell that is coated with antibody
Natural killer cells (NK or null cells)	Lymphocyte cells that detect and kill tumor cells and a broad range of foreign cells

other parasites; and trigger only those parts of the immune system necessary to act against these agents. Indeed, it is the viruses, fungi, and other parasites that produce the majority of opportunistic infections when the T4 cells have been depleted by the AIDS virus.

T4 Cell Function and HIV Disease

In general, individuals with partial or absolute defects in T cell function have infections or clinical problems for which there is no effective treatment. The T cell disorders are more severe than the B cell disorders.

The T cells are selectively deleted as a result of a series of events initiated by the binding of HIV to the CD4 molecule by means of the viral envelope protein gp120. Once HIV enters a T4 cell, it begins to lose normal function. This change, however, is not immediately apparent. HIV's takeover is a quiet event. The virus joins the host cell's DNA, then—nothing happens. Little or no viral replication takes place until the T4 cell is activated by some antigen. Then, instead of functioning normally, the T4 cell manufactures the invader's viral RNA strands. The activating antigen does not seem to be another HIV but some unrelated viral, fungal, or parasitic invader. It is the T4 cells which are destroyed by HIV. The loss of T4 cells severely reduces cell-mediated immunity, eliminates the T4 cell dependent production of antibodies by B cells, and eventually makes HIV-infected people susceptible to opportunistic infection and subsequent death. AIDS is diagnosed when the T4 cell count drops to less than 200/μL. (T4 counts from 600 to 1,200 are considered normal in adults.) T4 cell counts of less than 100 are associated with *profound* immunodeficiency and multiple or disseminated opportunistic infections (Crowe et al., 1991). (See Chapters 5 and 6.)

One of the most interesting findings has been the discovery of a subset of healthy, long-term survivors who have lived for years with T4 counts of less than 200. For the most part, they do not develop the secondary infections that are associated with AIDS, or if they do, they tend to recover. This means that there is a lot about the immune system that immunologists still do not understand. Some researchers believe these men managed to press other white blood cells into service to make up for the T4 deficiency.

B Cell Function and HIV Disease

The ultimate product of the B cells is immunoglobulin. Any abnormalities in the transition of the B lymphocyte from the stem cell level to the plasma cell may affect immuno- globulin synthesis. The earlier the rupture in the developmental pathway, the more extensive the loss in antibody-forming capacity.

The B lymphocytes can produce and secrete soluble antibodies in response to direct contact with an antigen (T cell-independent B cell response), or the B cell with the help of T4 cells can produce antibodies specific for a given antigen (T4 cell-dependent B cell response). The antibodies enter the circulatory system and are carried throughout the body.

HIV does not normally infect B cells. However, in laboratory experiments, HIV is able to infect B cells, if the B cells are first infected by the Epstein-Barr virus, which is the cause of infectious mononucleosis. The Epstein-Barr virus appears to change B cells in some way, allowing subsequent HIV infection. HIV can grow and replicate within B cells transformed by the Epstein-Barr virus, without destroying the host cell. Whether similar events occur in humans is not known. B cell function is almost normal in most HIV-infected persons. Small defects in B cell function exist, seemingly resulting from the disrupted communication with other cells, not from some internal B cell defect.

T8 Cell Function and HIV Disease

Together, T4 cells and T8 cells regulate the body's immune response to invaders. Also, T8 cells help the immune system recognize (and not attack) the cells of its own body. But some T8 cells are lost in HIV-infected persons. Depending on how many are lost, the immune system may not be properly suppressed and an autoimmune response (the immune system attacks self) may occur.

Summary: Immune Dysfunction Caused by HIV/AIDS

HIV enters the body via infected body fluids: blood, semen, and vaginal secretions. Once inside, HIV specifically infects a type of white blood cell called the T4 helper cell (also called CD4+ cells). These cells direct the body's immune response against infection. As HIV takes over the T4 cells, it alters their growth and reproduction through a complicated process that leads to the T4 cells' destruction. The ratio of T4 to other cells called T8 then changes. In healthy people, the number of T4 cells is greater than the number of T8 cells. In HIV-infected individuals, a decline in the T4 count signals the progress of immune system deterioration. The results are debilitating: the T4 cells are not as responsive to antigen identification, macrophages become less responsive, and B cells produce fewer specific antibodies and lose their normal responsiveness. At this point, the immune system becomes dysfunctional and vulnerable to attack from opportunistic infections that would normally be held in check by a healthy immune system. (A normal T cell count ranges from 600 to 1,200.)

ANTIBODIES AND VIRUSES

Twenty-four hours a day, 365 days a year, the body's lymphocytes must be on the lookout for harmful bacteria, viruses, and other pathogens. And these agents of disease don't look very different, biochemically, from most of the normal molecules lymphocytes normally encounter in the blood. Yet a mistake by these immune cells can leave the body open to infection.

But, the immune system has evolved antibodies for distinguishing the body's own molecular debris from potentially harmful material. Antibodies are Y-shaped molecules that bind to specific foreign proteins, or pieces of protein, called antigens. If the immune system mistakenly identifies the body's own proteins as foreign, an autoimmune disorder can result.

When antibodies on the surface of a B cell snag an undesirable or foreign protein, both disappear inside the cell. Eventually, a bit of the foreign protein may reemerge, attached to a "self" recognizable protein molecule called a class II protein (Figure 4.3). The pair, the small piece of foreign protein attached to a "self" class II protein, acts as a red flag to a special set of lymphocytes called T4 cells, which set off an aggressive immune response.

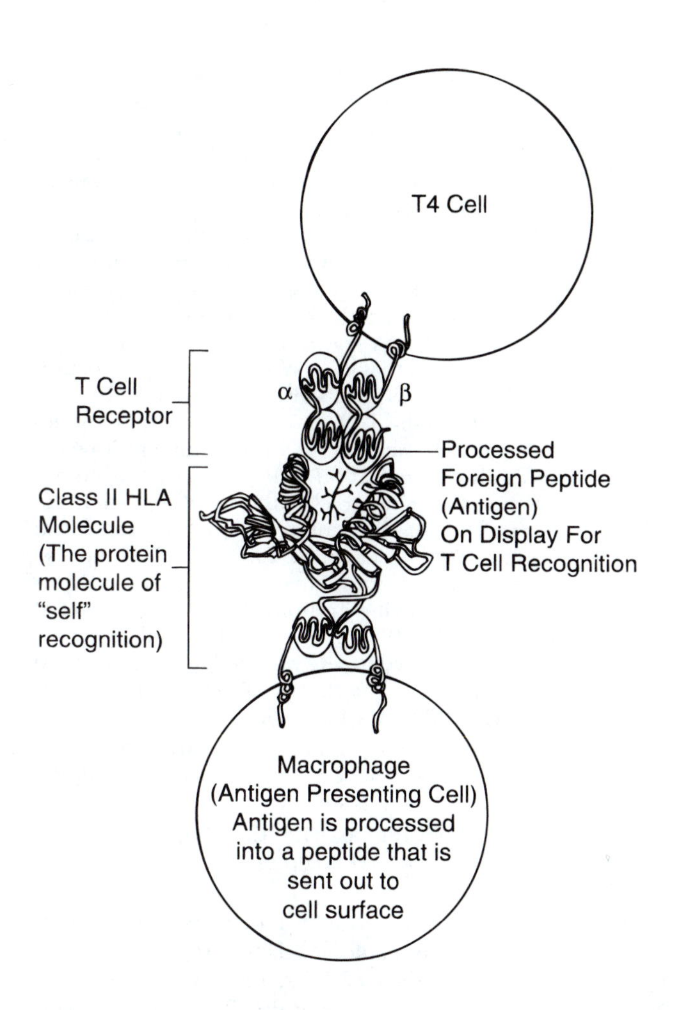

FIGURE 4.3 Interaction Between a Human Leucocyte Antigen "self" protein (HLA), a Foreign Peptide (Antigen, and a T Cell Receptor. The diagram represents the trimolecular interaction of a processed antigen into a peptide that is being presented on the surface of the antigen-presenting cell to a T4 cell. The presence of the class II HLA self identity marker and the presence of the foreign peptide stimulate the T4 cell into action. (*Adapted from Sinha, 1990*)

Until now, scientists did not know where the cell degraded this undesirable protein and attached it to a "self" recognizable protein.

In mid-1994, four research teams announced the discovery of a special compartment, or organelle, inside cells where this processing occurs. Using sophisticated biochemical and immunological techniques, they independently determined that both the "self" recognizable protein and the antibody-antigen complex wind up in this new compartment called an endosome (Amigorena et al., 1994; Pennisi, 1994; Schmid et al., 1994; Tulp etal., 1994).

The characterization of a specialized vesicle is an important step. It permits an understanding of the trafficking events and defines the intracellular event of antigen processing.

B Cells Make Antibodies and Release Them into the Bloodstream

After an antibody and virus join, they are digested by macrophages or cleared from the blood by the liver and spleen. Some B cells become **memory cells** which are stored by the immune system. Memory cells can remember the antigen they have previously encountered. If the same virus ever gets into the bloodstream again, these cells rapidly begin antibody production. However, if the virus has mutated (changed), as the flu virus does yearly, previous antibodies will not affect it. New antibodies must be created to neutralize the new mutant virus. While this antibody production is taking place, the viral invader has time to multiply and infect new cells, and the infected person suffers the symptoms of the flu.

ANTIBODIES AND HIV DISEASE

Resistance to HIV does not seem to be the same as more common examples of immunity. The body's protective countermeasures against measles and mumps are absolute. Years after exposure, there is no hint within the body of the foreign agents that cause those diseases. After children become immune to mumps, they can no longer infect other people.

The human body makes antibodies against HIV, but they apparently do not work effectively. In several experiments where HIV has been isolated from blood, large numbers of antibodies to HIV were also found. This indicates that, even though the HIV antibody is present, it has difficulty neutralizing the virus, and, therefore, provides little protection. Infected persons move on through HIV disease to AIDS.

HIV Protected from Human Antibodies

Humans create antibodies against a number of HIV proteins, namely the envelope proteins (gp120), the transmembrane protein (gp41), and the proteins of HIV's core (gp24). But, antibodies cannot enter cells. The antibody can only attack HIV in the plasma. Plasma is the fluid part of the blood and does not include the blood cells. Once inside a host cell, HIV is protected from antibody. Cells can generate antiviral chemicals within themselves, but these too seem ineffective against the hidden HIV.

Once HIV gets inside T4 or other cell types as a provirus, it is likely to remain there for the rest of the person's life unless some other antiviral mechanism within the body or some chemical agent is able to destroy the provirus. To date, no such drug has been found to be effective against the HIV provirus.

How HIV Enters the T4 Cell

The envelope of HIV is studded with proteins made by the virus. The major envelope protein is called gp120:

1. gp120 proteins protrude from the viral envelope. The gp120 region contains a conserved or **constant region** (in this region the sequence of amino acids remains constant from virus to virus) and a **variable region** (among HIV, the amino acid sequence is often different in this region). The variable region is made up of three hyper variable areas—each of the areas contain their own sequence on loops of amino acids. The regions are referred to as the V1, V2, and V3 loops. Each loop undergoes antigen change as its amino acids are replaced by different amino acids as genetic mutations occur in sections of HIV-RNA that code for the amino acid arrangement in the loop regions. Each loop acts as a separate antigen in that each stimulates the production of a loop-specific antibody. The V3 loop, the area that binds to the T4 lymphocyte (CD4 binding domain) is the principal site in the viral envelope for antibody neutralization (antibodies that inactivate HIV) and is believed to be the most important site responsible for HIV's infectivity (Belshe et al., 1994; Cohen, 1994; Ghiara et al., 1994). The V3 loop also contains the determinants responsible for the formation of T4 cell syncytium (fusion of uninfected T4 cells with HIV-infected T4 cells) (Bobkov et al., 1994). A more complete knowledge of the V3 loop should facilitate the design of new drugs and vaccines to inhibit HIV infection.

2. When HIV enters the body, it circulates in the blood until by chance it bumps into a cell with the CD4 receptor on its surface.

3. The viral protein gp120 then binds specifically and tightly to a CD4 receptor site.

Helper and inducer T cells express numerous CD4 molecules and are, therefore, most readily infected by HIV. A number of other cells, including monocytes and cells in the skin and nervous system (including the brain), express CD4 and can be directly infected by HIV. But, because they express less CD4 than T4 cells, they may be less readily infected. There is some evidence of primary HIV infection in organs such as the kidneys and the intestines that do not have CD4 receptors. Thus investigators have been searching for a second receptor since the late 1980s. The feeling has been that the CD4 receptor, on its own, is not sufficient for HIV entry. For example, when mouse cells in culture are genetically engineered to produce human CD4 on their surfaces, HIV is able to bind to the cells but not actually enter them. This and other results suggested that a second receptor is required for HIV entry into cells.

In October of 1993, Ara Hovanessian and colleagues of the Pasteur Institute announced

BOX 4.2

HIV REQUIRES A COMPATIBLE RECEPTOR SITE FOR INFECTION

For HIV/AIDS, a lethal sexually transmitted disease (STD), infection may be initiated by receiving the free AIDS virus within a body fluid or within infected cells. Once inside the body, HIV, because of its specific glycoprotein "spikes" (gp120) that extend out from the viral envelope, is attracted primarily to those cells that display the CD4 receptor site antigen. All cells that carry a CD4 or T4 receptor antigen are susceptible to HIV infection. Cell types other than T4 cells known to carry the CD4 or T4 receptor antigen are monocytes, macrophages, glial cells, chromaffin cells of the lower intestine and vaginal lining, and retinal cells in the eye.

Laboratory experiments show that HIV can replicate in a wide range of human cells if **injected into the cells artificially**. HIV's difficulty is in entering the cells. HIV's protein projections on its protein coat successfully unlock the membrane of a cell's CD4 receptor site, but not most membranes without CD4. Thus HIV infects only those cells it can enter. A major concern is that HIV might change such that it can attach to receptor sites other than CD4 with equal efficiency.

T suppressor cells carry a different antigen than that found on T4 cells. This antigen is referred to by the number 8, so suppressor/cytotoxic T cells are called T8 cells (CD8). Thus the ability to tell one type of T cell from another, in fact, depends on the type of receptor cell antigen found on the cell's membrane surface.

the discovery of the second receptor site, CD26. According to Hovanessian, CD26, is an enzyme that is specific for dipeptide bonds containing the amino acid proline. It is found on the surface of human T cells (the targets for HIV infection), and is essential for assisting the entry of HIV together with the T cell surface receptor CD4.

According to the French group, CD26 cleaves the HIV envelope protein gp120 at the V3 loop region as the virus attaches to the cell surface. They claim that enzyme inhibitors and antibodies to CD26 block the entry of HIV-1 and HIV-2 into human cells, and that expression of both CD4 and CD26 is needed for virus entry into mouse cells that do not normally express these molecules (Butler, 1993).

The reaction to Hovanessian's work in the United States is mixed with support and mild to severe criticism. Twenty-nine scientists from eight different laboratories disagree with CD26 being a second receptor site (Broder et al., 1994; Fantini et al., 1994; Werner et al., 1994; West et al., 1994). Some scientists believe the experiments involving gene transfers into mouse cells were technically flawed. For one reason, the mouse cell lines used in the experiments are not stable and the viral assay, the means by which the virus as were counted, does not indicate whether the virus as were replicated within the mouse cells or were the original viruses put into the culture to cause an infection (Balter, 1993).

The Circuitous Relationship of HIV to the Human Immune System

HIV prefers to attack a specific type of cell, the T4 lymphocyte. The body responds to HIV entry via the T4 lymphocytes and other CD4-bearing cells by producing both humoral and cell-mediated responses. However, HIV has also evolved with a response to the human immune defenses by infecting the very cells which govern the immune response, most importantly, the T4 lymphocytes and macrophages!

T4 CELL DEPLETION AND IMMUNE SUPPRESSION

An understanding of the mechanisms which by HIV reduces the number of CD4 cells is important. However, we do not yet understand just how the T4 helper cell is killed or impaired by HIV infection. Recent research using the **polymerase chain reaction** (a method of amplifying present but unmeasurable quantities of HIV DNA in T4 cells into measurable quantities) has revealed that about *one in every 10 to 100* T4 cells is HIV-infected in an AIDS patient. Thus T4 helper and inducer cells serve as reservoirs of HIV in the body (Schnittman et al., 1989; Cohen, 1993). Collectively, T4 cell depletion leads to cumulative and devastating effects on the cell-mediated and humoral parts of the immune system.

Filling CD4 Receptor Sites

There is evidence from in vitro studies that HIV can attack CD4 receptor sites in at least two ways. First, HIV can attach, via its gp160 "spikes," to CD4 receptor sites. Second, HIV is capable of releasing or freeing its exterior gp120 envelope glycoprotein, thereby generating a molecule that can actively bind to CD4-bearing cells (Gelderblom et al., 1985). As a result of filling the receptor sites on the T4 cells, the T4 cells lose their immune functions; that is, the T4 cell does not have to be infected with HIV to lose immune function. In addition, CD4-bearing cells that attach the free gp120 molecule then become targets for immune attack by antibody-mediated antibody-dependent cell cytotoxicity (ADCC) and nonantibody-mediated cytotoxic T cells. Both events can result in the destruction of uninfected CD4 cells. The extent to which this occurs in vivo depends on the level of gp120 synthesis, secretion, and shedding. Free gp120 has not yet been measured in the circulation, but this is not surprising given its powerful affinity for CD4 (Bolognesi, 1989).

Single-Cell Killing

Single-cell killing may result from the accumulation of unintegrated viral DNA or from the inhibition of cellular protein synthesis after HIV infection.

Syncytia Formation

The formation of syncytia involves fusion of the cell membrane of an infected cell with the cell membranes of uninfected CD4 cells, which results in giant multinucleated cells. A direct relation between the presence of syncytia and the degree of the cytopathic effect of the virus in individual cells has been demonstrated in vitro, and HIV isolated during the accelerated phase of infection in vivo has a greater capacity to induce syncytia in vitro. Syncytia have rarely been seen in vivo.

In the asymptomatic phase of HIV infection, predominantly nonsyncytium inducing (NSI), HIV variants can be detected. In about 50% of the cases SI HIV variants emerge in the course of infection, preceding rapid T4 cell depletion and progression to AIDS (Groenink et al., 1993).

Superantigens

Superantigens are microbial or viral antigens that are capable of binding to nearly all T cells that have a specific variable region of the β chain of the T cell antigen receptor. Unlike conventional antigenic peptides that bind in the groove of the MHC class II molecule, superantigens bind only to the variable β region of the T cell antigen receptor. Superantigens therefore induce massive stimulation and expansion of T cells bearing the specific variables β regions, followed by deletion or anergy. The superantigen hypothesis regarding HIV infection stems from the observations that endogenous or exogenous retroviral-encoded superantigens stimulate murine T4 cells in vivo, leading to the anergy or deletion of a substantial percentage of T4 cells that have the specific variable β regions (Pantaleo et al., 1993).

Apoptosis

Programmed cell death, or apoptosis (a-po-toe-sis), is a normal mechanism of cell death that was originally described in the context of the response of immature thymocytes to cellular activation. It is a mechanism whereby the body eliminates autoreactive clones of T cells. It has recently been suggested that both qualitative and quantitative defects in T4 cells in patients with HIV infection may be the result of activation-induced cell death or apoptosis. Since apoptosis can be induced in mature murine T4 cells after cross-linking CD4 molecules to one another and triggering the T4 cell antigen receptor, there has been speculation that cross-linking of the CD4 molecule by HIV gp120 or gp120-anti-gp120 immune complexes prepares the cell for the programmed death that occurs when a MHC class II molecule in complex with an antigen binds to the T4 cell antigen receptor. Thus activation of a prepared cell by a specific antigen or superantigen could lead to the death of the cell, without direct infection by HIV (Pantaleo et al., 1993). For an excellent review of Apoptosis and its role in human disease, see Barr et al., 1944.

BOX 4.3

COFACTORS EXPEDITE HIV INFECTION

(An excerpt from Michael Callen's article, "Everything Must Be Doubted," *Newsline*, July/August 1988, pp. 44–5.)

By the age of 27 (when I was diagnosed with crypto [cryptococcus infection] and AIDS) I had had over 3,000 different sex partners. Not coincidentally, I'd also had: hepatitis A, hepatitis B, hepatitis non-A, non-B; herpes simplex types I & II; syphilis; gonorrhea; non-specific urethritis; shigella; entamoeba histolitica; chlamydia; fungal infections; venereal warts; cytomegalovirus infections; EBV [Epstein-Barr virus] reactivations; cryptosporidium and therefore, finally, AIDS. For me, the question wasn't why I got AIDS, but how I had been able to remain standing on two feet for so long... If you blanked out my name and age on my pre-AIDS medical chart and showed it to a doctor and asked her to guess who I was, she might reasonably have guessed, based on my disease history, that I was a 65-year-old malnourished equatorial African living in squalor... I believe that a small subset of urban gay men unwittingly managed to recreate disease settings equivalent to those of poor Third World nations and junkies.

This quote details many of the disease cofactors which play a role in the development of immune dysfunction; while any one infection might not cause a problem for a healthy individual, repeated infection and exposure to foreign body fluids takes a cumulative toll. And certain infections are unquestionably more immune-suppressive than others—In particular, the sexually transmitted diseases.

Cellular Transfer of HIV

Infected macrophages, or antigen-presenting cells, which normally interact with the T4 cells to stimulate the immune function, can transfer HIV into uninfected T4 lymphocytes. **In any case, immediate viral or proviral replication, kills the T4 cell.**

Autoimmune Mechanisms

One of the older theories, namely that HIV tricks the immune system into attacking itself is back because of the recent work of Tracy Kion and Geoffrey Hoffmann (1991). Their work showed that mice immunized with lymphocytes from another mouse strain make antibodies to the HIV envelope protein gp120, as do autoimmune strains of mice, even though **none of the animals had ever been exposed to the AIDS virus.** One implication of these results is that some component on the lymphocytes resembles gp120 closely enough so that antibodies directed against it can recognize gp120 as well. The converse is that antibodies to gp120 should also recognize the lymphocyte component so that an immune response directed against HIV might also interfere with normal lymphocyte function. The autoimmune theory is consistent with results that show there is a selective loss of particular subsets of T cells in AIDS patients.

Cofactors May Help Deplete T4 Cells

HIV-infected people who are a symptomatic show a wide variation in HIV disease time and progression to AIDS. It is believed that cofactors may be responsible for some of the time variation with regard to disease progression.

Many agents may act as cofactors to activate or increase HIV production. Although, in general, it is not believed that any cofactor is necessary for HIV infection, cofactors such as nutrition, stress, and infectious organisms have been considered as agents that might accelerate HIV expression after infection. One human herpes virus (HHV-6) discovered in 1986 may be a cofactor and play a role in causing immune deficiency. HHV-6 has been shown to infect HIV-infected T4-bearing cells. In these doubly infected cells, HHV-6 activates the HIV provirus to increase HIV replication. When HHV-6 replicates alone in T4 cells, it kills those cells with a greater efficiency than does HIV. Thus in doubly infected people, there are two viruses capable of killing T4 cells (Thomson et al., 199). Paolo Lusso and colleagues (1993) have also shown that HHV-6 infects and kills natural killer cells of the immune system, cells that seek out and destroy virus-infected cells. This will also help suppress immune system activity. Cytomegalovirus and the Epstein-Barr virus have also been associated with increased HIV expression. Over time, investigators expect to find other sexually transmitted diseases that behave as cofactors associated with HIV infection and expression.

Shyh-Ching Lo and colleagues at the Armed Forces Institute of Pathology suggested in 1989 that a mycoplasma infection was a cofactor in HIV infection. Mycoplasma lack a cell wall, are simpler than bacteria, and are more complex than viruses. They are the smallest known organisms that can live outside a host cell. Lo identified the mycoplasma as *M. incognitus* (Lo et al., 1989, 1991).

At the Sixth and Eighth International AIDS Symposiums, Luc Montagnier, the discoverer of HIV, said that many lines of evidence led him to the conclusion that mycoplasmas play a role in increasing the pathogenicity of HIV.

Drugs may also be cofactors in infection. Used by injection drug users (IDUs), heroin and other morphine-based derivatives are known to reduce human resistance to infection and produce immunological suppression. *Pneumocystis carinii* pneumonia is about twice as frequent in heroin users as in homosexuals. It is believed that the heroin has an immunosuppressive effect within the lungs (Brown, 1987).

Blood and blood products may also act as cofactors in infection because they are immunosuppressive. Because blood transfusions save lives, their long-range effects are generally overlooked. Transfusions in hemophiliacs, for example, result in lowered resistance to viruses such as cytomegalovirus (CMV), Epstein-Barr (Berkman, 1984; Blumberg et al., 1985; Foster et al., 1985), and perhaps HIV. Seminal fluid (fluid bathing the sperm) may also act as a cofactor in infection because it also causes immunosuppression. One of its physiological functions is to immunosuppress the female genital tract so that the sperm is not immunologically rejected (Witkin et al., 1983; Baxena et al., 1985).

Epidemiologically, homosexuals at greatest risk of AIDS are those who practice passive anal sex, that is, anal recipients (Kingsley et al., 1987). It is generally considered that this sexual behavior is a cofactor that enables the AIDS virus to enter the bloodstream by means of traumatic lacerations of the rectal mucosa; Brown (1987) believes it is more likely that the immunosuppressed rectal mucosa facilitates the absorption of HIV. Mucous membrane immunosuppression is undoubtedly a factor in the incubation and transmission of other infections carried in seminal fluid.

Seminal fluid immunosuppression probably has a role in the maintenance and growth of amoebae, bacteria, parasites, fungi, and other microbes associated with "gay bowel syndrome." This is also a factor in the increased incidence of sexually transmitted diseases among heterosexuals (Brown, 1987). Last but not least of the agents that can suppress the immune system and thereby act as a cofactor in HIV infection is *stress*. Stress can be mental or physical; but it is easier to measure the effects of physical stress. For example, overtraining is blamed by top athletes and their coaches for the illnesses that afflict them with increasing frequency as the sports season progresses. These illnesses range from persistent colds, sore throats, and flu-like infections to severely debilitating states such as postviral fatigue syndrome, which can cause the athlete to miss an entire season, or even force him to give up competitive sports.

Although moderate exercise appears to stimulate the immune system, there is good evidence that intensive exercise can suppress the immune system. We still do not really know why (Fitzgerald, 1988; LaPierre et al., 1992). The effect of stress on the immune system is one of the reasons why physicians did not want Earvin "Magic" Johnson to play basketball (see BOX 8.3 in Chapter 8).

Impact of T4 Cell Depletion

The overall impact of T4 cell depletion is multifaceted. HIV-induced T4 cell abnormalities alter the T4 cells' ability to produce a variety of inducer chemical stimulants such as the interleukins that are necessary for the proper maturation of B cells into plasma cells and the maturation of a subset of T cells into cytotoxic cells (Figure 4-4). Thus the critical basis for the immunopathogenesis of HIV infection is the depletion of the *helper/inducer subset of T4 lymphocytes* which results in profound immunosuppression.

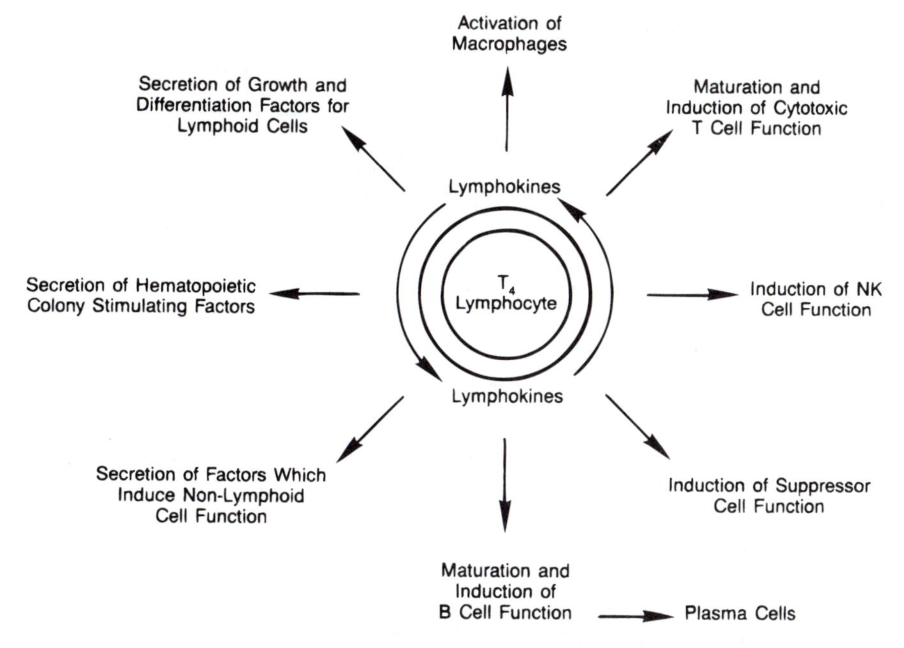

FIGURE 4-4 The T4 Cell Role in the Immune Response. T4 lymphocytes are responsible directly or indirectly for inducing a wide array of functions in cells that produce the immune response. They also induce nonlymphoid cell functions. T cell involvement is effected for the most part by the secretion of soluble factors or lymphokines that have trophic or inductive effects on the cells presented in the figure. Lymphokines serve to transfer control of the immune response from the external environmental proteins to the internal regulatory system consisting of ligands and receptors. (*Adapted from Fauci, 1991*)

Presumably, with time, the number of HIV-infected T4 cells increases to a point where, in terminal AIDS patients, few *normal T4 cells exist.*

ROLE OF MONOCYTES AND MACROPHAGES IN HIV INFECTION

Some scientists now believe that T4 cell infection alone does not cause AIDS because not enough T4 cells are destroyed. They believe that equally important to T4 cell infection is monocyte and macrophage infection (Bakker et. al., 1992). Monocytes change into various types of macrophages (given different names) in order to search and destroy foreign agents within tissues of the lungs, brain, and interstitial tissues, tissues that connect organs. Despite the name changes, all forms of macrophages basically work the same way: they eat things. Some macrophages travel around within the body, others become attached to one spot, digesting what comes by.

Macrophages are often the first cells of the immune system to encounter invaders, particularly in the area of a cut or wound. After engulfing the invader, the macrophage makes copies of the invader's antigens and displays them on its own cell membrane. These copies of the invader antigens sit right next to the self molecules. In effect, the macrophage makes a "wanted poster" of this new invader. The macrophage then travels about showing the wanted poster to T4 cells, which triggers the T4 cells into action. Macrophages also release chemicals which stimulate both T4 cell and macrophage production and draw macro- phages and lymphocytes to the site of infection.

Macrophages may play an important role in spreading HIV infection in the body, both to other cells and to HIV's target organs. First, HIV quietly spreads from macrophage to macrophage before the immune system is altered. Second, macrophages, in their different forms, travel to the brain, the lungs, the bone marrow, and to various immune organs, and bring HIV along with them.

HIV's ability to infect brain tissue is particularly important. The brain and cerebral spinal fluid (CSF) are vulnerable sites, and, consequently, are specially protected sites. CSF cushions the brain and the spinal cord from sudden and jarring movements. The brain–blood barrier, a chemical phenomenon, normally stops foreign substances from entering the brain and the CSF. But HIV-infected monocytes can pass through this barrier. For HIV, macrophages are Trojan horses, enabling HIV to enter the immune-protected domain of the central nervous system—the brain, the spine, and all the nerves.

HIV isolates taken from macrophages appear to grow better in macrophages than in lymphocytes. In human cell culture experiments, HIV isolates taken from lymphocytes appear to grow better in lymphocytes than in macrophages. These peculiarities of replication rates may be evidence of separate tissue-oriented HIV strains.

HIV-infected macrophages have proven to be a major problem in efforts to control and stop HIV infection.

Clinical Latency: Where Have All the Viruses Been Hiding?

The immunodeficiency syndrome caused by HIV is characterized by profound T4 cell depletion. Prior to the progressive decline of T4 cells and the development of AIDS, there is a symptom-free period which may last for 10 or more years, during which the infection is thought to be clinically latent. Scientists thought little if any viral replication occurred during this period. In recent years, a number of studies have offered an alternative view. Some investigations suggest that there is no real latency period in HIV infection. Instead, starting from the moment of infection, there appears to be a continuous struggle between HIV and the immune system, the balance of which slowly shifts in favor of the virus. These studies suggest that the virus invades the immune system and gradually reduces immune function without ever being present in high numbers (Tersmette et al., 1990; Fauci, 1991; Edgington, 1993). Cecil H. Fox of the Yale School of Medicine reported in December 1991 that HIV is not lying dormant at all but is continually infecting immune cells in the lymph nodes.

The lymph nodes, which are pea-sized capsules that trap foreign invaders and produce immune cells, are all over the body and are connected by vessels much like those that transport blood. Deep within the lymph nodes of 18 HIV-infected patients, researchers found millions of viruses. Based on those data, Fox suggested that the viruses use the lymph nodes as the places to meet up with most immune cells. Fox believes that HIV begins replication in T4 cells in the lymph nodes soon after it enters the body. Infected T4 cells leave the lymph nodes and new uninfected cells arrive to become infected. Years later, when enough immune cells have been killed, the patient's defenses become so impaired that he or she is vulnerable to any one of a wide array of opportunistic infections—AIDS has arrived.

Anthony Fauci (Figure 7-5), the head of the National Institute of Allergy and Infectious Diseases (NIAID), agrees that there are many more HIVs in the lymph nodes than in the blood. Studies in his laboratory have shown there are literally millions of HIV particles stuck to what are known as follicular dendritic cells in the lymph nodes of an infected individual.

The follicular dendritic cells, which have thousands of feathery processes emanating from them and whose normal function is to filter and trap antigens for presentation to antibody-producing B lymphocytes, serve as highly effective trapping centers for extracellular HIV particles. Virtually every lymphocyte in a lymph node is enmeshed in the processes of these cells. Although the follicular dendritic cells themselves do not seem to be susceptible to HIV infection, they appear to place huge numbers of virus particles into intimate contact with cells that are susceptible to HIV infection.

During the clinically latent phase, the lymph nodes of an infected individual are slowly destroyed.

In the final phase of an infection, the follicular dentritic network completely dissolves and the architecture of the lymph node collapses to produce what Fauci called a "burnt-out lymph node." With this collapse, large amounts of viruses are released into the circulatory system and an ever increasing number of peripheral cells are infected with HIV (Baum, 1992; Edgington, 1993).

Based on the recent works of Giuseppe Pantaleo (1993) and Janet Embretson (1993) and their colleagues, there is some proviral latency, but for the most part, HIV replicates at a slow but constant rate from the time of infection, giving the appearance of a clinical latency. One can conclude from the reports of Pantaleo and Embretson that the secondary lymphoid organs become heavily infected shortly after the initial HIV infection. Thus, until now, scientists have vastly **underestimated** the extent of virus activity in an HIV-infected person, particularly during the asymptomatic or "clinically latent" phase. These and other recent studies should satisfy the major unanswered question concerning HIV disease/AIDS, which **was**, "Where is the virus?" During the 1980s, it was difficult to find medium to high levels of infectious HIV in persons with HIV disease or even in those persons in the later stages of AIDS. We now know that there are large amounts of the virus present early in HIV-diseased people. Now, however, perhaps the most troubled group of researchers may be those currently developing AIDS vaccines. At present, vaccine strategies propose to introduce HIV antigen repeatedly during the long latent period to bolster B cell immunity. Vaccinated antigens, however, would wind up trapped in the lymph nodes, stimulating B cells to produce precisely the cytokines that stimulate T4 cell infection and speed lymph node architecture destruction. Thus the vaccine's effect could backfire, compressing the clinically latent period and causing a more rapid onset of AIDS.

SUMMARY

After a healthy person is HIV-infected, he or she makes antibodies against those viruses that are in the bloodstream, but not against those that have become integrated as HIV proviruses in the host immune cell DNA. Over time the immune system cells that are involved in antibody production are destroyed. Evidence is accumulating that cofactors such as nutrition, stress, and previous exposure to other sexually transmitted diseases that increase HIV expression are associated with HIV infection and HIV disease. Agents that suppress the immune system may also play a significant role in establishing HIV infection. There is some disagreement among HIV/AIDS investigators as to whether there is a true HIV proviral latency period after infection. In short, HIV infection is permanent. The virus may be latent, it does attack CD4-bearing cells and, as seen in Chapter 3, it undergoes rapid genetic change, and, as far as determined, attacks only human cells—mostly of the human immune system. It has recently become quite clear that large amounts of the virus are presented within weeks after HIV infection. The virus remains, for the most part, in the lymph nodes until very late in the disease process.

REVIEW QUESTIONS

(*Answers to the Review Questions are on page 479.*)

1. Which cell type is believed to be the main target for HIV infection? Explain the biological impact of this particular infection.

2. What is CD4, where is it found, and what is its role in the HIV infection process?

3. Is there a period of latency after HIV infection—a time when few or no new HIV are being produced?

4. True or False: HIV is the cause of AIDS.

5. True or False: HIV primarily affects red blood cells.

6. True or False: Lymphocytes have a major role in the immune response to antigens.

7. True or False: All T and B lymphocytes inhibit or destroy foreign antigens.

8. True or False: CD4 and CD8 molecules are antibodies.

9. True or False: HIV belongs to the family of retroviruses.

10. True or False: Cytotoxic and suppressor T lymphocytes are the main targets of HIV.

11. True or False: The latent period is that time between initial infection with HIV and the onset of AIDS.

12. True or False: HIV can spread to infect new cells after it buds out of infected cells.

13. True or False: HIV causes the gradual destruction of cells bearing the CD4 molecule.

REFERENCES

AMEISEN, JEAN CLAUDE. (1994). Programmed cell death capoptosis and cell survival regulation: relavance to cancer. *AIDS*, 8:1197–1213.

AMIGORENA, SEBASTIAN, et al., (1994). Transient accumulation of new class II MHC molecules in a novel endocytic compartment in B lymphocytes. *Natur*, 369: 113–120.

BAKKER, LEENDERT J., et al. (1992). Antibodies and complement enhance binding and uptake of HIV-1 by human monocytes. *AIDS*, 6:35–41.

BALTER, MICHAEL. Skepticism greets HIV coreceptor. *Science*, 262:843–844. BAUM, RANDY M. (1992). Progress fitful on understanding AIDS; Developing therapies. *Chem. Eng. News*, 70:26–31.

BARR, PHILIP, et al. (1994). Apoptosis and its role in human disease. *Bio/Technology*, 12:487–494.

BAXENA, S., et al. (1985). Immunosuppression by human seminal plasma. *Immunol. Invest.*, 14:255–269.

BELSHE, R. B., et al. (1994). Neutralizing antibodies to HIV in seronegative volunteers immunized with recombinant gp120 from the MN strain of HIV. *JAMA*, 272:475–480.

BERKMAN, S. (1984). Infectious complications of blood transfusions. *Sem. Oncol.*, 11:68–75.

BLUMBERG, N., et al. (1985). A retrospective study of transfusions. *Br. Med. J.*, 290:1037–1039.

BOBKOV, ALEKSEI, et al. (1994). Molecular epidemiology of HIV in the former Soviet Union: analysis of ENV V3 sequences and their correlation with epidemiologic data. *AIDS*, 8:619–624.

BOLOGNESI, DANI P. (1989). Prospects for prevention of and early intervention against HIV. *JAMA*, 261:3007–3013.

BRODER, CHRISTOPHER, et al. (1994). CD26 antigen and HIV fusion? *Science*, 264:1156–1165.

BROWN, RAYMOND KEITH. (1987). AIDS: A perspective. *Am. Chem. Prod. Rev.*, Nov.:44–47.

BUTLER, DECLAN. (1983). Publication by press conference under five. *Nature*, 366:6.

CALLEBAUT, CHRISTIAN, et al. (1993). T cell activation antigen, CD26 as a cofactor for entry of HIV in CD4+ cells. *Science*, 262:2045–2050.

COHEN, JOEL. (1994). The HIV vaccine paradox. *Science*, 264:1072–1074.

COHEN, JON. (1993). Keystone's blunt message: "It's the virus stupid." *Science*, 260:292–293.

COHEN, JON. (1993). HIV cofactor comes in far more heavy fire. *Science*, 262:1971–1972.

CROWE, S.M., et al. (1991). Predictive value of CD4 lymphocyte numbers for the development of opportunistic infections and malignancies in HIV-infected persons. *AIDS*, 48:770–776.

EDGINGTON, STEPHEN M. (1993). HIV no longer latent, says NIAID's Fauci. *BioTechnology*, 11:16–17.

EMBRETSON, JANET, et al. (1993). Massive covert infection of helper T lymphocytes and macrophages by HIV during the incubation period of AIDS. *Nature*, 362:359–362.

FAUCI, ANTHONY. (1991). Researchers dispute HIV latency. *Medical Tribune*, 32:20.

FITZGERALD, LYNN. (1988). Exercise and the immune system. *Trends genet.*, 2:1–12.

FOSTER, R,. et al. (1985). Adverse effects of blood transfusions in lung cancer. *Cancer*, 55:11951–12202.

FOX, CECIL H., et al. (1991). Lymphoid germinal centers for reservoirs of HIV type I RNA. *J. Infect. Dis.*, 164:1051–1057.

GELDERBLOM, H.R., et al. (1985). Loss of envelope antigens of HTLV III/LAV, a factor in AIDS pathogenesis. *Lancet*, 2:1016–1017.

GHIARA, JAYANT, et al. (1994). Crystal structure of the principal neutralization site of HIV. *Science*, 264:82–85.

GROENINK, MARTIJIN, et al. (1993). Relation of phenotype evolution of HIV to envelope V2 configuration. *Science*, 260:1513–1516,

KINGSLEY, L., et al. (1987). Risk factors for seroconversion to HIV among male homosexuals. *Lancet*, 8529:345–348.

KION, TRACY, et al. (1991). Anti-HIV and Anti-Anti-MHC antibodies in alloimmune and autoimmune mice. *Science*, 253:1138–1140.

LAPIERRE, A., et al. (1992). Exercise and health maintenance in AIDS, In Galantino, M.L. (Ed.), *Clinical Assessment and Treatment in HIV: Rehabilitation of a Chronic Illness*, Chap. 7. Slack, Inc. Thorofare NJ.

LO, SHYH-CHING, et al. (1989). A novel virus-like infectious agent in patients with AIDS. *Am. J. Trop. Med. Hyg.*, 40:213.

LO, SHYH-CHING, et al. (1991). Enhancement of HIV-1 cytocidal effects in CD4+ lymphocytes by the AIDS-associated mycoplasma. *Science*, 251:1074–1076.

LUSSO, PAOLO, et al. (1993). Infection of natural killer cells by human herpesvirus 6. *Nature*, 362:458–461.

Mountain-Plains Regional HIV/AIDS Curriculum, 4th ed. (1992). Mountain-Plains Regional AIDS Office, University of Colorado Health Sciences Center, Denver, CO 80262.

PANTALEO, G., et al. (1993). HIV infection is active and progressive in lymphoid tissue during the clinically latent stage of disease. *Nature*, 362:355–358.

PENNISI, ELIZABETH. (1994). A room of their own. *Science News*, 145:335.

SCHMID, SANDRA, et al. (1994). Making class II presentable. *Nature,* 369:103–104.

SCHNITTMAN, STEVEN M., et al. (1989). The reservoir for HIV-1 in human peripheral blood is a T cell that maintains expression of CD4. *Science,* 245:305–308.

SINHA, ANIMESH, et al. (1990). Autoimmune diseases: the failure of self-tolerance. *Science,* 248:1380–1387.

SPRENT, JONATHAN, et al. (1994). Lymphocyte lifespan and memory. *Science,* 265:1395–1400.

TERSMETTE, MATTHIJS, et al. (1990). Interactions between HIV and the host immune system in the pathogenesis of AIDS. *AIDS,* 4:S57–S66.

THOMSON, BRIAN J., et al. (1991). Acquisition of the human adeno-associated virus type-2 rep gene by human herpesvirus type-6. *Nature,* 351:78–80.

TULP, ABRAHAM, et al. (1994). Isolation and characterization of the intracellular MHC class II compartment. *Nature,* 369:120–126.

WITKIN, S., and SONNABEND, J. (1983). Immune responses to spermatozoa in homosexual men. *Fertil. Steril.,* 39:337–341.

CHAPTER 5

Opportunistic Infections and Cancers Associated with HIV Disease/AIDS

Chapter Concepts

- Suppression of the immune system allows harmless agents to become harmful opportunistic infections (OIs).
- OIs in AIDS patients are caused by viruses, bacteria, fungi, and protozoa.
- Cancer in AIDS patients is not caused by OIs.
- There are two types of Kaposi's sarcoma (KS): classic and AIDS-associated.
- KS is rarely found in hemophiliacs, intravenous drug users, and women with AIDS.

Humans evolved in the presence of a wide range of viruses, bacteria, parasites and fungi that do not cause disease in people with an intact immune system. But these organisms can cause a disease in someone with a weakened immune system, such as an individual with HIV disease. The infections they cause are known as **opportunistic infections**. Thus, opportunistic infections (OIs) occur after a disease-causing virus or microorganism, normally held in check by a functioning immune system, gets the chance to multiply and invade host tissue because the immune system has been compromised. For most of medical history, OIs were rare and almost always appeared in patients whose immunity was impaired by cancer or genetic disease.

With improved medical technology, a steadily growing number of patients are severely immunosuppressed because of medications and radiation used in bone marrow or organ transplantation and cancer chemotherapy. HIV disease also suppresses the immune system. And perhaps as a corollary to their increased prevalence, or because of heightened physician awareness, OIs seem to be occurring more frequently in the elderly, who may be rendered vulnerable by age-related declines in immunity. New OIs are now being diagnosed because the pool of people who can get them is so much larger, and, in addition, new techniques for identifying the causative organisms have been developed. However, most of the infections considered opportunistic are not reportable, which precludes any clear-cut count of their growing numbers.

Although OIs are still not commonplace, they are no longer considered rare—they occur in tens of thousands of patients each year. But despite this increase, physicians and their patients have reasons to be optimistic about their ability to contain these infections. The reasons are: (1) in a massive federal effort, driven by the HIV/AIDS epidemic, researchers are finding drugs that can prevent or treat many of the OIs; (2) various therapies have shown promise for warding off OIs by boosting patients' immune systems; and (3) drug studies suggest that organ transplant patients who are maintained on the experimental immunosuppressive drug FK-506 (Fujisawa) develop many fewer OIs than those treated with more conventional regimens.

PROPHYLAXIS AGAINST OPPORTUNISTIC INFECTIONS

Drug prophylaxis against OIs has become a cornerstone of treatment for AIDS patients. For example, the prevalence of *Pneumocystis carinii* pneumonia (PCP) dropped from about 80% in 1987 to about 50% by mid-1992 (Figure 5-1). The downside to OI prophylaxis is that it is difficult to find drugs that work without harmful side effects. In addition, viruses and organisms that cause OIs become resistant to the drugs over time. This is one of the primary reasons researchers are looking for ways in which to boost an immunosuppressed patient's immune system (Zoler, 1991).

OPPORTUNISTIC INFECTIONS IN HIV-INFECTED PEOPLE

AIDS is a devastating human tragedy. It appears to be killing everyone who demonstrates the symptoms. One well-known American surgeon said, "I would rather die of any form of cancer rather than die of AIDS." This statement was not made because of the social stigma attached to AIDS, or because it is a lethal condition. It was made in recognition of the slow, demoralizing, debilitating, painful, disfiguring, helpless, and unending struggle to stay alive.

Because of a suppressed and weakened immune system, viruses, bacteria, fungi, and protozoa that commonly and harmlessly inhabit the body become pathogenic (Figure 5-2). In addition, organisms and viruses from old infections that have lingered in the body reactivate. The suppression of the immune system presents an *opportunity* for the harmless to become harmful. This is called **opportunistic infection**. About 88% of deaths related to HIV infection and AIDS are caused by OIs, compared with 7% due to cancer and 5% due to other causes.

What makes HIV disease particularly horrible is that it leaves patients open to an endless series of infections that would not occur in people with healthy immune responses. *Pneumocystis carinii* pneumonia, toxoplasmosis, Kaposi's sarcoma, candidiasis, cytomegalovirus retinitis, cryptococcal meningitis, mycobacterium avium complex, herpes simplex, and herpes zoster are infections that sicken and disfigure, and some eventually kill most people with AIDS.

AIDS patients rarely have just one infection (Table 5-1). The mix of OIs may depend on life style and where the HIV/AIDS patient lives or has lived. Thus a knowledge of the person's origins and travels may be diagnostically helpful. (Note: a number of the symptoms listed in the CDC definition of HIV/AIDS can be found associated with certain of the OIs presented.)

Fungal Diseases

In general, healthy people have a high degree of innate resistance to fungi. But a different situation prevails with opportunistic fungal infections, which often present themselves as acute, life-threatening diseases in a compromised host (Medoff et al., 1991).

Because treatment seldom results in the eradication of fungal infections in AIDS patients, there is a high probability of recurrence after treatment (DeWit et al., 1991).

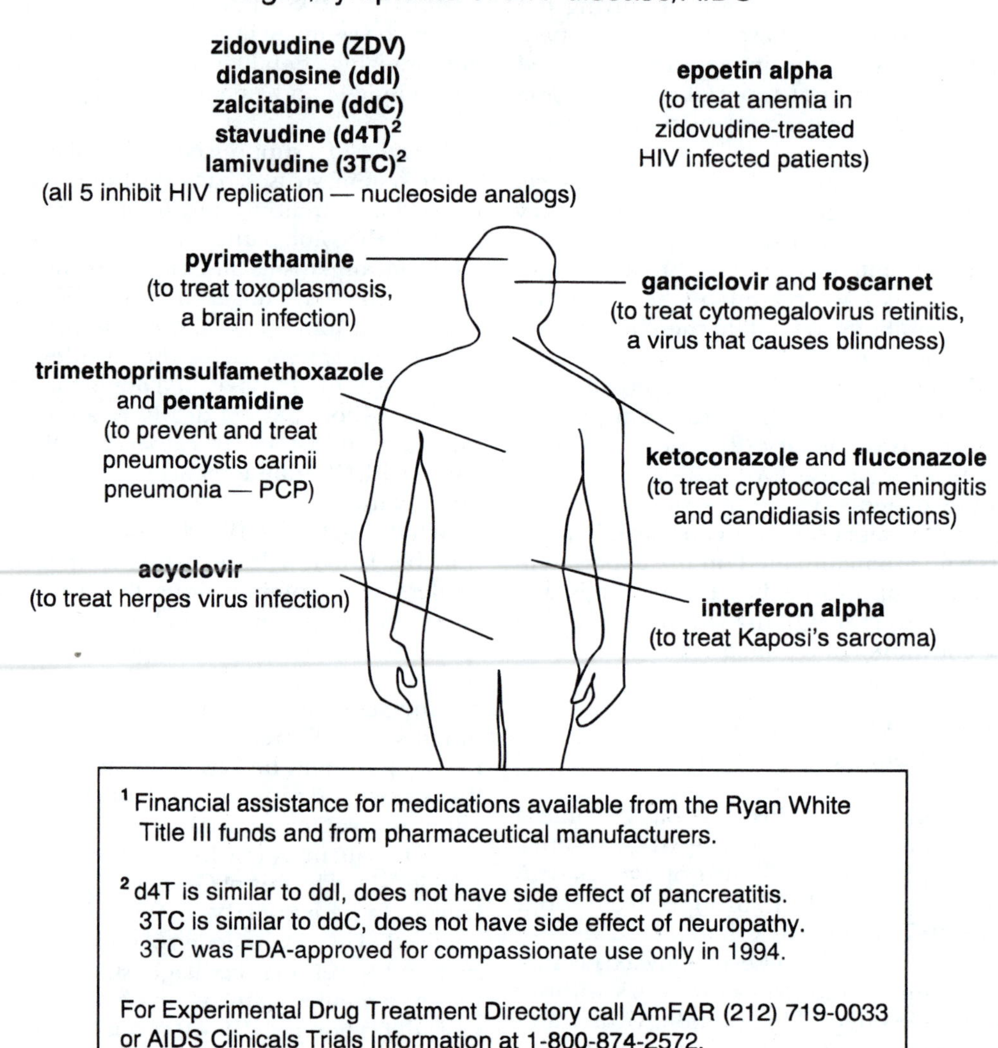

FIGURE 5-1 The More Common Drug Therapies for Treating HIV Disease, Some Opportunistic Diseases, and AIDS.

Fungal diseases are among the more devastating of the OIs and are most often regional in association. AIDS patients from the Ohio River basin, the Midwest, or Puerto Rico have a higher than normal risk of histoplasmosis *(his-to-plaz-mo-sis)* infection. In the Southwest, there is increased risk for coccidioidomycosis *(kok-sid-e-o-do-mi-ko-sis)*. In the southern Gulf states, the risk is for blastomycosis. Other important OI fungi such as *Pneumocystis carinii (nu-mo-sis-tis car-in-e-i), Candida albicans (kan-di-dah al-be-cans)*, and *Cryptococcus neoformans (krip-to-kok-us knee-o-for-mans)* are found everywhere in equal numbers. Because of their importance as OIs in AIDS patients, a brief description of histoplasmosis, candidiasis, *Pneumocystis carinii* pneumonia (PCP), and cryptococcosis are presented (Table 5-1).

TABLE 5-1 Some Common Opportunistic Diseases Associated with HIV Infection and Possible Therapy

Organism/Virus	Clinical Manifestation	Possible Treatments
Protozoa		
Cryptosporidium muris	Gastroenteritis (inflammation of stomach-intestine membranes)	Investigational only
Isospora belli	Gastroenteritis	Trimethoprim-sulfamethoxazole (Bactrim)
Toxoplasma gondii	Encephalitis (brain abscess), retinitis, disseminated	Pyrimethamine and leucovorin, plus sulfadiazine, or Clindamycin, Bactrim
Fungi		
Candida sp.	Stomatitis (thrush), proctitis, vaginitis, esophagitis	Nystatin, clotrimazole, ketoconazole
Coccidioides immitis	Meningitis, dissemination	Amphotericin B, fluconazole, ketoconazole
Cryptococcus neoformans	Meningitis (membrane inflammation of spinal cord and brain), pneumonia, encephalitis, dissemination (widespread)	Amphotericin B, fluconazole, itraconazole
Histoplasma capsulatum	Pneumonia, dissemination	Amphotericin B, fluconazole, itraconazole
Pneumocystis carinii	Pneumonia	Trimethoprim-sulfamethoxazole (Bactrim, Septra), Pentamidine, Dapsone
Bacteria		
Mycobacterium avium complex (MAC)	Dissemination, pneumonia, diarrhea, weight loss, lymphadenopathy, severe gastrointestinal disease	Rifampin + ethambutol + clofazimine + ciprofloxacin +/- amikacin; clarithromycin & azithromycin (both investigational)
Mycobacterium tuberculosis (TB)	Pneumonia (tuberculosis), meningitis, dissemination	Isoniazid (INH) + rifampin + ethambutol +/- pyrazinamide
Viruses		
Cytomegalovirus (CMV)	Fever, hepatitis, encephalitis, retinitis, pneumonia, colitis, esophagitis	Ganciclovir, Foscarnet
Epstein-Barr	Oral hairy leukoplakia, B cell lymphoma	Acyclovir
Herpes simplex	Mucocutaneous (mouth, genital, rectal) blisters and/or ulcers, pneumonia, esophagitis, encephalitis	Acyclovir
Papovavirus J-C	Progressive multifocal leukoencephalopathy	none
Varicella-zoster	Dermatomal skin lesions (shingles), encephalitis	Acyclovir, Foscarnet
Cancers		
Kaposi's sarcoma	Disseminated mucocutaneous lesions often involving skin, lymph nodes, visceral organs (especially lungs & GI tract)	Local injection, surgical excision or radiation to small, localized lesions; Chemotherapy with vincristine & Bleomycin
Primary lymphoma of the brain	Headache, palsies, seizures, hemiparesis, mental status, or personality changes	Radiation and/or chemotherapy
Systemic lymphomas	Fever, night sweats, weight loss, enlarged lymph nodes	Chemotherapy

Patients with compromised immune systems are at increased risk for all known cancers and infections (including bacterial, viral, and parasitic). Most infectious diseases in HIV-infected patients are the result of proliferation of organisms already present in the patient's body. Most of these opportunistic infections are not contagious to others. The notable exception to this is tuberculosis.

(**Disclaimer**: This table was developed to provide general information only. It is not meant to be diagnostic nor to direct treatment.)

(Adapted from Mountain-Plains Regional Education and Training Center *HIV/AIDS Curriculum*, 4th Ed., 1992)

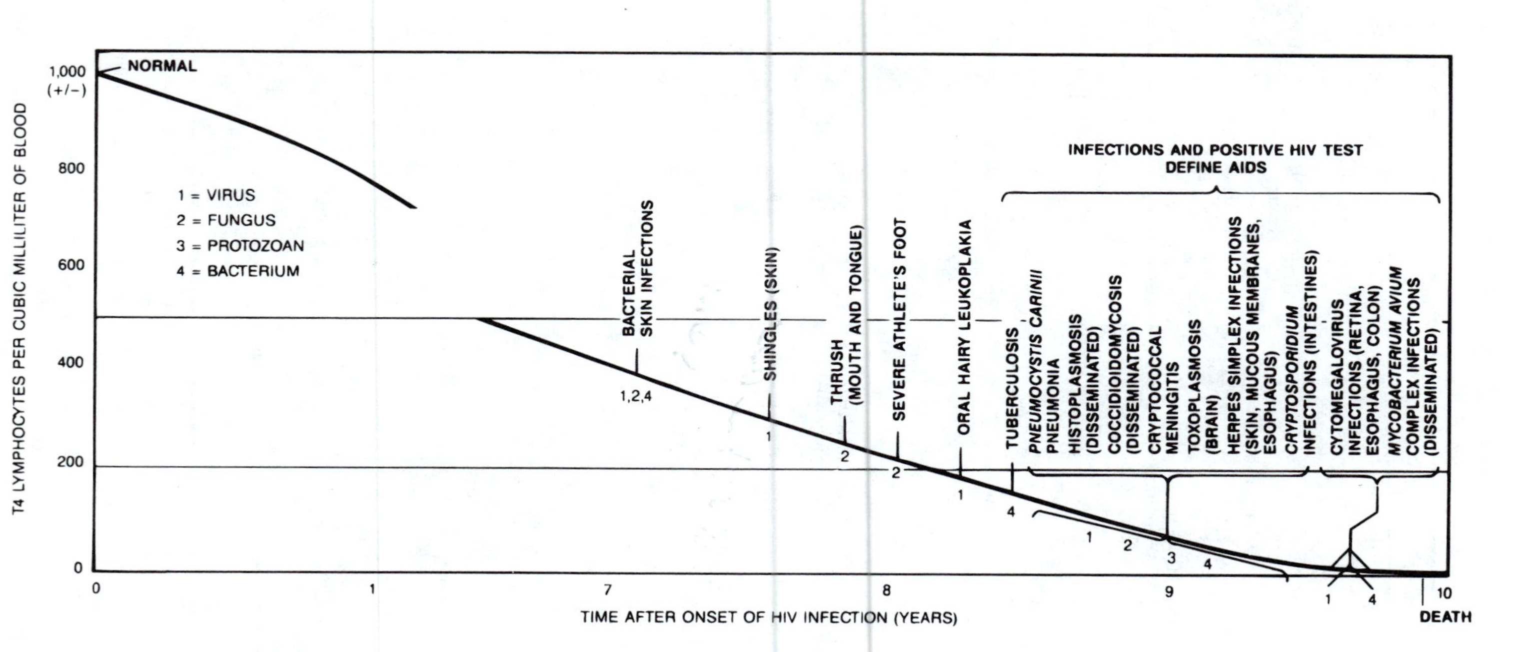

FIGURE 5-2 General Progression of Opportunistic Infections after HIV Infection. Normal T4 cell count in adolescent/adults is, on average, about 1,000/μL of blood. There is a relationship between the drop in T4 lymphocytes and the onset of opportunistic infections (OIs). The first sign of an OI begins under 500 T4 cells/μL. As the T4 cell count continues to drop, the chance of OI infection increases. Note the variety of OIs found in AIDS patients with 200 or less T4 cells/μL.

BOX 5.1

LIFE GOES ON!

by Wendi Alexis Modeste

What this epidemic has cost me is the complete faith I had in the medical profession. I was raised believing that doctors were second only to priests and God. They were never to be questioned. Whatever the doctor said was law. If a person didn't get well after seeing the doctor, somehow they (the patient) had done something wrong. This was pretty much standard thinking for middle-class African-Americans. For a variety of reasons (mainly no self-esteem) I became a drug addict, prostitute, convict, battered, homeless woman, in that order! With the exception of emergency room admissions (which are a joke and a whole `nother story) I had no access to health care.

Now, as a PWA (person with AIDS) fortunately/unfortunately on SSI, Medicaid pays for my nine different AIDS medications, clinic visits, treatment, tests, etc. When I received the "exciting news" that I was eligible for "all" Medicaid benefits, I was still under the impression doctors were those super-intelligent, gifted, Christian, saint-like people. Girlfriend, I am here to tell you, AIDS has totally shot that Marcus Welby theory straight to hell!

Early in my diagnosis, I went to my physician because my tongue was almost completely covered with what looked like cottage cheese. There was also a horrible pink lesion dead center. The first time I showed it to my doctor he said, "Ugh," and made a face. He told me to wait a month. If nothing changed or got worse when I returned he'd have someone look at it. Being ignorant about the disease at that time, and still blindly believing in the medical profession, I waited a month, then returned. Again I showed the doctor my tongue. He asked me if I wanted him to write me a prescription for codeine and Valium. I totally freaked! By this time, I'd done some reading and realized I probably had thrush and some sort of herpes. This physician was aware of my serostatus. He also knew that I was a person with a 20-year history of drug abuse. I'd been in recovery less than a year and this jerk wanted to prescribe for me two of the most addictive and abused prescription drugs. I'd never mentioned being in pain or that I was experiencing any type of anxiety. I contacted the Executive Director of this health facility and asked to have a different doctor assigned to me. In an attempt to make me feel guilty about requesting a change, I was told about the problems doctors have in getting Medicaid reimbursement. I was neither intimidated nor impressed. A new doctor was assigned. My new physician was very nice. After *I* told *him* what I thought my diagnosis was, he prescribed the appropriate medications. He was not trained in AIDS/HIV. I could have dealt with his ignorance because I knew he was trying. His nurse, however, was a different story. Every time she came to do my vitals she'd say the same thing: "I always get nervous when taking the temperature of you guys." She'd then force a little chuckle and go on to say, "Oh, well, I figure we all have to die of something." (I assume this was to show me what a courageous Florence Nightingale she was.)

Let me tell you, when you are burning up with a 103 degree temp. and your bowels haven't stopped running for a week, causing your butt to feel like it's on fire, it's real hard to be the patient, understanding AIDS educator. I really get crazy when the person I'm forced to educate is someone whose been privileged to more information than myself.

But life goes on!

One day I had a toothache. I go to the dentist. After waiting half the day, I'm brought into the treatment room for an X-ray. At first I thought the dental assistant had made a mistake. Surely this room had been prepared for a paint job. Everything was draped in white towels. The entire dental unit, including where my head, arms and feet went, was completely covered. The seat of the unit was securely wrapped up, as was the metal extension arm that holds the overhead dental lamp. All surfaces of the walls were also draped. When I asked the reason for this "painter preparation," I was informed it was done because I have AIDS, and they had to protect their other patients from coming into contact with my contaminated blood. Needless to say, I saw red! I knew I had to protect myself. I mean, what kind of dentistry were they practicing if they were concerned about my blood splattering that far and wide? What was even more frightening was that they'd done all this unnecessary draping and I was only having an X-ray. I filed a complaint with the Human Rights Dept.

I became a patient at the AIDS Care Center in Syracuse. My physician, a woman (need I say more?), is a caring person and well-educated about AIDS/HIV. My nurse/social worker is excellent, but as all of us living with AIDS know, shit happens. One day I awaken with enough yeast in my body to make all the baked goods in Central New York rise. My doctor isn't in. I wait a couple of days but can no longer stand the discomfort. I beg to see a doctor in the AIDS Care Unit. I'm assigned the doctor who sees the HIV-infected prisoners. (My heart and soul truly go out to those guys.) First he talks with me over the phone to find out if I can possibly wait another week when my doctor is due to return. I tell him my tongue is unrecognizable, the yeast in my esophagus is burning like a heart attack, and the Roto-Rooter service couldn't satisfy the itch caused by the yeast in my vagina. HELL NO, I can't wait another week! I go in to see him. I show him my tongue. I can't believe it, but like the first doctor, he uses that medical term, "Ugh," then says, "That does look nasty." At this point I'm ready to French kiss this idiot. But it gets worse. He won't touch me, let alone examine anything. He asks me what I think will work. I feel too badly to curse, so I tell him Mycelex, Myastatin suspension, Monistat 7. He writes the prescriptions and for good measure increases my acyclovir. For this he gets paid? He did nothing!

I'm now as educated as a lay person can be about HIV disease/AIDS. In addition to my doctor at the AIDS Care Center, I have a private primary care physician. Sometimes it's easier to get in to see this doctor. I call his office one day because there is swelling and burning on the sides of my tongue. I cannot eat. My regular doctor isn't in, but one of his associates assures me if I come in to the office he'll see me right away and give me something to ease the pain so I can at least eat. As a fat person who proudly admits a genuine fondness for food, I can tell you not being able to eat registers serious panic in my soul. Nothing stops me from eating. I was probably the only overweight homeless dope addict living on the streets of NYC. Being scared is putting it mildly. I scrape up the carfare and go to the office. After waiting an unreasonably long time, Doogie Howser's twin comes in to see me and announces he's Dr. Jones, whom I spoke to on the phone. OK, I know not to judge a book by its cover. I mean, Doogie is pretty good on TV. Dr. Jones looks at my tongue and proceeds to ask a zillion questions, all of which are answered in my chart. Finally he says he's never seen an HIV-infected person or a person with AIDS, and frankly he doesn't know what to do. He then suggests I eat popsicles for a few days because the cold will soothe the pain and the sugar should help give me energy. I kid you not, this actually happened. This jerk prescribed me popsicles. I truly wished I could transmit the virus by biting at this point. He used me so he could write in his journal or resume (or somewhere) that he'd treated a person with AIDS. He could also charge Medicaid for nothing.

But this type of quackery must stop.

The last gripe I'm going to list is this patient statement I hear all the time when I get an unexplained fever or infection and no one can determine its origin. I'm told, "there hasn't been enough studies done on the paths this disease takes in women. Even less has been done on the effects of different AIDS medications on people of color." This is said to me as if it's my fault they don't know. This disease has been documented for ten years in both men and women. I know African-Americans were dying of AIDS long before the gay white community mobilized and, thank God, refused to lay down and die quietly. There is no excuse for the fact that there's no studies done on these populations.

I am thankful to Dr. Sallie Klemmens and nurse/clinician/social worker Judith Swartout at University Hospital's designated AIDS Care Center here in Syracuse. I am thankful for Dr. Barbara J. Justice who with God's help kept me alive when I lived on the streets of NYC. They are all examples of what the medical profession should be about. Dr. Justice made me feel that I counted and should be assertive about my health care. Though no longer my surgeon, she continues to be a source of inspiration and a fountain of information for me. These three are gems in a field I think is greatly overrated, overpaid, and run by capitalist male chauvinist pigs.

Though medical people wear white, that absence of color symbolizing purity and goodness, I beg you all, "Don't believe the hype!" We need a national health care system for everyone. As PWAs we must be assertive about our health care. Good health care is a right not a privilege.

As a child I cried when I learned there was no Santa Claus. When my illusion about the medical profession was shattered I got angry. I decided to fight with the only ammunition I had, education! Knowledge gives one power. A close friend of mine told me I shouldn't submit this article because I might offend some members of the medical profession. He also felt because I'm on Medicaid I'm not supposed to complain, I should be grateful. To his comments I respond, raised with two college-educated parents, never wanting or needing anything, I wasn't supposed to be a drug addict. Unfortunately I was. After 20 years of addiction, I wasn't supposed to be able to stop. I've been in recovery almost two years now. I'm not supposed to be living with AIDS, but with God's help I'm happy and living large (as the kids say now).

The best things I do have always been what I'm not supposed to do!

Power to all PWAs!

Wendi Alexis Modeste a PWA who was diagnosed in 1990, died August 25, 1994.

Source: MODESTE, W.A., August 1991, Issue 68, *PWA Coalition Newsline.* Reprinted with permission.

Histoplasmosis (Histoplasma capsulatum)— Spores are inhaled and germinate in or on the body (Figure 5-3). Signs of histoplasmosis include prolonged influenza-like symptoms, shortness of breath, and possible complaints of night sweats and shaking chills. In AIDS patients there is a multisystem involvement: the liver, central nervous system, lymph nodes, and gastrointestinal tract are affected, while mucosal ulcers and enlarged spleen may also occur. Histoplasmosis in an HIV-positive person is considered diagnostic of AIDS. In about two-thirds of AIDS patients with histoplasmosis, it is the initial OI. Over 90% of cases have occurred in patients with T4 cell counts below 100/µL (Wheat, 1992).

FIGURE 5-3 Anal Histoplasmosis. Histoplasmosis is caused by *Histoplasmosis capsulatum* and causes infection in immunocompromised patients. (*Courtesy CDC, Atlanta*)

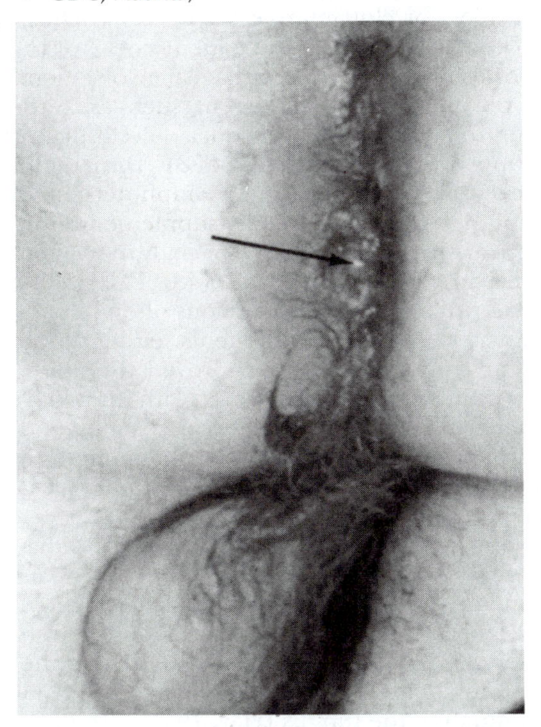

In non-HIV-infected patients, amphotericin B is almost always successful in treating histoplasmosis (Table 5-1). Only 50% to 80% of AIDS patients respond, however, and relapse is common during maintenance therapy. Nonetheless, amphotericin B followed by weekly maintenance therapy remains the recommended strategy. Earlier reports suggested ketoconazole as a potential alternative for initial or maintenance therapy, but it had an even higher failure rate than amphotericin B and is no longer recommended in HIV-infected patients.

Itraconazole (Sporanox) has recently been approved for treating histoplasmosis and some now consider it the drug of choice for HIV-related histoplasmosis (Daar et al., 1993).

Candidiasis (Candida albicans)— This fungus is usually associated with yeast infections of the vagina. It is a fungus quite common to the body and in particular inhabits the alimentary tract. It is normally kept in check by the presence of bacteria that live on the linings of the alimentary tract. However, in immunocompromised patients, especially those who have received broad spectrum antibiotics, candida multiplies rapidly. Because of its location in the upper reaches of the alimentary tract, if unchecked, it may cause mucocutaneous candidiasis or thrush, an overgrowth of

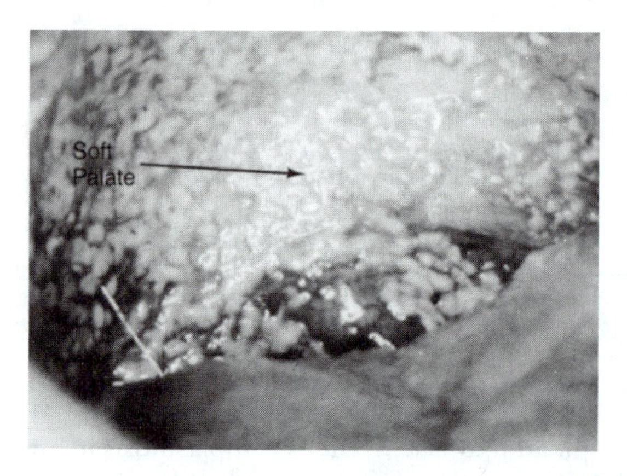

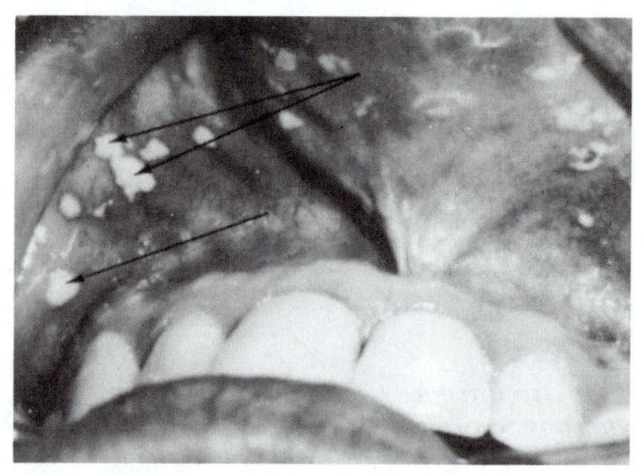

FIGURE 5-4 Thrush. **A,** An overgrowth of *Candida albicans* on the soft palate in the oral cavity of an AIDS patient. **B,** Creamy patches of candida that can be scraped off leaving a red and sometimes bleeding mucosa. (**A,** *Courtesy CDC, Atlanta;* **B,** *Courtesy of Drs. M. Schiodt, D. Greenspan, J.S. Greenspan, Oral AIDS Center, University of California, San Francisco, and* Journal of Respiratory Diseases, *1989, 10:91-109)*

candida in the esophagus and in the oral cavity (Figure 5-4A & B). Mucosal candidiasis was associated with AIDS patients from the very beginning of the AIDS pandemic (Powderly et al., 1992). In women, overgrowths of candidiasis also occur in the vaginal area.

Gynecological conditions in women with HIV disease have been found to be more aggressive and to occur with a greater frequency than in noninfected women. Vaginal candidiasis (VC) is generally caused by *C. albicans.* VC is seen at all stages of HIV disease, with increasing frequency in conjunction with PCP and genital herpes in patients with <200 T4 cells per µL. It is sometimes associated with the use of birth control pills, chemotherapeutic regimens, corticosteroids, and immune suppression related to pregnancy. Common symptoms include a thick, whitish discharge; severe itching; localized, sometimes severe pain; and infrequently, the development of lesions. Vaginal manifestations of the disease are thought to precede esophageal and/or oral thrush. HIV-related vaginal candidiasis may be characterized by resistance to standard therapy. Candida infections should be monitored for frequency and response to antifungal treatments (Table 5-1). If candidiasis is limited to the mouth and oropharynx and the patient is not debilitated, treatment with topical nystatin (Mycostatin Pastilles) or clotrimazole (Mycelex Troches) is often sufficient. If the patient does not respond adequately, or esophageal involvement is possible, a systemic agent such as ketoconazole (Nizoral) or fluconazole (Diflucan) is appropriate (Daar et al., 1993). Difficult to treat cases may require IV amphotericin B (Fungizone). Acidopholis supplementation appears to be beneficial, especially in women receiving PCP prophylaxis with TMP/SMX (Bactrim or Dapsone). Persons often self-administer alternative treatments, either alone or in conjunction with approved therapies. These include changes in diet, with the avoidance of foods containing yeast, sugar, and dairy products. Vitamin C supplementation and herbal products are often used (Willoughby, 1989).

Some people with oropharyngeal candidiasis may experience a sore mouth. This is particularly painful when acidic foods and juices are taken. In addition, the taste of food is often altered. Treatment is aimed at relieving the symptoms, as therapy is rarely successful at eliminating the fungus (Hay, 1991).

Impaired cell-mediated immunity, as occurs in people with HIV disease, may allow for a disseminated infection (distributed to other areas of the body). Oral or **esophageal candidiasis** causes thick white patches on the mucosal surface and may be the first manifestation of AIDS. Because other diseases can cause similar symptoms, candidiasis by itself is not sufficient for a diagnosis of AIDS.

***Pneumocystis carinii*—** This fungus, until recent reclassification, was considered a protozoan (Edman et al., 1988). The life cycle and reproductive characteristics of *P. carinii* are not completely understood because the organism is difficult to culture for laboratory study. However, the molecular biology and molecular taxonomy are now being rapidly constructed (Walzer, 1993). Virtually everyone in the United States by age 30 to 40 has been exposed to *P. carinii.* It lies dormant in the lungs, held in check by the immune system. Prior to the AIDS epidemic, *P. carinii* pneumonia was seen in children and adults who had leukemia or Hodgkin's disease and were receiving chemotherapy. In the AIDS patient, the onset of *P. carinii* pneumonia is insidious—patients may notice some shortness of breath and they cannot run as far. It causes extensive damage within the alveoli of the lung.

FIGURE 5-5 **A,** A concentration of *Pneumocystis carinii* cysts. (See text for details.) **B,** Scanning electron microscope image of *P. carinii* attached to lung tissue. Note the tubular extensions through which it extracts nutrients from host lung tissue. (*Courtesy of Linda L. Pifer, St. Jude Children's Research Hospital, Memphis and* Pediatric Research, *1977, 11:305-306*)

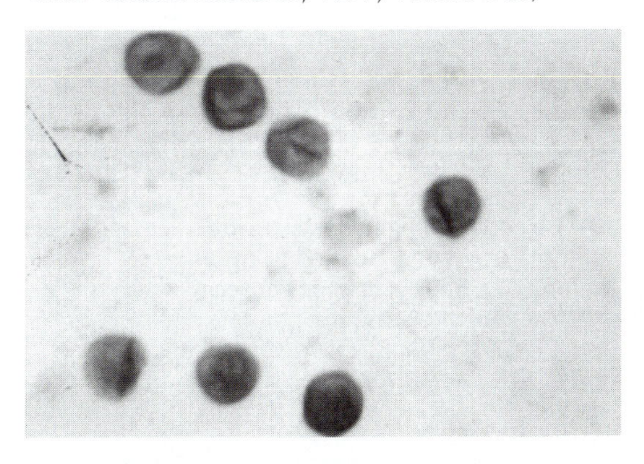

A

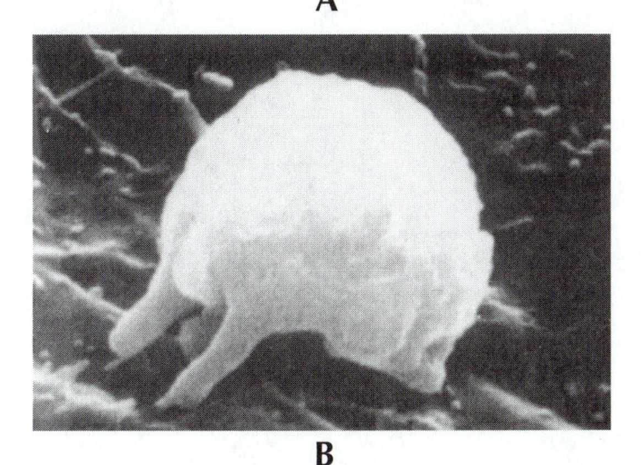

B

The *P. carinii* fungus develops from a small unicellular trophozoite into a cyst containing eight sporozoites (Figure 5-5A). These sporozoites are disseminated throughout the body, but they show a greater affinity for the lungs, where they multiply in the spaces between the lung sacs and cause pneumonia (Figure 5-5B). Prior to 1981, fewer than 100 cases of *P. carinii* infection were reported annually in the United States; yet 80% of AIDS patients develop *P. carinii* pneumonia at some time during their illness. This is one of the few AIDS-related conditions for which there is a choice of relatively effective drugs. The first of these to be made available was the intravenous and aerosolized versions of pentamidine. There are frequent recurrences of this infection. With treatment, about 7% of first PCP episodes result in death (Montgomery, 1992). PCP accounts for a diagnosis of AIDS in over 65% of AIDS cases (Ernst, 1990). The triad of symptoms that almost always indicates the onset of PCP during HIV disease is fever, dry cough, and shortness of breath (Grossman et al., 1989). *P. carinii* pneumonia is unlikely to develop in people with HIV disease unless their T4 cell count drops below 200 (Phair et al., 1990).

The antifolate (blocking action to folic acid) drugs pentamidine and trimethoprim/sulfamethoxazole are currently treatments of choice for *P. carinii* pneumonia (Zackrison et al., 1991).

Cryptococcosis (Cryptococcus neoformans)— Since its discovery in 1894, *C. neoformans* has been recognized as a major cause of deep-seated fungal infection in the human host. The infection can affect many sites, including skin, lung, kidney, prostate, and bone. However, symptomatic disease most often represents infection of the central nervous system. Cryptococcal meningitis is the most common form of fungal meningitis in the United States (Ennis et al., 1993). This fungus is shed in pigeon feces, the spores of which enter the lung. If the lung does not eliminate it, it gets into the bloodstream, travels to the brain, and can cause cryptococcal meningitis.

In a healthy person, *C. neoformans* may cause pulmonary problems or meningeal infection (infection of the membranes that envelop the brain and spinal cord). It is more commonly seen in people with immunosuppression, especially in HIV/AIDS cases. *C. neoformans* is a fatal OI that occurs in about 13% of AIDS patients (Brooke et al., 1990). It is acquired through the respiratory tract and most commonly causes cryptococcal meningitis. Disseminated *C. neoformans* (Figure 5-6A) infection may involve bone marrow, the central nervous system (CNS), and the lungs, causing cryptococcal pneumonia. In AIDS patients, *C. neoformans* also causes infection of the skin (Figure 5-6B), lymph nodes, and kidneys. *Cryptococcus* cannot be cured and it does recur. What drugs should be used is a subject of controversy. Eric Darr and colleagues (1993) report that fluconazole and itraconazole are effective in treating cryptococcal meningitis (Table 5-1).

Viral Diseases

Because of a depleted T4 cellular component of the immune system, AIDS patients are at particularly high risk for the herpes family of viral infections: cytomegalovirus, herpes simplex virus types 1 and 2, varicella-zoster virus, and Epstein-Barr virus.

Cytomegalovirus (CMV)— This virus is a member of the human herpesvirus group of viruses. CMV is the consummate parasite. It

FIGURE 5-6 *Cryptococcus neoformans.* **A,** Large, budding, and encapsulated *C. neoformans* shows white against an India ink stain. Isolated from the cerebral spinal fluid of a patient with meningitis. **B,** Skin lesions caused by *C. neoformans* may be single or multiple. The "ulcer" is usually painless but is an early sign of infection. (**A,** *Courtesy CDC, Atlanta.* **B,** *Courtesy of Ronald P. Rappini, University of Texas Medical School and reprinted with permission from* Cutis, *1988, Vol. 42:125-128)*

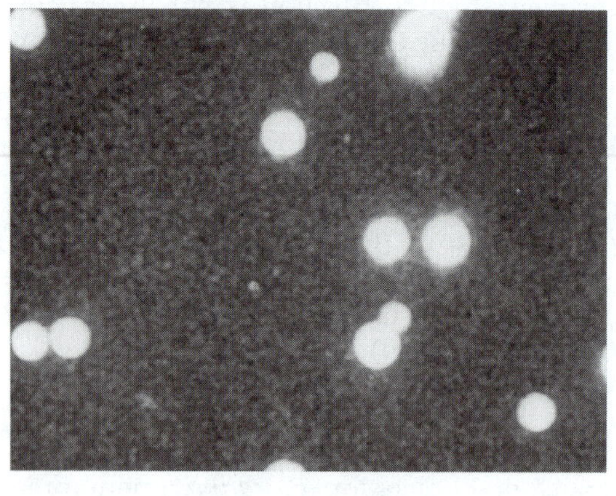

A

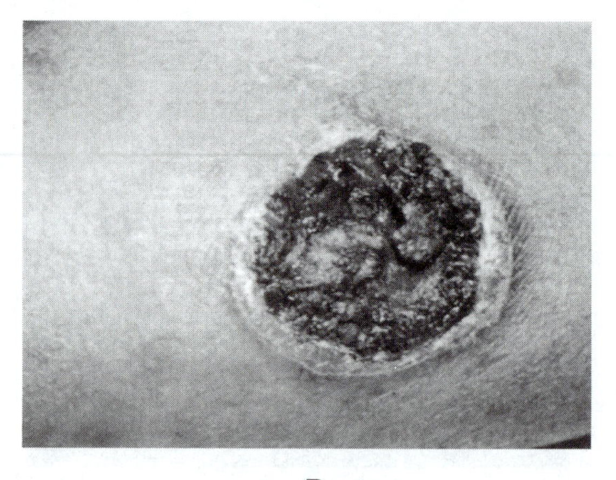

B

BOX 5.2

A PHYSICIAN'S AGONIZING DILEMMA

Opportunistic infections are the primary threat to patients with AIDS; they are the main causes of illness and death. The cruel irony is that although there are 26 or more FDA approved drugs to treat these infections, most cannot be used in patients receiving zidovudine (ZDV) *because the combination drug therapy is devastatingly toxic to bone marrow.*

EXAMPLE:

Cytomegalovirus (CMV) Retinitis

CMV retinitis is one of the *worst* of the opportunistic infections and it develops in 90% of AIDS patients (Gottlieb et al., 1987). Both the patient who contracts CMV retinitis and the treating physician confront an almost impossible dilemma: whether to continue the zidovudine and risk blindness or to treat the retinitis and risk death from another infection. A physician recently said, "In my experience, I have never yet been able to combine zidovudine with the experimental drug ganciclovir (DHPG), which is the only recognized treatment for CMV retinitis, because the combination destroys the bone marrow. I therefore face the virtually impossible task of asking a 25-year-old person: 'Which of these options do you prefer: to take zidovudine and keep on living but go blind, or to preserve your sight by having retinitis treatment but risk dying?' That is a truly terrible question to ask of any patient, especially a young one." He continued, "Recently, I treated just such a young patient. He had been taking zidovudine for AIDS when he contracted CMV retinitis. When I presented him with this agonizing choice, he told me, 'I definitely don't want to go blind. I want to be treated for this retinitis.' So he stopped taking zidovudine and was started on DHPG treatment. He started to have seizures, which were a consequence of the toxoplasmosis brain abscess that eventually ended his life. Just before he died, he told me that the worst decision he ever made was to stop taking zidovudine. 'I should have stayed on it,' he said, 'and gone blind.'" (Robert J. Awe, M.D., 1988)

Cryptococcal Meningitis

The situation for AIDS patients with cryptococcal meningitis is similarly depressing. Because of the severe bone marrow toxicity, it is virtually impossible to use amphotericin B, the effective treatment for this meningitis, at the same time as zidovudine. Besides, the use of amphotericin B has its own side effects as can be noted from this excerpt from Paul Monette's *Borrowed Time: An AIDS Memoir:*

> Amphotericin B is administered with Benadryl in order to avoid convulsions, the most serious possible side effect. It was about nine or ten when they started the drug in his veins, and I sat by the bed as nurses streamed in and out. A half hour into the slow drip, the nurse monitoring the IV walked out, saying she'd be right back, and a couple of minutes later Roger began to shake. I gripped him by the shoulders as he was jolted by what felt like waves of electric shock, staring at me horror-struck. Though Cope [the physician] would tell me later, trying to ease the torture of my memory, that "mentation" [mental activity] is all blurred during convulsions, I saw that Roger knew the horror. (Page 336)
>
> When the nurse returned she looked at him in dismay: "How long has this been going on?" Then she ordered an emergency shot of morphine to counteract the horror. When at last he fell into a deep sleep they all told me to go home, saying they would try another dose of the ampho in a few hours. I was so ragged I could barely walk. So I left him there with no way of knowing how near it was [Roger's death], or maybe not brave enough to know.

Whichever option is chosen, the patient is bound to suffer, and perhaps die, either of cryptococcal meningitis or of some other infection.

infects most people asymptomatically. When illness does occur, it is mild and nonspecific. There have been no epidemics to call attention to the virus. Yet CMV is now considered the most common infectious cause of mental retardation and congenital deafness in the United States.

A latent state follows initial infection, with CMV probably located in the white blood cells and involving many organs and organ systems. Later it is reactivated, usually by some form of immunosuppression such as organ or bone marrow transplantation, cancer chemotherapy, or HIV disease (Jacobson et al., 1992).

The virus is very labile and survives only a few hours outside a human host. It can be found in saliva, tears, blood, stool, cervical secretions, and in especially high levels in urine and semen. Transmission occurs primarily by intimate or close contact with infected secretions. The incidence of CMV infection varies from between 30% and 80% depending on the geographical community tested. However, over 90% of homosexual males have tested positive for CMV (Jacobson et al., 1988). CMV causes the more important viral infections in AIDS patients (Figure 5-7). This virus causes a broad spectrum of diseases in HIV-infected people, ranging from mild or severe gastrointestinal problems to infections of the brain, the liver (hepatitis), and the onset of fulminant (sudden and severe) pneumonia. Gastrointestinal infection may result in severe ulceration of the esophagus, stomach, small intestines, and colon. CMV pneumonia occurs in 10% to 20% of AIDS patients and can be lethal because therapy is unsuccessful.

FIGURE 5-7 Cytomegalovirus. This is an electron micrograph magnified 49,200 times. (*Courtesy CDC, Atlanta*)

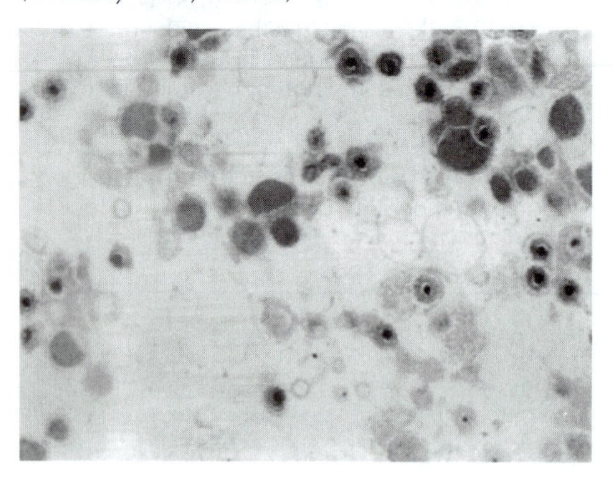

CMV infection of AIDS patients usually results in prolonged fever, anemia (too few red blood cells), leukopenia (too few white blood cells), and abnormal liver function. CMV also causes severe diarrhea and HIV-associated retinitis resulting in eventual blindness (*Emergency Medicine,* 1989; Lynch, 1989).

Perhaps 75% of AIDS patients have an eye disease, with the retina the most common site (Russell, 1990). The retina, which is a light-sensitive membrane lining the inside of the back of the eye, is also part of the brain and is nourished by blood vessels. AIDS-related damage to these vessels produces tiny retinal hemorrhages and small **cotton wool spots**—early indicators of disease that are often detected during a routine eye examination.

Symptoms of CMV retinitis may be subtle, such as blurred vision, haze or floaters, or small dim spots in side vision. In unusual circumstances, the virus can produce dramatic symptoms, such as loss of vision within 72 hours.

In August 1991, the United States Food and Drug Administration (FDA) approved the use of **foscarnet** (Foscavir) and **ganciclovir** (Cytovene) for the treatment of CMV retinitis (Table 5-1). The drugs slow the progression of CMV retinitis (Palestine et al., 1991; Jacobson et al., 1992). In mid-1992, Foscavir, the drug of choice, was priced at $21,500/year wholesale; $58.62/250 mL, enough for one day's treatment.

Herpes Viruses Types 1 & 2 (HSV 1 & 2)— Both viruses cause *severe* and progressive eruptions of the mucous membranes. HSV 1 affects the membranes of the nose and mouth. Also, when herpetic lesions involve the lips or throat, 80% to 90% of the time they either precede or occur simultaneously with **herpes-caused pneumonia** (Gottlieb et al., 1987). Bacterial or fungal superinfections occur in more than 50% of herpes-caused pneumonia cases and are a major contributory cause of death in AIDS patients.

Mortality from HSV pneumonia exceeds 80% (Lynch, 1989). Herpes may also cause blindness in AIDS patients. The following is from Paul Monette's *Borrowed Time*:

> I woke up shortly thereafter, and Roger told me—without a sense of panic, almost puzzled—that his vision seemed to be losing light and detail. I called Dell Steadman and made an emergency appointment, and I remember driving down the freeway, grilling Roger about what he could see. It seemed to be less and less by the minute. He could barely see the cars going by in the adjacent lanes. Twenty minutes later we were in Dell's office, and with all the urgent haste to get there we didn't really reconnoiter till we were sitting in the examining room. I asked the same question—what could he see?—and now Roger was getting more and more upset the more his vision darkened. I picked up the phone to call Jamiee, and by the time she answered the phone in Chicago he was blind. *Total blackness, in just two hours!*
>
> The retina had detached. (An operation on retinal attachment was successful and sight was restored. The cause of the retinal detachment was a herpes infection of the eyes.)

HSV 2 also affects the membranes of the anus, causing severe perianal and rectal ulcers primarily in homosexual men with AIDS (Figure 5-8A & B). Herpes of the skin can generally be managed with oral **acyclovir** (Zovirax) or Foscavir (Table 5-1).

Herpes Zoster Virus (HZV)— Like herpes simplex, this virus has the potential to cause fulminant pneumonia in AIDS patients.

FIGURE 5-8 Perirectal Ulcer in an AIDS Patient. **A,** This ulcer was caused by the herpes type II virus. Herpes infections out of control in AIDS and other immunocompromised patients are a serious threat. **B,** The chronic expression of herpes type II virus on the scrotum of an AIDS patient. (*Courtesy of Ronald P. Rappini, University of Texas Medical School and reprinted with permission from* Cutis, *1988, Volume 42:125-128*)

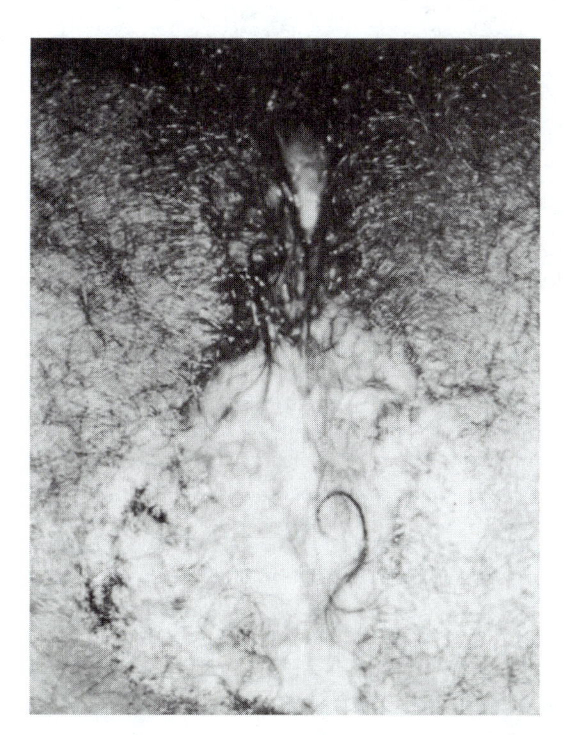

A

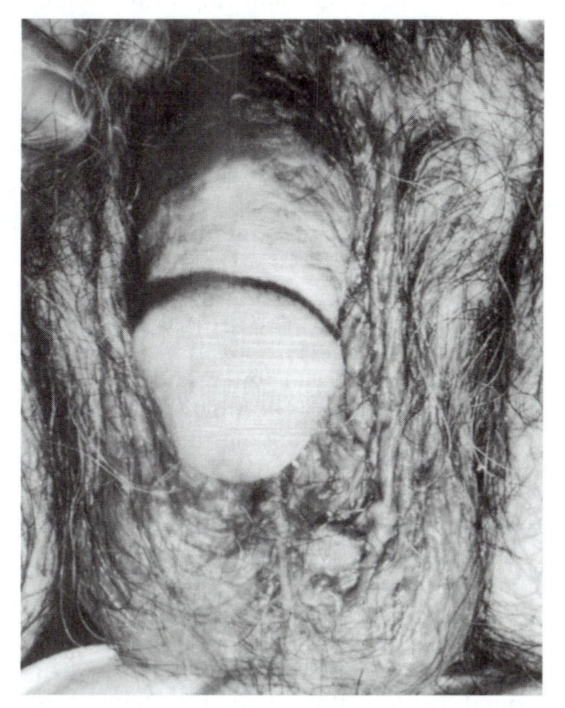

B

Untreated HZV pneumonia has a mortality rate of 15% to 35%. HZV is now monitored as an early indicator that HIV-positive people are progressing toward AIDS.

Protozoal Diseases

An increasing number of infections *which have not been observed in immunocompromised* patients are being found in AIDS patients. Three such infections are caused by the protozoans *Toxoplasma gondii, Isospora belli,* and *Cryptosporidium muris.*

Toxoplasma gondii— *T. gondii* is a small intracellular protozoan parasite that lives in vacuoles inside host macrophages and other nucleated cells. It appears that during and after entry, *T. gondii* produces secretory products that modify vacuole membranes so that the normal *fusion* of cell vacuoles with lysosomes containing digestive enzymes is blocked. Having blocked vacuole-lysosome fusion, *T. gondii* can successfully reproduce and cause a disease called **toxoplasmosis** (Joiner et al., 1990). It can infect any warm-blooded animal, invading and multiplying within the cytoplasm of host cells. As host immunity develops, multiplication slows and tissue cysts are formed. Sexual multiplication occurs in the intestinal cells of cats (and apparently only cats); oocysts form and are shed in the stool (Sibley, 1992). Transmission may occur transplacentally, by ingestion of raw or undercooked meat and eggs containing tissue cysts or by exposure to oocysts in cat feces (Wallace et al., 1993).

In the United States, 10% to 40% of adults are chronically infected but most are asymptomatic. *T. gondii* can enter and infect the human brain causing **encephalitis** (inflammation of the brain). Toxoplasmic encephalitis develops in over 30% of AIDS patients at some point in their illness (Figure 5-9). And, is the initial opportunistic infection is 10% to 38% of AIDS patients (Harden et al., 1994). The signs and symptoms of cerebral toxoplasmosis in AIDS patients have been presented in detail by Rossitch and colleagues (1990). Based on the projected incidence of AIDS cases in the United States in 1992, 40,000 to 70,000 cases of toxoplasmic encephalitis were expected to

POINT OF INFORMATION 5.1

PET GUIDELINES FOR PERSONS WITH HIV DISEASE

Cats

The results of a study presented at the Eighth International Conference on AIDS, the summer of 1992, on whether cat ownership increases the risk of infection with toxoplasmosis in HIV-infected persons suggests that cat ownership does not predispose HIV-positive people to becoming infected with *T. gondii.* In fact, the authors conclude that toxoplasmosis antibody seroconversion in adult HIV-infected population is unusual and unrelated to cat ownership.

With regard to Cat-Scratch Fever, while cat-scratch disease seems to be a relatively rare complication of AIDS, it may be worth taking a special skin test of suspicious skin lesions. If appropriate, antibiotic therapy yields good lesion resolution. HIV-positive people should keep their cat's nails trimmed short and may wish to discuss the pros and cons of declawing with a veterinarian.

Birds

Parrots and parakeets can acquire a rare but serious disease called psittacosis. Transmission of this infection from birds to humans has been traced to contact with pigeons, ducks, turkeys, and chickens. The disease causes severe headaches, high fever, chills, dry cough, and chest pains in humans. Tetracycline is an effective treatment for the disease.

General Rules for Pet Care:

1. Keep your animal clean and well-groomed and stay up-to-date on vaccinations.
2. Control fleas and ticks for your pet's health and your own.
3. Minimize contact with pet saliva, urine, feces, and vomit, especially if you have sores on your skin. (Clean up body fluids that come in contact with sores on your hands and face with a solution of one ounce of bleach to a quart of water.
4. Feed your animals commercial pet foods only. Especially avoid feeding pets raw or undercooked meat, eggs, or unpasteurized milk.
5. Don't let your pet drink from the toilet.
6. If possible, keep your pets inside, or on a leash when outside, to stop them from eating infected rodents, birds, feces, soil, and garbage.
7. Avoid sick or stray animals and exotic or wild animals.

(Coalition News, 1993)

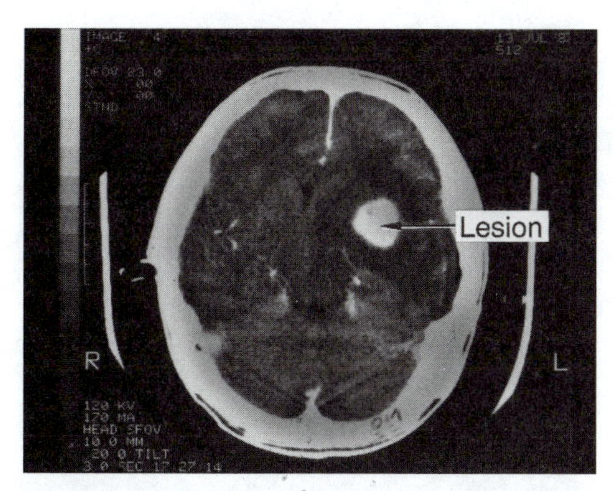

FIGURE 5-9 *Toxoplasma gondii* Lesions in the Brain. Radiographic imaging shows a deep ring-enhancing lesion located in the basal ganglia. *(By permission of Carmelita U. Tuazon, George*

occur (Dannemann et al., 1989). Similar to a variety of other OIs manifested in HIV-infected people, toxoplasmosis appears to represent a reactivation of an earlier infection. In the United States, 30% of the population between the ages of 10 and 19 demonstrate serological evidence (antibody) to *T. gondii* exposure. *T. gondii* lies dormant in the reticuloendothelial system until it becomes reactivated within the immunocompromised host. Thus, for most AIDS patients, it is believed that *T. gondii* is latent within their bodies and is reactivated by the loss of immune competence. Once activated, symptoms can be as mild as chills, headaches that do not respond to common pain killers, low fevers, and delusions; or as severe as hard seizures, coma, and death. Arthur Ashe, tennis champion who died in February of 1993, was being treated for *T. gondii* infection.

Current treatment (Table 5-1) is with pyrimethamine combined with sulfadiazine or clindamycin and with trimethoprim/sulfamethoxazole (Bactrim) or dapsone (Daar et al, 1993).

Cryptosporidium— *Cryptosporidium* is the cause of cryptosporidiosis, and is a member of the family of organisms that includes *Toxoplasma gondii* and *Isospora.* Its life cycle is similar to that of other organisms in the class Sporozoa. Oocysts are shed in the feces of infected animals and are immediately infectious to others. In humans, the organisms can be found throughout the GI tract, including the pharynx, esophagus, stomach, duodenum, jejenum, ileum, appendix, colon, and rectum. Various case reports of patients with AIDS describe infection in the gallbladder and pulmonary dissemination which clinically resembles *Pneumocystis carinii* pneumonia. *Cryptosporidium* causes profuse watery diarrhea of six to 26 bowel movements per day with a loss of 1 to 17 liters of fluid (a liter is about 1 quart). It is an infrequent infection in AIDS patients, usually occurring late in the course of disease as immunological deterioration progresses.

Studies of transmission patterns have shown infection within families, nursery schools, and from person to person, probably by the fecal-oral route. The infection is particularly common in homosexual men, perhaps as a consequence of anilingus (oral-anal sex). Cryptosporidiosis made headlines in March and April 1993 when an outbreak of the infection in Milwaukee resulted in diarrheal illness in more than 400,000 people. Following that outbreak, testing for *Cryptosporidium* in people with diarrhea increased substantially in some areas of Wisconsin. As a result of the investigations, *Cryptosporidum* contamination was found in several public swimming pools. At this time, there are no effective prophylaxes against cryptosporidiosis (Church, 1992). The prevention of transmission rests on good hygiene, hand washing, and awareness of the risks of direct fecal-oral exposure (Wofsy, 1991).

Isospora belli— *Isospora belli* enters the body via feces-contaminated food and drink or is sexually transmitted (DeHovitz, 1988). This organism infects the bowels. Isosporiasis is characterized by an acute onset of profuse watery diarrhea (eight to 10 stools per day), fever, malaise, cramping, abdominal pain, and in some cases significant weight loss and anorexia. According to the 1987 revised definition for AIDS, isosporiasis persisting for longer than 1 month and a positive test for HIV is indicative of AIDS.

Treatment (Table 5-1) calls for high doses of trimethoprim-sulfamethoxazole, furazolidone, and pyrimethamine-sulfadiazine (Wofsy, 1991).

Bacterial Diseases

There is a long list of bacteria that cause infections in AIDS patients. These are the bacteria that normally cause infection or illness after the ingestion of contaminated food, such as species of *Salmonella.* Others, such as *Streptococci, Haemophilus,* and *Staphylococci are* common in advanced HIV disease. A number of other bacterial caused sexually transmitted diseases such as syphilis, chancroid, gonorrhea, and chlamydial diseases are also associated with HIV disease.

One difference between AIDS and non-AIDS individuals is that bacterial diseases in AIDS patients are of greater severity and more difficult to treat. In fact, drug treatments for HIV/AIDS patients have been associated with an increase in the incidence of bacterial infections (Rolston, 1992). Two bacterial species, *Mycobacterium avium intracellulare* and *Mycobacterium tuberculosis* are of particular importance as agents of infection in AIDS patients (Table 5-2).

TABLE 5-2 Categories of Organism and Viral Involvement in Opportunistic Diseases

Symptoms	Causative Agent
Generally Present	
Fever, weight loss, fatigue, malaise	*Pneumocystis carinii* Cytomegalovirus Epstein-Barr virus *Mycobacterium avium intracellulare* *Candida albicans*
Diffuse Pneumonia	
Dyspnea, chest pain, hypoxemia, abnormal chest X-ray	*Pneumocystis carinii* Cytomegalovirus *Mycobacterium tuberculosis* *Mycobacterium avium intracellulare* *Candida albicans* *Cryptococcus neoformans* *Toxoplasma gondii*
Gastrointestinal Involvement	
Esophagitis (sore throat, dysphagia)	*Candida albicans* Herpes simplex Cytomegalovirus (suspected)
Enteritis (diarrhea, abdominal pain, weight loss)	*Giardia lamblia* *Entamoeba histolytica* *Isospora belli* Cryptosporidium *Strongyloides stercoralis* *Mycobacterium avium intracellulare*
Proctocolitis[a] (diarrhea, abdominal pain, rectal pain)	*Entamoeba histolytica* Campylobacter Shigella Salmonella *Chlamydia trachomatis* Cytomegalovirus
Proctitis[a] (pain during defecation, diarrhea, itching and perianal ulcerations)	*Neisseria gonorrhoeae* Herpes simplex *Chlamydia trachomatis* *Treponema pallidum*
Neurological Involvement	
Meningitis, encephalitis, headaches, seizures, dementia	Cytomegalovirus Herpes simplex *Toxoplasma gondii* *Cryptococcus neoformans* Papovavirus *Mycobacterium tuberculosis*
Retinitis (diminished vision)	Cytomegalovirus *Toxoplasma gondii* *Candida albicans*

[a]Especially in those persons practicing anal sex.
Adapted from Amin, 1987)

Mycobacterium avium intracellulare (MAI)— Over the past 40 years, MAI has gone from a rare, reportable infection to something that is common in most large American communities. Unlike tuberculosis, which is almost exclusively spread person-to-person, MAI is, in most instances, environmentally acquired. One theory is that MAI exists in water supplies and enters people's lungs as an aerosol when they take showers.

When an elderly person develops MAI infection, it is invariably confined to his or her lungs. In contrast, MAI infections in AIDS patients run rampant and are clearly systemic (Zoler, 1991).

The fact that MAI produced disseminated disease in AIDS cases was recognized in 1982. The epidemiology of MAI continues to evolve. MAI has been implicated as the cause of a nonspecific **wasting syndrome**. AIDS patients demonstrate anorexia (inability to eat), weight loss, weakness, night sweats, diarrhea, and fever. Some patients also experience abdominal pain, enlarged liver or spleen, and malabsorption. In contrast to viral infections, this bacterium rarely causes pulmonary or lung problems in AIDS patients. Among persons with AIDS, the risk of developing disseminated MAI increases progressively with time. AIDS patients surviving for 30 months had a 50% risk of developing disseminated

MAI. It appears most HIV-infected persons will develop disseminated MAI if they do not first die from other OIs (Chin, 1992). Some new drugs in use are clofazimine, amikacin, azithromycin (Zithromax), and calithromycin (Biaxin), but their effectiveness is limited—resistance to these drugs develops quickly (Table 5-1).

Mycobacterium tuberculosis— Tuberculosis (TB) is an infectious disease caused by the bacterium *Mycobacterium tuberculosis*, which is spread almost exclusively by airborne transmission. TB has been observed in elephants, cattle, mice, and other animal species. In 1993, TB was transmitted from an infected seal to its trainer in Australia. In the United States, monkeys are the primary source of animal-to-human transmission.

The disease can affect any site in the body, but it most often affects the lungs. When persons with pulmonary TB cough, they produce tiny droplet nuclei that contain TB bacteria, which can remain suspended in the air for prolonged periods of time. Anyone who breathes air that contains these droplet nuclei can become infected with TB. It has been suggested that there is a minimal chance of inhaling HIV in blood-tinged TB sputum (Harris, 1993).

During the 19th century, the spitting of blood was considered a sure sign of impending doom, although in the elite circles it was thought to be the mark of a delicate tragedy. For those who succumbed, death before 40 was perceived to be the sad, sweet consequence of an exquisitely sensitive nature.

Keats, Chopin, Elizabeth Barrett Browning, and many other illustrious persons languished and died of "the white plague" or phthisis or consumption, as tuberculosis was then called. Byron reportedly felt deprived because he remained stubbornly free of the disease. The less romantic victims in Europe and America, who would have gladly declined the honor of such company, died in great numbers. Early in the century it was estimated that in England, some 10,000 children/young adults died of the disease each year. And as the century wore on, the toll was calculated at 185 per 100,000 in the United States (Bendiner, 1992).

A person who becomes infected with the TB bacillus remains infected for years. Usually a person with a healthy immune system does not become ill, but is usually not able to eliminate the infection without taking an antituberculosis drug. This condition is referred to as "latent tuberculosis infection." Persons with latent tuberculosis infection are asymptomatic and do not spread TB to others. Generally, a positive TB skin test is the only evidence of infection. The test involves placing a TB "protein derivative" beneath the skin of the forearm. There is no risk of acquiring TB from the test, which may create a small bubble on the skin within 48 to 72 hours of the test if there are antibodies that show evidence of previous TB infection. The important thing about knowing the results of the skin test is so that one can get preventive therapy immediately.

About 10% of otherwise healthy persons who have latent tuberculosis infection will become ill with active TB at some time during their lives (*MMWR*, 1992). With HIV disease the risk is 10% per year (Daar et al., 1993).

Tuberculosis is not generally considered to be an OI because people with healthy immune systems contract TB. After infection with *M. tuberculosis* about 5% of immunocompetent individuals will develop TB (Daley, 1992). But, people with a depressed immune system are much more likely to develop the disease (Zoler, 1991). Tuberculosis in people with AIDS does not look like ordinary tuberculosis. In the usual presentation of the disease, TB is usually restricted to a given area in the chest. People with AIDS may have tuberculosis throughout the chest cavity.

The tubercule bacilli is the world's single largest cause of bacterium-associated deaths. There are *1.7 billion* people infected with *tuberculosis (TB)*; some *20 million* of them are sick and *3 million* a year die. There are 8 million new TB cases worldwide annually and the World Health Organization predicts that TB will kill over 30 million people within the next decade unless moves are made to stop the spread. Up to 80% of adult/adolescents in the poor and overcrowded cities in the developing nations carry the tubercule bacilli. In the United States about 15 million people are infected with *M. tuberculosis*. There are some 27,000 new active cases diagnosed each year

BOX 5.3

NURSE SAYS HER TB WAS AVOIDABLE (FROM *AIDS WEEKLY*, APRIL 26, 1993)

Laura Hopkins has spent the past year battling a fatal form of tuberculosis, and the past four months in a hospital more than 1,500 miles from family and friends. She has undergone treatment after treatment that proved to be unsuccessful—including surgical removal of a part of her lung—and she will remain on a battalion of widely toxic drugs for some time.

And though she is scheduled to return to her home in upstate New York in late April 1993, the 47-year-old nurse faces an uncertain future with the ever-present threat of disease recurrence. "None of this had to happen," Hopkins said in an interview with *AIDS Weekly's* companion newsletter, *TB Weekly*, April 12, 1993. "This all happened because I was doing my job, and it could easily happen to others in the health care profession."

Hopkins' personal TB nightmare began in the summer of 1991 soon after taking a job at an upstate New York teaching hospital. While still undergoing orientation she came into contact with an AIDS patient who had a highly contagious form of multidrug-resistant TB (MDR-TB). As many as 60 hospital employees are believed to have been infected with tuberculosis from this one patient.

Hopkins said the patient was placed on her floor in a room without negative pressure ventilation or ultraviolet lighting.

"This guy had been on the floor for about three weeks to a month," she said. "There is no way they didn't know how infectious he was because sputums are done regularly and charts are reviewed by the doctors.

"I don't know how or why he was allowed to be on that floor, and I don't think I ever will. We had negative pressure rooms in the hospital and my guess is that they were all full. I do know it was a major, major error leaving him there."

For the next eight months the hospital supervised the nurse's treatment. Even though the strain of MDR-TB that Hopkins has is resistant to all the first-line treatments and only partially susceptible to about half of available second-line treatments, doctors did not believe her disease was life-threatening.

"When I got the disease I was dealing with a lot of ignorance regarding MDR-TB," she said. "Basically the people who had it were all immunosuppressed and all dead—they hadn't treated anybody with a normal immune system. I was told by the doctors that because I had a normal immune system my chances for recovery were really good. That's what I wanted to hear, so I believed them.

"I was concerned, though, because there wasn't any agreement about what kind of treatment I should be on. That's when I started doing a lot of research on my own."

Hopkins said the more she read, the more she learned about Denver, Colorado's National Jewish Center for Immunology and Respiratory Medicine. She was the one who suggested the facility to her doctors.

"That name kept coming up, so I wrote them a letter and sent them my files." she said. "By the time I went there in January of 1993, my TB had become active again and I had developed cavities in my lungs—both signs that things aren't going well."

In her four months at National Jewish the nurse has received a six-drug regimen of therapy including the experimental agents ofloxacin and clofazimine (most widely used in drug-resistant leprosy). She has also undergone the surgical removal of the right upper lobe of her lung.

"Really, I was fortunate because the TB was localized in my lungs in an area which made surgery a viable option," she said. "If it had spread through two lung fields there would have been a real problem."

Hopkins' biggest problem now, as she prepares to return home to New York, is uncertainty regarding her future and whether or not she will have a job to return to.

She has been receiving workman's compensation from the hospital, including two-thirds of her salary. Although all of her medical bills have been paid, Hopkins said the compensation system has really worked against her.

"Comp doesn't go on forever, and at this stage I have no idea what's going to happen as far as whether or not I can even be employed again," she said. "I don't see how I can return to nursing and they now have the right to terminate me."

Hopkins said that in New York state if a person accepts workman's compensation they lose the right to sue their employer.

"Workman's comp originally came about to protect employees who had no health insurance and were at their employer's mercy, but it has also evolved to be a disadvantage in cases like mine because employers can hide behind it to keep from being sued. If they decide to terminate me, which I guess they will, I will lose my health insurance, my prescription plan, everything."

Hopkins said she was extremely angry at the beginning of her illness, but that the rage has given way as she has become active, through her union, in educating health care workers about the risk of contracting TB in the workplace.

She said at the very minimum those working in hospitals should become familiar with the policy regarding isolation of tuberculosis patients, and make sure that the policy is followed. If hospital officials are uncooperative, she said, workers should contact their unions or even go outside the hospital community to the media.

"I'm not the only health care worker who has this, and it's only going to get worse if changes are not made," she said.

"Tuberculosis was a disease of the past, but it is now a disease of the future. People have to become knowledgeable in order to protect themselves."

by Salynn Boyles, News Editor, *TB Weekly*

and 1,800 deaths from this disease (Ravikrishnan, 1992). There is a strong association between HIV disease and TB: HIV infection is the highest risk factor for progression from latent *M. tuberculosis* infection to TB (Bermejo et al., 1992).

Prior to 1950, TB killed about 100,000 people a year in the United States. Antibiotics brought this epidemic under control. But TB re-emerged in HIV/AIDS patients in about 1985. In 1991, 26,283 cases were reported to the CDC (*MMWR*, 1992). And from 1989 through early 1992, at least seven major outbreaks of multidrug-resistant TB occurred. Most of these cases have been in AIDS patients. But researchers fear that these drug-resistant strains of mycobacteria may spread to the non-HIV/AIDS population. Mortality among patients with drug resistant TB in the seven outbreaks ranged between 72% and 89%. The median interval between TB diagnosis and death ranged from 4 to 16 weeks (*MMWR*, 1992).

HIV infection is now considered to be the single most important risk factor in the expression of TB. HIV disease is associated with the reactivation of a dormant or inactive TB infection (Stanford et al., 1993).

M. tuberculosis infection occurs in about 35% of HIV-infected individuals, usually as the result of *M. tuberculosis* reactivation from a latent prior infection (Brooke et al., 1990). The CDC defines extrapulmonary TB combined with an HIV-positive test as diagnostic of AIDS.

Drugs used to treat TB are isoniazid, rifampin, pyrazinamide, streptomycin, and ethambutol. Ethambutol is used in combination with the other four drugs when the infecting organism is suspected to be drug-resistant (Bernardo, 1991; Dannenberg, 1993). However, health officials state that between 40% and 60% of those developing multidrug resistant TB will die (Ezzell, 1993).

Early in 1994, a study by Banerjee reported on the discovery of a gene in *M. tuberculosis* called inhA, for isonicotinic acid hydrazide. The gene directs the production of an enzyme that the researchers suspect helps chain lipids to each other to make mycolic acid. The drug isoniazid blocks the manufacture of mycolic acid, which is present in the cell wall of *M. tuberculosis.*

Tuberculosis Testing Hampered by HIV Infection— The tuberculin skin test is the standard method of identifying individuals infected with TB. However, with human immunodeficiency virus (HIV) infection, cell-mediated immune function is imparied and anergy, unresponsiveness to skin test antigens, occurs. It is possible, therefore, that an individual may have a negative reaction to the tuberculin skin test yet be infected with TB (Zoloth et al., 1993).

Other Opportunistic Infections

Other opportunistic infectious organisms and viruses and the diseases they cause and possible therapies are listed in Table 5-1. Table 5-2 separates OIs into the body parts most affected by a particular organism or virus.

BOX 5.4

William "Skip" Bluette (continued from page 18) 3 weeks before he died. Treatment to maintain Skip was failing—the multiple opportunistic infections were defeating the best medicine had to offer.

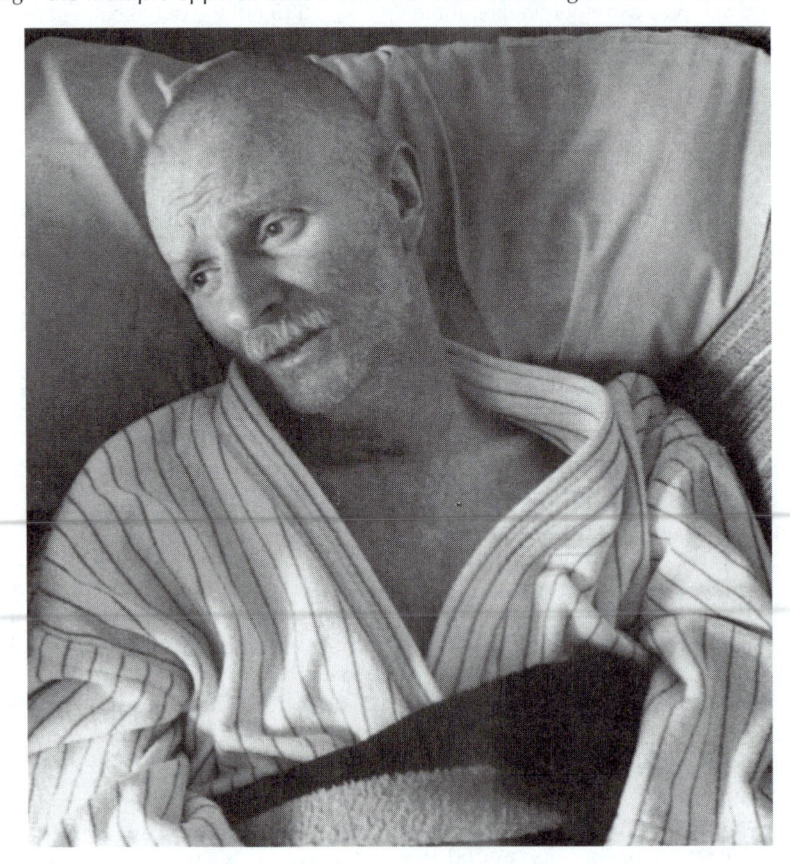

FIGURE 5-10 Drug Therapy for William `Skip' Bluette. Skip's treatment included amphotericin B, an antifungal drug, to combat meningitis. Starting in July 1986, he had to visit one of the hospital's clinics at least once a week to receive his treatments, which were given over several hours. Skip started taking zidovudine, a drug known to slow the progress of the disease, during the summer of 1987. Unfortunately, zidovudine also made it difficult for his body to produce blood cells. Skip stopped taking zidovudine when this occurred. In June of 1988, Skip started cleaning out his closets. He said it was part of the dying process to give belongings away "so you know where they're going." Partly in jest, he said he wanted his ashes scattered on 42nd Street in New York—he thought that's where he got AIDS.

He was hospitalized July 5, 1988. It was presumed that he had *Pneumocystis carinii* pneumonia, which Skip called "the killer." His breathing and speaking were labored. He had inflammation of the pancreas, for which he received morphine, and his kidneys began to fail. (*By permission of Mara Lavitt and* The New Haven Register)

BOX 5.5

AUTOPSY DIAGNOSES OF DISEASES IN AIDS PATIENTS

Between 1984 and 1991, autopsy diagnos is of AIDS-defining diseases as determined in 250 AIDS patients. Forty-seven percent of diseases found at autopsy had not been diagnosed during life. Examples of diseases found at autopsy but not in life were CMV visceral infection, mycoses, HIV-specific brain lesions, cerebral lymphomas, and progressive multifocal leukoencephalopathy. Another important finding was that only a small number of AIDS-diagnostic diseases present at some point during life were *not* observed at autopsy. This indicates that AIDS-related diseases are seldom cured (Monforte et al., 1992).

From diagnosis until death, the AIDS battle is *not just against its cause,* HIV, but against those organisms and viruses that cause OIs. Opportunistic infections are severe, tend to be disseminated (spread throughout the body), and are characterized by multiplicity. Fungal, viral, protozoal, and bacterial infections may be controlled for some time but are rarely curable.

CANCER IN AIDS PATIENTS

Because of the severe and progressive impairment of the immune system, host defense mechanisms that normally protect against certain types of cancer are lost. Four kinds of cancer are occurring with increased frequency among AIDS patients: progressive multifocal leukoencephalopathy, squamous cell carcinoma (oral and anal), non-Hodgkin's lymphoma, and HIV/AIDS-associated Kaposi's sarcoma (KS).

TABLE 5-3 Malignancies Associated with HIV/AIDS

Kaposi's sarcoma (epidemic form)
Burkitt's lymphoma
Non-Hodgkin's lymphomas
Hodgkin's disease
Chronic lymphocytic leukemia
Carcinoma of the oropharaynx
Hepatocellular carcinoma
Adenosquamous carcinoma of the lung

None of these cancers, except for KS, is considered to be an opportunistic infection because they are not infections. They are cancers arising from cells that have lost control of their division processes. Of the eight types of AIDS-associated cancers, KS occurs with the greatest frequency and is discussed in some detail. Lymphomas are briefly described (Table 5-3).

Kaposi's Sarcoma (cap-o-seas sar-comb-a)

KS, as it occurs in HIV/AIDS patients, may not be an opportunistic infection. Its cause is still unknown. It is uncertain whether KS is really a cancer because unlike cancer, which arises from one cell type, KS arises from several cell types. KS lesions are made up of an overgrowth of blood vessels.

In the United States, Kaposi's sarcoma is at least 20,000 times more common in people with HIV/AIDS than in the general population, and 300 times more common than in other immunosuppressed groups (Beral et al., 1990).

KS was first described by Moritz Kaposi in 1877 as a cancer of the muscle and skin. Characteristic signs of early KS were bruises and birthmark-like lesions on the skin, especially on the lower extremities. KS was described as a slow growing tumor found primarily in elderly Mediterranean men, with a more aggressive form found among Africans.

Kaposi's sarcoma as described by Moritz Kaposi is called classic KS and it differs markedly from the KS that occurs in AIDS patients (Figure 5-11A & B). Classic KS has a variable prognosis (forecast), is usually slow to develop, and causes little pain (**indolent**). Patient survival in the United States ranges from 8 to 13 years with some reported cases of survival for up to 50 years (Gross et al., 1989). Symptoms of classic KS are ulcerative skin lesions, swelling (**edema**) of the legs, and secondary infection of the skin lesions.

The AIDS epidemic has brought a more virulent and fatal form of KS marked by painless, flat to raised, pink to purplish plaques on the skin and mucosal surfaces which may spread to the lungs, liver, spleen, lymph nodes, di-

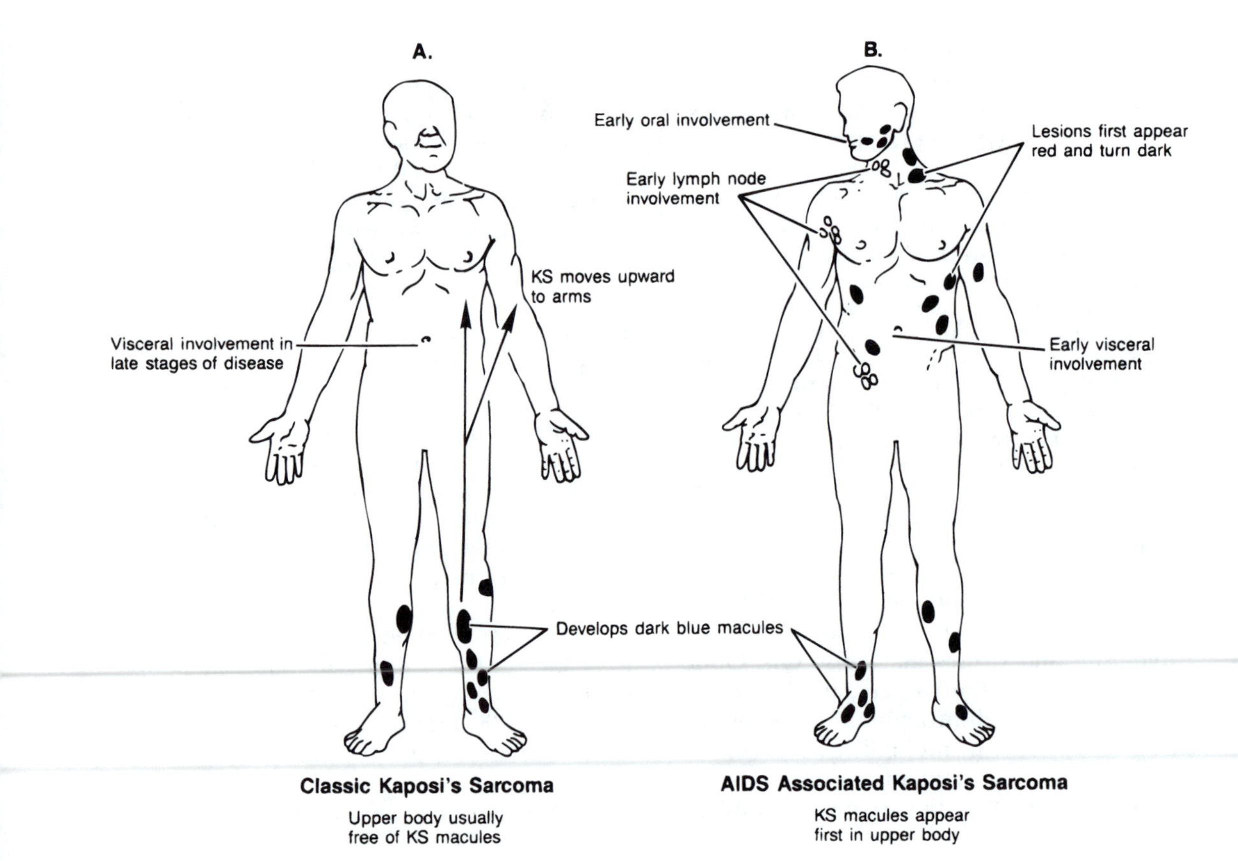

FIGURE 5-11 Classic and AIDS-Associated Kaposi's Sarcoma. **A,** Patients with classic KS (non-AIDS-related) demonstrate violet to dark blue bruises, spots, or macules on their lower legs. Gradually, the lesions enlarge into tumors and begin to form ulcers. KS lesions may, with time, spread upward to the trunk and arms. The movement of KS appears to follow the veins and involves the lymph system. In the late stages of the disease, visceral organs may become involved. **B,** For AIDS patients, initial lesions appear in greater number and are smaller than in classic KS. They first appear on the upper body (head and neck) and arms. The lesions first appear as pink or red oval bruises or macules that, with time, become dark blue and spread to the oral cavity and lower body, the legs, and feet. Visceral organs may be involved early on and the disease is aggressive. However, death is usually caused by opportunistic infection.

gestive tract, and other internal organs. In its advanced stages it may affect any area from the skull to the feet (Figure 5-12, A–C). In the mouth, the hard palate is the most common site of KS (Figure 5-13) but it may also occur on the gum line, tongue, or tonsils.

KS in AIDS patients is fulminant; it comes on swiftly and spreads aggressively. However, there have been *no reported* AIDS deaths due to KS. Most AIDS deaths are due to opportunistic infections.

The prevalence of KS among gay men in 1981 was 77%; by 1987, it had fallen to 26%. This drop in KS among gay men was paralleled by a fall in CMV cases. However, as reasons for these drop-offs remain unknown, KS continues to decline in frequency. Now, less than 20% of patients with AIDS who die have this disease.

Two questions provide differing views of the basic nature of the KS lesion: Is KS merely a polyclonal proliferation of blood vessel cells?

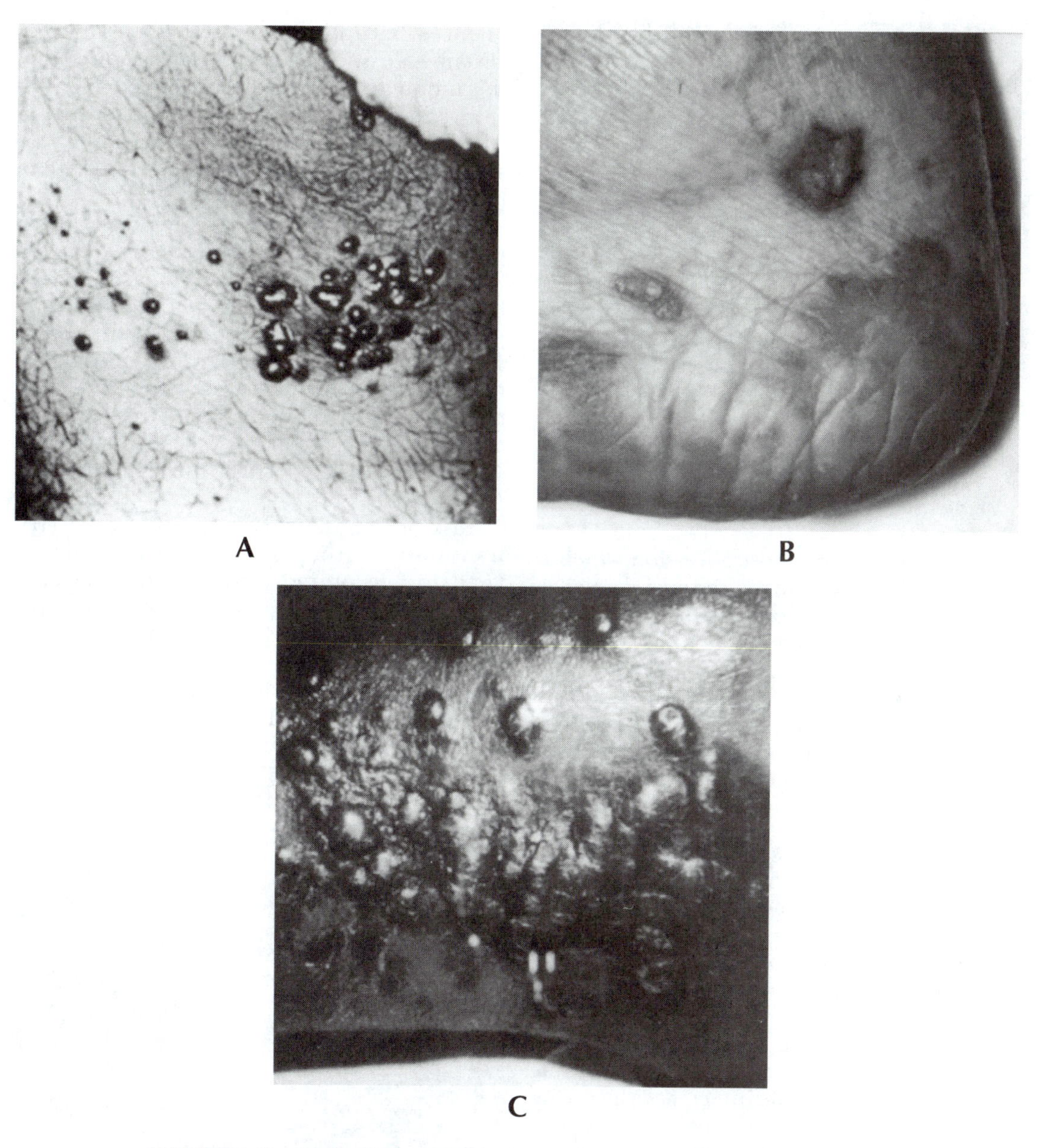

FIGURE 5-12 Kaposi's Sarcoma in AIDS Patients. **A,** KS on the right thigh. **B,** On heel and foot. **C,** On lower leg. (**A** *and* **C**, *courtesy of Nicholas J. Fiumara, M.D., Boston;* **B**, *courtesy of CDC, Atlanta*)

Or is it a true neoplastic process? Whatever the answer, there must be additional host factors modulating the expression of KS to explain its *male predominance* both in mice and in humans and, among AIDS patients, its preferential occurrence among gays (*Hospital Practice,* 1989). It has a low rate of incidence in hemophiliacs, intravenous drug users, women with AIDS, and in pediatric AIDS cases. In summary, KS does *not* appear to be caused

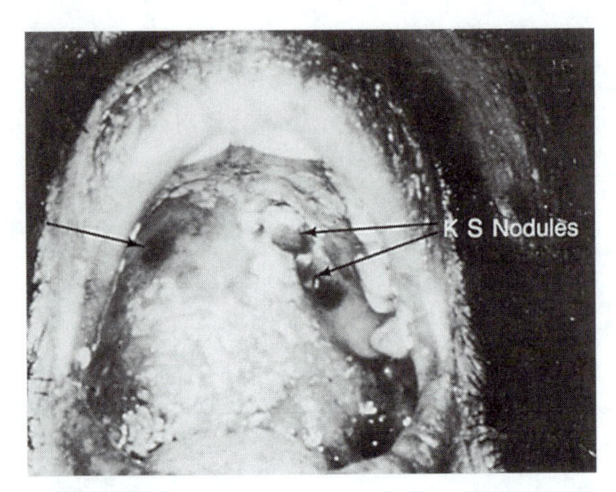

FIGURE 5-13 Oral Kaposi's Sarcoma. KS can be seen on the hard palate and down the sides of the oral cavity. *(Courtesy of Nicholas J. Fiumara, M.D., Boston)*

by HIV, but the immunosuppression which is caused by HIV infection may be an essential element in the evolution of this disease. In October of 1991, investigators found new drugs called SP-PG and AGM-1470. SP-PG and AGM-1470 are drugs that block the development of new blood vessels (angiogenesis) which tumors need to nourish themselves. These drugs have blocked the development of KS in mice. Trials in humans are in progress.

Proposed Kaposi's Virus— Some researchers suspect that the AIDS virus is not the primary pathological agent for Kaposi's sarcoma. Beral and colleagues (1990) at the Centers for Disease Control and Prevention concluded that the epidemiological data on Kaposi's distribution suggest that it is caused by a sexually transmitted pathogen other than HIV. They found, for example, that KS was more common in people infected with HIV by sexual contact (gay males) than those infected by contaminated needles or blood (Palca, 1992).

Friedman-Kien and colleagues believe that human papillomavirus-16 (HGPV-16) is a major cofactor, if not the direct cause of KS. They have detected HPV-16 DNA in 95% of KS cells tested (Palca, 1992). Other scientists believe the cause of KS is another retrovirus. In December of 1994, Yuan Chang and colleagues reported that they found DNA sequences that appear to represent a *new* herpes virus in KS tissue. Preliminary data showed that this unique DNA sequence occurred in KS tissue of 25 out of 27 gay men who had died of AIDS, but was found in only 6 of 39 non-KS tissues from AIDS patients. Investigations are in progress (Schulz et al., 1995).

KS is rare in Caucasian women, but those who acquired HIV through *heterosexual contact* were more likely to have it if their partners were bisexual men than if their partners were injection drug users (3% vs. 0.7%) (Gorin et al., 1991). For men and women who acquired HIV through heterosexual contact, Kaposi's sarcoma was more frequent among those born in the Caribbean, Mexico, Central America, or Africa than those born in the United States (6% vs. 2%).

Risk of Kaposi's sarcoma within each HIV transmission group was not consistently related to age or race and varied across the United States. Kaposi's sarcoma in AIDS patients decreased 50% between 1983 and 1988, a trend that could be due to changes in reporting, the short incubation period for Kaposi's sarcoma, and a declining exposure to the causal agent (Beral et al., 1990).

FIGURE 5-14 HIV/AIDS Patient Demonstrating a Lymphoma of the Neck. *(Courtesy CDC, Atlanta)*

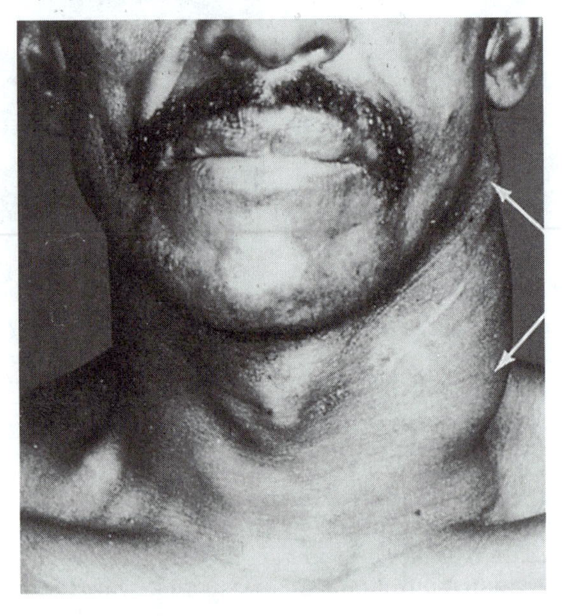

The theoretical "Kaposi's virus" may have entered the same population in which the AIDS virus is endemic, which would explain why the two are often transmitted together. HIV may produce the right conditions for Kaposi's development by causing growth factor production, and possibly by suppressing the body's immune defenses against cancer.

Lymphoma (lim-fo-mah)

Like KS, lymphoma is not an opportunistic infection. A lymphoma is a neoplastic disorder (cancer) of the lymphoid tissue (Figure 5-14). *B cell* lymphoma occurs in about 1% of HIV-infected people, but makes up about 90% to 95% of all lymphomas found in people with HIV disease (Herndier et al., 1994). Although it occurs most often in those demonstrating persistent generalized lymphadenopathy (swollen lymph glands), the usual site of lymphoma growth is in the brain, the heart, or the anorectal area (Brooke et al., 1990). The most common signs and symptoms are confusion, lethargy, and memory loss. Lymphomas are increasing in incidence primarily due to the extension of the life span of AIDS patients, by medical therapy (Table 5-1).

There were approximately 36,000 cases of non-Hodgkin's lymphoma (NHL) diagnosed in 1992, between 8% and 27% occurred in individuals infected with HIV. A recent large prospective observational study indicated an incidence of approximately 1.6% per year in a population with advanced HIV infection treated with zidovudine. It is clear that as HIV infection increases in the population and as individuals infected with HIV survive for longer periods because of more successful treatment, NHL cases will continue to rise (Kaplan, 1992).

HIV Provirus: A Cancer Connection

In early 1994 AIDS investigators reported that HIV, on entering lymph cell DNA, activated nearby cancer-causing genes (oncogenes). The evidence suggests that HIV itself can trigger cancer in an otherwise normal cell (Figure 5-15).

These findings may mean that a variety of retroviruses that infect humans may also cause cancer (McGrath et al., 1994). Such findings raise concerns for developing an HIV vaccine. Using a weakened strain of HIV to make the vaccine may, when used, increase the incidence of lymphoma and other cancers.

NEUROPATHIES IN HIV DISEASE/AIDS PATIENTS

Neuropathies are functional changes in the peripheral nervous system, therefore, any part of the body may be affected. Although neuropathies are not OIs, they may result from the presence of certain OIs. Peripheral neuropathy is caused by nerve damage and is usually characterized by a sensation of pins and needles, burning, stiffness, or numbness in the feet and toes. It is a common, sometimes painful, condition in HIV-positive patients, affecting up to 30% of people with AIDS. Neuropathy has been a continuous problem for patients throughout the HIV/AIDS epidemic. It is most common in people with a history of multiple opportunistic infections and low T4 cell counts. There is a wide range of expression among patients with neuropathy, from a minor nuisance to a disabling weakness. The kinds of neuropathies occurring in people with HIV/AIDS are numerous and must be identified before appropriate treatment can be prescribed. The underlying cause of the most common type of peripheral neuropathy remains elusive. What was a common complaint early in HIV infection of severe neuropathy—usually, burning feet, causing patients to walk on their heels—has diminished. The decrease in such complaints may be attributable to the antiviral effects of the drug ZDV. On the other hand, new varieties of drug-induced nerve damage (neuropathies) have been recognized in the use of antivirals like dideoxyinosine (didanosine) (ddI) and dideoxycytosine (zalcitabine) (ddC). Researchers have also identified cytomegalovirus as a contributing factor in some different kinds of neuropathies in HIV disease.

HIV/AIDS SURVEILLANCE CHECKLIST/REPORT

A few of the most prevalent OIs found in HIV/AIDS patients have been discussed. Figure 5-16 lists those OIs and cancers that are used in

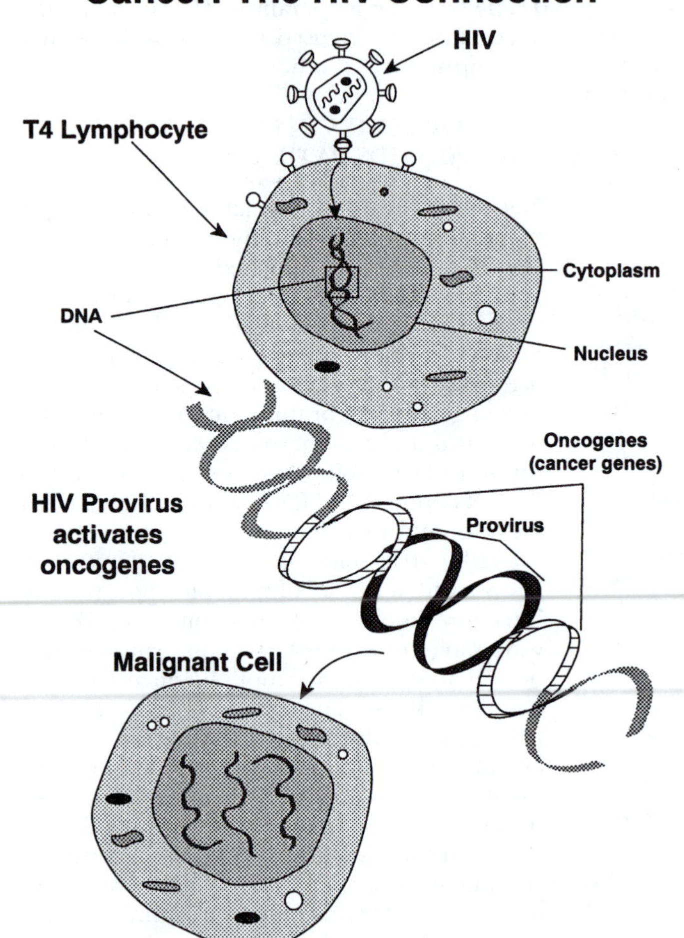

FIGURE 5-15 An HIV-AIDS cancer connection. HIV invades the lumph cell. Its RNA-produced DNA enters lymph cell DNA, becoming an HIV provirus. Sometime during or after intergration into host cell DNA, dormant oncogenes, located nearby, become activated and a cancer results. In lumph cells the cancer becomes a lymphoma.

the CDC criteria for defining AIDS. The report form presented in Figure 5-16 is in use at a public health HIV/AIDS clinic in Florida.

DISCLAIMER

This chapter is designed to present information on opportunistic infections in HIV/AIDS patients. It is not intended to provide medical advice. Consult proper health care providers for medical advice before undertaking any treatment discussed herein.

SUMMARY

One of the gravest consequences of HIV infection is the immunosuppression caused by the depletion of the T4 helper cell population; suppressed immune systems allow for the expression of opportunistic diseases and cancers. It is the OI that kills AIDS patients, not HIV per se. The major OIs are listed in Table 5-1. It is the cumulative effect of several OIs that creates the chills, night sweats, fever, weight loss, anorexia, pain, and neurological problems.

HIV/AIDS SURVEILLANCE CHECK LIST/REPORT FORM

A person will have CDC defined AIDS (MMWR Vol. 36, No. 1S, Aug. 14, 1987) if they have a positive test result for Human Immunodeficiency Virus (HIV) and at least one of the following:

(If HIV test is not performed or inconclusive, please refer to the MMWR for additional criteria)

Disease

(Please indicate definitive diagnosis (D) with laboratory data or presumptive diagnosis (P) where option exists)

___Candidiasis, bronchi, trachea, or lungs
___Cervical cancer
___Coccidiodomycosis, dissem. or extrapul.
___Cryptosporidiosis, chronic intestinal
___Cytomegalovirus retinitis with vision loss (D or P)
___Herpes Simplex, chronic ulcers
>1 month duration, or bronchitis, pneumonitis, or esophagitis
___Isosporiasis, chronic intest.
>1 month duration
___Lymphoma, Burkitt's or equivalent
___Lymphoma, primary in brain
___M.Tuberculosis, dissem. or extrapul. (D or P)
___Pneumocystis carinii pneumonia (PCP)(D or P)
___Salmonella septicemia, recurrent
___Wasting (>10% baseline body weight + diarr or fatigue)

Disease

___Candidiasis, esophageal (D or P)
___Cryptococcosis, extrapulmonary
___Cytomegalovirus, other than liver, spleen, nodes
___HIV Encephalopathy (AIDS Dementia Complex)
___Histoplasmosis, dissem. or extrapul.
___Kaposi's Sarcoma (D or P)
___Lymphoma, immunoblastic or equivalent
___Mycobacterium avium, M. kansasii, dissem. or extrapul. (D or P)
___Mycobacterium tuberculosis, any site (pulmonary or extrapul.)
___Mycobacterium, other, dissem. or extrapul. (D or P)
___Pneumonia, recurrent
___Progressive multifocal leukoencephalopathy
___Toxoplasmosis of brain

Pediatrics (<13 years of age) include:

___Bacterial infections, multiple, recurrent
___Lymphoid interstitial pneumonia and/or pulmonary lymphoid hyperplasia

HIV+ Test/Laboratory Date ____/____/____ Current CD4 cell count ______ Diagnosed as Inpatient ______ or Outpatient ______?
Risk Factor: male/male sex ______ IVDU ______ Transfusion/Hemophilia ______ male/female sex with HIV infected person ______
Mom to Baby ______ none of the above ______ other ____________________

Patient Name: ____________________ Date of Birth: ____/____/____ Male/Female: _____ Race: ____________
Address: ____________________ Zip: ____________ Country of Birth: ____________________

Clinic/Hospital Name: ____________________ Med. Record #: ____________ SS Number #: ____/____/____
Physican Name: ____________________
Name of person notifying Surveillance Office: ____________________ Date sent/called: ____/____/____

Instructions: Place form in chart of each HIV+ patient. When at least one of the opportunistic infections listed is diagnosed, complete the form and either call the Surveillance Office, or mail a copy of this form in an envelope marked "CONFIDENTIAL" to:

AIDS Surveillance Office

Keep the original in each medical record for documentation of having reported to the Surveillance Office.
Thank you!

*** THIS FORM WAS ALTERED TO REFLECT THE JANUARY, 1993 CDC AIDS DEFINITION. THE MAJOR CHANGE IS THAT ALL PERSONS WITH A T4 CELL COUNT OF LESS THAN 200/mm^3 HAS AIDS. THREE MORE DISEASES WERE ADDED TO THE LIST (See Table 1-3.)**

FIGURE 5-16 HIV/AIDS Surveillance Report Form. The form is completed and sent to an AIDS Surveillance Office. The information is then sent on to the CDC in Atlanta.

One tragic disease that does not result from an OI is Kaposi's sarcoma (KS), a cancer (?) that can spread to all parts of an AIDS patient's body. About 20% of AIDS patients, mostly gay men, have KS. It is not usually found in hemophiliacs, intravenous drug users, or female AIDS patients.

REVIEW QUESTIONS

(Answers to the Review Questions are on page 479.)

1. Define opportunistic infection (OI).

2. Which OI organism expresses itself in 80% of AIDS patients? Where is it located and what does it cause?

3. Which of the protozoal OI organisms causes weight loss, watery diarrhea, and severe abdominal pain?

4. Which of the bacterial OIs causes "wasting syndrome," night sweats, anorexia, and fever?

5. True or False: Kaposi's sarcoma (KS) is caused by HIV. Explain.

6. Name the two kinds of KS.

7. True or False: KS affects all AIDS patients equally. Explain.

8. True or False: Candidiasis and ulceration may be present in patients with HIV infection.

9. True or False: Oral candidiasis occurs frequently with HIV infection.

REFERENCES

AMIN, NAVIN M. (1987). Acquired immunodeficiency syndrome, Part 2: The spectrum of disease. *Fam. Pract. Recert.,* 9:84-118.

AWE, ROBERT J. (1988). Benefits, promises and limitations of zidovudine (AZT). *Consultant,* 28:57-72.

BANERJEE, ASESH, et al. (1994). InhA, a gene encoding a target for isoniazid and Ethionamide in *Mycobacterium tuberculosis. Science,* 263:227-230.

BENDINER, ELMER. (1992). Albert Calmette: A vaccine and its vindication. *Hosp. Pract.,* 27:113-132.

BERAL, VALERIE, et al. (1990). Kaposi's sarcoma among persons with AIDS: A sexually transmitted infection? *Lancet,* 335:123-138.

BERMEJO, ALVERO, et al. (1992). Tuberculosis incidence in developing countries with high prevalence of HIV infection. *AIDS,* 6:1203-1206.

BERNARDO, JOHN. (1991). Tuberculosis: A disease of the 1990s. *Hosp. Pract.,* 26:195-220.

BROOKE, GRACE LEE, et al. (1990). HIV disease: A review for the family physician Part II. Secondary infections, malignancy and experimental therapy. *Am. Fam. Pract.,* 42:1299-1308.

CHANG, YUAN, et al. (1994). Identification of Herpes virus-like DNA sequences in AIDS-Associated Kaposis Sarcoma. *Science,* 266:1865–1869.

CHIN, DANIEL. (1992). Mycobacterium avium complex infection. *AIDS File: Clinical Notes,*6:7-8.

CHURCH, DEIRDRE L. (1992). Fatal diarrhea in an AIDS patient. *Patient Care,* 26:280-283.

Coalition News. (1993). Pet guidelines for people with HIV. 2:4-5.

DAAR, ERIC S., et al. (1993). The spectrum of HIV infection. *Patient Care,* 27:99-128.

DALEY, CHARLES L. (1992). Epidemiology of tuberculosis in the AIDS era. *AIDS File: Clinical Notes,* 6:1-2.

DANNEMANN, BRIAN R., et al. (1989). Toxoplasmic encephalitis in AIDS. *Hosp. Pract.,* 24:139-154.

DANNENBERG, ARTHUR M. (1993). Immunopath-ogenesis of pulmonary tuberculosis. *Hosp. Pract.,* 28:51-58.

DEHOVITZ, JACK A. (1988). Management of *Isospora belli* infections in AIDS patients. *Infect. Med.,* 5:437-440.

DEWIT, STEPHANE, et al. (1991). Fungal infections in AIDS patients. *Clinical Advances in the Treatment of Fungal Infections,* 2:1-11.

EDMAN, JEFFREY C., et al. (1988). Ribosomal RNA sequence shows *Pneumocystis carinii* to be a member of the fungi. *Nature,* 334:519-522.

ENNIS, DAVID M., et al. (1993). Cryptococcal meningitis in AIDS. *Hosp. Pract.,* 28:99-112.

Emergency Medicine. (1989). Fighting opportunistic infections in AIDS. 21:24-38.

ERNST, JEROME. (1990). Recognize the early symptoms of PCP. *Med. Asp. of Human Sexuality,* 24:45-47.

EZZELL, CAROL. (1993). Captain of the men of death. *Science News,* 143:90-92.

GORIN, ISABELLE, et al. (1991). AIDS-associated Kaposi's sarcoma in female patients. *AIDS,* 5:877-880.

GOTTLIEB, MICHAEL S., et al. (1987). Opportunistic viruses in AIDS. *Patient Care,* 23:139-154.

GROSS, DAVID J., et al. (1989). Update on AIDS. *Hosp. Pract.,* 25:19-47.

GROSSMAN, RONALD J., et al. (1989). PCP and other protozoal infections. *Patient Care,* 23:89-116.

HARDEN, C.L., et al. (1994). Diagnosis of central nervous system toxoplasmosis in AIDS patients confirmed by autopsy. *AIDS* 8:1188–1189.

HARRIS, CHARLES. (1993). TB and HIV: The boundaries collide. *Medical World News,* 34:63.

HAY, R.J. (1991). Oropharyngeal candidiasis in the AIDS patient. *Clinical Advances in the Treatment of Fungal Infections,* 2:10-12.

HERNDIER, BRIAN, et al. (1994). Pathogenesis of AIDS lymphomas, *AIDS,* 8:1025–1049.

Hospital Practice. (1989). Probing the pathogenesis of Kaposi's sarcoma. 24:320-321.

HUGHES, WALTER. (1994). Opportunistic infections in AIDS patients. *Postgrad. Med.,* 95:81-86.

JACOBSON, MARK A., et al. (1988). Serious cytomegalovirus disease in the acquired immunodeficiency syndrome (AIDS): Clinical findings, diagnosis, and treatment. *Ann. Intern. Med.,* 108:585-594.

JACOBSON, MARK A., et al. (1992). CMV disease in patients with AIDS: Introduction. *Clinical Notes,* 6(2):1-11.

JOINER, K.A., et al. (1990). Toxoplasma gondii: Fusion competence of parasitophorous vacuoles in Fe receptor-transfected fibroblasts. *J. Cell Biol.,* 109:2771.

KAPLAN, LAWRENCE. (1992). HIV-associated lymphoma. *Clinical Notes,* 6(1):1-11.

LYNCH, JOSEPH P. (1989). When opportunistic viruses infiltrate the lung. *J. Resp. Dis.,* 10:25-30.

MCGRATH, MICHAEL, et al. (1994). Identification of a common clonal human immunodeficiency virus integration site in human immunodeficiency virus-associated lymphomas. *Cancer Res.,* 54:2069.

MEDOFF, GERALD, et al. (1991). Systemic fungal infections: An overview. *Hosp. Pract.,* 26:41-52.

MONETTE, PAUL. (1988). *Borrowed Time: An AIDS Memoir.* New York: Avon Books.

MONFORTE, ANTONELLA D'ARMINIO, et al. (1992). AIDS-defining diseases in 250 HIV-infected patients; A comparative study of clinical and autopsy diagnoses. *AIDS,* 6:1159-1164.

MONTGOMERY, BRUCE A. (1992). *Pneumocystis carinii* pneumonia prophylaxis: Past, present and future. *AIDS,* 6:227-228.

Morbidity and Mortality Weekly Report. (1992). National action plan to combat multidrug-resistant tuberculosis. 41:1-70.

Morbidity and Mortality Weekly Report. (1993). Estimates of future global TB morbidity and mortality. 4:961-964.

PALCA, JOSEPH. (1992). Kaposi's sarcoma gives on key fronts. *Science,* 255:1352-1354.

PALESTINE, A.G., et al. (1991). Foscarnet delays progression of CMV retinitis. *Ann. of Intern. Med.,* 115:665-673.

PHAIR, JOHN, et al. (1990). The risk of *Pneumocystis carinii* among men infected with HIV-1. *N Engl J Med.,* 322:161–165.

POWDERLY, WILLIAM G., et al. (1992). Molecular typing of Candida albicans isolated from oral lesions of HIV-infected individuals. *AIDS,* 6:81-84.

RAVIKRISHNAN, K.P. (1992). Tuberculosis. *Postgrad. Med.,* 91:333-338.

ROLSTON, KENNETH. (1992). Changing pattern of bacterial and fungal infections in patients with AIDS. *Primary Care and Cancer,* 12:11-15.

ROSSITCH, EUGENE, et al. (1990). Cerebral toxoplasmosis in patients with AIDS. *Am. Fam. Pract.,* 41:867-873.

RUSSELL, JAMES. (1990). Study focuses on eyes and AIDS. *Baylor Med.,* 21:3.

SCHULZ, THOMAS, et al. (1995). Karposi's Sarcoma; A finger on the culprit. *Nature,* 373:17.

SIBLEY, L. DAVID. (1992). Virulent strains of *Toxoplasma gondii* comprise single clonal linage. *Nature,* 359:82–85.

STANFORD, J.L., et al. (1993). Old plague, new plague, and a treatment for both? *AIDS,* 7:1275–1276.

TUAZON, CARMELITA, et al. (1991). Diagnosing and treating opportunistic CNS infections in patients with AIDS. *Drug Therapy,* 21:43–53.

WALLACE, MARK R., et al. (1993). Cats and toxoplasmosis risk in HIV-infected adults. *JAMA,* 269:76–77.

WALZER, PETER D. (1993). *Pneumocystis carinii:* Recent advances in basic biology and their clinical application. *AIDS,* 7:1293–1305.

WHEAT, L. JOSEPH. (1992). Histoplasmosis in AIDS. *AIDS Clin. Care,* 4:1–4.

WILLOUGHBY, A. (1989). AIDS in women: Epidemiology. *Clin. Obste. Gynecol.,* 32:15–27.

WOFSY, CONSTANCE. (1991). Cryptosporidiosis and isosporiasis. *AIDS Clin. Care,* 3:25–27.

ZACKRISON, LEILA H., et al. (1991). *Pneumocystis carinii:* A deadly opportunist. *Am. Iam. Pract.,* 44:528–541.

ZOLER, MITCHELL L. (1991). OI's widening realm. *Medical World News,* 32:38–44.

ZOLOTH, STEPHEN, et al. (1993). Anergy compromise screening for TB in high-risk populations. *Am. J. Public Health,* 83:749–751.

CHAPTER

6

A Profile of Biological Indicators for HIV Disease and Progression to AIDS

CHAPTER CONCEPTS

- Clinical signs and symptoms of HIV infection and AIDS are presented.
- Stages of HIV disease vary substantially.
- From infection, HIV replication is rapid and continuous.
- AIDS Dementia Complex presents as mental impairment.
- Clues to adult AIDS diagnosis are listed.
- Diarrhea is the most common gastrointestinal sign and symptom of HIV/AIDS infection.
- Pathological brain changes in pediatric cases of AIDS are described.
- Clues to pediatric AIDS diagnosis are presented.

HIV DISEASE DEFINED

The CDC feels that enough has now been learned about HIV infection to call it a disease. This makes sense, as the vast majority of those who become infected become ill. HIV infection leads to the loss of T4 cells, which in turn produces a variety of signs and symptoms of a *nonspecific disease* with initial acute febrile illness or mononucleosis-like symptoms which may last up to 4 weeks or longer. After the initial symptoms most individuals enter a clinically asymptomatic phase. This means the infected person feels well while his or her immune system is slowly compromised. It has been shown that long-lasting symptomatic primary HIV infection predicts an increased risk of rapid development of HIV-related symptoms and AIDS, but it is not known whether the different responses to HIV infection are caused by viral or host factors. Virulent strains of HIV have been characterized by their rapid replication, **syncytium-inducing (SI)** capacity, and tropism for various types of T cells. It is known that the biological properties of HIV strains in asymptomatic HIV-infected individuals with normal T4 cell counts may predict the subsequent development of HIV-related disease, and that patients who harbor SI isolates develop immune deficiency more rapidly. It is not clear whether the appearance of more virulent strains during the chronic phase of the infection is a cause or an effect of progressive immune deficiency (Nielson et al., 1993). Several studies have demonstrated that a long period of fever around the time of seroconversion is associated with more rapid development of immune deficiency (Pedersen et al., 1989).

Spectrum of HIV Disease

Because the immune system slowly falters, HIV disease is really a spectrum of disease. At one end of the spectrum are those infected with HIV who look and feel perfectly healthy. At the opposite end are those with AIDS who are visibly sick and require significant medical and psychosocial support (Figure 6-1). Between these two extremes, HIV-infected people may develop illnesses that range from mild to serious. The interval between initial HIV infection and the presence of signs and symptoms that characterize AIDS is variable and may range from several months to a median duration of 10 or more years (Figure 6-2).

POINT OF INFORMATION 6.1

ONE MISTAKE COST HIM HIS LIFE

I held my son today while he died from AIDS. There is no pain like the pain in a mother's heart. He was 28 years old, and now, he is dead.

This wonderful young man will never have a family. He will never again have a chance to do the things he enjoyed so much — water ski, snow ski, travel. He loved *Star Trek* and music. He loved working for the airlines and traveling all over the world. He was delightful and smart — a computer whiz — could take one apart and put it back together.

He wasted away from a handsome young man to a skeleton — nothing more than skin and bones. His weight dropped from 160 pounds to 80 pounds. His hair fell out. His beautiful teeth fell out. Sores broke out all over his body. He couldn't hold down any food, and eventually, he starved to death.

No, young people, he was not gay, nor was he a drug user. He just went to bed with a girl he didn't know.

His Mom

(Source: Ann Landers, Syndicated Columnist, 1994)

STAGES OF HIV DISEASE

The course of the disease in the infected individual varies substantially. At the extremes are individuals who show either little evidence of progression (loss in T4 cells) 10 to 15 years following infection (1% to 3%) or extremely rapid progression and death within less than 2 to 3 years. In general, HIV-infected adults experience a variety of conditions, categorized into four stages: acute infection, asymptomatic, chronic or symptomatic, and AIDS.

Acute Stage

The acute stage usually develops in 3 to 8 weeks after initial infection or exposure to the virus. Up to 70% of infected individuals develop a brief illness similar to influenza or mononucleosis: fever, sore throat, head-aches, and swollen lymph nodes. The symptoms last about 2 to 4 weeks and resolve spontaneously (Table 6-1). It is during this time that most individuals first begin to produce antibodies to the virus. The acute phase is marked by high levels of virus production. During this phase, large numbers of viral particles spread throughout the body, seeding themselves in various organs, particularly lymphoid tissues such as the lymph nodes, spleen, tonsils, and adenoids. A true state of **microbiological latency,** according to the work of Xiping Wei and co-workers (1995) and David Ho and co-workers (1995), does not exist at any time during the course of HIV infection. The investigations of Wei and Ho show that from the time of infection HIV replication is rapid and continuous, and within 2 to 4 weeks the infecting HIV strain is replaced by drug-resistant mutants. Each day up to 1 billion HIV are produced and mostly destroyed and up to 1 billion T cells are infected, dying, and replaced. Over time the immune system fails to replace its losses and HIV disease progresses. Also, over time, many T4 cells in the lymphoid organs probably are activated by the increased secretion of certain

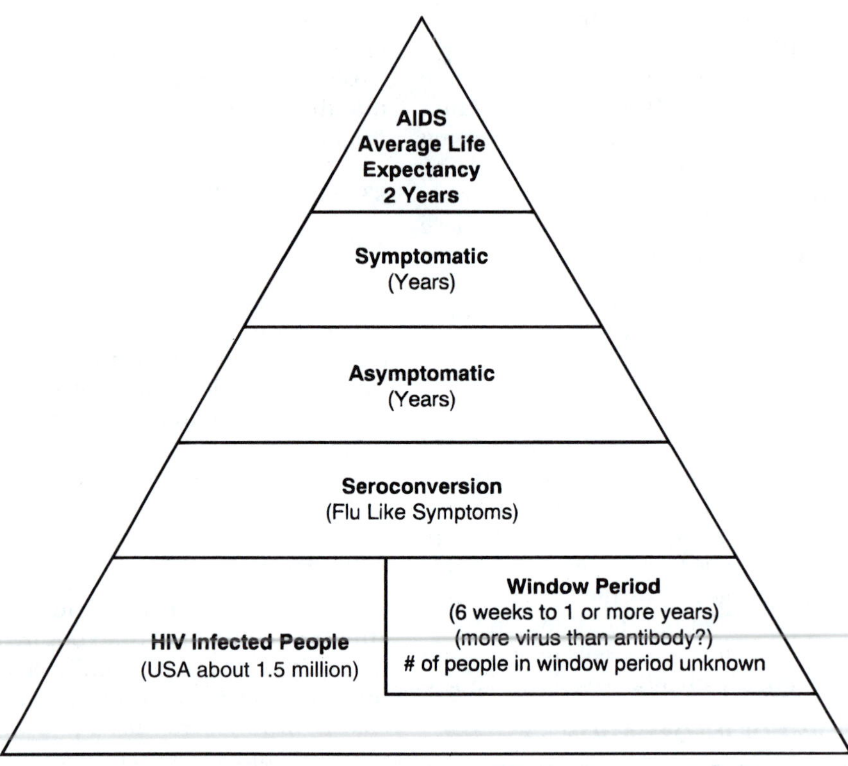

FIGURE 6-1 The HIV/AIDS Pyramid for the United States. This figure demonstrates that current AIDS cases are coming from an existing pool of HIV-infected persons living in the United States. Most of those infected (about 80%) do not yet know they are HIV positive. Although both the asymptomatic and symptomatic periods may last for years, once diagnosed with AIDS the average life expectancy is 2 years. Drug therapy has not changed the outlook for AIDS patients.

cytokines such as tumor necrosis factor-alpha and interleukin-6. Activation allows uninfected cells to be more easily infected and causes increased replication of HIV in infected cells. Other components of the immune system also are chronically activated, with negative consequences that may include the suicide of cells by a process known as programmed cell death or apoptosis (pronounced a-po-toe-sis) and an inability of the immune system to respond to other invaders.

Asymptomatic Stage

Following acute illness, an infected adult can remain free of symptoms from 6 months to a median time of 10 years or more. During the asymptomatic period, the virus continues to replicate and continues to destroy T4 cells within the lymph nodes and the body continues to produce new T4 cells and antibodies to the virus (Figure 6-3). An asymptomatic individual appears to be healthy and can assume normal activities of daily living.

Chronic or Symptomatic Stage

The chronic phase can last for months or years before a diagnoisis of AIDS occurs. During this phase, as viral replication continues, T4 cells become depleted. As the number of immune system cells decline, the individual develops a variety of symptoms such as fever, weight loss, malaise, pain, fatigue, loss of appetite, abdomi-

Adult/Adolescent HIV Disease Continuum to AIDS

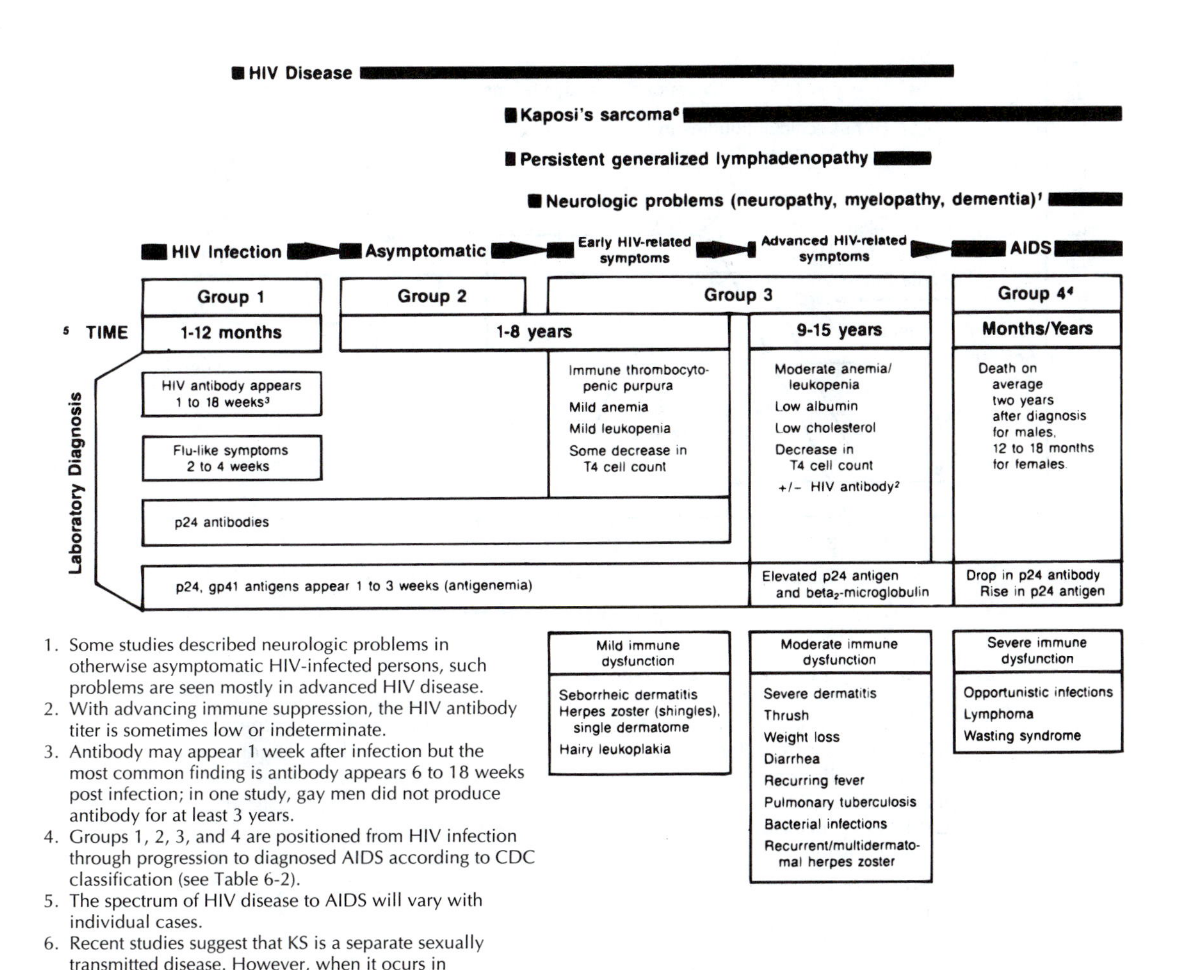

1. Some studies described neurologic problems in otherwise asymptomatic HIV-infected persons, such problems are seen mostly in advanced HIV disease.
2. With advancing immune suppression, the HIV antibody titer is sometimes low or indeterminate.
3. Antibody may appear 1 week after infection but the most common finding is antibody appears 6 to 18 weeks post infection; in one study, gay men did not produce antibody for at least 3 years.
4. Groups 1, 2, 3, and 4 are positioned from HIV infection through progression to diagnosed AIDS according to CDC classification (see Table 6-2).
5. The spectrum of HIV disease to AIDS will vary with individual cases.
6. Recent studies suggest that KS is a separate sexually transmitted disease. However, when it ocurs in HIV/AIDS patients, it ocurs during this time frame.

FIGURE 6-2 Spectrum of HIV Infection, Disease, and the Expression of AIDS. Seroconversion means that HIV antibodies are measurably present in the person's serum. With continued depletion of T4 cells, signs and symptoms appear announcing the progression of HIV disease to AIDS. Although HIV antibodies have been found as early as 1 week after exposure, most often seroconversion occurs between weeks 6 and 18; 95% within 3 months, 99% within 6 months (see Figure 6-3). The early stage of HIV infection can be separated from the symptomatic stage by years of clinical latency. Early infection is characterized by a high number of infected cells and a high level of viral expression. AIDS is characterized by increased levels of viremia and p24 antigenemia, activation of HIV expression in infected cells, an increased number of infected cells, and progressive immune dysfunction.

(continued on next page)

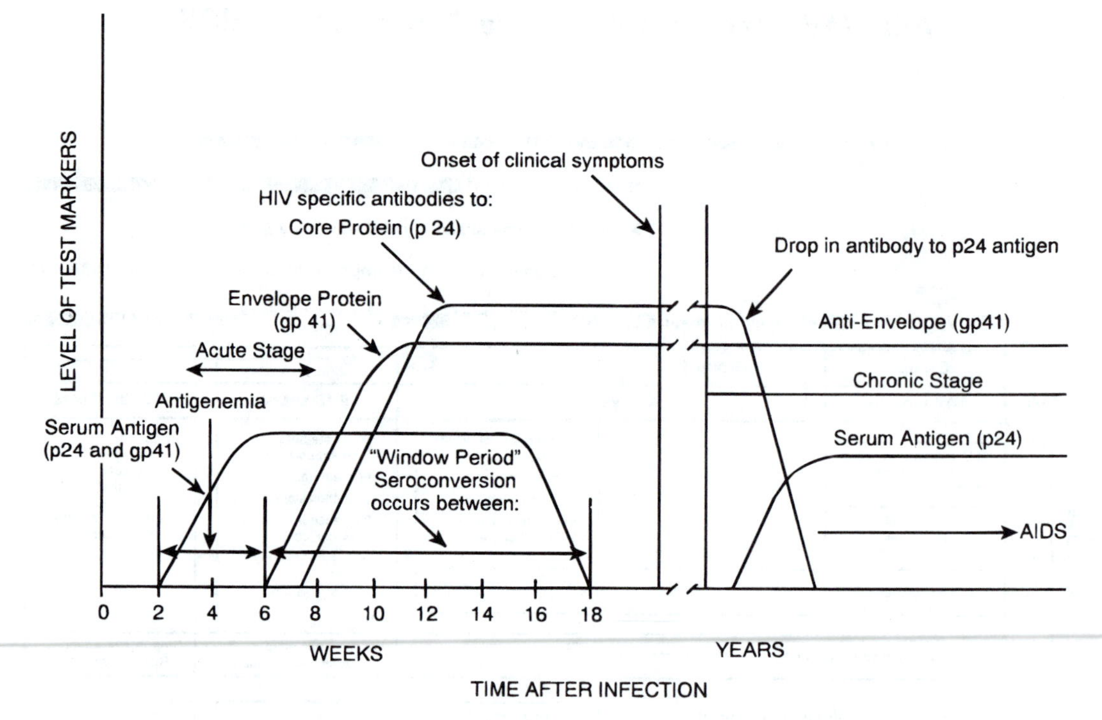

FIGURE 6-3 Profile of Serological Changes after HIV Infection. The dynamics of antibody response to HIV infection was determined by enzyme immunoassays (EIA). Note that during antigenemia, specific HIV proteins (antigens) can be detected before seroconversion occurs. Perhaps other HIV proteins will allow even earlier detection of HIV infection. Once antibodies appear, some antigens disappear only to show up again later on. Note also that although antibody production is a sign that the immune system is working, in HIV-infected people, it is not working well enough. Although envelope and core protein antibodies are being produced as clinical illness begins, as the p24 antibody drops, the illness becomes more serious. *(Adapted from Coulis et al., 1987)*

(continued)

Stages of HIV disease blend into a continuum ranging from the asymptomatic with apparent good health, to increasingly impaired health, to the diagnosis of AIDS. Thus the spectrum of HIV disease ranges from the silent infection to unequivocal AIDS. Clinical expression moves from one condition to another, often without a clear-cut distinction. The level of an individual's infectiousness cannot be correlated with the stage of the disease, the level of antibody, or any other clinically identifiable factor. Therefore, people who are HIV-infected can transmit the virus at any time.

TABLE 6-1 Clinical and Laboratory Analyses an Acute HIV Infection

Signs
Erythematous truncal maculopapular rash
Generalized urticaria, roseola-like exantham, palm and sole desquamation
Generalized lymphadenopathy, splenomegaly
Acute meningo-encephalitis
Myelopathy, Guillain-Barre syndrome
Radiculopathy (brachial or sacral plexopathy)
Peripheral neuropathy
Myopathy
Pharyngitis
Hepatitis
Mental changes
Oral or esophageal ulcerations
Weight loss
Symptoms
Fever, night sweats, chills, malaise, fatigue
Arthralgias, myalgias
Anorexia, nausea and vomiting, abdominal cramps, diarrhea
Headache, retro-orbital pain, photophobia, lethargy
Sore throat, dry cough
Laboratory Analysis
Mild-moderate neutropenia, relative monocytosis
Lymphopenia to lymphocytosis/atypical lymphocytes
Elevated erythrocyte sedimentation rate
Appearance of HIV antibodies
HIV in serum and/or CSF
Abnormal liver function tests
Raised levels of beta-2 microglobulin

nal discomfort, diarrhea, night sweats, headaches, and swollen lymph glands. Ultimately, HIV overwhelms the lymphoid organs. The follicular dentritic cell networks break down in late-chronic stage disease and virus trapping is impaired, allowing spillover of large quantities of virus into the bloodstream. The destruction of the lymph node structure seen late in HIV disease may stop a successful immune response against not only HIV but other pathogens as well, and heralds the onset of the opportunistic infections and cancers that characterize AIDS. Individuals at this stage often develop thrush, oral lesions, and other fungal, bacterial, and/or viral infections. The duration of these symptoms varies, but it is common for HIV-infected individuals to have them for months at a time. Of those persons in the chronic stage, about 30% developed AIDS-associated infections within 5 years.

BOX 6.1

DESCRIPTION OF AN AIDS PATIENT

Cecilia Worth is a registered nurse and author. In a recent edition of The New York Times Magazine she wrote:

> Clustered near the bed, framed photos show a burly athlete who placed in the triathlon, a handsome man who grins disarmingly, an arm slung around his wife's shoulders. Now, transformed into a skin and bones caricature of himself, he is ruled by fatigue. After an interminable struggle to reach the bathroom, knees buckling, leg muscles barely able to hoist his feet forward over the floor, a heroic effort of will, he collapses back in bed, exhausted, motionless, glaring from huge, haunted eyes when I speak to him.
>
> Only in his wife's presence is he calm, though no less armored. She is angry, too, and afraid of him. She cooks for him but will not touch him. His children, parents, brother visit often, struggle for words, and leave without embracing.
>
> He rejects kindness in any form. To my cordial first greeting, he responds with silence, slamming shut his eyes. To suggestions of television, music, back rubs, his response is emphatic, curt: "No!"

Worth vividly describes some of the agony of this terrible disease. She also describes the mental and emotional strain that tears at family life.

There is a point at which sickness and dying cease to offer insights into the human condition and become instead an unbearable, unredeemable absurdity. This is most often how AIDS appears to those who know it.

An alarming feature of HIV infection is that you cannot look at someone and determine whether he or she is infected—a person can be infected and transmit the virus to others for years before becoming ill. Like other disease-causing organisms and viruses, HIV does not recognize age, race, religion, ethnic group or gender. The virus is very democratic.

AIDS Stage

In the final stage of HIV infection, called the crisis or AIDS, continued rapid viral replica-

BOX 6.2

EVOLUTION OF HIV DURING HIV DISEASE

HIV is a unique retrovirus. For example, mitosis, a form of cell dividion, is a requirement for the nuclear entry of most retroviral nucleic acids. In contrast, mitosis does not appear to be required for nuclear entry of HIV nucleic acids, particularly in terminally differentiated cells (e.g., macrophages and dendritic cells) (Freed et al., 1994). And second, HIV lacks any mechanism to correct errors that occur as its genetic material is being duplicated. This means that every time the virus makes a copy of itself there will be, on average, at least one genetic "mistake" incorporated in the new virus. So a few days or weeks after initial infection, there may be a large population of closely related, but not identical, viruses replicating in an infected individual. Simon Wain-Hobson (1995) suggests that because of 24-hour-a-day HIV replication, as shown by Wei and co-workers (1995), an HIV-infected asymptomatic person can harbor at least 1 million distinct HIV variants and an AIDS patient more than 100 million HIV variants. While the immune system will recognize most members of this population of viruses, some mutants will evade the immune response for a time. Until they are brought under immune control, these so-called escape mutants will attack T4 cells. It is these cells that are key to orchestrating the overall immune response, and once they are gone the immune system collapses.

As the virus multiplies and continues to produce mutant forms, the immune system responds to these new forms. But ultimately the sheer number of different viruses to which the immune system must respond becomes overwhelming. It's a bit like the juggler who tries to keep too many balls in the air: The result is disastrous. Once the immune system is overwhelmed, the latest escape mutant—which may not necessarily be the most pathogenic one to come along—will predominate.

tion finally upsets the delicate balance of HIV production/T cell infection to T cell replacement and the virus largely depletes the cells of the immune system. It has been suggested that during the crisis stage, serious immunodeficiency occurs when viral diversity exceeds some threshold beyond which the immune system is unable to control viral replication (Nowak et al., 1990; Wei et al., 1995; Cohen, 1995).

In addition to the symptoms and conditions caused by HIV, opportunistic infections, and malignancies, HIV-infected patients often experience side effects from various drugs they are taking for primary conditions. In many instances, the toxic side effects of the drugs are life-threatening.

In the symptomatic stages of HIV disease, an individual's ability to carry on the activities of daily living is impaired. The degree of impairment varies considerably from day to day and week to week. Many individuals are debilitated by the symptoms of the disease to the point where it becomes difficult to hold steady employment, shop for food, or do household chores. However, it is also quite common for people with AIDS to experience phases of intense life-threatening illness, followed by phases of seemingly normal functioning, all in a matter of weeks. For a good review on the mechanisms of HIV disease, read "The Immunopathogenesis of HIV Infection" by Giuseppe Pantaleo et al. (1993).

HIV Can Be Transmitted During All Four Stages

A person who is HIV-infected, even while feeling healthy, may unknowingly infect others. Thus the term HIV disease more appropriately describes the entire scope of this public health problem than does the term AIDS.

HIV DISEASE WITHOUT SYMPTOMS, WITH SYMPTOMS, AND AIDS

A person may have no symptoms (asymptomatic) but test HIV-positive. This means that the virus is present in the body. Although he or she has not developed any of the illnesses associated with HIV disease or AIDS, it is possible to pass the virus on to other people.

Persons may develop some symptoms early on in HIV disease such as swollen lymph glands, night sweats, diarrhea, or fatigue. (This stage used to be called ARC for AIDS-

Related Complex; the term is no longer used by the Centers for Disease Control and Prevention.)

In time, most, if not all, people with HIV disease progress to AIDS. (This is sometimes referred to as full-blown AIDS. This term is not used in this text; one either is or is not diagnosed with AIDS.) A person has HIV/AIDS when the defect in his or her immune system caused by HIV disease has progressed to such a degree that an unusual infection or tumor is present or when the T4 cell count has fallen below 200/µl of blood. In AIDS patients, a number of diseases are known to take advantage of the damaged immune system. These include opportunistic infections usually caused by viruses, bacteria, fungi, or protozoa; or tumors such as Kaposi's sarcoma, a form of skin cancer (?), or lymphoma, a malignancy of the lymph glands. It is the presence of one of the opportunistic diseases, or a T4 cell count of less than 200, along with a positive HIV test that establishes the medical diagnosis of AIDS. Thus the disease we call AIDS is actually the end stage of HIV disease. It is important to remember that AIDS itself is not transmitted—the virus is. AIDS is the most severe clinical form of HIV disease.

BOX 6.3

DEVELOPMENT OF AIDS OVER TIME

The San Francisco Department of Public Health reported that in a 10 year follow-up of a group of HIV-infected gay men, 4% developed AIDS after 3 years, 9% after 4 years, 14% after 5 years, 22% after 6 years, 34% after 7 years, 38% after 8 years, 42% after 9 years, and 50% after 10 years. Such epidemiological data indicate that about 100% of HIV-infected persons, should develop AIDS within 17 years. To date, because the first known cases were reported in 1981, known HIV-infected persons still alive from 1981 may live to the year 1998 and still be within statistical expectations. Those who outlive the statistical limits will gain recognition for their resistance to the virus and its biological effects.

The morbidity figures for gay males appear to hold for all HIV-infected individuals regardless of their risk group, exposure rate, race, or ethnic background.

Philip Rosenberg and colleagues (1994) reported that the length of incubation, progression from HIV infection to AIDS, varied acording to the age at the time of infection. Younger ages were associated with a slower progression to AIDS. The estimated median treatment-free clinical incubation period was 12 years for those infected at age 20, 9.9 years for infection at age 30, and 8.1 years for infection at age 40.

The Clinical Course of AIDS Among Men and Women

Andrew Phillips and colleagues (1994) compared the development of AIDS-defining diseases between 566 women and 1988 men with AIDS who were HIV-infected via similar routes, mainly by sharing IDU equipment and by heterosexual sexual contact. They concluded that there was little if any difference between men and women in the clinical course of AIDS.

INCREASES IN THE NUMBER OF HIV/AIDS CASES

Prior to 1988, there were between 5 and 10 million HIV-infected people worldwide, an estimated 1.5 million of them living in the United States. Relatively few of these people were actually sick. The majority of these people were infected by HIV in the early 1980s. But from 1988 on (there is an average clinical latency period of about 10 years), the number of new HIV infections, new AIDS cases, and AIDS-related deaths began to rise rapidly; and by the end of 1995, over 280,000 reported AIDS patients in the United States out of an accumulated 509,000 AIDS cases will have died. (AIDS cases are still being underreported by 15% to 20% in the United States.) The point is that the number of AIDS cases and deaths will rise rapidly in the 1990s because those who became infected by HIV in the 1980s will progress to AIDS. In addition, the CDC estimated that there were at least 40,000 to 80,000 new HIV infections in the United States for each year from 1991 through the 1990s.

ASPECTS OF HIV INFECTION

HIV infection depends on a variety of events, for example, the amount and strain of HIV that enters the body (some strains of HIV are known to be more pathogenic than others), perhaps where it enters the body, the number of exposures, the time interval between exposures, the immunological status of the exposed person, and the presence of other active infections. These are referred to as cofactors that contribute to successful HIV infection.

Post Infection

Estimating the date of initial HIV infection helps predict the likely timing of disease progression. The task is easiest when there has been a known blood exposure, but even in other cases, the patient may have experienced a limited number of high-risk sexual or drug-use exposures—or perhaps only one such exposure.

The virus may be present in the bloodstream or within cells for various lengths of time prior to antibody formation. (Normally it takes 7 to 10 days after antigen exposure for the first antibody to appear.) When the antibody appears it is called **seroconversion** (sero = serum of the blood; conversion from antibody negative to antibody present or positive). Seroconversion for HIV may occur as early as 1 week, but most often is detected between 6 and 18 weeks after infection.

Immunosilent HIV Infection: Time Before Seroconversion

The period after HIV infection necessary to induce production of specific antibodies, immunological defect, and AIDS is variable and probably depends on the characteristics of both the virus and the host. It has been estimated that approximately 95% of infected individuals seroconvert (produce HIV antibodies) within 6 months of infection (Horsburg et al., 1989). However, according to some investigators, antibodies may not appear for up to 36 months or more (Ranki et al., 1987; Imagawa et al., 1989; Ensoli et al., 1990, 1991). However, the actual frequency and duration of these late seroconversions and the mechanism by which HIV may escape immune surveillance are yet to be established. In fact, in other studies, the presence of the HIV genome in seronegative individuals is rare or absent. It is therefore of great importance to determine to what extent individuals who remain seronegative for prolonged periods can transmit HIV through blood cells or cell-free body fluids.

Several studies of seronegative gay males have reported intermittant presence of HIV nucleic acid *prior to* seroconversion. These findings were based on the use of a very sensitive test called the polymerase chain reaction or PCR test (this test is explained in Chapter 12). Using the PCR test, over 80% of seronegative persons actually carried HIV nucleic acid in their T4 cells. The findings suggest that seroconversion from HIV negative to HIV positive may average 18 months and occasionally take up to 42 months (Lee et al., 1991). Other investigators have, however, found little or no evidence of infection in groups of high-risk, seronegative individuals, similar to those groups in which frequent silent infections were reportedly detected.

The results of Ensoli and others should not be taken lightly because, if true, they will have profound public health implications as well as important ramifications for HIV pathogenesis. It is therefore imperative that stringent confirmation of their results be obtained before acceptance.

The time from HIV infection to the first signs and symptoms of HIV disease is called the clinical incubation period. Evidence suggests that the route or manner of HIV infection may influence the **incubation period**. For example, exposure through sexual intercourse has a mean incubation time of 6 months. Infection by transfusion has a mean incubation time of 2.5 years. It appears that for unknown reasons, **free viruses** (those not inside cells) present at the time of infection do not stimulate the immune system. Infected cells in the transfused blood have a *latent* (inactive) proviral state and antibody will not be made until new viruses are produced which then engender HIV disease symptoms. Infected newborns have a mean incubation period of 10 months. (Newborns in general begin making their own antibody about 3 to 6 months after birth, but may not make antibody against HIV for several years.)

The time between infection and the presence of first HIV antibody or seroconversion is called the **window period**. Because it can be quite lengthy, HIV antibody tests performed

BOX 6.4

ARE THERE LONG-TERM AIDS SURVIVORS—YES!

A 39-year-old San Francisco artist has beaten the odds against him by living with the virus that causes AIDS for 15 years. He has only routine medical complaints: the stuffiness of an occasional head cold or the aches and pains of a flu. He has never taken a drug to fight HIV. His own immune system seems to have held the virus at bay. "It feels good to be on the winning side of HIV," he says. Looking to the future, he hopes to fix up the Victorian house that he shares with his HIV-negative companion of 10 years.

Susan Buchbinder and colleagues (1992, 1994) reviewed 588 HIV-infected gay men. Thirty-one percent were still AIDS-free 14 years after infection. They attempted to determine why these men lived while others died of HIV/AIDS. Why certain HIV-infected males remain healthy remains a mystery. Some long-term survivors have low T4 cell counts, some have never taken antiviral therapy, and some have high T4 cell counts. The question is, what is keeping them healthy? If it can be determined why or how their bodies have delayed the progression of HIV disease, then perhaps new approaches to treating all HIV-infected persons will follow. Understanding their defense may help in preventing HIV infection per se.

Buchbinder and colleagues have found that three aspects of the healthy survivors' immune system appear to delay HIV disease progression.

1. Survivors have strong cytotoxic lymphocyte activity,

2. Survivors have strong suppressor or T8 cell activity,

3. Survivors have higher levels of antibodies against certain HIV proteins.

It is also possible that long-term survivors carry a less pathogenic virus or that these men have not been reexposed to the virus through unprotected sexual activities. One thing found in the studies that leads to confusion is that, in general, the healthy long-term positives in the study are living very healthy lifestyles, but so are many of the other men who are not doing as well. In addition, physicians who treat HIV/AIDS persons do not notice any trends that would lead one to recognize the type of patient or factors that would lead to long-term survival. It was concluded that, at the moment, there is a dire lack of advice for longer life for persons who have become HIV-infected. AIDS investigators at the National Institute of Allergy and Infectious Diseases are studying the immune systems of 14 people who have been HIV positive for 12 or more years. And a separate study has shown that 10% of 260 female prostitutes who work in Nairobi have not developed antibodies to HIV. They have remained seronegative for 3 years despite ongoing unprotected sexual exposure to HIV-infected men.

During the past few years it has become clear that apparently harmless, and possibly protective, encounters with HIV can occur. Some individuals who have been exposed to the virus and are therefore at high risk for HIV infection remain apparently uninfected; they do not have antibodies to HIV in their blood, and neither HIV nor its nucleic acids can be detected in blood samples. In one study of 97 HIV-exposed individuals who were seronegative for HIV, 49% exhibit cell-mediated immunity to HIV (their T cells respond to HIV peptides in vitro), whereas only 2% of 163 individuals not known to be exposed to HIV exhibit responses to these peptides. Such HIV-specific, cell-mediated responses have been seen in gay men with known sexual exposure, injection drug users, health care workers exposed by accidental needlestick, and newborn infants of HIV-positive mothers. HIV-specific lymphoproliferation or cytotoxic T lymphocyte (CTL) activity, hallmarks of cell-mediated responses, have also been observed by other investigators in some exposed, but apparently uninfected subjects (Salk et al., 1993). Mario Clerici and colleagues (1994) have also reported on HIV-specific T-helper cell activity in six (75%) of eight HIV-negative health care workers with exposure to HIV-positive body fluids. Potent HIV-specific T-helper activity was detectable 4 to 8 weeks after the exposure and was lost in individuals followed up for 8 to 64 weeks. Three health care workers remained responsive at 8, 19, and 24 weeks. Exposure to HIV without evidence of subsequent infection appears to result in activation of cellular immunity without activation of antibody production.

Parade Magazine, January 31, 1993, carried a review of 16 long-term AIDS survivors who date back to 1982. *Time Magazine*, March 22, 1993, says there are at least 70 documented cases of long-term male AIDS survivors. Investigators have recently found long-term AIDS survivors among women and children. Such news is good news and provides hope that more people will survive AIDS than previously expected.

One of the most striking things about the healthy survivors is that after the initial drop, their T4 count stabilizes—usually above 500. Assaulted but not overwhelmed, they no longer lose any ground against HIV. One possible explanation is that these men were exposed to a strain of the virus that is natually weaker than most. The immune system subdues the less lethal virus, allowing the body to fend off attacks by more dangerous strains. In the same way, English milkmaids who suffered from cowpox in the 18th century developed an immunity to cowpox that also protected them against its more lethal related smallpox.

during the window period that are negative may be falsely negative (Figure 6-3).

PRODUCTION OF HIV-SPECIFIC ANTIBODIES

During the 12 years since the discovery of HIV, scientists have constructed a serological or antibody graph of HIV infection and HIV disease. The graph reveals how soon the body produces HIV-specific antibodies after infection and about when the virus begins its reproduction. Different parts of the graph (Figure 6-3) have been filled in by Paul Coulis and colleagues (1987), Dani Bolognesi (1989), and Susan Stramer and colleagues (1989). The chronology of the HIV antibody is not yet complete, but the order of appearance and disappearance of antibodies specific for the serologically important antigens over the course of HIV disease has been described.

The time period from seroconversion to the presentation of clinical symptoms is quite variable and may last for 10 or more years in adults and adolescents, but occurs earlier in children and older persons with HIV disease. The time period for moving from clinical symptoms of HIV disease to AIDS is also quite variable (Figure 6-2). Much depends on the individual's genetic susceptibility and his or her response to medical intervention. The average time from HIV infection to AIDS from 1990 through 1994 was 11 years. Note that Figure 6-3 shows that HIV plasma viremia (the presence of virus in blood plasma) and antigenemia (an-ti-je-ne-mi-ah—the persistence of antigen in the blood) can be detected as early as 2 weeks after infection. This demonstrates that viremia and antigenemia occur prior to seroconversion. Using HIV proteins produced by recombinant DNA methods (making synthetic copies of the viral proteins), antibodies specific for gp41 (a subunit of glycoprotein 160) are detectable prior to those specific for p24 (a core protein) and persist throughout the course of infection. Levels of antibody specific for p24 rise to detectable levels between 6 and 8 weeks after HIV infection but may disappear abruptly. The drop in p24 antibody has been shown to occur at the same time when there is a rise in p24 antigen in the serum. This strange phenomenon is thought to be due to the loss of available p24 antibody in immune complexes—too little p24 antibody is being made to handle the new virus being produced. It is believed that this imbalance is one of the important factors that moves the patient towards AIDS. Thus a sudden decrease in anti-p24 is considered by many scientists to be a prognostic indicator that people with HIV disease are moving towards AIDS.

It is believed by some AIDS researchers and health care professionals that 95% to 99% of those persons infected with HIV will eventually develop AIDS. It has been estimated that approximately 20% to 50% of people with HIV disease will progress to AIDS within 5 years after infection. At 10 years, 50% to 70% will have developed AIDS. After that, an additional 25% to 45% of the remainder will develop AIDS. It is *most improbable* that 100% of those infected will develop AIDS.

AIDS Survival Time Has Nearly Doubled

A National Institute of Allergy and Infectious Diseases study followed more than 5,000 homosexual and bisexual men with HIV infection or who were at risk of infection from 1984 through 1991. For men diagnosed with AIDS during the years 1984 and 1985, 50% had a survival time of less than 11.6 months. For men diagnosed with AIDS in 1990 or 1991, a large percentage had survived for nearly 2 years. The greatest gain in survival time occurred among those whose AIDS-defining illness was *Pneumocystis carinii* pneumonia (PCP). Survival time following the diagnosis of AIDS among the participants who developed *P. carinii* increased from a median of 12.8 months in 1984 and 1985 to a median of 26.3 months in 1990 and 1991. The increase in survival time is related to effective PCP therapy. The survival estimate of persons classified with AIDS using the 1993 definition will be considerably longer than for those diagnosed with AIDS using the 1987 definition. Using the 1987 definition, the median survival for patients enrolled in the registry was 24 months; using the new definition, 53% were still alive after 57 months. These findings have important implications for health planners as well as for those involved in providing care and counseling for patients with AIDS (Vella et al., 1994).

TABLE 6-2 CDC Classification of HIV-Related Diseases

HIV Disease

Group 1: Acute infection—HIV antibodies absent; asymptomatic or if symptomatic mononucleosis-like symptoms which subside in most cases

Group 2: Asymptomatic infection—HIV antibodies present; eventually moves on to

Group 3: Persistent generalized lymphadenopathy; eventually moves on to group 4

AIDS

Group 4:

Subgroup A: Constitutional symptoms (previously called ARC, aids-related complex) and <200 T4 cells/μl of blood.

Subgroup B: Neurologic, symptoms (AIDS dementia complex, neuropathy)

Subgroup C

Category C-1: Secondary infections listed in the CDC surveillance definition for AIDS: *Pneumocystis carinii* pneumonia, recurrent pneumonia, chronic cryptosporidiosis, CNS toxoplasmosis, extraintestinal strongyloidosis, isosporiasis, esophageal candidiasis, cryptococcosis, histoplasmosis, *Mycobacterium avium intracellulare* or *Mycobacterium kansasii*, cytomegalovirus, chronic or disseminated herpes simplex, progressive multifocal leukoencephalopathy

Category C-2: Other specified secondary infections: oral hairy leukoplakia, multidermatomal herpes zoster, recurrent *Salmonella* bacterium, nocardiosis, pulmonary tuberculosis, oral candidiasis

Subgroup D: Secondary cancers: Kaposi's sarcoma, non-Hodgkin's lymphoma (small, noncleaved lymphoma; immunoblastic sarcoma), primary brain lymphoma

Subgroup E: Other conditions: lymphocytic interstitial pneumonitis, neoplasms, infections not previously listed

Classification of HIV/AIDS Progression

There are several classifications that spell out the progression of signs and symptoms from HIV infection to the diagnosis of AIDS. The classifications were developed to provide a framework for the medical management of patients from the time of infection through the expression of AIDS. All classification systems are fundamentally the same—they group patients according to their stage of infection, based on signs that indicate a failing immune system (Royce et al., 1991).

The Walter Reed Army Medical Center System (WRS) classifies HIV infection through six stages. The stages are based on signs and symptoms associated with immune dysfunction. Although individual parts of the immune system appear to function independently of one another, all parts appear to depend on the function of T4 cells (see Chapter 4).

A second classification, the most widely accepted because of its greater clinical applicability, comes from the CDC (Table 6-2). The CDC classification uses four mutually exclusive groupings (Figure 6-4). The groupings are based on the *presence* or *absence* of signs and symptoms of disease, and clinical and/or laboratory findings and the chronology of their occurrence. Group 1, acute infection, means the person is **viremic** (i.e., many virus particles are present in his or her blood or serum). There are *no measurable antibodies*; one is HIV-positive but lacks HIV antibodies and signs and symptoms of HIV disease.

The majority of people in Group 1 remain asymptomatic. Some may experience flu- or mononucleosis-like symptoms that generally disappear in a few weeks. In relatively few cases

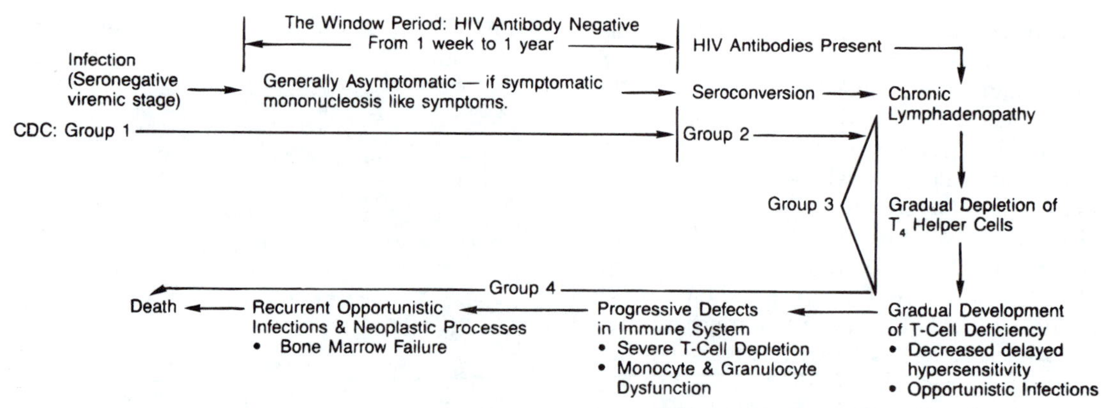

FIGURE 6-4 Clinical History of HIV Infection According to Centers for Disease Control and Prevention Groupings. Seroconversion means that HIV antibodies are measurably present in the person's serum. With continued depletion of T4 cells, various signs and symptoms appear announcing the progression of HIV disease (prodromal AIDS period) into AIDS. Although HIV antibodies have been found as early as 1 week after exposure, most often seroconversion occurs between weeks 6 and 18 but may not occur for up to 1 year.

the patient moves rapidly from mild symptoms into severe opportunistic infections and is diagnosed with AIDS.

In Group 2, antibodies are present but most patients remain free of HIV disease symptoms. Regardless of the lack of outward clinical symptoms, 90% of those who are asymptomatic experience some form of immunological deterioration within 5 years (Fauci, 1988).

In Group 3, asymptomatic people from Groups 1 and 2 become symptomatic and demonstrate lymphadenopathy in the neck, armpit, and groin areas (Figure 6-5). Although a number of other diseases may cause the lymph nodes to swell, most swelling declines as the other symptoms of illness fade. However, with HIV infection, the lymph nodes remain swollen for months, with no other signs of a related infectious disease. Consequently, lymphadenopathy is sometimes called **persistent generalized lymphadenopathy** (PGL). People with PGL may experience night sweats, weight loss, fever, on and off diarrhea, fatigue, and the onset of oral candidiasis or thrush (a fungus or yeast infection of the oral cavity) (Figures 6-6 and Figures 5-4). Such signs and symptoms are prodromal (symptoms leading to) for AIDS. Studies have shown that people in group 3 appear to become more infectious as the disease progresses.

People in Group 4 have been diagnosed with AIDS. They fit the 1987 CDC criteria for AIDS diagnosis (The CDC AIDS diagnostic criteria are listed in Tables 6-2 and 1-1). Hairy leukoplakia Figure 6-7, Table 6-2 Category C-2) is virtually diagnostic of AIDS in group 4 patients. Statistics show that about 30% of all the newly HIV-infected will progress to group 4 (AIDS) every 5 years, so that about 90% will have been diagnosed with AIDS within 15 years. Not all of the opportunistic diseases (OIs) or cancers will appear in any one AIDS patient. But some OIs, like *Pneumocystis carinii* pneumonia occur in some 80% of AIDS patients prior to their deaths.

NEED FOR REPRESENTATIVE INDICATORS TO TRACK HIV DISEASE PROGRESSION

Because infection with HIV causes a chronic, progressive disruption of the immune system that is usually asymptomatic (unless punctuated by episodes of opportunistic infections or tumors), there is a great need for accurate bio-

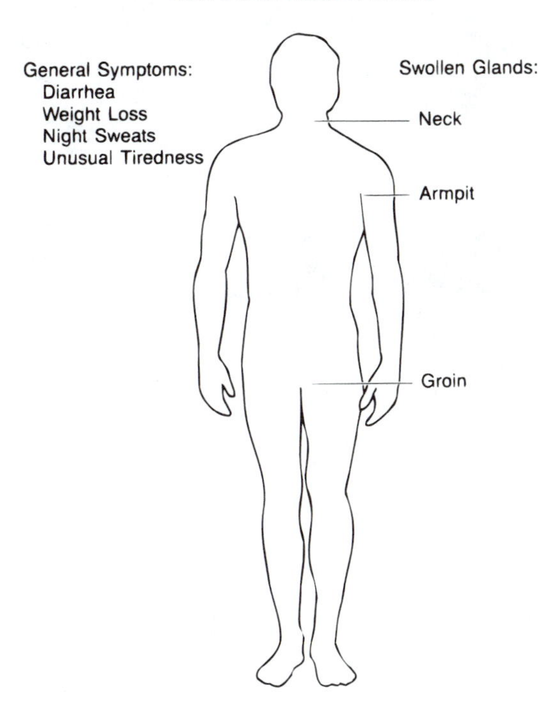

FIGURE 6-5 HIV-Infected Symptomatic People. HIV-infected individuals demonstrating these symptoms would be listed in group 3 of the CDC classification system (see text for CDC groupings). Swollen glands persisting over several weeks or months denote persistent lymphadenopathy.

logical indicators that will predict the development and progression of HIV disease. The use of appropriate indicators or biological markers can expedite the evaluation of what stage of the disease is present, which will then determine medical treatment to some degree. Researchers hope that biological indicators will reflect the step-by-step progression from symptomless HIV infection to AIDS. If the markers are good, they can be exploited as substitutes for clinical end points such as AIDS symptoms or death. There are at present a limited number of useful biological markers that are considered in an HIV-infected person: the levels of p24 antigen and p24 antibody levels, the level of beta-2 microglobulin, neopterin, and interferon; delayed type hypersensitivity reaction; and the number of circulating T4 and T8 lymphocytes and the latest marker measuring the levels of HIV messenger RNA in the blood (Holden, 1994).

Prognostic Biological Markers: p24 Antigen and Antibody Levels Related to AIDS Progression

p24 Antigen Levels— p24 is a specific protein located in the core or inner layer of HIV. Because the immune system produces antibody against foreign protein, antibody is made against p24. A positive test for p24 antigen in

FIGURE 6-6 Erythematous Candidiasis. An inflammation of the tongue caused by the growth of *Candida albicans*. Note fungal (yeast) growth affects the dorsum (upper or top surface of the tongue) where it causes a loss of filiform papillae (conical projections on the top surface of the tongue). *(Courtesy of Drs. M. Schiodt, D. Greenspan, J.S. Greenspan, Oral AIDS Center, University of California, San Francisco* and Journal of Respiratory Diseases, *1989, 10:91–109*).

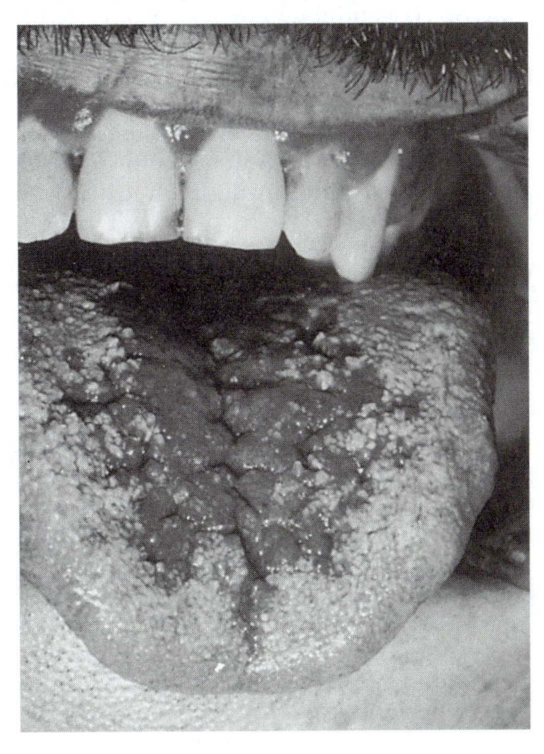

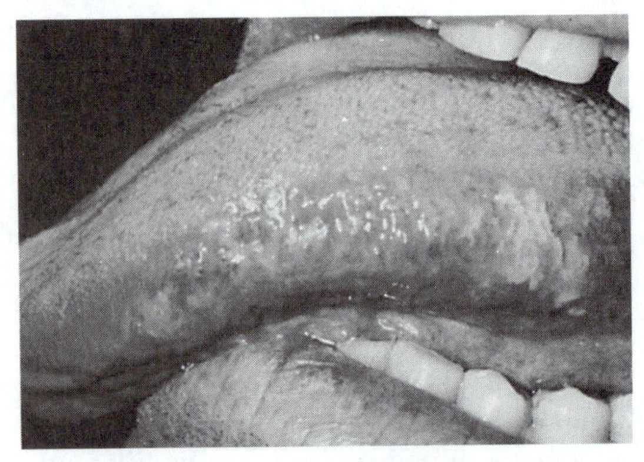
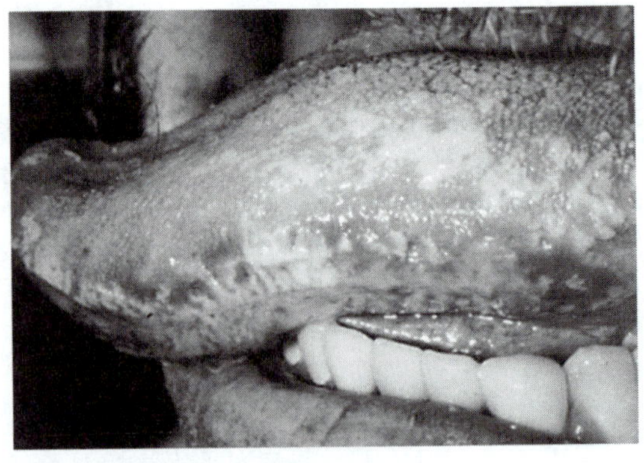

FIGURE 6-7 Oral Hairy Leukoplakia (lu-ko-pla-ki-ah) of the Tongue. An early manifestation, it is virtually diagnostic of AIDS. The white patches are not caused by OIs and the white plaques cannot be removed. **A,** A milder form of the disease. **B,** A more severe manifestation of the disease. Note that the white plaques may cover the entire tongue. (*Courtesy of Drs. M. Schiodt, D. Greenspan, and J.S. Greenspan, Oral AIDS Center, University of California, San Francisco* and Journal of Respiratory Diseases, *1989, 10:91–109*).

the blood means that HIV production is so rapid that it overcomes the available antibody (Figure 6-3). That is, there is more HIV antigen than antibody to neutralize it. During this state of HIV-antibody imbalance, HIV is believed to spread into uninfected cells. This raised p24 antigen level condition occurs at least twice; once shortly after infection and again during the AIDS period when the immune system is rapidly deteriorating and unable to produce sufficient antibody to deal with newly produced HIV.

Those who, during the early stage of HIV infection, test p24 antigen positive are likely to progress to AIDS earlier than those who test p24 negative. Thus, a positive p24 test is an early and serious warning sign for HIV-infected people (Escaich et al., 1991; Phillips et al., 1991a).

p24 Antibody Levels— High levels of p24 antibody indicate that the immune system is functioning well and clearing the body of free HIVs. High antibody levels appear to slow the progression toward AIDS. Typically, p24 antibody levels are high during a person's asymptomatic or latent stage (Figure 6-3). However, antibody levels begin to decrease over time. As measurable antibody falls, p24 antigen levels rise, indicating a loss of immune function. When both p24 antigen and antibody levels are high, the body may be expressing an autoimmune disorder—the immune system is attacking its own body cells. Why this occurs is not understood.

Beta-2 Microglobulin and Neopterin Levels Related to AIDS Progression

Beta-2 microglobulin (B-2M) is a low molecular weight protein that is present on the surface of almost all nucleated cells. As cells die, this compound is released into body fluids. Thus there is always some B-2M in the blood because of normal cell degeneration and replacement. However, in a chronic illness with increased cell destruction, as in HIV infection, B-2M increases beyond normal levels.

A 3-year follow-up study of the San Francisco General Hospital cohort (a population group) revealed progression to AIDS in 69% of HIV-seropositive patients with baseline serum B-2M concentrations of more than 5 mg/L. To date, a B-2M level of 5.0 or higher is the best available indicator of progression to AIDS within 3 years. Levels below 2.6 are considered normal. Similar to p24 antigen, B-2M protein increases dramatically shortly after infection occurs, then declines, and finally rises again with

AIDS. But unlike p24, it can be measured in the blood of any HIV-infected person. Research shows B-2M can be used with T4 counts to foretell which HIV-positive individuals face the greatest immediate risk of progressing to AIDS.

Neopterin is a metabolite of guanosine triphosphate which is produced in stimulated monocytes and macrophages and is found in increased levels in HIV disease. In some studies, the presence of these two compounds have been better HIV disease progression indicators than T4 cell counts (Cohen, 1992).

Interferon is a protein that transfers chemical signals between subtypes of lymphocytes (white blood cells). Levels are generally increased in proportion to the stage of HIV disease.

Delayed type hypersensitivity (DTH) means that persons with HIV disease progressively lose their ability to respond to antigens. DTH is a gauge of functioning cell-mediated immunity rather than antibody response.

T4 and T8 Lymphocyte Levels Related to AIDS Progression

The use of accumulated data on levels of p24 antigen/antibody and B-2M help identify individuals at increased risk for progression to AIDS. However, the most extensive data for AIDS progression risk identification involve the number of T4 and T8 cells circulating in the blood (Anderson et al., 1991; Burcham et al., 1991; Phillips et al., 1991b).

T4 cells and the ratio of T4 cells to T8 cells found in the blood are widely used as prognostic indicators for AIDS progression (Hecht et al., 1990). Table 6-3 presents the **probability** of progression to AIDS based on T4 cell counts. However, T4 counts are not ironclad predictors of HIV disease progression. In some cases persons with HIV disease and very low (less than 50 or 100) T4 counts remain healthy; conversely some HIV-diseased persons have relatively high counts (over 400) and are quite ill. T4 counts are notoriously fickle, they can vary widely between labs or because of a person's age, the time of day a measurement is taken, and even whether the person smokes. Yvonne Rosenberg, investigating the number of T4 to T8 cells in Macaque monkey blood versus the lymph organs, revealed that even a drastic drop of T4 cells in the blood had no influence on the level of T4 cells found in the lymph nodes. She found that as the level of T4 to T8 cells declined in the blood, the ratio remained stable in the lymph nodes. Only much later was there a decline in T4 cells in the lymph nodes. This pattern leads Rosenberg to suspect that initial declines in T4 cells in the blood are deceptive. T4 cells are

TABLE 6-3 T4 Cell Counts in HIV-Infected Men and Probability of Developing AIDS

T4 cells (no/μL)	Probability[a] (%)
100	58
200	33
300	16
400	8
500	4

[a] Of developing AIDS within 18 months
(Adapted from Fahey et al., 1986)

BOX 6.5

THE MEANING OF T4 CELL COUNTS

The lower the T4 cell count, the more likely a person is to begin developing symptoms, because the lower the T4 count, the harder it is for the body to fight disease and infection. When the T4 count falls to 200, a patient is at risk of developing *Pneumocystis carinii* pneumonia (PCP), the leading cause of death among AIDS patients. For that reason, physicians begin prescribing drugs, such as trimethoprim/sulfamethoxazole and aerosolized pentamidine. Symptoms that patients may develop at this stage include fever, fatigue, weight loss, loss of appetite, diarrhea, and infections of the skin and mucous membranes.

As the T4 cell count continues to fall, the risk of developing deadly infections increases. With a T4 count of 50 or lower, brain infections, lymphomas, and other life-threatening conditions may be diagnosed.

The federal Centers for Disease Control and Prevention in Atlanta has revised its definition of AIDS in January of 1993 to include patients with a T4 count of less than 200.

not all disappearing, some are being sequestered in the lymphoid tissue. This could have some major implications for clinical treatment of HIV disease, because it raises the possibility that to prevent onset of AIDS, researchers should focus on preventing the decline of T4 levels in the lymph nodes, not in blood (Cohen, 1993).

In summary, quantifying T4 cells is useful in staging HIV disease and, therefore, in deciding when to recommend HIV treatment or prophylactic antibiotics. More controversial, however, is the sole use of T4 cell counts as an AIDS—qualifying diagnosis. Also, T4 cell number has been disappointing as a surrogate marker of the clinical benefits of antiretroviral drugs. Of particular concern is that T4 cell depletion is a distal effect of HIV infection and may be influenced by other cofactors.

HIV Levels of Messenger RNA in the Blood

David Baltimore, the Nobel Prize-winning retrovirologist, believes he and his co-workers may have found a useful new clinical predictor: levels of HIV messenger RNA (mRNA) in the blood. The mRNA carries the genetic information needed for the virus to copy itself. More mRNA means faster replication and more HIV, and that, proposes the Baltimore group, makes patients get sicker sooner. They believe mRNA is a more sensitive measure than other assays and may detect the virus earlier than it would be seen otherwise.

When the researchers analyzed mRNA levels in 18 HIV-positive men being monitored at the New York Blood Center, they found that mRNA—but not CD4 counts—tightly correlated with AIDS progression (Holden, 1994).

Regardless, T4 counts are still being used as the most important marker of HIV disease status. Using repeat counts at 3- and 6-month intervals, T4 counts still provide more meaningful information than any other single marker test to date.

An interesting study by Schechter et al, (1990) suggested that one's progression to AIDS may be determined very early in HIV infection. They documented HIV seroconversion in 119 gay males. Eighteen cases progressed to AIDS. Their clinical and laboratory results following seroconversion were compared to 54 men who were HIV-infected but remained AIDS free. The authors concluded that factors responsible for rapid progression to AIDS are present before or shortly after infection. Their detailed analysis revealed two points of interest: first, that elevated T8 cell counts appeared to be associated with progression; and second, that those patients who had a symptomatic seroconversion fared worse than those who did not, a finding which is in agreement with other studies.

No single test or cell count, or measure of p24 antigen, antibody, B-2M, T4 cells, or T4-T8 ratios can give a complete picture of the immune system's function at any given moment. Taken together, however, they are important diagnostic indicators of HIV progression to AIDS.

In summary, a good biological marker should improve quickly with an effective treatment, and the change in the marker's status should be directly correlated with improvements in the person's clinical condition. To date, all biological markers used in following the progression of HIV disease to AIDS fail in this respect.

HIV INFECTION OF THE CENTRAL NERVOUS SYSTEM

A wide variety of central nervous system (CNS) abnormalities occur during the course of HIV infection. They result not only from the opportunistic infections and malignancies in the immunodeficient individual, but also from direct HIV infection of the CNS. Certain brain cells have surface molecules similar to the CD4 antigen on T4 lymphocytes and are receptive to HIV infection. In other brain cells, an alternative receptor for HIV has recently been identified. It was shown that a glycolipid in these cells can mediate HIV infection. In addition, HIV-infected monocytes can migrate to the brain, become tissue macrophages, and release HIV to infect adjacent cells. Although the precise mechanisms by which HIV gains entry into the CNS and produces nerve cell dysfunction are still undetermined, infection of the brain is an integral component of the biology and natural history of HIV infection; the resulting clinical manifestations are summarized in Table 6-4.

TABLE 6-4 Neurological Manifestations Associated with Direct HIV Infection of the Nervous System

AIDS dementia complex
Asymptomatic infection
Acute encephalitis
Aseptic meningitis
Vacuolar myelopathy
Inflammatory demyelinating polyneuropathy
Radiculopathy
Mononeuropathies
Distal sensory neuropathy

AIDS Dementia Complex

In addition to cancers and opportunistic diseases, a progressive dementia (mental deterioration) due to HIV infection of the central nervous system develops in over half of AIDS patients. Pathological changes in the CNS are observed in up to 80% of those autopsied (McGuire, 1993). Investigators have found that this dementia is solely associated with HIV infection and progression to AIDS. HIV-caused dementia has a unique set of clinical and pathological features. Some authorities estimate that 90% of AIDS patients in the terminal stages of the disease have AIDS Dementia Complex (ADC) (Hanley et al., 1988). Information presented by the National Institute of Allergy and Infectious Diseases in June 1989 indicated that *asymptomatic* HIV-infected persons *do not demonstrate mental impairment* (Figure 6-8). Therefore, the onset of mental impairment must begin sometime after the HIV-infected person becomes symptomatic (Update, 1989). Initially, investigators thought that OIs caused ADC, but it was later discovered that HIV is carried into the brain by HIV-infected macrophages.

Early Symptoms— Early symptoms of cognitive (quality of knowing or reasoning) dysfunction include forgetfulness, recent memory loss, loss of concentration and slowness of thought, social withdrawal, slurring of speech, loss of balance (inability to walk a straight line), deterioration of handwriting, and impaired motor function. An early diagnosis of ADC in AIDS patients is difficult be-

FIGURE 6-8 Central Nervous System Events after HIV Infection. Note that aseptic meningitis (an inflammation of the membrane of the brain and spinal cord in the absence of viral or bacterial infection), when it occurs, occurs early after HIV infection. Although usually apparent later, AIDS dementia complex may begin during the early–late phase. The late phase represents the period during which major AIDS-defining opportunistic infections occur. The headings acute, latent, early-late and late refer to periods after HIV infection. It appears that OI infection of the brain occurs after the onset of ADC. (*Adapted from Price et al., 1988*)

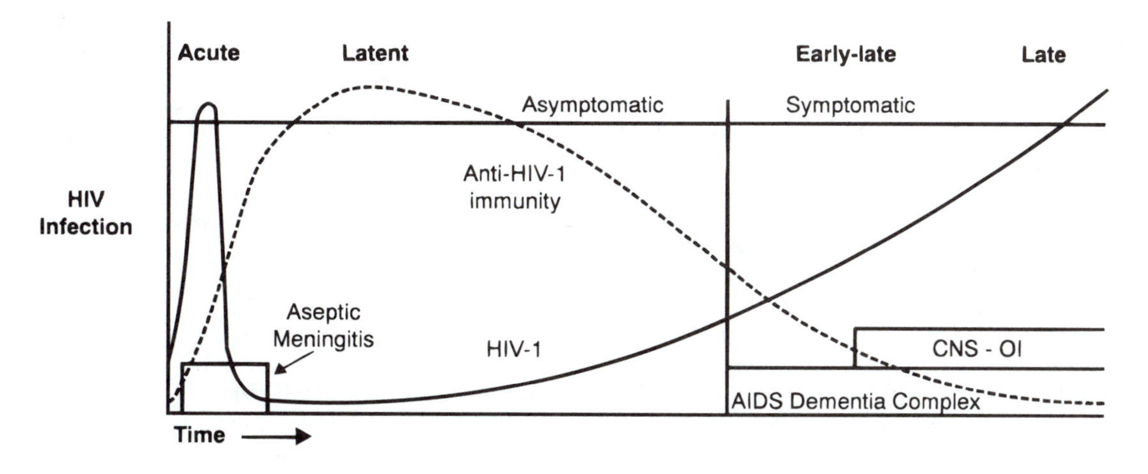

cause the early signs of neurological disease are very similar to those symptoms used to identify emotional depression. However, neurological symptoms may be the first sign of illness in about 10% of adult AIDS patients.

It is unclear just how HIV causes brain damage. Do virus-laden macrophages within the brain secrete a toxin; or does the HIV itself or its gene-coded products interfere with nervous cell function? A cytotoxic factor secreted by some HIV-infected macrophages has recently been demonstrated. This factor may be responsible for some of the neurological damage.

Late Symptoms— These symptoms are characterized by loss of speech, great fatigue, muscle weakness, bladder and bowel incontinence (loss of control), headache, seizures, coma, and finally death. About 95% of patients with ADC have HIV antibodies in their cerebral spinal fluid.

Therapy for HIV-Related Central Nervous System Infection

The blood–brain barrier has been a significant hurdle in the management of HIV-related CNS infection. To date, only zidovudine, which possesses some ability to penetrate the CNS, has been effective in slowing the progress and occasionally even reversing AIDS dementia complex and distal sensory neuropathy (Figure 6.9) (Hanley et al., 1988).

OTHER CLINICAL INDICATORS TO AIDS DIAGNOSIS

Dermatology

Dermatology is the branch of medicine concerned with the study of the skin. Many different cutaneous (skin) disorders have been reported in HIV-infected patients progressing towards AIDS. The six major skin disorders associated with HIV infection are Kaposi's sarcoma, oral hairy leukoplakia, condylomata acuminata (genital warts), seborrheic dermatitis (excessive sebum—a product of the sebaceous glands), molluscum contagiosum, and oral candidiasis (Table 6-5).

All HIV-infected individuals at some time during their illness suffer from one or more cutaneous diseases. These diseases cause significant discomfort, morbidity, and frustration because of their chronicity and lack of response to therapy.

Kaposi's Sarcoma

Kaposi's Sarcoma (KS) is a well known skin manifestation of HIV infection (Figure 6-10). About 10% of KS is found in the patient's peripheral lymph nodes, about 50% in the mouth or gastrointestinal (GI) tract. KS lesions are generally multicolored and range from violet to brown in color. Externally, KS usually appears on the face and chest, although it may be expressed anywhere on the body. Internally, KS may enlarge to block the airways or cause GI dysfunction. KS may be treated with vincristine, vinblastine, or irradiation. Table 6-5 lists a number of other HIV-associated skin disorders and some of the OIs that may also cause severe skin disorders in AIDS patients.

Ocular Lesions

Ocular abnormalities in HIV-infected individuals may provide an important clue to the presence of disseminated infections and in some instances lead to a diagnosis of AIDS.

The most common eye lesions in AIDS patients are cotton wool spots (CWS) and cytomegalovirus retinitis (CMV).

Cotton Wool Spots— Cotton wool spots appear as white fluffy lesions with indistinct borders on the surface or inner layer of the retina. CWS indicate a diminished localized blood supply (ischemia) in the retina. They may spontaneously resolve. CWS have been noted in 42% to 92% of AIDS patients during their first examination, but they are *not dangerous* (Kauffmann, 1989). CWS may also be seen in patients with diabetic or hypertensive retinopathy, severe anemia, autoimmune or collagen-vascular diseases, sarcoidosis, and malignant infiltration of the retina, especially in conjunction with leukemia.

Cytomegalovirus Retinitis— CMV retinitis causes mild to severe damage to the retina that can lead to blindness. CMV retinitis does

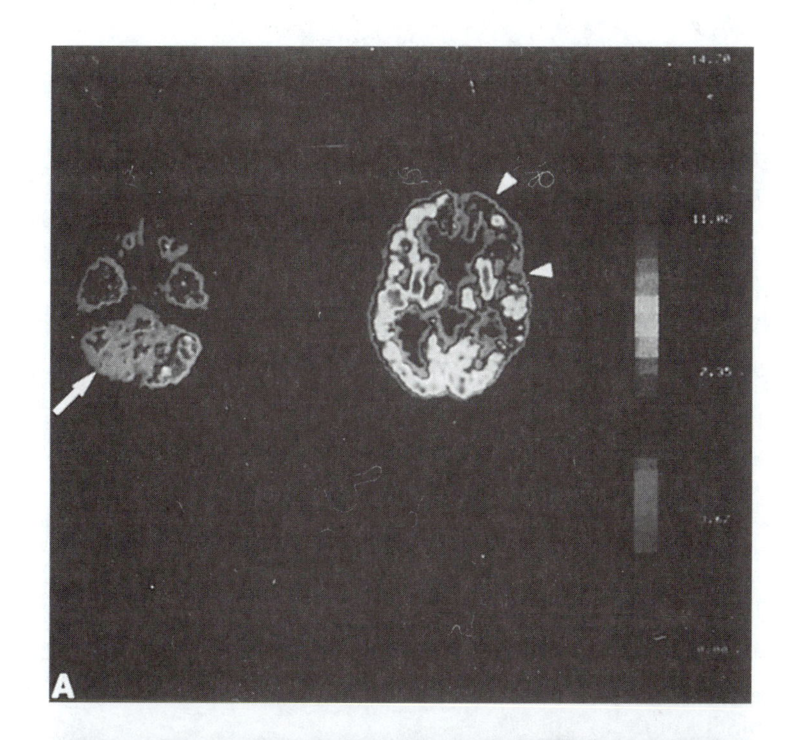

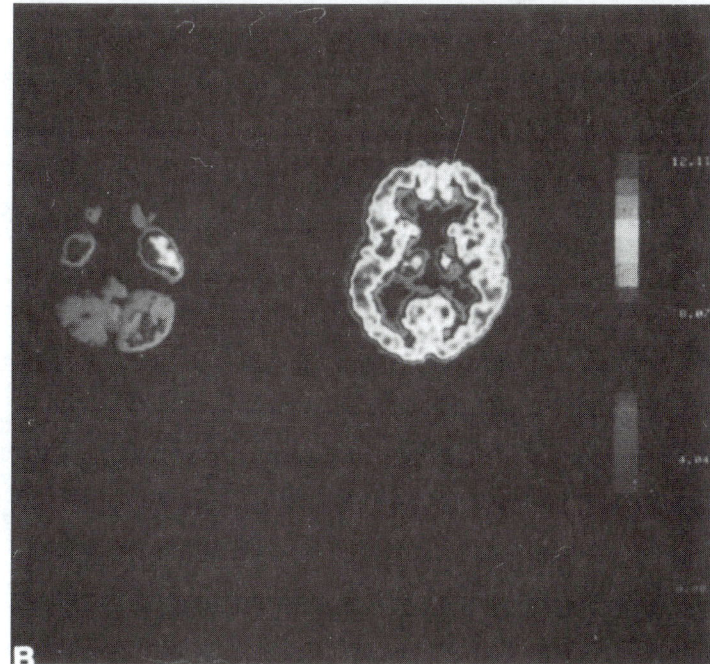

FIGURE 6-9 Improved Brain Function Following Zidovudine Therapy. Brain glucose metabolism was evaluated in patients demonstrating AIDS dementia complex using fluorodexoxglucose (FDG) and positron emission tomography (PET) scan images at the level of the cerebellum (left) and the basal ganglia (right). **A,** The baseline PET image shows left cerebellar (*arrow*) and right front-temporal (*arrowheads*) hypometabolism prior to zidovudine therapy. **B,** The post treatment PET image shows a normal cortical metabolic pattern. (*Courtesy of A. Brunetti, G. Berg, G. DiChiro, and R.M. Cohen, Journal of Nuclear Medicine,* 1989, 30:588.)

TABLE 6-5 Some Cutaneous Noninfectious Manifestations in AIDS Patients

HAIR	
AIDS Trichopathy	Hair becomes smoother, lighter, softer, and silkier.
MOUTH	Thrush (candida overgrowth), Kaposi's sarcoma, and hairy leukoplakia (white "hairy" surfaces mainly on the top and laterial borders of the tongue, Figure 6-7)
NAILS	Nails turn yellow; if patient is on zidovudine, nail bands become purple.
SKIN	
Kaposi's sarcoma	Purple blotches, "cancer" growths
Psoriasis	Reddened skin patches covered by white scales. Can occur on any region of the skin or mucous membrane surfaces. Development of explosive psoriasis or a sudden flare-up of preexisting psoriasis should raise suspicion of underlying HIV infection.
Severe and inflammatory seborrheic dermatitis	May have an abrupt onset, is often severe and may be an early marker of AIDS.Seborrheic dermatitis in AIDS patients is histologically distinct from that seen in non-HIV patients. It occurs on the central face, mid-chest, mid-back, groin, and armpit.
Hives and "itchy red bump disease"	A skin problem that may develop in an otherwise healthy HIV-infected person is a widespread itching condition of the skin with tiny red bumps.
Folliculitis	A condition resembling acne, folliculitis occurs in many HIV-infected persons around the hair follicules on the chest, back, face, scalp, legs, and buttocks.
Ichthyosis	Fishlike scaling of the skin

not resolve spontaneously; it must be vigorously treated to save the patient's vision. Recently, a purine nucleoside analog, 9-(1,3 dihydroxy-2-propoxymethyl) guanine (ganciclovir or DHPG), has been reported to arrest the course of CMV retinitis in AIDS patients. Actually, a considerable number of ocular diseases may occur in AIDS patients due to disseminated OIs. For example, both the herpes simplex and herpes zoster viruses can cause a rapidly progressive tissue necrotizing (killing) retinitis.

FIGURE 6-10 Kaposi's Sarcoma. This patient clearly shows pigmented Kaposi's sarcoma spots over his face. (*Courtesy of Nicholas J. Fiumara, M.D., Boston*)

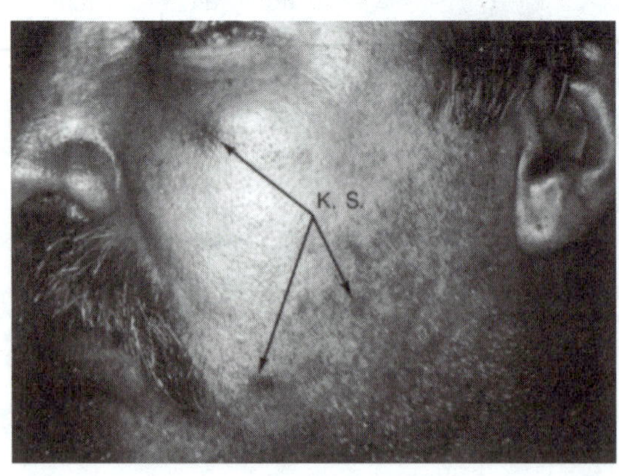

Oral Lesions

Over 70% of all AIDS patients develop one or more HIV-related oral infections during their illness (Kelly etal., 1991). These oral lesions overlap with lesions of the skin. For persons with HIV disease, AIDS can often be diagnosed by the presence of certain oral lesions. These include Kaposi's sarcoma, oral hairy leukoplakia, candidiasis or thrush, and herpes (Figures 6-6 and 6-7).

Oral thrush alone is not sufficient for AIDS diagnosis, but if it is located in the esophagus (throat) it is diagnostic of AIDS. Thrush is easily treated with clotrimazole lozenges, nystatin, ketoconazole, or low-dose amphotericin B. Oral hairy leukoplakia may respond to acyclovir, an antiviral agent, but it reappears after therapy is stopped. Usually no treatment is given for KS. If it becomes aggressive and causes discomfort, treatment varies from low dose irradiation to surgical or laser excision. Oral ulcers caused by the herpes virus can be treated with acyclovir.

Pulmonary Disease

Pulmonary diseases are the most frequent cause of morbidity and mortality in HIV/AIDS patients. However, pulmonary diseases are the most common *treatable* diseases in HIV/AIDS patients.

Pneumocystis carinii pneumonia (PCP) is the most common and treatable pulmonary disease. Although several treatments are available, aerosol pentamidine is the drug of choice.

Other fairly common lung infections that may result in severe complications are caused by cytomegalovirus (effective therapy not yet available), *Mycobacterium avium intracellulare* (widely disseminated in HIV/AIDS patients; therapy not yet available), and *Mycobacterium tuberculosis,* the agent that causes tuberculosis (excellent treatment available). Less often found bacteria that cause lung infections are *Legionella pneumophila, Haemophilus influenzae,* and *Streptococcus pneumoniae.* The herpes virus can also cause lung infection.

Renal Disease

Renal diseases associated with HIV infection occur in 10% to 30% of individuals, most commonly in black injection drug users (IDUs). Acute renal failure secondary to acute tubular necrosis due to toxins is frequent in AIDS patients with active infections; patients will respond to hemodialysis, which removes the toxins.

Gastrointestinal Disease

There are a number of gastrointestinal (GI) diseases that begin as the HIV-diseased person becomes symptomatic and progresses toward AIDS. Some of these disorders occur at both ends of the GI tract; in the mouth and throat, and in the anal canal and rectum. Generally, these disorders, mainly thrush of the mouth and throat and warts or herpes of the rectum, are treatable. Gastric diseases include ulcers or diffuse gastritis associated with cymegalovirus, herpes simplex virus, *Mycobac-terium avium intracellulare,* and *Cryptosporidium. Candida albicans* has been reported as causing a gastric mass and gastric inflammation. The stomach is the most common gastrointestinal site affected with Kaposi's sarcoma. Gastric non-Hodgkin's lymphoma is usually multifocal, but large central tumor masses causing gastric obstruction have been described.

Of the lower gastrointestinal tract diseases in HIV/AIDS patients, the most common is **diarrhea.** Diarrhea occurs in about 65% of American patients and in about 95% of Haitian and African patients (Forsmark, 1993).

PEDIATRIC CLINICAL SIGNS AND SYMPTOMS

Currently between 80% and 90% of pediatric AIDS cases are newborns and infants who received HIV from mothers who were injection drug users or the sexual partners of IDUs. For those who become HIV-infected during gestation, clinical symptoms usually develop within 6 months after birth. Few children infected as fetuses live beyond 2 years and survival past 3 years used to be rare; but with better therapy for opportunistic diseases now available, some children born with HIV are still alive at 5, 10, and 12 years old (personal communications).

The clinical course of infants diagnosed with AIDS is marked by failure to thrive, persistent lymphadenopathy, chronic or recurrent oral candidiasis, persistent diarrhea, enlarged liver and spleen (hepatosplenomegaly), and chronic pneumonia (interstitial pneumonitis). Bacterial infections are common and can be life-threatening. Bacterial infection and septicemia (the presence of a variety of bacterial species in the bloodstream) was the leading cause of death in one group of affected infants in Florida. An excess of gamma globulin and depressed cell-mediated immunity and T cell function are frequently encountered.

Less than 25% of AIDS children express the kinds of OIs found in adult AIDS patients. Kaposi's sarcoma occurs in about 4% of them. Young AIDS children experience delayed development and poor motor function. Older AIDS children experience speech and perception problems.

SUMMARY

The clinical signs and symptoms of HIV infection and AIDS have been addressed in the previous chapters. However, there are two major classification systems used to diagnose patients as they progress from HIV infection to AIDS. The first is the Walter Reed System. It recognizes six stages of signs and symptoms which a person passes through to AIDS. The CDC uses four groupings that identify the stage of illness from infection to AIDS. Both systems revolve around the recognition of a failing immune system, persistent swollen lymph nodes, and opportunistic infections. Mysteries still to be resolved are exactly why and how HIV attacks the body cells, and why some people stabilize after the initial symptoms of HIV infection while others move directly on to AIDS.

One disorder that was not immediately recognized in AIDS patients is AIDS dementia complex (ADC), a progressive mental deterioration due to HIV infection of the central nervous system. ADC develops in over 50% of adult AIDS patients prior to death. Research has shown that some of the symptoms of this dementia can be reversed with the use of the drug zidovudine.

With regard to signs and symptoms of AIDS, almost every major organ can be affected. Most often the onset of AIDS can be detected by the occurrence of one or more skin disorders. The most notable of these is Kaposi's sarcoma, which manifests as dark colored skin blotches or blotches in the mouth or intestines. Ocular lesions may also indicate the onset of AIDS. The most common are cotton wool spots on the retina and cytomegalovirus caused retinitis. The most common oral lesions are thrush and hairy leukoplakia. The most common pulmonary disease is pneumocystic pneumonia caused by the fungus *Pneumocystis carinii.* Other signs and symptoms of AIDS occur as a result of kidney disorders and gastrointestinal diseases such as severe forms of diarrhea that cause weight loss.

REVIEW QUESTIONS

(Answers to the Review Questions are on page 479.)

1. Name the two major AIDS classification systems in use in the United States.
2. What percent of HIV-infected individuals will progress to AIDS in 5 years; in 15 years?
3. What is the neurological set of behavioral changes in AIDS patients called?
4. Name three body organs and their associated AIDS related diseases.
5. True or False: Currently the single most important laboratory parameter that is followed to monitor the progress of HIV- infection is the T4 cell count.
6. True or False: The average time from infection to seroconversion is 2 weeks. Explain.
7. True or False: Being infected with HIV and being diagnosed with AIDS are the same thing. Explain.
8. True or False: The average length of time from infection with HIV to an AIDS diagnosis is approximately 2 years.

REFERENCES

ANDERSON, ROBERT E., et al. (1991). CD8 T lymphocytes and progression to AIDS in HIV-infected men: Some observations. *AIDS,* 5:213–215.

BOLOGNESI, DANI P. (1989). Prospects for prevention of and early intervention against HIV. *JAMA,* 261:3007–3013.

BUCHBINDER, SUSAN P., et al. (1992). Healthy long-term positives: Men infected with HIV for more than 10 years with CD4 counts of 500 cells. *Eighth International Conference on AIDS,* Amsterdam, July 1992. Abstr. TUCO572.

BUCHBINDER, SUSAN P., et al. (1994). Long-term HIV infection without immunologic progression. *AIDS* 8:1123–1128.

BURCHAM, JOYCE, et al. (1991). CD4 % is the best predictor of development of AIDS in a cohort of HIV-infected homosexual men. *AIDS,* 5:365–372.

CLERICI, MARIO, et al. (1994). HIV-specific T helper activity in seronegative health care workers exposed to contaminated Blood. *JAMA,* 271:42–46.

COHEN, JON. (1992). Searching for markers on the AIDS trail. *Science,* 258:387–390.

COHEN, JON. (1993). Keystone's blunt message: It's the virus stupid. *Science,* 260:292–293.

COHEN, JON. (1995). High turnover of HIV in blood revealed by new studies. *Science,* 267:179.

COULIS, PAUL A., et al. (1987). Peptide-based immunodiagnosis of retrovirus infections. *Am. Clin. Prod. Rev.,* 6:34–43.

ENSOLI, F., et al. (1990). Proviral sequences detection of human immunodeficiency virus in seronegative subjects by polymerase chain reaction. *Mol. Cell Probes,* 4:153–161.

ENSOLI, F., et al. (1991). Plasma viraemia in seronegative HIV-1 infected individuals. *AIDS,* 5:1195–1199.

ESCAICH, SONIA, et al. (1991). Plasma viraemia as a

marker of viral replication in HIV-infected individuals. *AIDS,* 5:1189–1194.

FAHEY, J.L., et al. (1986). Diagnostic and prognostic factors in AIDS. *Mt. Sinai J. Med.,* 53:657–663.

FAUCI, ANTHONY S. (1988). The scientific agenda for AIDS. *Issues Sci. Technol.,* 4:33–42.

FORSMARK, CHRIS E. (1993). AIDS and the gastrointestinal tract. *Postgrad. Med.,* 93:143–152.

FREED, ERIC, et al. (1994). HIV infection of nondividing cells. *Nature* 369:107–108.

HANLEY, DANIEL F., et al. (1988). When to suspect viral encephalitis. *Patient Care,* 22:77–99.

HECHT, FREDERICK M., et al. (1990). Care of the asymptomatic patient. *Sexually Transmitted Dis. Bull.,* 10:3–10.

HO, DAVID, et al. (1995). Rapid turnover of plasma virons and CD4 lymphocytes in HIV infection. *Nature,* 373:123–126.

HOLDEN, CONSTANCE. (1994). New tool for predicting AIDS onset. *Science,* 263:606.

HORSBURG, C.R., et al. (1989). Duration of HIV infection before detection of antibody. *Lancet,* ii:637–639.

IMAGAWA, D.T., et al. (1989). Human immunodeficiency virus type I infection in homosexual men who remain seronegative for prolonged periods. *N. Engl. J. Med.,* 320:1458–1462.

KAUFFMANN, DANNY J.H. (1989). Ocular manifestations of AIDS. *Med. Aspects Human Sexuality,* 23:86–92.

KELLY, MAUREEN, et al. (1991). Oral manifestations of human immunodeficiency virus infection. *Cutis,* 47:44–49.

LEE, TZONG-HAE, et al. (1991). Absence of HIV-1 DNA in high-risk seronegative individuals using high input PCR. *AIDS,* 5:1201–1207.

MCGUIRE, DAWN. (1993). Pathogenesis of brain injury in HIV disease. *Clini. Notes,* 7:1–11.

NATIONAL INSTITUTE OF ALLEGY AND INFECTION DISEASES. (1989). Tests confirm lack of mental impairment in asymptomatic HIV-infected homosexual men. June:1–2

NIELSON, CLAUS, et al. (1993). Biological properties of HIV isolates in primary HIV infection: Consequences for the subsequent course of infection. *AIDS,* 7:1035–1040.

NOWAK, M.A., et al. (1990). The evolutionary dynamics of HIV-1 quasispecies and the development of immunodeficiency disease. *AIDS,* 4:1095–1103.

PANTALEO, GIUSEPPE, et al. (1993). The immunopathogenesis of HIV infection. *N. Engl. J. Med.,* 328:327–335.

PEDERSEN, C., et al. (1989). Clinical course of primary HIV infection: Consequences for subsequent course of infection. *Br. Med. J.,* 299:154–157.

PHILLIPS, ANDREW N., et al. (1991a). p24 Antigenaemia, CD4 lymphocyte counts and the development of AIDS. *AIDS,* 5:1217–1222.

PHILLIPS, ANDREW N., et al. (1991b). Serial CD4 lymphocyte counts and development of AIDS. *Lancet,* 337:389–392.

PHILLIPS, ANDREW, et al. (1994). A sex comparison of rates of new AIDS-defining disease and death in 2554 AIDS cases. *AIDS* 8:831–835.

PRICE, RICHARD W. (1988). The brain in AIDS: Central nervous system HIV infection and AIDS dementia complex. *Science* 239:586–593.

RANKI, A., et al. (1987). Long latency precedes overt seroconversion in sexually transmitted human immunodeficiency virus infection. *Lancet,* ii:589–593.

ROSENBERG, PHILIP, et al. (1994). Declining age at HIV infection in the United States. N. Engl. J. Med., 330:789–790.

ROYCE, RACHEL A., et al. (1991). The natural history of HIV-1 infection: Staging classifications of disease. *AIDS,* 5:355–364.

SALK, JONAS, et al. (1993). A strategy for prophylatic vaccination against HIV. *Science,* 260: 1270–1272.

SCHECHTER, M.T., et al. (1990). Susceptibility to AIDS progression appears early in HIV infection. *AIDS,* 4:185–190.

STRAMER, SUSAN L., et al. (1989). Markers of HIV infection prior to IgG antibody seropositivity. *JAMA,* 262:64–69.

VELLA, STEFANO, et al. (1994). Differentiated survival of patients with AIDS according to the 1987 and 1993 CDC case definitions. *JAMA,* 271:1197–1199.

WAIN-HOBSON, SIMON. (1995). Virological mayhem. *Nature,* 373:102.

WEI, XIPING, et al. (1995). Viral dynamics in HIV type 1 infection. *Nature,* 373:117–122.

CHAPTER

7

Therapy for HIV Disease and Opportunistic Diseases

CHAPTER CONCEPTS

- Treatment for an opportunistic infection is lifelong because of relapse if it is stopped.
- By mid-1995 there were at least 185 antiviral and antiinfection drugs, immunomodulators, and vaccines in development in the United States.
- Investigational new drugs (IND) may be used in patients with terminal illnesses.
- New drugs normally go through three Food and Drug Administration (FDA) phases of investigation.
- Zidovudine therapy slows mental deterioration in children.
- Zidovudine, didanosine, zalcitabine and stavudine are four FDA-approved nucleoside antiviral drugs. All four inhibit HIV replication.
- Other nucleoside analogs in experimental trials
- The first zidovudine-resistant mutants were found in 1988.
- Zidovudine-resistant mutants occur by chance and are selected for survival because the drug does not inactivate them.
- Immunomodulators are compounds that may revitalize an immunosuppressed system.
- Soluble CD4 is the first recombinant product that has been used to neutralize HIV.
- Decoy CD4 molecules attach to HIV gp120.
- A three-dimensional structure for HIV protease has been determined.
- Knowledge of protease structure can be used to design a drug that will inhibit its activity, thereby inhibiting HIV production.
- Macrobiotics is the use of diet to promote health and prevent disease.

We are constantly humbled by the devastation that something so small can cast upon something so large. This chapter provides no final

POINT OF VIEW 7.1

MEDICAL SOLACE: A CURE?

Many diseases cause death. "We can cure those diseases," people say, "but we can't cure AIDS." Tell me, how many diseases can we cure? We cannot cure very many viral diseases, nor can we cure many of the diseases that kill people, like heart disease and forms of cancer. The concept of curing people is relatively new. The strength of physicians used to come from their capacity to accompany. Accompanying a person through an illness towards health or towards death was central to the practice of medicine, but it disappeared when the issue became one of curing.

—*Jonathan Mann,* in Thomas A. Bass, *Reinventing the Future: Conversations with the World's Leading Scientists* (Addison-Wesley, 1994)

answers; there are still debates about the details of the standard of care for HIV/AIDS patients. Additional diagnostic procedures and therapies may become available in the coming months and years. The information given herein will be revised and augmented as knowledge improves.

POINT OF VIEW 7.2

STANDARD OF TREATMENT

Access to treatment information and better health care is a political issue as well as a medical one. The more people living with HIV know about available treatments, the better equipped we are to redefine AIDS as a chronic, manageable disease and to transform our health care systems.

Treatment standards change and evolve as new drugs are tested and become available and as we learn more about HIV and how it affects the immune system. Living with HIV and AIDS means having to make important treatment decisions based on incomplete information, and adjusting those decisions over time. Know the treatments that are out there,learn about your own health status and work with your health care practitioners to support you in your treatment decisions. Don't rely exclusively on any single information source for your treatment decisions. Read widely, monitor the available information sources and adjust your treatment accordingly.

Regardless of the patient's history, there is no certain way to restore a failing immune system, so the reasonable way to manage HIV/AIDS is to treat its symptoms.

Various governmental health care agencies have estimated that between one and two million Americans are HIV-infected. Once infected, people do not get well; there is no cure. Most, but not all, will ultimately develop AIDS within an average of 9 to 16 years after HIV infection. Thus an effective HIV-directed therapy is essential. Because HIV becomes integrated within our cells' DNA (called a provirus), most likely any therapy developed will have to be administered for the rest of the patient's life.

GENERAL CONCEPT FOR ANTIMICROBIAL THERAPY: HOW IT DIFFERS FROM VIRAL THERAPY

Antimicrobial therapy usually capitalizes on some biochemically unique life cycle event or structure of a living infecting organism. It serves as a target for intervention by weakening the pathogen but not the host and altering the host's immune system to control the infection. This approach has been highly successful in the discovery and development of antibacterial chemotherapy, and has also been successful to lesser degrees for other life forms that are biochemically less distinct from man (e.g., fungi).

Viral diseases present very difficult problems because they depend largely on host cellular machinery for their existence. Interference with these processes almost always interferes with other important host physiological processes. HIV poses other challenges as well because its pathogenic properties include destruction of the human immune system.

GOALS FOR HIV AND AIDS THERAPY

Because of the complexity of HIV disease, science and society must establish both short- and long-range therapeutic goals (Figure 7-1). In the short run, the goal must be to improve both

POINT OF INFORMATION 7.1

THE BEGINNING OF ANTIBIOTIC THERAPY

It all began in the spring of 1942. A young woman was dying of blood poisoning in the Yale-New Haven Hospital after experiencing complications following a miscarriage. With her fever raging at 106°F, her doctors decided to gamble on a last-ditch measure—a new experimental drug. A courier from the Merck Pharmaceutical Company arrived carrying a brown paper bag. It contained 5.5 grams of crystalline penicillin—about a teaspoonful—representing half the wartime supply then available in the United States. The drug was passed through a filter for purification and dissolved in a saline solution for intravenous injection. Penicillin, in development for 14 years, was about to be tried in a human being.

The penicillin targeted in on the *Streptococcus* organisms causing septicema and collapsed their cell walls in much the same way that a pin deflates a balloon. By midnight, her temperature had fallen from 106°F to 100°F; by morning, it was down to normal for the first time in a month. She made a full recovery. Her month-long hospitalization cost $10 a day; the penicillin that cleansed her blood of bacteria was free.

WHERE DID THIS ANTIBIOTIC COME FROM?

In 1928, a rare airborne fungus, *Penicillium notatum,* came in through the open window of Alexander Fleming's London research lab and landed on an agar plate containing a culture of bacteria. The fungus killed the bacteria, a very significant event, but it required 10 years to produce enough of the drug to prove that it destroyed disease-causing bacteria in animals. Nazi bombing raids had relocated the historic quest for a human antibiotic from Oxford, England to America.

FROM THE MIRACLE TO AIDS

This woman's miracle began the modern war on disease. Overnight, doctors became optimists. Dr. Lewis Thomas, the distinguished medical essayist, would later note, "The realization that disease could be turned around by treatment was a totally new idea in 1942." Soon, penicillin and its 200 cousins, the "wonder drugs," had proven that medicine could control most bacterial diseases.

And yet . . .

Spring, 1993: Anthony Fauci, MD, Director of the National Institute of Allergy and Infectious Diseases at the National Institutes of Health (NIH), was born in 1940. Today, Fauci is the leader of the U.S. war on AIDS, the virus-caused disease that is beyond cure by penicillin—and so far, all other drugs (Breo, 1993).

The discovery of penicillin and numeous other antibiotics led us into a false sense of security—"we met the enemy and they are ours." Perhaps it would be better to say, we have met the enemy and they are us. Because of the wonder drugs, attention to basic research on the real issues of how bacteria, protozoa, and viruses cause disease and why they cause a disease in humans or other species was diverted to other things of importance. Mechanisms of pathogeneicity were for the most part neglected in the grand scheme of things. AIDS has brought the need for basic research back into focus as no other event has over the last 40 to 50 years.

---

the social response to those who have HIV disease and the duration and quality of life of those with AIDS. In the long run, therapeutic drugs must be found that will control the provirus and stop viral penetration of the central nervous system and the production of mutant HIV. In addition, therapy should be accessible to *all* who need it.

The ideal solution would be to prevent HIV from causing an infection. However, there is no means available to stop HIV from entering the body and infecting a limited number of cell types—primarily those cells displaying CD4 antigen receptor sites. Following infection, there is a depletion of cells carrying CD4, especially T4 cells. With T4 cell loss, over time immunological response is lost. Loss of immunological response leads to a variety of opportunistic infections (OIs). The suppression of the immune system and increasing susceptibility to OIs and cancers give HIV/AIDS a multidimensional pathology. Because HIV/AIDS is a multidimensional syndrome, it is unlikely that a *single drug* will provide adequate treatment or a cure. Many scientists worldwide are testing potential therapies for HIV-

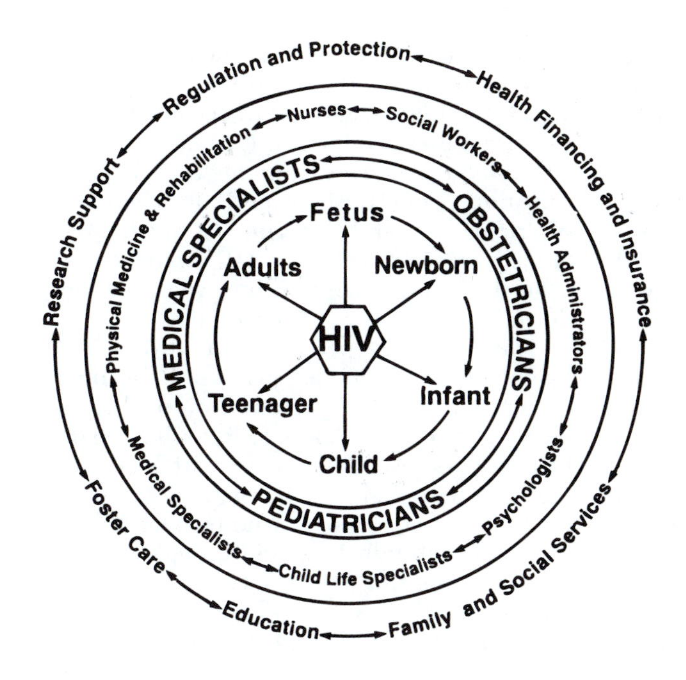

FIGURE 7-1 HIV/AIDS Presents a Challenge to Investigators, Health Care Workers, and Society. The AIDS virus is, in many ways, unlike any other human virus. There is no evidence that anyone is immune to HIV infection. All facets of society are involved in HIV/AIDS care. (*Adapted from Phillip A. Pizzo*)

infected and AIDS patients. Some of those therapies are discussed in this chapter.

TREATMENT VS. CURE

While everyone wants a cure for HIV disease and AIDS, researchers speak only of treatment. The difference between cure and treatment appears, at this moment, to be as night is to day. An effective treatment (therapy) means finding drugs *with acceptable side effect levels* that will prevent opportunistic infections, control the proviral state, and bolster the diminishing functions of a damaged immune system. At the moment there is not a single Food and Drug Administration (FDA)-approved drug (or any other drug) that is without adverse side effects, nor does it appear that such a drug will be available soon. Existing therapy for those with HIV disease and opportunistic infections or AIDS is lifelong. Stopping treatment for any disease in an AIDS patient means eventual relapse.

Can HIV Infection Be Cured?

An effective cure means cleansing the body of the AIDS virus. To find a cure, HIV incorporation into human DNA and subsequent reproduction of new virus must be understood. Without interference, the **HIV provirus** will remain in host cell DNA for the individual's lifetime. The provirus can, at any time, become activated to mass produce HIV which leads to cell death and eventually to the individual's death. As of this writing there is no way to prevent either the proviral state or proviral activation. We must learn about the molecular mechanisms the virus and cell use to govern the proviral state.

Examples of Unproven AIDS Drug Therapies

With the pandemic spread of HIV/AIDS and no cure in sight, many patients diagnosed with HIV disease or AIDS are seeking drug treatments that are not approved by the FDA. Such treatments are available through the underground network.

A University of Pennsylvania study presented in June, 1991, at the Seventh International Conference on AIDS in Florence, Italy claimed that 30% to 50% of AIDS patients use unproven alternative treatments. Members of the gay community—the largest group affected by AIDS in the United States—share treatment information by word of mouth and through community newsletters and the gay press.

There are lipid solutions—mixtures of fatty acids that promoters claim are absorbed through the intestine and work as antiviral agents. There are Chinese herbs and vitamin supplements. Many AIDS patients travel to Japan and other countries to get dextran sulfate. Some has been smuggled in from Mexico. Its side effects are painful. One user said, "It did nothing but give me diarrhea for a year and it was expensive."

Another controversial treatment is made from a Chinese cucumber and is called Compound Q (trichosanthin). A user of Compound Q said, "Q has all the side effects of chemotherapy. The pain, insomnia, dizziness—it takes you out for a couple of days after each treatment. If Q were the miracle it was held out to be, no one would hesitate to put up with its effects."

Another patient says Compound Q is an example of an underground drug gone wrong. "After the second treatment, I felt small pains in my feet, then in my ankles and then in my legs. It's 17 months later, and I'm still in pain."

At least one doctor in New York City is treating AIDS patients with ozone—a gas that he claims "kills" the AIDS virus. He claims his ozone treatment is less toxic than other drugs used on AIDS patients.

Alternative AIDS drugs are sold underground through buyers' clubs—small storefronts that sell supplemental or alternative products to people with HIV disease and AIDS. In most cities, a recorded message details what's new, what's out of stock, and how to place an order by mail. The buyers' clubs also provide mainstream health products at low prices. Some of the drugs are made in underground labs, but most are smuggled into the United States from other countries.

The FDA has given no indication that it will move to shut down the underground. The underground poses an unsolvable regulatory challenge because those whom it harms do not want their source of solace closed to them.

Alternative treatments fall into three categories:

First, there are treatments that claim to enhance the immune system. Coffee enemas and Freon enemas are popular treatments at a few holistic clinics in Mexico. These are the same Mexican clinics that sold laetrile to cancer patients from the 1950s through the 1970s. They are now selling the same extract of apricot pits to AIDS patients (Hodgin, 1991).

Second, there are treatments that focus on nutrition. They push macrobiotics, mineral supplements, and vitamin C megadoses. Nutrition is important for AIDS patients, but there is no evidence that intravenous megadoses of vitamins are effective.

Third, there are people who tell you it is all psychology, and if you just think beautiful thoughts you will get better. One of the best known therapists with a large following of HIV-positive patients is Louise L. Hay, who tells people through her books, tapes, seminars, workshops, and videos how to heal both mind and body through New Age thought. In her book *You Can Heal Your Life,* Hay prints a list of illnesses, their potential causes, and a "new thought pattern" to be repeated to heal oneself. For example, when the problem is AIDS, she writes that the probable cause is "denial of the self. Sexual guilt. A strong belief in not being 'good enough'." The recommended thought pattern to solve this problem is to repeat several times: "I am a divine magnificent expression of life. I rejoice in my sexuality. I rejoice in all that I am. I love myself." (Hodgin, 1991).

Underground Drug AL-721

INGREDIENTS.

6 1/3 tablespoons of butter
5 tablespoons of lecithin (PC-55*)
3/4 cup of water

DIRECTIONS.

1. Melt butter in a saucepan.
2. Mix PC-55 and water in a blender.
3. Very slowly add the melted butter to the PC-55–water mixture.
4. Blend the mixture for 3 to 5 minutes or until an even color is obtained.
5. Pour mixture into an ice cube tray and freeze.
6. These cubes can be sucked or broken into fragments and ingested.

*PC-55 is a commercially available lecithin (posphatidylcholine) concentrate.

BOX 7.1

UNDERGROUND DRUGS AND BUYING CLUBS

The court documents do not reveal much about Mark. He was young, he had AIDS, and he was desperate to live—so desperate that he was willing to try just about any cure, no matter how unconventional; and to trust any physician who offered one. That trust may have killed him and other desperate AIDS patients like him.

Mark began treatment in late 1988. The treatments recommended by his physician varied widely. He had injections of typhoid vaccine and of a homemade chemical concoction called Viroxan, manufactured by another physician in his kitchen sink, packaged in nonsterile vials and sold at $300 for a month's supply. Mark was told it would have a long-term effect in arresting the AIDS virus and had been tested and found nontoxic and effective against a wide spectrum of diseases.

Mark had a device called a Hickman catheter surgically implanted into his chest, allowing the Viroxan to be injected into the bloodstream directly above his heart. He was not informed that the implant itself could cause an infection—especially when used to inject a nonsterile fluid. Two weeks after the implant he began vomiting and having trouble breathing. Five days later Mark experienced total body numbness and pain. He was given an antibiotic and more Viroxan. When admitted to a medical center 3 days later, Mark was diagnosed with blood poisoning, meningitis, dehydration, pneumonia, and staphylococcal infections throughout his body. He died 4 days later.

A medical board has charged Mark's physicians with unprofessional conduct. The case against the two doctors highlights a growing problem: The number of desperate patients seeking a cure has created a frightening new market for questionable remedies.

What is this concoction? A mixed drink to which someone forgot to add the bourbon or scotch? NO; THIS IS AN UNDERGROUND FORMULA FOR MAKING **AL-721**. The claim is that AL-721 will restore health to AIDS patients. AL-721 is a lipid mixture containing glycerides, lecithin, and phosphatidylethanolamine (fos-fa-tiddle-eth-an-ol-ah-mean) in a 7:2:1 ratio.

The compound extracts cholesterol from cell membranes. This may alter the cell enough to alter the lipid content of HIV as it buds out of the cell, thus blocking the attachment of HIV to cells displaying CD4 antigen receptor sites. In early test trials, AL-721 reduced HIV reverse transcriptase activity and appeared to improve clinical symptoms. AL-721 has not yet been approved by the FDA.

HIV/AIDS Drugs in Development and FDA Approved

The **gold standard** for determining the efficacy of a new treatment is that it objectively alters the natural history of the disease in a way that is beneficial to the patient. Therefore the end points most often used in clinical trials of therapies for a chronic disease such as HIV include prolongation of life or the time to a significant disease complication.

But, studies using these end points require large numbers of patients and/or the passage of considerable amounts of time. **Surrogate markers** (i.e., physiological measurements that serve as substitutes for these major clinical events) can eliminate this problem if their validity and correlation with clinical outcome can be confirmed. The use of surrogates has the potential to shorten significantly the duration of clinical trials and expedite the development of new therapies.

The T4 or CD4 cell number is the best studied and most commonly used surrogate for clinical efficacy of antiretroviral therapies. It is imperfect, however, because changes following nucleoside antiretroviral therapy are only partially explained by the therapy. Furthermore, it exhibits a high degree of day-to-day variation in individual patients, and the assays are difficult to standardize and control for quality.

Fourteen FDA-approved medicines are presented in Table 7-1. From the end of 1988 to the end of 1991, 12 new medicines were FDA approved. Since the first AIDS medicine, zidovudine (ZDV), was approved in 1987, 13

TABLE 7-1 HIV/AIDS Opportunistic Disease FDA-Approved Medicines

Drug Name	Indication
Amphotericin B	Oral and internal fungal infections
Zithromax	Toxoplasmosis, cryptosporidosis
Azithromycin	*Mycobacterium avium*—intracellulare?
Bactrim™* trimethoprim and sulfamethoxazole	PCP prophylaxis
Biaxin Clarithromycin	Similar to zithromax
Mepron	PCP, toxoplasmosis, and cryptosporidiosis prophylaxis
Neutrexin (trimetrexate glucuronate)	PCP prophylaxis (FDA approved 1993)
Cytovene® ganciclovir (IV)	CMV retinitis
Daraprim®* pyrimethamine	Toxoplasmosis
Diflucan® fluconazole	Cryptococcal meningitis, candidiasis
Doxorubicin	AIDS-related Kaposi's sarcoma
Foscavir® foscarnet sodium	CMV retinitis
HIVID* dideoxycytosine (ddC)	For patients that cannot tolerate zidovudine; inhibits HIV replication
3TC-Cytosine Lamivudine	Works similar to ddC—FDA compassionate use approved 1994; expecting full FDA approval 1995
Intron® A* interferon alpha-2b (recombinant)	Kaposi's sarcoma; hepatitis B and C viruses; human papillomavirus
NebuPent® aerosol pentamidine isethionate	PCP prophylaxis
Pentam® 300 IM & IV pentamidine isethionate	PCP
PROCRIT®* epoetin alpha	Anemia in Retrovir-treated HIV-infected patients
Retrovir® zidovudine (ZDV)	HIV-positive asymptomatic and symptomatic, pediatric and adults; inhibits HIV replication
Marinol delta-9-tetrahydrocannabinal	Active ingredient in marijuana—FDA approved 1993 to treat anorexia in AIDS persons
Mycobutin ribabutin	Prevents *Mycobacterium avium* complex infection
Roferon® -A* interferon alpha-2a, recombinant	Kaposi's sarcoma
Stavudine (d4T) didehydrothymidine	Works similar to ddI—FDA approved June 1994.
Septra®* trimethoprim and sulfamethoxazole	PCP
VIDEX®	Treatment of adult and pediatric patients didanosine (ddI) (over 6 months of age) with advanced HIV infection, who are intolerant or who have demonstrated significant clinical or immunological deterioration during Retrovir® therapy; inhibits HIV replication
Zovirax® acyclovir	Herpes simplex, varicella zoster
Valacyclovir	Valine ester of acyclovir; near FDA approval; much better than acyclovir

*Denotes medicines that have been approved by the FDA for other conditions.
(Source: Pharmaceutical Manufacturers Association, 1991)

more therapies for AIDS and AIDS-related conditions have gone on the market. In 1991, three medicines were approved. One of them, didanosine or dideoxyinosine (ddI), is the second medicine that prevents HIV reproduction to be approved. The other drugs approved were Epoetin alpha for the treatment of anemia in ZDV-treated AIDS patients, and foscarnet for CMV retinitis. In April 1992, the FDA-approved zalcitabine or dideoxycytosine (ddC), the third nucleoside drug that prevents HIV reproduction.

Much research is committed to developing compounds that will inactivate the virus. Two means of attacking the virus are: (1) to destroy or block the virus's glycoprotein that fits the CD4 receptor sites (Figure 7-2); and (2) to block the activity of the reverse transcriptase enzyme, thus allowing host cell enzymes to degrade viral DNA. Other parts of the HIV reproductive cycle that may be interrupted to prevent infection and viral reproduction can be seen in Figure 7-2. Drugs that perform some of these functions are being studied in human clinical trials. However, into 1995 only four drugs, all nucleoside analogs, that interfere with reverse transcriptase activity have been FDA approved for treating HIV disease and AIDS. They are *zidovudine* (ZDV), often mistakenly called AZT (*3′-azido-2′,3′-deoxythymidine*), trade name *Retrovir*; *didanosine* or *ddI* (*2′,3′-dideoxyinosine*), trade name *VIDEX*; *dideoxycytosine*, zalcitabine, or *ddC* (*2′,3′-dideoxycytosine*), trade name *HIVID;* and stavudine or d4T, trade name zerit. A fifth nucleoside analog, lamivudine or 3CT, has been FDA approved but for compassionate use only. Full approval is expected in 1995.

Drug Approval Processes

Drug approval in the United States is a rigorous and often controversial process. With the Kefauver amendments to the Food and Drug Act adopted by Congress in 1962, a drug's sponsor is required to prove not only that a drug is safe, but also efficacious—it must work. Drug companies must prove their drug meets FDA standards before approval is granted. Testing is required—sometimes double-blind, placebo-controlled, multicenter trials—and the outcome must be statistically significant.

This stringent standard was established in the United States after the thalidomide incident. The drug, widely prescribed in Europe, was in the process of being evaluated by the FDA in the early 1960s when one official, Frances Kelsey, concerned by reports of peripheral neuropathy associated with thalidomide use, delayed its approval. In the interim, the link between thalidomide and birth defects (typically, warped limbs) became apparent. Although a major catastrophe had been averted, some 3,750 women of child-bearing age (624 of whom were reportedly pregnant) had already taken thalidomide on an experimental basis.

Model for Research and Approval of a New Drug— The general model for research and development of a drug is fundamentally a two-stage process. In the first stage, discovery, a potential new treatment is initially identified. The second stage, development, includes a series of preclinical and clinical studies as well as production steps in which the treatment is progressively characterized for use in routine clinical care. This model of research and development is usually applied to single drugs, but its conceptual features are equally useful for other pharmacological approaches (e.g., combination chemotherapy) or modalities (e.g., immune reconstitution). Logistically, it results in a series of decision points where progressively accumulating data are used to determine or design the next set of experiments or production steps; this process thereby ensures participants' safety while permitting the most efficient utilization of resources. This approach is widely employed by the pharmaceutical industry to identify and implement the critical path studies, which lead to a new drug's licensure.

However, AIDS and cancer interest groups, along with an increasing number of scientists and laypeople, argue that in determining drug approval or a drug's worth, more than just life or death should be considered. For example, improvement in the quality of life while using the drug should be of importance. For example, although existing antiretroviral drugs are not curative and their duration of effectiveness

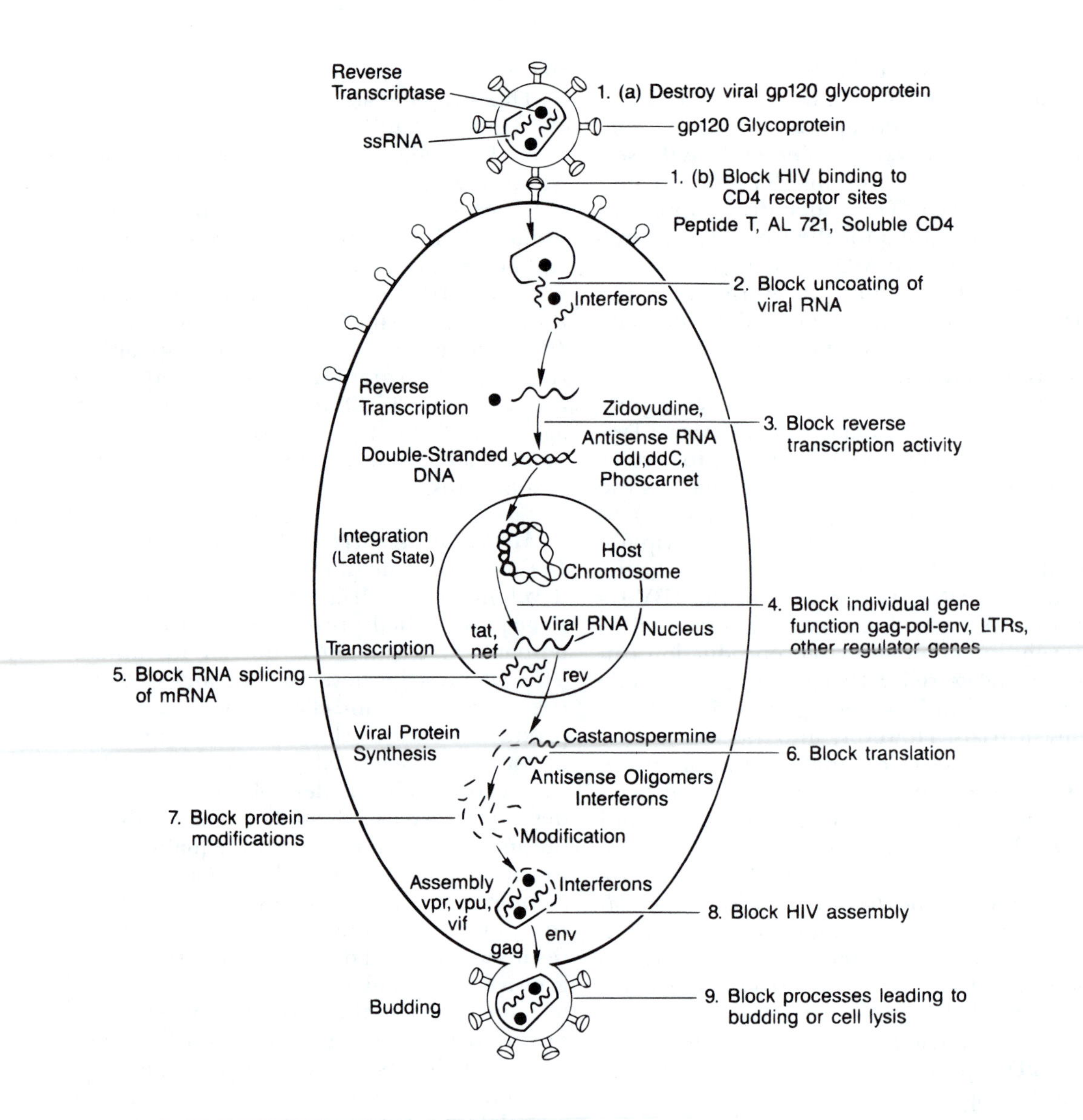

FIGURE 7-2 Blocking HIV Infection and Viral Reproduction. AIDS research is involved in producing drugs that can stop the virus from CD4 receptor cell attachment, HIV budding, or, in some cases, cell lysis. Antibodies have been developed to block CD4 cell receptor sites. Expression of HIV genes is controlled by a complex network. The genes in the diagram are at the positions where their products are involved in HIV replication. *Tat,* located in the nucleus, increases transcription by *tat* protein binding to newly synthesized RNA. *Rev,* also located in the nucleus, is necessary for the export of partially spliced mRNA from the nucleus. The role of the *nef* gene remains controversial. *Vif,* *vpu,* *vpr,* and *gag* gene products are all found in the cytoplasm. *Vpu* and *vif* are essential in virus assembly. How other gene products bring about HIV reproduction is in question.

is limited because they have dose-limiting toxicities, they have been shown to extend life and prolong disease-free survival in defined patient populations.

Both the National Institutes of Health (NIH) and the FDA have been accused by AIDS activists of slowing the approval process on new experimental therapies. They claim that American AIDS patients are being denied promising treatments available elsewhere in the world. This has been a rallying point for a group of AIDS patients who first called themselves Persons With AIDS (PWA). They are now referred to as Persons Living With AIDS (PLWA). PLWA groups have repeatedly interrupted scientific presentations through the first nine international AIDS conferences.

Federal officials counter that the "promising treatments" lack scientific proof of safety and efficacy. According to Martin Hirsch, an AIDS investigator, "Never have so many antiviral drugs been developed this rapidly and never have so many clinical trials been begun for viral diseases so rapidly." There are 185 antiviral drugs, immunomodulators, and vaccines currently under development and investigation in the United States. Ninety-one of them pertain solely to AIDS.

According to many scientific investigators, research on AIDS treatment has moved further and faster than research on virtually any other fatal and/or sexually transmitted disease. For example, tuberculosis had been known for centuries before the causative agent was found in 1882; and an effective treatment was not discovered until 1944, some 64 years later. It took 57 years to find an effective treatment for influenza, 75 years for cholera, 30-plus years for polio, many hundreds of years for the black plague, and over 2,000 years for smallpox.

The reason for the delay in bringing effective treatments to the general population has been the strict FDA regulations for general drug use approval. The FDA believes that it is prudent to deny approval before *all* precautionary investigative criteria have been satisfied.

The American system, which uses three-phase testing for new drug approval, is perhaps the most rigorous in the world (Table 7-2). Only one of every 4,000 compounds screened will be licensed as a new drug (Breo, 1991). It takes, on average, 12 years and 231 million dollars in research and development for an experimental drug to reach the market (Pharmaceutical Mfg. Assoc., 1991).

Change in FDA Policy— Perhaps for the first time since the FDA set its operational drug approval guidelines, nonscientists, with the help of scientists, have forced the FDA to reevaluate and change its policy.

In 1988, the FDA adopted an interim rule, a policy aimed at speeding drug approval for treatment to patients with AIDS and other life-threatening or debilitating diseases.

Parallel Tracking (Fast Tracking)— In 1991, the FDA established a new drug approval program called parallel tracking (some refer to this as fast tracking). In parallel tracking, data for any new drug used in clinical trials are collected on a few hundred people over a limited time span—a few months. Promising new drugs are made available to physicians in exchange for an agreement that they will continue to collect data and report back to the FDA. This procedure represents a fundamental shift in the accepted mode of drug testing—a shift in which patients assume far more of the risk involved in the testing of unproved drugs. Not all patients want to shoulder the additional risk.

The potential downside of moving to the more rapid approval of new drugs was recently demonstrated by the findings of the European Concorde study of zidovudine in asymptomatic patients with HIV. That 3-year investigation has brought into question the briefer, 1-year study conducted in the United States on which clinical recommendations were made. The Concorde studies are presented later in this chapter.

FDA Approval of Zidovudine— From 1985 to 1987, while the FDA was being encouraged to alter its traditional three-phase investigational policy, zidovudine (ZDV) was shown to generate anti-HIV activity. In 1985, ZDV rapidly completed phase I trials. In 1986, ZDV investigators terminated phase II trials before completion because of the significant drop in mortality among those receiving it. (Only one person receiving ZDV died, com-

TABLE 7-2 Drug Development and Approval Process

	Preclinical Testing	Phase I	Phase II	Phase III	FDA Review	Final Approval
Years	3.5	1	2	3	2.5	Total = 12
Test population	Laboratory and animal studies	20 to 80 healthy volunteers	100 to 300 patient volunteers	1,000 to 3,000 patient volunteers		Postmarketing safety monitoring
Purpose	Assess safety and biological activity	Determine safety and dosage	Evaluate effectiveness Look for side effects	Verify effectiveness, monitor adverse reactions from long-term use	Review process	Large-scale manufacturing
			Expedited Review: Phases II and III combined to shorted approval process on new medicines for serious & life-threatening diseases			Distribution Education
% of all new drugs that pass		70% of INDs	33% of INDs	27% of INDs	20% of INDs	

It takes 12 years on average for an experimental drug to travel from lab to medicine chest. Only 5 in 4,000 compounds screened in preclinical testing make it to human testing. One of these five tested in humans is approved.
(Source: Pharmaceutical Manufacturers Association, 1990)

pared to 19 deaths in the placebo groups over the same time period. Thus drug trials stopped in this case for compassionate reasons after the first sign that the drug worked.) In just 14 months, ZDV was made available to physicians under an investigational new drug program. ZDV was approved by the FDA in March 1987.

FDA Approval of Dideoxyinosine and Dideoxycytosine— In 1989 and 1991, the drugs dideoxyinosine and dideoxycytosine, respectively, were made available in phase I trials to people with signs and symptoms of AIDS and to AIDS patients who could not tolerate ZDV. This was an example of parallel tracking. Like ZDV, ddI and ddC stop HIV replication while producing fewer side effects. These were the first FDA-unapproved drugs to become widely available so early in the FDA testing protocol. In October 1991, ddI was FDA approved and ddC was approved for use in combination with ZDV, for those with advanced HIV disease, in April 1992. (Approval of ddC was based on limited data from two studies, each involving fewer than 100 persons.)

Backlash to FDA Policy— Despite the FDA's willingness to change policy, there are laypeople and scientists who feel that the FDA has not gone far enough fast enough to release experimental drugs to HIV/AIDS patients. From the very beginning of the AIDS epidemic, AIDS patients have grasped at any "treatment" that might offer relief from the symptoms of AIDS. Drugs of all varieties were and are, to some degree, still being smuggled into the United States from Europe and Mexico. In 1988, the FDA advised its agents in writing to ignore the importation of certain unapproved drugs by patients for their own use (Freedman et al., 1989). Drugs that are taken on the basis of potential benefit but have not been either accepted or rejected by the experts of the medical community are called nonvalidated drugs. Nonvalidated drugs, along with, for example, specific diets said to offer great health benefits to AIDS patients, are called nonvalidated therapies.

Nonvalidated Therapies— Nonvalidated therapies are not customary or medically accepted treatments, but neither are they considered "quack medicine." They are drugs, diets, and lifestyle changes that benefit some patients some of the time, but have not had sufficient support to be formally investigated. Investigation of a nonvalidated therapy with respect to human response under all types of conditions would require trained personnel and a great deal of time and money.

POINT OF INFORMATION 7.2

PREMATURE CONSEQUENCES: AIDS ACTIVISTS NOW FAVOR A MORE DELIBERATE APPROACH FOR AIDS DRUG APPROVAL

Across the country, thousands of people with HIV/AIDS read with disbelief the headline on the cover of the August 15, 1994 issue of Barron's Magazine—"Do We Have Too Many Drugs for AIDS?"—and the article within. Some say they wept. Others were more angry than they had ever been before.

The Treatment Action Group (TAG), an organization of the country's most powerful AIDS treatment activists, had written to Dr. David Kessler, the Commissioner of the Food and Drug Administration (FDA). TAG urged Kessler to withhold accelerated approval for a drug called Saquinavir—the first of a new class of anti-HIV compounds called *protease inhibitors*—because the data to prove that it works was incomplete.

Whether intended or not TAG's letter was an unexpected bombshell dropped into the heart of the FDA's accelerated approval system. Never, before had AIDS activists said that the government should prevent the distribution of a promising new AIDS drug. Moreover, TAG's objection to Saquinavir had less to do with the drug itself than with the limitations of the kind of research that makes it possible to have an accelerated approval system in the first place.

It sounded unthinkable. Long-time AIDS activists were saying that the Food and Drug Administration's accelerated drug approval system, widely regarded as their greatest accomplishment, was a mistake. They said that a new generation of AIDS drugs should be kept off the market until researchers can test them in "large simple trials" that may take two years or longer to complete. Most astonishing of all, they said that one third of the participants in those trials—as many as 6,000 people—should receive a placebo. "We were naive," admits same members of the TGA, "there are standards for a reason." People at TAG and many drug investigators now believe that testing of new drugs has been so inadequate, that no one can tell if the drugs work and that with the way things now are, no one will ever know.

Some people at the FDA may wish to point to the activists' change in philosophy as proof that their earlier zeal was misguided and dangerous to their cause. But the entire AIDS research and medical community has been undergoing an intense period of reassessment. Activists were not the only people who assumed AIDS would quickly fall before some magic bullet molded by science. As that illusion fades, more realistic—and successful—strategies are emerging.

To AIDS patients, time is of the essence and they are willing to try anything. However, there are some practical and moral issues to consider in providing treatment, even in desperate situations. Two sides of the dispute are presented here in point-counterpoint fashion.

Point. In keeping with AIDS patients' needs, Mathilde Krim, founding chairman of the American Foundation For AIDS Research (AmFAR), proposed maintaining FDA regulations with respect to asymptomatic HIV-infected individuals and those in AIDS-related

BOX 7.2

YOU CALL IT

A new drug has just been developed that might improve the immune systems of people with HIV/AIDS. So far it has only been tested on animals. No one knows whether it actually is effective or what its side effects may be. Furthermore, if it is effective, no one knows the minimum effective dosage or the maximum tolerated dosage. On what basis should people with HIV/AIDS begin to receive this drug? Should access to the drug be restricted at first to people who are willing to participate in carefully controlled, randomized, blind studies where they do not know whether they are receiving the drug or a placebo; or should it be given to the patients of physicians who will administer the drug, record the results, and report the results back to the FDA? Perhaps it should be given to those who ask for it, after they sign a malpractice release for the physician. You make the decision or provide an acceptable alternative.

BOX 7.3

The vigil for William "Skip" Bluette (continued from page 94) 48 hours before he died. Time and therapy were running out on "Skip." His last wish was to have his sisters Arlene and Nancy near when he died and they were there. On July 15, 1988 the doctors told Nancy and her mother that Skip's kidneys had failed—this time Skip would not recover. He died on July 17. He was 42 years old.

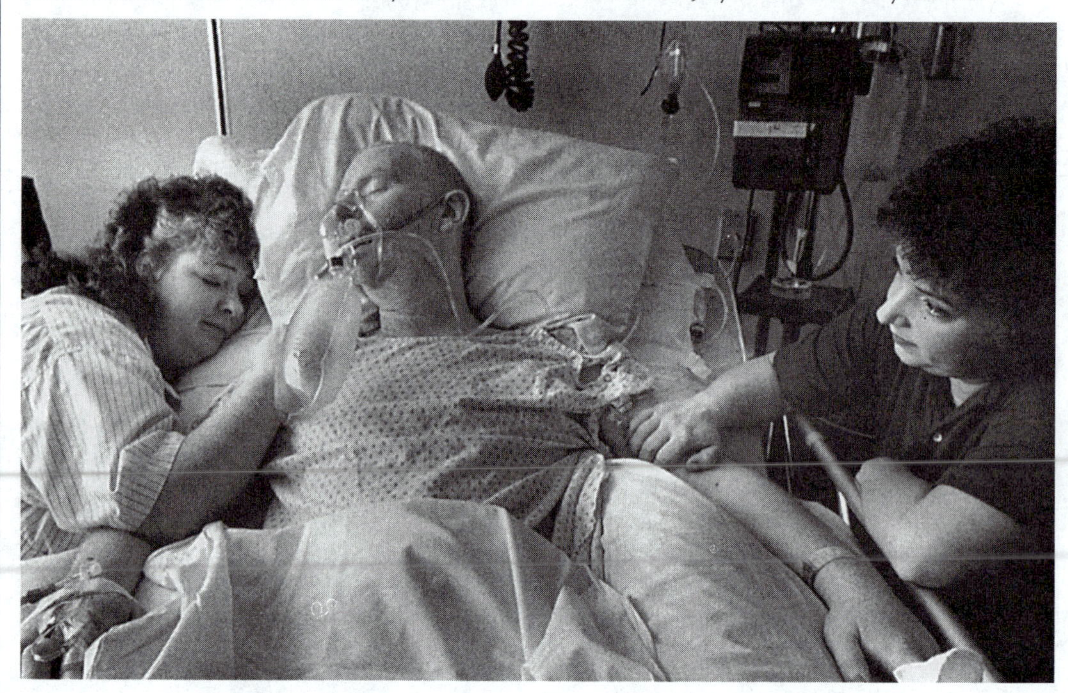

FIGURE 7-3 The Vigil for William "Skip" Bluette. The Bluette family rallied around Skip from the moment they found out he had AIDS. In April 1988, his mother had a heart attack but she survived it. Skip celebrated his 42nd birthday on May 18; it was his second birthday since his diagnosis. (*By permission of Mara Lavitt and* The New Haven Register)

complex (ARC) but *eliminating all restrictions to free access, under the supervision of a physician, to any substance proposed for treatment for a person with AIDS.* Krim feels that offering such treatment is ethically imperative. She says, "Permitting physicians to use experimental drugs to treat patients whose lives are in immediate jeopardy should not be done out of a wishful belief that the treatment would work. It should be done out of respect for the patient's right to fight for life with whatever tools we can offer" (Krim, 1986).

COUNTERPOINT. Because the AIDS patient is terminal and nothing is going to save his or her life, does it follow that he or she is beyond being hurt, beyond having the suffering increased by the use of untried or unproven drugs or nutritional regimes? It has already been demonstrated that some experimental drugs can, when used at the wrong time or without supervision, actually hasten the patient's death. For example, ZDV can be beneficial to AIDS patients, but the harm-to-benefit ratio changes with time. Early on, ZDV is so toxic to some patients that it most likely enhances opportunistic infections by causing loss of overall stamina. Studies on the drug *suramin* clearly showed it to be toxic to AIDS patients and to increase their immune disorders and loss of adrenal function. In 1985, cancer patients found hope in the announcement that interleukin-2, a molecule derived from the human immune system, could be used to stop several types of cancer. Before the ink was dry, it was reported that four out of 157 patients were killed by use of the compound.

The death of any patient should never be considered to be so imminent that misguided treatment is allowed. One should never believe that the quality of the AIDS patient's life cannot be impaired regardless of treatment. Oliver Wendell Holmes, Sr. once said, "If all of the unproven remedies doctors carry in their saddle bags were to be dumped into the ocean, it would be so much the better for their patients and so much the worse for the fish" (Freedman, 1989). Hippocrates (460–350 BC) said, "I shall use treatment for the good of the sick to the best of my ability and judgment, and I shall refrain from using it for either harm or wrongdoing."

Eight years after Krim's first quote, in 1993, Krim stated, with respect to experimental drug use, that "People have to be warned that this [experimental drug tests] has all been done in test tubes—not in human beings. Drugs in human beings can have toxicity that you cannot see in the laboratory. Nobody should try to medicate themselves."

SUMMARY. One of the great challenges is to achieve a balance between the rights of incurably ill patients who want access to drugs of unproven efficacy and the obligation of society to protect medical consumers from unproven drugs. It will lead us to new formulations of social practice and policy that go far beyond AIDS.

Focus on Zidovudine (ZDV), Dideoxyinosine (ddI), Dideoxycytosine (ddC), and Stavudine (d4T)

Each of the four drugs (Figure 7-4) has limited effectiveness. The principal limitations are: (1) they will not cure HIV disease; (2) positive medical effects are short term, they are not sustained; (3) each drug has its own set of toxic side effects; and (4) their ability to delay the onset of AIDS was brought into question by the European Concorde studies.

UNITED STATES VS. ANGLO-FRENCH FINDINGS ON THE USE OF ZIDOVUDINE TO DELAY PROGRESSION TO AIDS

United States

During 1988–1989, United States investigators conducted a large, 1-year study which suggested that the drug zidovudine (ZDV) could delay the onset of symptomatic disease. These results led the FDH to approve the use of ZDV in asymptomatic people infected with HIV. FDA approval was given based on two separate clinical trials in which those subjects receiving ZDV had fewer progressions to AIDS over an average of 12 months than those on placebo (inert medication). Therapy with ZDV was recommended for all HIV-infected persons, even those who were totally asymptomatic, once their T4 cell counts fell below 500/mm^3. An entire program of early intervention was built around the use of ZDV, resulting in a dramatic increase in HIV antibody testing, standards for monitoring disease progression through T4 counts, and aggressive use of immunizations and *Pneumocystis carinii* pneumonia (PCP) prophylaxis. Virtually all trials of antiviral drugs used ZDV as **the standard** in the United States (and to a lesser extent in Europe and Australia) and specific studies were launched to test its efficacy in children, in pregnant women (to interrupt vertical transmission), and for postexposure prophylaxis. The fact that ZDV caused a transient rise in T4 cell number resulted in the use of this surrogate marker to screen other promising agents for efficacy, and as a replacement for clinical end points for drug approvals, in order to speed additional agents to patients with advanced disease.

Thus, for clinical investigators and practitioners attending the Ninth International Conference on AIDS in June, 1993, the news of the Anglo-French Concorde studies, which

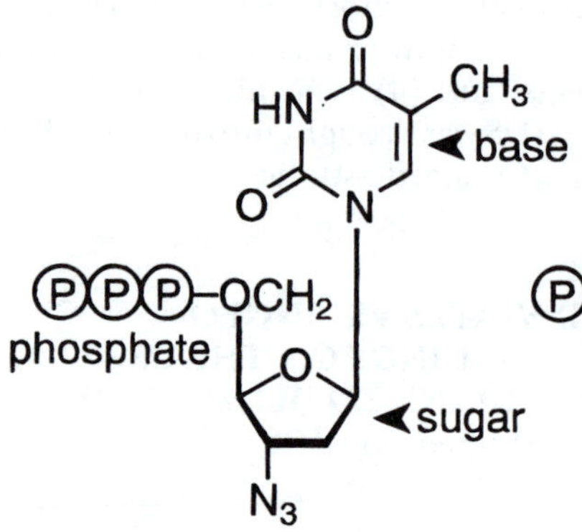

AZT-TP
(azidothymidine)
(zidovudine)

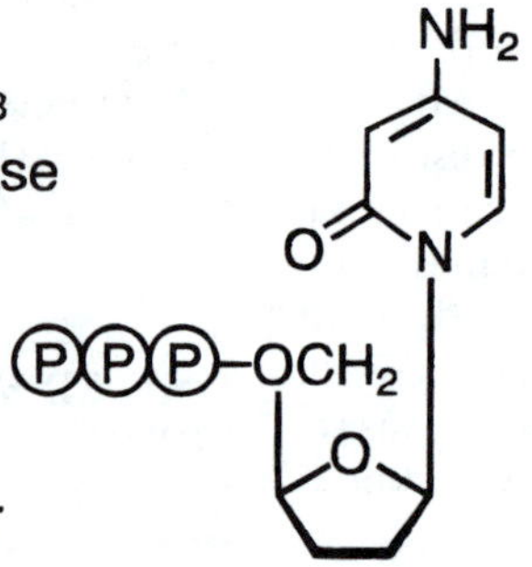

ddC-TP
(dideoxycytosine)
(zalcitabine)

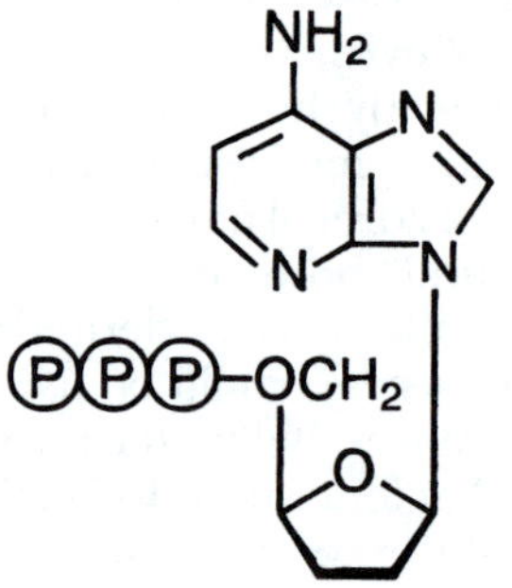

ddA-TP
(dideoxyinosine)
(active form of didanosine)

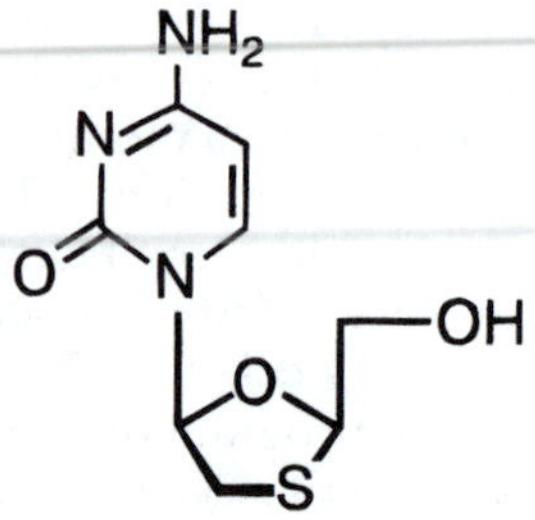

3TC
(lamivudine)

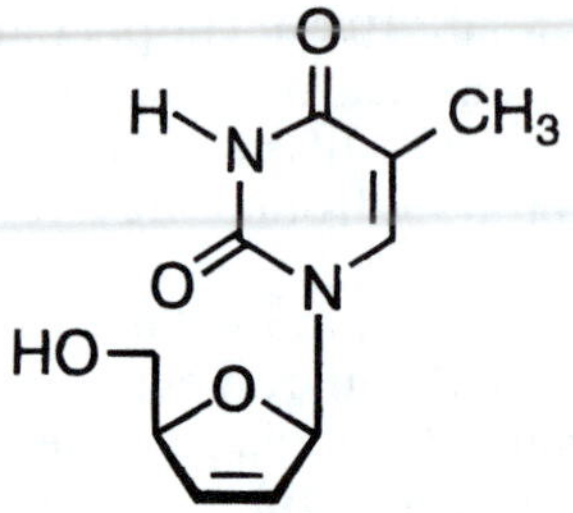

d4T
(stavudine)

FIGURE 7-4 Structure of Five FDA-Approved Drugs for HIV/AIDS. The drug 3TC has been FDA approved for compassionate use only. Full Approval of 3TC is expected in 1995. These nucleoside analog agents competitively inhibit physiological deoxynucleoside triphosphates (part of the HIV proviral DNA chain) when incorporated by HIV reverse transcriptase, causing DNA chain termination. Azidothymidine triphosphate (AZT-TP) competes with deoxythymidine triphosphate (dTTP), dideoxycytidine triphosphate (ddC-TP) competes with deoxycytidine triphosphate (dCTP), and dideoxyinosine (ddI, not shown) is converted to dideoxyadenosine triphosphate (ddA-TP), which competes with deoxyadenosine triphosphate (dATP). Stavudine (d4T) competes with deoxythmidine triphosphate (dTTP).

showed that **ZDV did not prolong life or delay the onset of AIDS**, was clearly unsettling. Data were presented which raised serious questions about the extent to which ZDV truly benefits those early in disease, the value of T4 counts as a surrogate marker of drug effect, the true efficacy of other nucleoside analogs such as ddC and ddI, and the likelihood that much publicized newer drugs will result in clinically useful approaches in the near future.

Anglo-French Concorde Studies

The Concorde trial was a multicenter, randomized, double-blind, placebo-controlled trial conducted in Europe, designed to determine whether HIV-infected adults benefit from starting ZDV therapy while still asymptomatic rather than deferring therapy until symptoms develop. The investigators analyzed data from 1,749 patients randomized to early or delayed treatment between October 1988 and October 1991 and followed through December 1992 (mean follow-up, 3 years).

Publication of the preliminary analysis of the Concorde trial data dominated discussion of antiretroviral treatment during the 1993 Ninth International Conference on AIDS. The subsequent presentations in Berlin on the trial corroborated its conclusion that a strategy of starting zidovudine in the asymptomatic stage of HIV infection, rather than deferring such therapy until symptoms develop, does not prolong life or delay the onset of late HIV symptoms or AIDS.

The Concorde analysis was based on the use of asymptomatic HIV-infected individuals, randomized to receive ZDV (4 × 250 mg/day; n = 877) or matching placebo (n = 872). The end points of the trial were based on one or more minor opportunistic infections, death, or severe drug toxicity (Aboulker et al., 1993).

The Concorde results seem at first sight to conflict with those from a large U.S. trial [AIDS Clinical Trial Group (ACTG) 019] published in April, 1990. ACTG 019 showed that ZDV treatment of asymptomatic HIV-infected individuals with T4 cell counts of less than 500/mm^3 did slow HIV disease progression to AIDS. However, the Concorde trial lasted approximately 3 years—about three times that of ACTG 019. All studies conducted in comparable populations of asymptomatic HIV-infected subjects show that ZDV delays disease progression after 1 year of follow-up, but that this effect **disappears with prolonged follow-up**. Possible explanations for this waning of effect are many and complex. Many investigators now believe that the time-limited effect of ZDV is most likely related to the development of HIV-ZDV-resistant strains.

It is clear from Concorde and other studies presented (Hamilton, 1992; Jacobsen 1993; Lundgren, 1994; Phair, 1994; Volberding, 1994) that the nucleoside analogs—such as ZDV, zalcitabine (ddC), and didanosine (ddI)—are relatively weak anti-HIV drugs, even when used in combination, and that they are not going to provide the final answer for the management of HIV infection.

FUTURE USE OF ZDV, DDI, AND DDC ANTIVIRAL THERAPY

The results of the combined United States and Anglo-French studies have left investigators puzzled about the use of ZDV therapy. Data presented on the effects of antivirals later in disease course were perhaps even more difficult to interpret. Data presented from a later (1993) study, AIDS Clinical Trial Group (ACTG) 118, compared three different doses of ddI in patients with advanced disease who were unable to tolerate ZDV, or were clearly progressing to AIDS while on ZDV. This study demonstrated no difference in these three treatment groups in death rates or in time to death.

Since the Concorde study report, clinicians are faced with a difficult set of questions: What is the optimal time to begin ZDV therapy, if at all? If a patient has been on ZDV therapy for a long time and has dropping T4 cell counts, should the drug be stopped, switched for another or given in addition to another drug? For late-stage disease, is there any real role for antiviral therapy, and if so, which one? Is combination therapy worthwhile, at least in the group of patients with T4 counts between 150 and 300 cells, and is it worth the extra toxicity? (Cotton, 1993). After over 9 years of studies and use of ZDV, it would appear that investigators are almost back to square one with regard to antiviral drug therapies.

New Physician Guidelines on the Use of Zidovudine

In June of 1993, an independent panel of HIV drug-use experts created by the United States government recommended a major shift in strategy for treating HIV-infected persons. The panel's view is that physicians should no longer automatically prescribe the antiviral drug ZDV to HIV-infected individuals whose immune systems have begun to deteriorate but who have not yet developed AIDS symptoms.

The recommendations emphasize that patients and doctors should decide together about when and how to treat HIV by focusing on the patient's views about drug therapy, personal health, and other factors that vary in each case. The guidelines recognize that individuals respond to ZDV differently and that before starting ZDV therapy, in each case, the drug's benefits and risks, like bleeding and anemia, should be fully discussed.

Treatment guidelines for symptomless, HIV-infected people are no longer solely based on T4 cell counts!

Conclusion

Clearly there are take-home messages from the combined United States–Anglo-French studies. They are as follows:

1. The present generation of antiviral agents is weak, and new and novel drugs must be found.
2. There is need for a greater understanding of the virus itself and of the pathogenesis of the disease.
3. Clinical trials may need to revert to the use of traditional clinical end points.
4. Scientists should probably reconsider whether, with this great uncertainty about antiviral drug use, some placebo-controlled trials should be initiated.
5. There is a need for increased emphasis on prevention and treatment of opportunistic infection because of the increasing pessimism over the value of antiviral therapies.
6. Given the uncertainty created by the present drug situation, the wisdom of providing early access to drugs which have not been rigorously tested may be seen as questionable, even in life-threatening disease.

It can be seen from the Concorde studies that many questions remain about the optimum use of these drugs when used singly or in combination. Improving treatment for HIV disease and AIDS will require that new agents be found. Whatever drug or drugs are developed, the ideal agent should provide **curative** therapy. To do so the agent should meet three criteria: (1) Restore full-term life expectancy to HIV-positive individuals; (2) eliminate the carrier state of HIV (that is, eliminate the ability of HIV-positive individuals to infect others with the virus); and (3) eradicate functional HIV genetic information (the provirus) in people infected with the virus.

All three criteria are important. Restoring the health of HIV-positive individuals without eliminating their ability to infect others would be a disaster because it would increase the spread of HIV.

The problem is we know what we need in the way of a drug but lack the knowledge, at the moment, necessary to find it. And that is where the problem begins. Over the years, scientists and the lay press have given people the idea that, with respect to disease, whatever comes can be dealt with swiftly and successfully (see Point of Information 7.1). But this is not true, and never has been; most things are not possible in the battle between medicines and disease. Most of the human diseases are self-cured—we don't even know in most cases that we have been exposed to a disease-causing agent. Over time, certain drugs have been developed that save lives, but millions more die from disease each year than surgery or medications such as antibiotics save. Anthony Fauci, Director of the National Institute of Allergy and Infectious Diseases, (Figure 7-5) states that "HIV disease is extraordinarily complex. The disease has many components and is characterized by multiple and overlapping phases of active viral replication, inappropriate immune activation, elevated secretion of immune system proteins called cytokines, and immune deficiency. This complexity suggests that therapeutic strategies for the treatment of

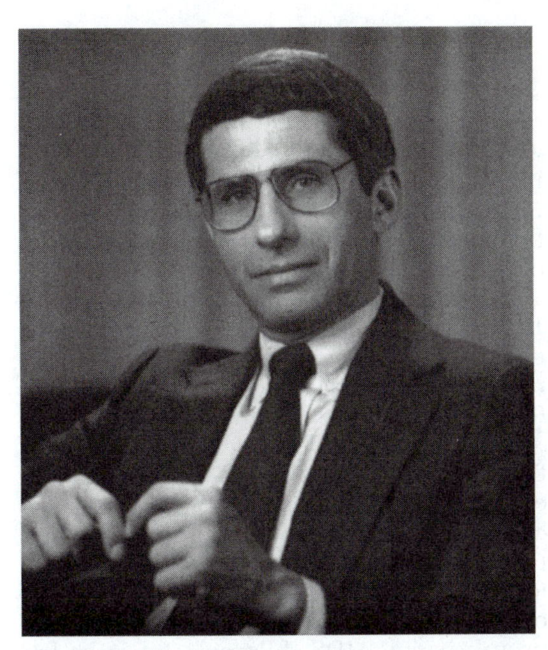

FIGURE 7-5 Anthony S. Fauci, M.D. (1989). Director, National Institute of Allergy and Infectious Diseases, National Institutes of Health; Associate Director of NIH for AIDS Research.

people with HIV must be multidimensional and comprehensive, addressing all of HIV's known pathogenic mechanisms."

ZIDOVUDINE THERAPY

Cost of Zidovudine

The yearly cost for ZDV in mid-1989 was about $10,000. In September 1989, the manufacturer reduced the price from $3.00 to $1.20 per capsule, which lowered the overall cost to about $6,400 (Anderson et al., 1991). Five capsules of ZDV, a day's supply, contain an estimated 15 cents worth of ingredients, but cost about $1.00 to $2.00 to manufacture. They did sell for about $6.00 to $9.00 at the drugstore. In 1993, ZDV cost $250/gram or $113,500/pound. Patient cost per year was down to $3,000/year.

Side Effects of Zidovudine

This drug, long the standard of AIDS therapy, is now believed to be of only limited value for a limited time and can be highly toxic. Patients may first experience nausea, rash, insomnia, vomiting, malaise, and headaches, which will lessen with dose reduction. In addition, loss of red blood cells leads to severe macrocytic anemia in 40% of AIDS patients and requires dosage reduction or blood transfusion. Only 60% of AIDS patients can tolerate ZDV therapy for more than 1 year. Prolonged use of ZDV has also been associated with symptomatic myopathy similar to that produced by human immunodeficiency virus.

Zidovudine Therapy for the HIV-Infected

The drawback to using ZDV is that most often it produces grave toxic side effects. Treatment of AIDS patients with ZDV during the first 6 months leads to a significant reduction in disease progression and in the number of HIVs present in the blood. At between 6 and 18 months, the number of HIVs rises. Two mechanisms have been proposed to explain the failure of ZDV therapy: the occurrence of ZDV-resistant mutants and the location of ZDV within cells where the virus replicates (McLean et al., 1991).

The potential for an expanded role for ZDV in HIV infection is being investigated worldwide. Preliminary evidence suggests that ZDV may be effective in AIDS-associated dementia, HIV-associated thrombocytopenia (abnormally low number of platelets in the blood), and HIV-associated psoriasis (a scaly red rash most prevalent at the joints). These findings may eventually apply to all or most of the millions of HIV-infected and many thousands of AIDS patients in the world. This raises the important question of funding for massive use of ZDV therapy. If all HIV-infected people were to receive ZDV, the costs would run into billions of dollars.

Preliminary Results of Zidovudine and Intravenous Immunoglobulin Therapy in Children

By mid-1995, over 6,500 cases of pediatric AIDS were reported in the United States. Information from the Centers for Disease Control and Prevention (CDC) indicates that the real number may be three or four times greater. Over 80% of these children acquired the virus from their mothers before or during birth, either through the placenta or within the birth canal. Seventy percent of the mothers were injection drug users or the sexual partners of injection drug users (*AIDS Newslink*, 1992). There are several reports of children becoming HIV-infected shortly after birth, possibly from the mother's breast milk. In other cases, children have been infected through blood transfusion or blood products. Now that all blood is screened for HIV, transfusion and hemophilia treatment pose only a very small risk. (HIV transmission via breast milk is discussed in Chapter 8.)

AIDS tends to present differently in children than in adults. While both suffer frequent opportunistic infections, children have more visible brain disease. Several studies suggest that brain damage will eventually occur in all AIDS-afflicted children. AIDS also progresses much more rapidly in children than in adults. The most frequent OI, especially in those under 1 year of age, is *Pneumocystis Carinii* pneumonia (Crain, 1991).

Based on 1987 data from patients who acquired AIDS from blood transfusions, British scientists reported that children under the age of 5 at the time of HIV infection developed their first symptoms of AIDS *about 2 years after transfusion.* This is at least four times earlier than the 10-year clinical latency period seen in adult patients.

Pediatric Zidovudine Therapy— In late 1988, Phillip Pizzo and colleagues reported on treatment of children with ZDV (Pizzo et al., 1988). Most of the children experienced improved appetites, weight gain, and increased T4 cell counts. They also experienced reduction in the size of swollen lymph nodes, enlarged livers, and spleens.

The most prevalent characteristic of AIDS in children—loss of mental function and verbal and motor skills due to AIDS encephalopathy—showed a marked improvement. Prior to the initiation of therapy, about two-thirds of the children in the study showed mental deterioration. All of the children improved according to serial measurement of IQ scores after 3 and 6 months of continuous therapy. One 11-year-old whose IQ had dropped 28 points after HIV infection returned to 99 after 9 months of treatment. Equally significant changes were seen in younger children who regained the ability to walk, talk, or exhibit other developmental achievements. Pizzo suggests that impaired cognitive function may be among the earliest manifestations of pediatric AIDS.

In contrast with previously published data, a 12-month study, by Molly Nozyce and co-workers (1994) demonstrated no improvement in neurodevelopmental functioning in 54 HIV-infected children treated with oral zidovudine.

Several new studies have shown, however, that children with advanced HIV disease tolerate ZDV well and respond by showing clinical improvement in their immune systems and the reduction of measurable virus in their bodies (McKinney et al., 1991). Because drugs for children must go through a separate FDA approval system, AIDS children tend to be left out of the network of new drug therapies such as ddI and ddC.

Intravenous Immunoglobulin— Immunoglobulins are proteins produced by B lymphocytes. The immunoglobulins are, in effect, antibodies. Intravenous immunoglobulins (IVIGs) have been used as therapeutic agents in a variety of immunodeficiency conditions, in infected low-birth-weight infants, bone marrow transplants, and so on (National Institutes of Health Conference, 1990).

After preliminary studies on HIV-infected pediatric cases, the National Institute of Child Health and Human Development (NICHD) announced in 1990 that IVIGs impede development of serious bacterial infections in children with HIV. Bacterial infections occur because of these patients' impaired immune systems; these infections may result in prolonged hospitalization and can be life-threatening. Monthly administration of IVIGs results in less time spent hospitalized for children with symptoms of HIV infection.

Pregnancy and ZDV Therapy

Giving ZDV to pregnant women implies that if the number of viral particles circulating in the mothers' blood can be reduced, then transmission of HIV to their fetuses will be less likely to occur. This may be a reasonable assumption, but there is no animal model in which to test it. And testing the drug on pregnant women has created much controversy. The controversy is centered on the dangers of exposing fetuses to a highly toxic drug, particularly as the majority of babies born to HIV-infected women would not become infected. Protests come from AIDS researchers working with adults. They view ZDV as a treatment for HIV infection, and one that should not be applied when not strictly necessary because of its toxic effects.

Worldwide, perinatal (i.e., mother-to-infant) transmission accounts for most human immunodeficiency virus (HIV) infections among children. In the United States, approximately 7,000 infants, 1,000–2,000 of whom are HIV infected, are born to HIV-infected women each year. In the United States, HIV is currently the seventh leading cause of death in children 1–4 years of age and the fourth among women 25–44 years of age.

The recently reported interim results of the Acquired Immunodeficiency Syndrome (AIDS) Clinical Trials Group (ACTG) Protocol 076, a clinical trial sponsored by the National Institutes of Health in collaboration with the National Institute of Health and Medical Research and the National Agency of Research on AIDS in France, indicate that zidovudine (ZDV) administered to a selected group of HIV-infected pregnant women and their infants can reduce the risk for perinatal HIV transmission by approximately two-thirds (MMWR, 1994a; Goldschmidt et al., 1995). This use of ZDV has the potential to substantially reduce the rate of perinatal transmission, which would reduce overall child mortality. However, the results of this study are directly applicable only to HIV-infected women with characteristics similar to those of the women who entered the study, and the long-term risks of ZDV used in this manner are not known.

Summary of Results of ACTG Protocol 076— On February 21, 1994, the National Institute of Allergy and Infectious Diseases (NIAID) and the National Institute of Child Health and Human Development announced the interim results of a randomized, multicenter, double-blind, placebo-controlled clinical trial, ACTG Protocol 076. Eligible participants were HIV-infected pregnant women at 14–34 weeks of gestation who had received no antiretroviral therapy during their current pregnancy had no clinical indications for antepartum antiretroviral therapy, and had T (before childbirth) lymphocyte counts ≥ 200/μL at the time of entry into the study. The study began in April 1991; as of December 20, 1993, the time of the interim analysis, 477 women had been enrolled and 421 infants born. The racial/ethnic distribution of the HIV-infected women enrolled in the trial was similar to that of the total population of HIV-infected women in the United States.

Enrolled women were assigned randomly to receive a regimen of either ZDV or placebo. The ZDV regimen included oral ZDV initiated at 14–34 weeks of gestation and continued throughout the pregnancy, followed by intravenous ZDV during labor and oral administration of ZDV to the infant for 6 weeks after delivery. The placebo regimen was administered identically. Blood specimens were obtained for HIV culture from all infants at birth and at 12, 24, and 78 weeks of age. A positive viral culture was considered indicative of HIV infection. Sera from the infants at 15 and 18 months of age also were tested for HIV antibody.

The estimated transmission rate was 25.5% among the 184 children in the placebo group compared with 8.3% among the 180 children in the ZDV group. ZDV treatment did not appear to delay the diagnosis of HIV infection.

Observed toxicity specifically attributable to ZDV was minimal among the women in this study. Adverse effects such as anemia, neutropenia, thrombocytopenia, and liver chemistry abnormalities were reported as frequently among women receiving placebo as among women receiving ZDV. Six women—three in each treatment group—discontinued therapy because of toxicity attributed to the study drug. The women were evaluated at 6 weeks and 6 months postpartum. A statistically significant increase in CD4+ T-lymphocyte count from baseline to 6 weeks postpartum was observed for women in both ZDV and placebo treatment groups; this increase was greater among women in the ZDV group. At 6 months postpartum, the CD4+ T-lymphocyte counts for both groups had decreased to similar levels. CD4+ T-lymphocyte counts decreased to < 200/µL in only four women, including one receiving ZDV and three receiving placebo. No women died during the study.

Birth parameters (gestational age; birth weight, length, and head circumference; and Apgar scores) were similar among infants born to women in either group. No statistically significant difference was observed between the ZDV and placebo groups in the number of infants with birth weight < 2,500 g, who were small or large for gestational age, or who were born prematurely. The occurrence of major or minor congenital abnormalities was approximately equal between the two groups, and no pattern in the type of abnormalities was observed.

The infants in the study tolerated the ZDV therapy well. The only adverse effect observed more frequently among infants in the ZDV treatment group was mild, transient anemia. The hemoglobin values of infants receiving ZDV were similar to those of placebo recipients by 12 weeks of age. The incidence of neutropenia and serum chemistry abnormalities was similar between ZDV and placebo groups of infants, and no difference in the pattern of chemistry abnormalities was observed.

Based on these interim findings, NIAID accepted the recommendation of its independent data and safety monitoring board to terminate enrollment into the trial and to offer ZDV to women in the placebo group who had not yet delivered and to their infants up to 6 weeks of age. Follow-up of patients enrolled in the study is ongoing.

Limitations in Interpretation and Extrapolation of ACTG Protocol 076 Results— This clinical trial demonstrated that the ACTG Protocol 076 ZDV regimen can substantially reduce perinatal HIV transmission. However, several important limitations should be noted. First, perinatal HIV transmission was still observed despite drug therapy. Second, the efficacy of this therapy is unknown for HIV-infected pregnant women who have advanced disease, who have received prior antiretroviral therapy, or who have ZDV-resistant virus strains. Third, although the ZDV regimen used in this trial was not associated with serious short-term adverse effects, such effects may be observed when this use of ZDV becomes more widespread. Fourth, the long-term risks for the child associated with exposure to ZDV in utero and early infancy have not been determined. Fifth, it is not known if use of ZDV during pregnancy will affect the drug's efficacy for the woman when it becomes clinically indicated for her own health.

Further complicating the incorporation of this ZDV regimen into clinical practice is the fact that some HIV-infected women seek medical care late in pregnancy or when they are already in labor, when the full ZDV regimen used in ACTG Protocol 076 cannot be administered. Moreover, many pregnant women are not aware that they are HIV infected, are not tested before or during pregnancy, and remain undiagnosed. As a result, they do not receive information about therapy that could reduce the risk for HIV transmission to their infants.

Potential Long-Term Adverse Effects of ZDV Administered During Pregnancy— The long-term effects of ZDV treatment during pregnancy solely to reduce perinatal transmission or of fetal and neonatal exposure to ZDV are not known. ZDV is a nucleoside analog that inhibits HIV replication by interfering with HIV RNA-dependent DNA polymerase. ZDV triphosphate also can inhibit human cellular DNA polymerases, but only at concentrations much higher than those required to inhibit HIV polymerase. However, gamma DNA polymerase, which is required for mitochondrial replication, may be inhibited by ZDV at concentrations nearer to those that can be achieved in vivo.

Conclusion— The decision by an HIV-infected pregnant woman to use ZDV to reduce the risk for perinatal transmission requires a complex balance of individual benefits and risks that is best accomplished through discussions with her health-care provider. Such discussions should be noncoercive, linguistically and culturally appropriate, and tailored to the patient's educational level. (MMWR, 1994b).

PHARMACOLOGY OF DRUG THERAPIES

Zidovudine (Retrovir)

ZDV is a nucleoside analog of thymidine, one of the four bases used in the structure of DNA (Figure 7-6). This means that the structure of ZDV is so similar to thymidine that when present in an HIV-infected cell, it is used in place of thymidine as the reverse transcriptase enzyme synthesizes complementary DNA from its RNA. ZDV should not harm DNA replication in cells that are *not* HIV-infected because it takes a viral gene to make an enzyme which adds a phosphate group to ZDV. This makes the drug structurally ready for incorporation into DNA in place of thymidine. Uninfected cells do not make this enzyme. Therefore, ZDV, ddI, and ddC are *selective poisons* for HIV reproduction.

Zidovudine Stops HIV RNA from Making HIV DNA— ZDV must be phosphorylated within the host cell to inhibit HIV reproduction (Figure 7-7). After ZDV is incorporated into DNA at sites where there should be thymidine, the azide group of ZDV (N_3), located in the 3′ position of the sugar molecule where there should be an hydroxyl (OH) group, stops the next nucleotide from attaching at the 3′ position. Because the next nucleotide cannot attach, the nucleotide chain stops and production of a DNA copy of HIV RNA, necessary for insertion into host cell DNA, is prevented (Figure 7-8).

Experiments show that the reverse transcriptase enzyme itself remains functional, but it cannot continue placing nucleotides in the DNA it is making (Matthes et al., 1987). Although ZDV has proven its value in HIV therapy, it is not 100% effective in stopping all HIV replication (Merluzzi, 1990).

Other Nucleoside Analogs

The majority of agents undergoing clinical trials are nucleoside analogs because they have an antiviral effect. The nucleoside analogs all lack the 3′ hydroxy group and inhibit HIV replication by slightly different mechanisms even though they interact with a common target: HIV reverse transcriptase. They exert their inhibitory effect through their resemblance to natural nucleoside building blocks of DNA. Once the nucleoside analog enters the cell and is phosphorylated, it competes with the natural nucleosides for incorporation into the growing viral DNA strand. The altered DNA structure prevents additional natural nucleosides from being added to the growing DNA strand (Figure 7-8).

Dideoxyinosine: Didanosine (ddI) or VIDEX— The rapid FDA approval of this drug addressed the need for alternatives to ZDV. It has been used in trials, mostly in cases where patients could not take ZDV or had lost their tolerance to ZDV. As of mid-1995, indications for the use of didanosine were still vague. When and how much didanosine should be given? When should ZDV therapy be stopped and didanosine started? The clinical effectiveness of this drug is also still in question.

Didanosine is a purine dideoxynucleoside that is converted to an active metabolite, dideoxyadenosine triphosphate (ddATP), with prolonged intracellular activity (half-life, 8 to 24 hours) allowing for oral administration twice a day. In vitro, didanosine is active against HIV in both T cells and monocytes and has a relatively low toxicity profile. In trial studies, doses ranged from 0.8 mg to 66 mg/kg/day (milligrams of drug per kilogram of body weight per day). The highest tolerated dose was defined in relation to clinical toxicity and ranged between 12 and 20 mg/kg/day. The cost of treatment is about $2,000 per year.

TOXICITY. Unlike ZDV, didanosine does not cause severe anemia. Didanosine's two principal forms of toxicity are pancreatitis (inflammation of the pancreas) in 3% and peripheral neuropathy in 20% of ddI users, both of which are more likely to occur in patients who have had them before. Neuropathy is a tingling sensation or pain in the hands, feet, or other parts of the body. Some HIV-infected people develop a temporary neuropathy which goes away on its own. This type of neuropathy is caused by the body's natural response to HIV or other virus such as

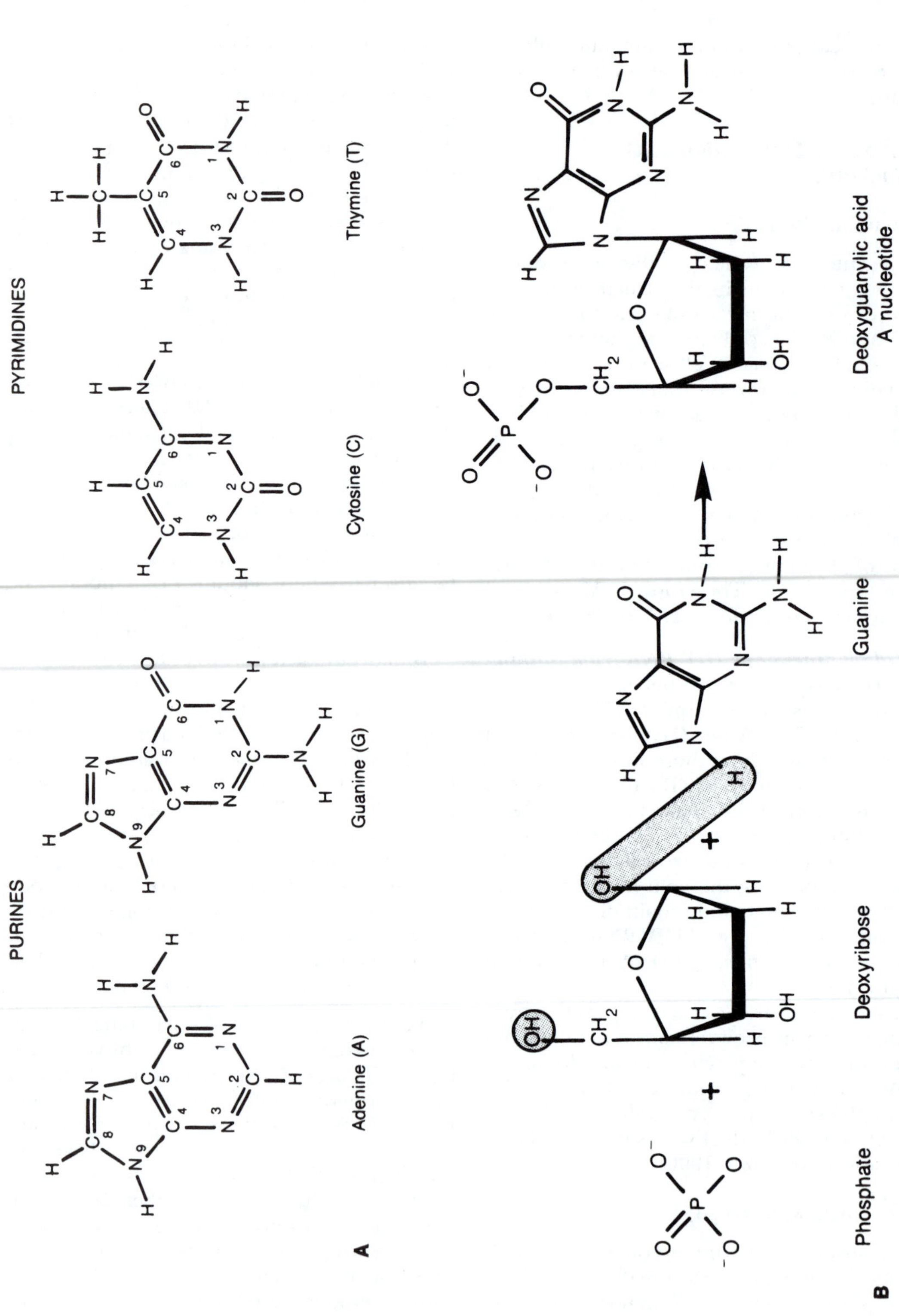

PURINES

PYRIMIDINES

A

Adenine (A)

Guanine (G)

Cytosine (C)

Thymine (T)

B

Phosphate

Deoxyribose

Guanine

Deoxyguanylic acid
A nucleotide

FIGURE 7-6

DNA Replication

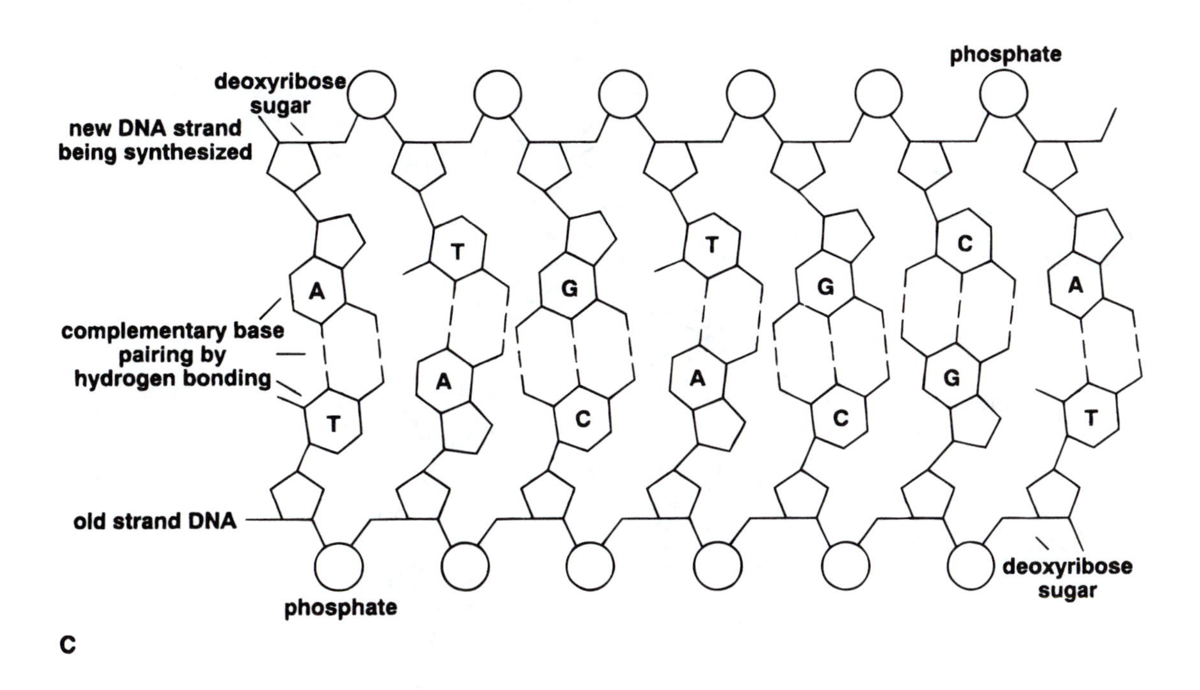

FIGURE 7-6 (pages 150–153) The Four Bases in the Structure of DNA. **A**, In the structure of DNA, the base adenine (A) chemically pairs in a complementary fashion with the base thymine (T); and the base guanine (G) pairs with cytosine (C). Bases A and G are purines; T and C are pyrimidines. A purine pairs with a pyrimidine. Each base is attached to a molecule of sugar and a molecule of phosphate. The combination of phosphate + sugar + base is referred to as a nucleotide. The structure of a nucleotide is presented. **B**, Complementary nucleotides linked together in a linear fashion make up a polymer of DNA. **C**, A single strand of DNA being replicated into a double-stranded molecule by the complementary addition of nucleotides. **D**, Nucleotides are linked to each other in both a linear and complementary fashion. To replicate, DNA strands separate from each other and each nucleotide complementary pairs with a new nucleotide. **E**, Note that zidovudine (in Figure 7-4) has a chemical structure similar to thymine. Thus zidovudine becomes incorporated into the new DNA strand in place of the thymine nucleotide. The incorporation substitution of zidovudine for thymine stops the replication process which in turn stops the production of new HIV. Note that dideoxycytosine and dideoxyinosine in Figure 7-4 also have chemical structures similar to DNA bases and act to inhibit the production of HIV in a manner similar to zidovudine.

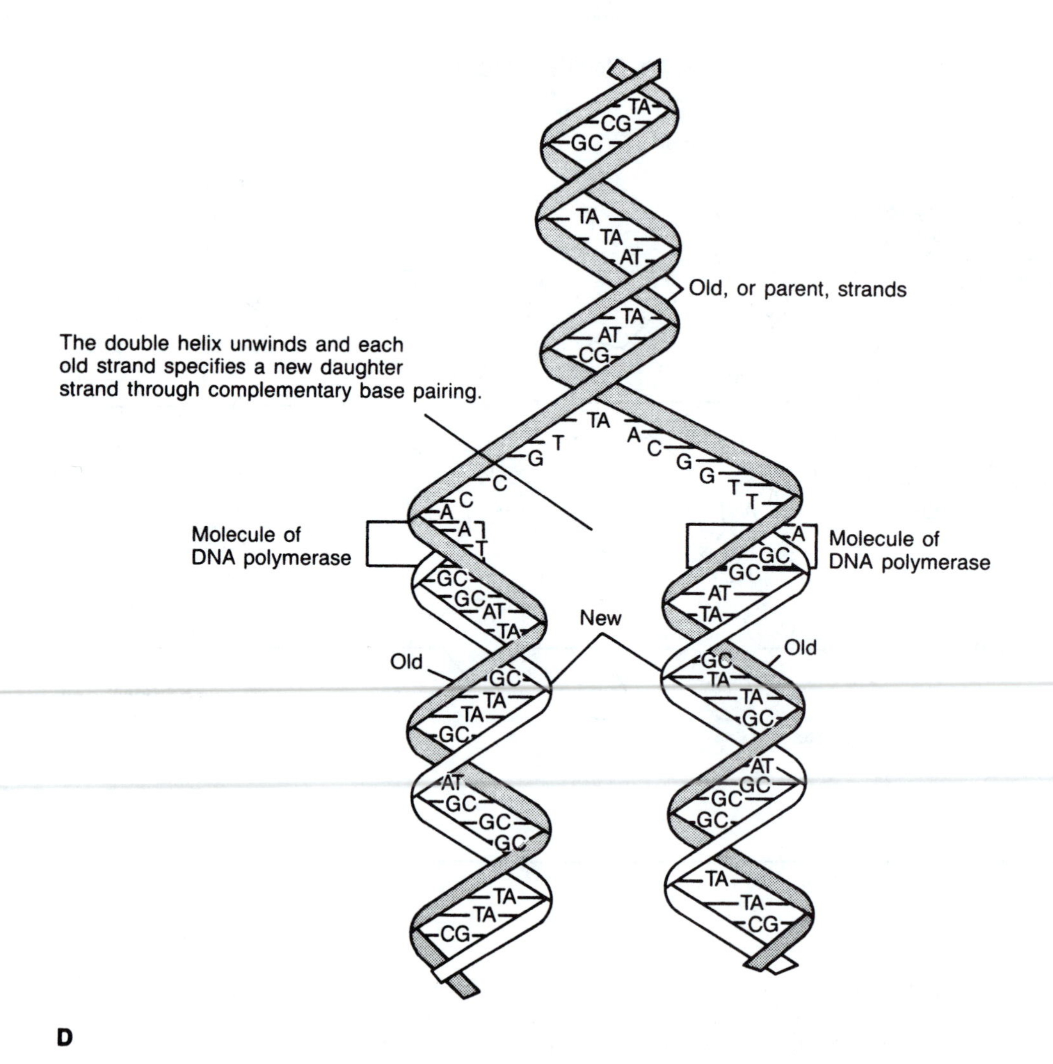

FIGURE 7-6 *(Continued)*

herpes. It can cause muscle weakness and difficulty in walking and balancing. However, as HIV can also cause a painful neuropathy which affects nerve fibers, ddI-attributed neuropathy may be the result of the spread of HIV, other infections, or other drugs. ZDV, didanosine, and dideoxycytosine (ddC) have been used to treat neuropathy successfully. Ironically, these drugs can also cause neuropathy in people who have been taking them for a long time.

PREGNANCY. There are no adequate studies to evaluate the safety of ddI or ddC during pregnancy. Therefore, the manufacturers suggest that "these drugs should be used during pregnancy only if clearly needed." It is not known if either drug is secreted in breast milk and so it is suggested that mothers should be instructed to discontinue nursing when taking ddI or ddC (Kahn, 1991).

In early 1994, a report from the CDC stated that HIV-positive women who took ZDV after their 14th week of pregnancy reduced the risk of HIV transmission into the fetus by 20%.

Dideoxycytosine (ddC) or Zalcitabine (HIVID)— A third FDA-approved nucleoside is chemically similar to ddI.

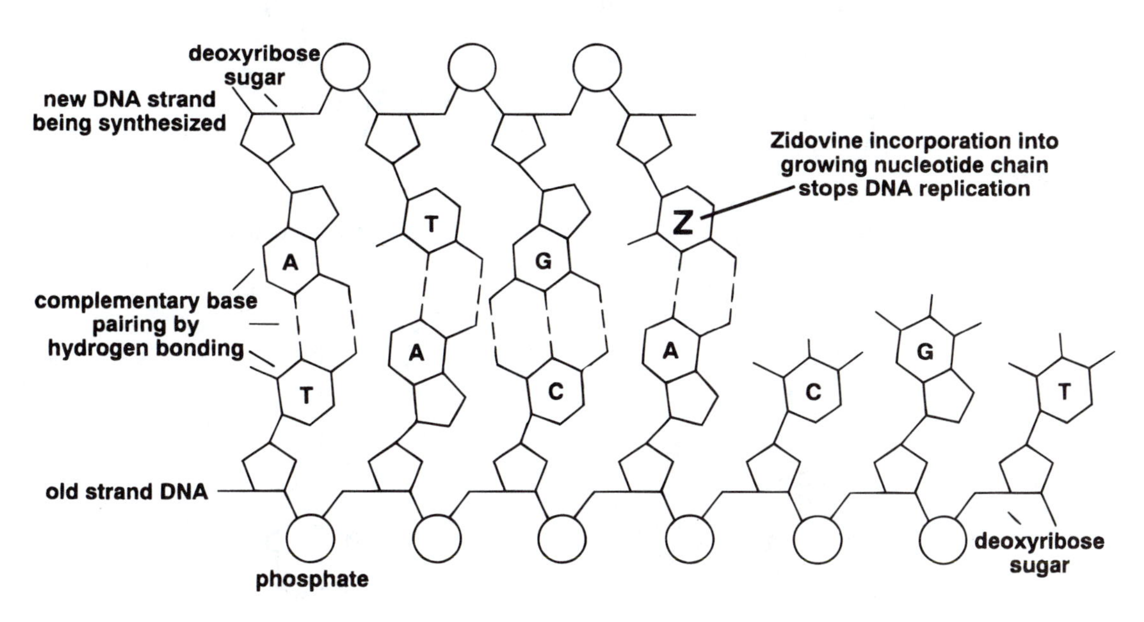

FIGURE 7-6 *(Continued)*

BOX 7.4

A PERSONAL TESTIMONY TO THE USE OF DIDANOSINE

I hate ddI. I have taken AZT [ZDV] and ddC, and neither of them bothered me nearly as much. Yes, I got headaches at the beginning from AZT, but the headaches soon disappeared and I took the stuff without noticeable problems for 18 months.

Though I have only used ddC for about 3 months (sometimes in combination with AZT), it seems the gentlest of all the nucleoside analogs: I never felt anything at all from it.

But ddI is a different story. From the beginning it caused diarrhea and mood swings. The fact of not being able to eat before and after taking it is extremely inconvenient, as is the mixing process.

Most unsettling of all is how ddI makes my extremities tingle and "fall asleep" quickly—the beginnings, I suspect, of peripheral neuropathy. When I take it before bedtime, chances are I won't be able to sleep. Odd spasms and ticks occur in my upper belly, the corners of my eyes and mouth, and the veins in my arms. Sometimes it feels as if little bugs are crawling under my skin. After about two months on ddI my neck, shoulders, and arms were constantly stiff and I had frequent backaches. Shooting, burning pains in muscles were also common. Pancreatitis is much more likely from ddI than ddC (it is not a side effect from AZT) so, aside from other symptoms of tension which I am sure come from it, there is this very real fear for all of us taking ddI.

Since I am in a clinical trial comparing ddI to AZT, I will not sign this letter. I just wanted to let all of you know how ddI makes one PWARC feel [Person With AIDS-Related Complex].

With permission: *PWA Coalition Newsline*, August 1991.

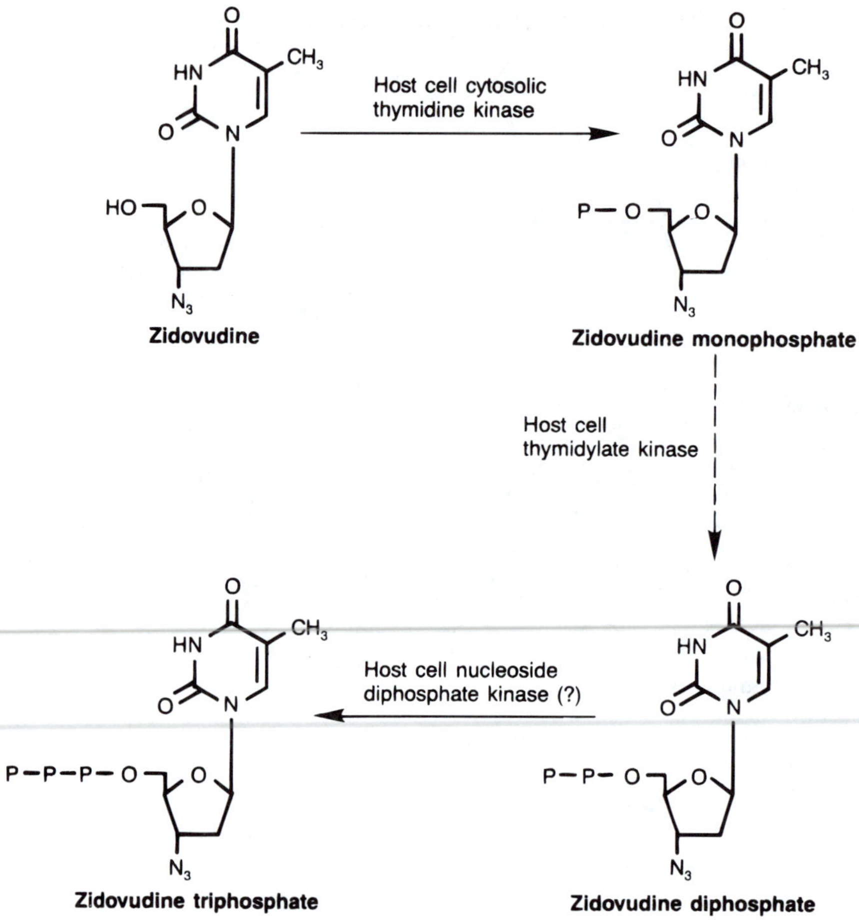

Host cell cytosolic thymidine kinase

Zidovudine

Zidovudine monophosphate

Host cell thymidylate kinase

Host cell nucleoside diphosphate kinase (?)

Zidovudine triphosphate

Zidovudine diphosphate

FIGURE 7-7 Enzymatic Phosphorylation of Zidovudine to the Monophosphate, Diphosphate, and Triphosphate Derivatives. Zidovudine triphosphate is the active form of the drug.

Like ddI, ddC can cause pancreatitis and peripheral neuropathy, but the manufacturer asserts that the pancreatitis can be controlled by adjusting dosage. The cost of ddC runs about $2,000/year. Because of painful neuropathy, ddC is used in doses of approximately 0.01 mg/kg of body weight every 8 hours (Skowron, 1992).

Comparing ZDV, ddI, and ddC

The three nucleoside analogs all inhibit viral reverse transcriptase activity and all have similar effectiveness. The main difference to date is their toxicity profiles and acquired viral resistance to each. The value of the three drugs appears to lie in their use in combination. HIV is less likely to become resistant to three drugs than to one.

Other Nucleoside Analogs in Experimental Trials

Other nucleoside analogs are dideoxydidehydrothymine or stavudine (d4T); 3TC, 1[2R,5S)-2-hydroxymethyl-1,3-oxathiolan-5-Yl] cytosine, a novel dideoxynucleoside analog and azidouridine (AZdU), all in early phase II clinical trials. d4T received FDA approval in June of 1994. 3TC should receive FDA approval in 1995.

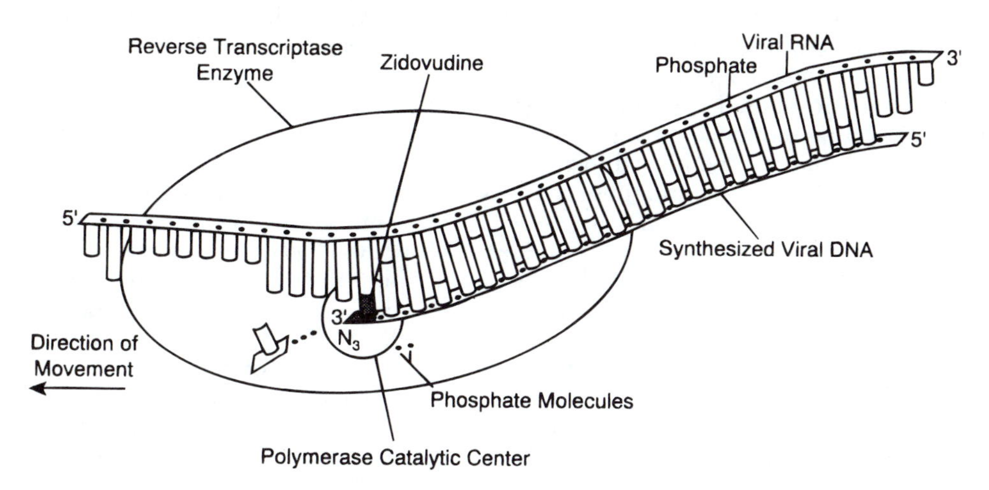

FIGURE 7-8 Incorporation of Zidovudine on HIV Replication. The incorporation of zidovudine-triphosphate into HIV DNA by the action of HIV reverse transcriptase terminates DNA chain extension because polymerization opposite the azide (N_3) group cannot occur. Similar events occur when ddI or ddC is used. All three nucleoside analogs terminate reverse transcriptase activity.

In summary, the nucleoside analogs are the cornerstone of therapy for HIV/AIDS. Of the three that have been approved for clinical use, none have clearly shown that they prolong survival. ddI is used in persons who have developed toxicity or resistance to ZDV. Current data do not support the use of ddC by itself.

ZIDOVUDINE-, DIDANOSINE-, AND ZALCITABINE-RESISTANT MUTANTS OF HIV

HIV Resistance to Zidovudine

HIV investigators fear that the early use of ZDV may over time produce HIV-resistant mutants. A successful mutation for drug resistance may be defined as a mutation that permits the organism or, in this case, HIV to replicate normally in the presence of the inhibitor.

The Burroughs Wellcome Company announced that prolonged use of ZDV can lead to the appearance of ZDV-resistant mutants of HIV (Marx, 1989). HIV isolates taken from five out of 15 patients in ZDV treatment for 6 months were as much as 100 times more resistant to ZDV than HIV isolates taken from AIDS patients who took ZDV for less than 6 months. Land and colleagues (1992) reported that HIV resistance to ZDV therapy increased over time; after 5 months on ZDV, 12% of 362 HIV isolates were resistant; after 36 months, 93% were resistant.

Investigators studying the therapeutic benefits of ZDV state that although patient response to ZDV is dramatic, it is relatively short-lived. The drug is clearly effective for 6 to 18 months, after which a noticeable deterioration in health begins. However, by mid-1989, through altering the dose and combining it with other drugs, the effectiveness of ZDV has been extended from 12 to 36 months.

At the moment there is no indication that AIDS patients who carry mutant or resistant HIV experience symptoms that are any different from those in AIDS patients not carrying mutant HIV. However, the implications, although unclear, are sobering. The appearance of ZDV-resistant mutants implies that HIV in some patients has found a way to evade the best single-drug treatment available. It has yet to be determined whether ZDV-resistant mutants can be or have already been transmitted to others.

Brendan Larder and colleagues (1991) reported that HIV resistance to ZDV is caused by multiple nucleotide changes in the viral gene that codes for its reverse transcriptase enzyme. The protein enzyme, RT, is put together with the wrong amino acids. Thus an alteration in viral RNA coding sequence changes the kind of amino acids that can be placed in the protein that makes the enzyme; and these changes make the enzyme resistant to ZDV.

One report lists six patients who demonstrated clinical failure using standard doses of ZDV. HIV isolated from these patients had developed resistance to the drug. The patients were put on dideoxyinosine and showed immediate signs of improvement as clinical signs of infection disappeared. The study suggests that the development of HIV resistance to ZDV can be correlated with deteriorating health in HIV-infected individuals. HIV ZDV-resistant mutants have also been isolated from patients during prolonged therapy (Larder et al., 1989; Land et al., 1992).

HIV Resistance to Didanosine and Zalcitabine

Mid-1991 reports indicated that ddI- and ddC-resistant HIV strains had occurred (McLeod et al., 1992). Research at the University of Rochester revealed that six of 14 patients receiving didanosine for 1 year lost the therapeutic effect of the drug. This finding was later confirmed by M.H. St. Clair and colleagues (1991). This study also suggests that resistance to didanosine develops more slowly than resistance to ZDV.

HOW DO MUTANT HIVS OCCUR?

Drug resistance occurs in viruses by random chance mutations in their genetic codes, that is, in their DNA, or in HIV, in its RNA or proviral DNA. The occurrence of individual mutations is infrequent, but when a treatment like ZDV destroys or selects against most of the drug-sensitive HIV viruses, it allows the mutant or drug-resistant variant to survive.

The discovery of ZDV mutants should not have been a major surprise. Mutations to antibiotics and other drugs are known to occur in all species. It is a natural part of the evolutionary process. During the years following World War II, it briefly seemed as if DDT and other pesticides would win the ages-old human war on insect crop pests and disease vectors. Such dreams overlooked the way the natural world has been shaped by evolutionary challenges and responses—the challenge of chemical pesticides soon evoked the response of resistant genotypes of arthropods. Today, more than 500 species of insects and mites that are pests in crops or orchards have evolved resistance, often to a wide range of different pesticides. Overall, more than one-third of all agricultural production is still lost to pests, the same proportion as a century ago (May, 1993).

The discovery of ZDV mutants does complicate the medical response to the AIDS pandemic. With about 200,000 AIDS patients alive in the United States and over seven million cases expected worldwide through 1995, tremendous pressure is being placed on scientists to come up with alternative single or combination drug therapies.

NATIONAL TASK FORCE ON AIDS DRUG DEVELOPMENT

Because of the recent setback in the use of the three FDA-approved anti-HIV drugs and the fact that as of December 1, 1993, not a single new antiviral drug application was before the FDA, Secretary of Health and Human Services, Donna Shalala, set up a National Task Force, in February of 1994, to develop new HIV/AIDS drugs. The task force consists of 15 representatives from government, industry, academia, and AIDS-affected communities. The task force idea builds on a late-1993 15-drug-company collaboration attempting to streamline the AIDS drug development process. But, to date (mid-1995), the task force has little to show for its effort.

UNCONVENTIONAL COMBINATION THERAPIES

Early in 1993, Yung-Kang Chow and colleagues used three drugs, each a reverse transcriptase inhibitor to stop HIV replication in a test tube. The drugs are ZDV, ddI (nucleoside analogs), and either pyridinone or nevirapine (non-nucleoside analogs). Chow and colleagues determined that the test tube strategy prevented infection of healthy cells and successfully treated HIV in cells that had been infected. Chow's strategy is to force HIV to mutate to the three drugs simultaneously against a single target or protein, the reverse transcriptase enzyme. The idea is that the three mutations in one area would damage the virus's ability to replicate; the virus would mutate itself out of function. Chow has been unable to reproduce his work and has since retracted his published data.

POINT OF VIEW 7.4

ARE ALL MEDICAL STUDIES CREDIBLE?—NO!

Almost daily, somewhere in the United States an investigator or group headlines their new and promising advance against some disease. All too often, reputations, fortunes, and hope rise and fall with each tantalizing news release or rumor. True break-throughs are often lost in the presence of the large number of short-lived claims of medical success. People, in general, must be more skeptical of all the medical advances that they hear and read about. Questions must be raised because medical studies of value must be big enough to find real trends; small ones are easily swayed by bias or chance. Studies that prove death or survival rates, in particular, require huge numbers of subjects. To be statistically significant, there must be less than 1-in-20 probability that any medical result happened by chance.

Often patients get better or worse on their own. Therefore a control group is needed to compare a new drug with standard treatment or a placebo. Was the therapeutic effect of a drug substantial compared to conventional treatment? Was the test fair? Were people in the study group and in the control group equally old, sick, or poor (factors that could skew the study's outcome)? Did the scientists tell the whole story or just offer a glimpse of selected results? And who's paying them? Also important is the fact that test-tube results or tests done on animals, while important, don't guarantee a drug will work on humans. In fact, 90% of drugs in development fail somewhere along the road between the lab bench and FDA approval.

TIBO Derivatives Inhibit HIV Replication

In 1990, a team of researchers in Belgium and the United States found a series of compounds they said were "the most specific and potent inhibitors of HIV-1 replication studied so far" (Pauwels et al., 1990).

The new antiviral agents are members of a class of compounds called tetrahydroimidazo[4,5,1-jk][1,4]benzodiazepin-2(1H)-one and -thione (TIBO) derivatives. Remarkably, they inhibit the replication of HIV-1 but not HIV-2 or any other DNA or RNA viruses.

Certain TIBO derivatives have been found to inhibit HIV replication by inhibiting reverse transcriptase activity in cell culture at nanomolar (billionths of a liter) concentrations 20,000 to more than 30,000 times lower than those levels that impair the viability of uninfected human lymphocytes. By contrast, ZDV inhibits HIV replication at a level only about 6,000 times below its cytotoxic concentration. For newer anti-HIV agents such as dideoxyinosine and dideoxycytosine, the margin of safety is even smaller.

One highly potent TIBO derivative, R82150 (Figure 7-9), was well tolerated when given to dogs and six healthy male volunteers. However, more derivatives are being synthesized as the research team searches for the one most suitable for clinical studies in HIV-infected patients.

FIGURE 7-9 TIBO Derivative that Inhibits HIV Replication.

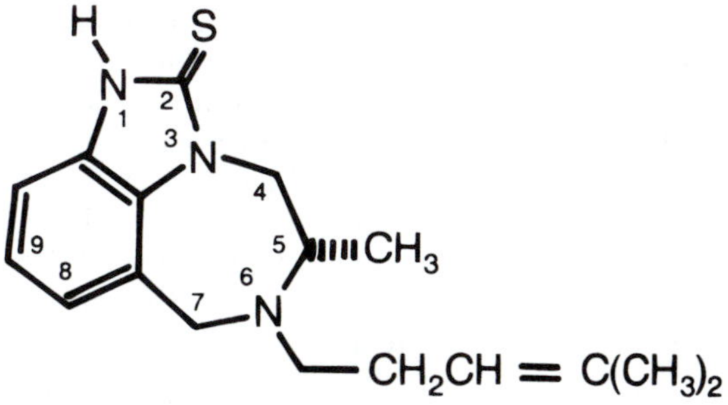

COMBINATION DRUG AIDS THERAPY

The concept of combination therapy is not new. For AIDS patients, combination therapy (CT) involves the use of other drugs in combination with ZDV. CT is designed for two purposes: (1) to decrease the toxicity of ZDV; and (2) to enhance its antiviral or immunorestorative effects. ZDV combined with erythropoietin (a protein made in the kidneys that stimulates the production of red blood cells) or granulocyte macrophage stimulating factor (GMSF) may lessen bone marrow suppression. In 1990, the FDA approved epoetin alpha, a genetically engineered form of erythropoietin, to treat anemia in AIDS patients using ZDV.

Alternating CT treatment cycles with antiviral marrow-sparing drugs such as dideoxycytosine (Figure 7-4) may allow patients to continue to receive therapy for longer periods and at higher doses.

The antiviral and immunorestorative activities of ZDV may be enhanced when combined with other antivirals such as acyclovir or foscarnet; or immunomodulators such as alpha, beta, or gamma interferons; interleukin-2; or ampligen (Table 7-3). There are studies currently in progress to evaluate each of these therapeutic possibilities.

RECONSTITUTION OF THE IMMUNE SYSTEM

Nothing illustrates the necessity of a healthy immune system more dramatically than the consequences of its loss. Of all the human diseases that are known to suppress the immune system, few can compare to the damage caused by HIV disease/AIDS. Many opportunistic infections and cancers can affect HIV/AIDS patients within a relatively short time. These diseases do occur in patients with non-AIDS-suppressed immune systems, but they do not experience the collective devastation of so many recurrent infections. This must mean that the level of immune system impairment in HIV disease/AIDS is greater than in the other immune suppression diseases or immune suppression caused by drug therapy.

What is needed is a way to renew, rehabilitate, and resurrect the immune system in HIV/AIDS patients.

Immunological Reconstitution

Different approaches to *immunological reconstitution* depend on the degree of immune impairment that is present. For patients with severe depletion of T4 cells, augmentation of the immune system is not sufficient. These patients require replacement therapy—that is, lymphocyte transfer (T cells), bone marrow transplantation (stem cells, T progenitor cells, and T cells), and, for patients with recurrent bacterial infections, immunoglobulins. Those patients with some residual immunological function need to augment their defenses with biological response modifiers. To this end, scientists are researching compounds that appear to enhance the function of a severely damaged immune system such as interleukin-2, interferons, colony-stimulating factors, and other cytokines. Salk has been trying to boost the immune response to HIV infection by challenging infected patients with inactivated HIV. It appears to have reacted in some but not all of those tested.

Immunomodulators

Compounds that appear to have a stimulatory effect on the immune system are called **immunomodulators** (Table 7-3). The starting point for using immunomodulators can be based on T4 cell counts. When the count is sufficiently high, there are enough T4 cells to trigger an effective immune response. When the count falls too low, however, it is very difficult to get it back up again, even with immunomodulators. In short, you must have something left of an immune system to rebuild it.

T4 Cell Ranges

Lowest (under 200)	Low (200–500)	High (500 plus)

High Range— In general, a T4 count of 500 or above suggests no immediate danger. The 500 level is often cited as the bottom of the "normal" range, but this can be mislead-

TABLE 7-3 Immunomodulator Compounds Under Investigation

Compound	Description	Possible or Known Effects
Alpha interferon	A human protein	Approved in November 1988 for use against Kaposi's sarcoma. Early studies in 1988: produces partial or complete tumor regression in some AIDS patients with KS. New studies in 1989–1990 stops HIV budding from infected cells; being used in combination with zidovudine.
Ampligen	Mismatched RNA molecule	Reported to increase interferon production and activation of natural killer cells. 1988 studies proved negative.
Anti-interferon immunoglobulin	Antibody specific for interferon	Reduces high levels of acid labile alpha interferon that may be upsetting immune system balance.
AS-101	Ammonium trichloro (dioxyethylene-O,O') tellurium	Enhances production of CSF[a] and IL-2[b] in human leukocytes in culture. Improved T4 cell counts. Adverse effects include vomiting diarrhea.
Bropirimine (ABPP)	2-amino-5-bormo-6-phenyl-4 (3H)-pyrimidine	Induces interferon production, stimulates natural killer cells and macrophage-mediated killing, enhances B cell response.
CL246, 738	(3,6-bis(2-piperidinoethyloxy)-acridine trihydrochloride	Induces interferon production and natural killer cell activity in animals. Improved immune function in experimentally immunodeficient animals.
GM-CSF	Recombinant granulocyte-macrophage colony stimulating factor	Human glycoprotein from lymphocytes; regulates growth and function of immune system cells including granulocytes and macrophages. In trials it raised leukocyte counts in all patients. Mild side effects noted.
Imreg-1	A mixture of 2 human peptides obtained from lymphocytes	Stimulates production of IL-2, gamma interferon, and improves T4 cellfunction. Studies showed clinical improvement—slowed AIDS progress. No side effects observed.
Imuthiol	Sodium diethyldithiocarbonate	Metal chelating agent. Induces T cell maturation; increased number of T4 cells in some AIDS patients.
Interleukin-2 (IL-2)	A glycoprotein produced by T cells	Used alone did not restore T cell immune function. Now being tested in combination with zidovudine.
Isoprinosine	Inosine pranobex	Produced natural killer cell activity and T4 cell counts in AIDS patients; now being phase II tested.
Methionine-enkephalin	Opiod pentapeptide, stress produced by adrenal glands	Limited test results: increased natural killer cell activity, IL-2 production and T cell counts, patient weight gain.
MTP-PE	Muramyl tripeptide-dipalmit-olyphosphatidylethanolamine conjugate	A macrophage activator; being studied in AIDS and KS[c] patients.
Naltrexone	17-(cyclopropylmethyl)-4,5,-epoxy-3,14-dihydroxymorphinan-6-one	A licensed heroin antagonist; lowers alpha interferon levels. Responding patients had fewer OIs.[d]
Soluble CD4	Genetically engineered form CD4 receptor protein of T4 cells	Has reduced levels of HIV-like virus in monkeys, improved of bone marrow protein of RBC[e] and WBC[f] in animals. Is being used as an HIV decoy. First 45 humans showed minimal side effects, 1989.
Thymopentin	TP-5, a pentapeptide, may be the "active site" of a thymic hormone	Limited study; some AIDS patients showed immunological improvement.
Tumor Necrosis Factor (TNF)	Macrophage-derived protein	Kills tumor cells, reason unknown; being studied in AIDS and KS. Used with gamma interferon, the combination showed antiviral and immunological effects. Now in phase II study.

[a]CSF = colony stimulating factor; [b]IL-2 = interleukin-2—both immune system regulators;
[c]KS = Kaposi's sarcoma; [d]OI = opportunistic infections; [e]RBC = red blood cells; [f]WBC = white blood cells.

ing. While an occasional drop to 500 may be normal, a steadily or slowly falling count to 500 or even 600 is not normal and indicates suppressed immunity (but no immediate danger of AIDS). With counts this high, many people feel little motivation to begin immunomodulator treatment. A growing number of researchers, however, believe it may be the best time to do so.

Lowest Range— T4 counts below 200 indicate the greatest risk of opportunistic infections. This level is common among AIDS patients. There are exceptions, but even people in this range who seem healthy have greater difficulty combating OIs when they occur. Treatment includes preventative therapy against common opportunistic infections. While some people have additional warning signs in the form of symptoms before major infections occur, this is not always the case. Some individuals progress directly from apparent sound health to serious OIs.

A number of immunomodulator compounds hold promise, but they are expensive and can be dangerous. For example, interleukin-2 (IL-2), one of the lymphokines produced by the T leukocytes of the immune system, costs about $80,000 for one course of treatment. It is also dangerous. Patients have died during IL-2 treatment. Until now, IL-2 treatment was reserved for patients with advanced cancer. Early in 1995, 27 immunomodulators were in development by 25 companies.

Soluble CD4 Protein— On August 10, 1988, a new and different immunomodulator was used for the first time in humans. It was also the first product of recombinant DNA technology to be used specifically against HIV. The product is called recombinant soluble CD4 protein or rsCD4. CD4 is the receptor site to which HIV most often binds to infect CD4-bearing cells, especially T4 helper cells. CD4 protein, when experimentally released from the T4 cell membrane, is soluble in solution. The theory is that if enough soluble CD4 is injected into the bloodstream, the decoy rsCD4 molecules will attach to the HIV, thereby preventing its infecting CD4-bearing immune system cells (Figure 7-10). The use of decoy rsCD4 molecules is not envisioned as a cure for AIDS, but as a means of controlling the level of HIV infection, thereby extending patients' lives.

One problem encountered in using rsCD4 is its short half-life in the human bloodstream—about 1 hour when injected intravenously (Ezzell, 1989). There is hope of increasing the half-life of CD4 by attaching the CD4 molecule to human immunoglobulin-G

FIGURE 7-10 Soluble CD4: A Decoy for HIV Attack. Recombinant DNA methodology (genetic engineering) was used to produce large quantities of soluble CD4 receptor protein units. Glycoprotein 120 of HIV attaches to the CD4 receptor sites on a variety of CD4-bearing immune cells, most importantly, the T4 helper cell. Once HIV attaches to the CD4 site, it is taken inside the cell, thereby causing HIV infection. **A**, HIV attaching to a CD4-containing cell. **B**, HIV being decoyed away from CD4 immune cells by HIV attachment to the many copies of soluble CD4 receptors available in the system. Soluble CD4 units actually intercept the virus by chance. In clinical use, many millions of copies of CD4 are injected into and float freely within the bloodstream.

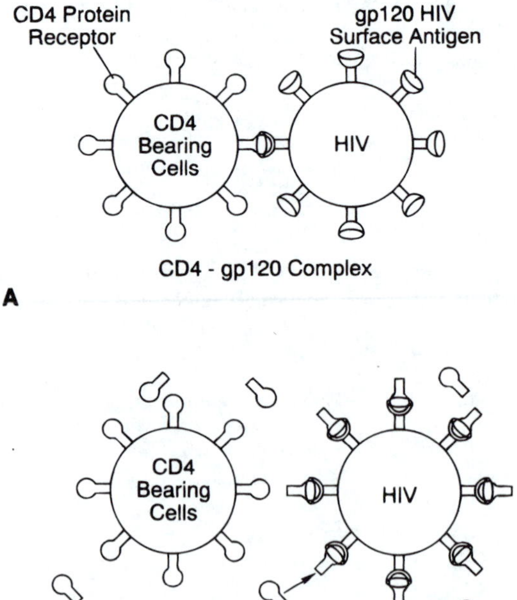

or IgG. The reason for attaching CD4 to the IgG molecules is threefold: (1) IgG has a much longer half-life in humans and might protect CD4 from early destruction; (2) IgG itself may contribute to neutralizing or attaching to HIV; and (3) IgG may carry the CD4 molecule across the placenta and protect the developing fetus from HIV infection.

NEW THERAPEUTIC APPROACHES

Protease (Proteinase)

New therapies are focusing on protease or proteinase enzyme function, hyperthermia, and diet. In 1989, Tom Blundell and colleagues reported on the work of Irene Weber and colleagues (1989), who performed X-ray analysis of retroviral *protease* of the Rous sarcoma virus, and Manuel Navia and colleagues (1989), who X-rayed the HIV protease. Recall that the retroviral genes code for reverse transcriptase (RT) integrase and protease. The reproductive cycle of retroviruses requires a specific protease to process the precursor GAG and POL polyproteins into mature retroviral components (Erickson, 1990). If protease is missing or inactive, noninfectious retroviruses are produced. Therefore, inhibitors of protease enzyme function become potential therapeutic blocking agents of retroviral infections.

X-ray studies on the proteinase enzyme have allowed for replicating its three-dimensional structure. This is the opening salvo in what may be the second front of the therapeutic war on AIDS. To date, several research groups have found chemicals that inhibit proteinase or protease in test tube experiments, but these chemicals are too large to enter human cells. Whatever chemical protease blocker is found, it will have to survive in the bloodstream where many drugs and chemicals are destroyed. Because of its low survival rate in the bloodstream, after an effective protease blocker is found, it will have to be taken three times a day for the rest of one's life & it will be an expensive drug!

As research progresses, scientists have found that **HIV protease is distinctly different from other protease enzymes in the body, so a drug that blocks the enzyme in HIV probably will not affect the normal cells**. This means a protease blocker would be very specific to HIV and that would help minimize dangerous side effects. As of early 1995, 11 protease inhibitors are under study. Each inhibitor is a polypeptide made up of a small number (up to 15) of amino acids. Each has shown the ability to block aspartyl protease, whose function is to cut viral protein precursors into individual functional lengths of protease. Studies on one specific protease inhibitors-Saquinavir, began in humans in 1993/1994 in France, United Kingdom, Italy and the United states (AIDS Clinical Trials Group 229). Saquinavir is the first of this new class of protease/proteinase inhibitors to undergo extensive clinical evaluation for the treatment of HIV infection. Its potent antiviral activity and low potential toxicity suggest it will have a wide therapeutic index.

The three European trials and the American trials have shown that saquinavir is very well tolerated, both as monotherapy and in combination with zidovudine. Adverse effects related to saquinavir were mild and rare. The 600-mg dose of the drug was the most clearly associated with a positive effect on the CD4 cell count in the French and United Kingdom monotherapy studies. Moreover, the combination of saquinavir and zidovudine gave higher and more sustained improvements in the CD4 cell count than either drug alone. Further long-term studies in a large number of patients are now being initiated in Europe and the United States to confirm the clinical relevance of the observed increase in CD4 cell counts. These studies will investigate both monotherapy and combination therapy (Vella, 1994).

But, as this work continues, David Ho and collegues have reported the occurrence of protease-resistant HIV (Ho et al., 1994). HIV has mutated or changed so that the protease block does not work (Ho et al., 1994). However, new studies by Ho and colleagues (1995) using agent ABT-538 successfully and dramatically inhibited HIV protease. Currently, 15 companies are working on protease inhibitors.

HIV Integrase

HIV controls the production of new HIV as it resides with the DNA of the host cell. HIV inserts itself inside host DNA by using an enzyme called HIV integrase. The enzyme cuts the host-cell DNA and allows the viral DNA to become spliced into the host-cell DNA. Researchers have long realized that if they could find a way to block this enzyme, they might be able to prevent the virus from infecting new cells and thereby defeat it. But they have faced a difficult problem: The search for HIV integrase inhibitors has been a hit-or-miss operation because the precise shape of the enzyme was not known. But that may be about to change. In December of 1994, Fred Dyda and co-workers reported the three-dimensional structure of this enzyme. Now that they know the shape of the enzyme, researchers have a better basis for designing drugs to block its activity, for example by tailoring molecules that will bind to and obscure the enzyme's catalytic site.

Now, with the structure of the third of the trio of key HIV enzymes in hand (reverse transcriptase and protease being the other two), researchers are hoping that they may ultimately be able to develop a cocktail of inhibitors for the three enzymes that would be used together. Such a combined attack would help reduce the chances that HIV could mutate and become resistant to drug therapy. Mutations that resist reverse transcriptase and protease inhibitors have already turned up.

Anti-*tat* Therapy

The *tat* gene of HIV produces a protein that promotes the expression of other HIV genes whose proteins are essential for HIV reproduction. The *tat* gene protein has also been associated with fostering the spread of Kaposi's sarcoma and damaging immune function. HIVs that contain a mutant *tat* gene appear normal but are incapable of infecting cells. If scientists could block *tat* gene function, there could be many benefits. Thus several pharmaceutical companies are in the process of screening agents that might inhibit the function of the *tat* gene protein.

Alpha-Trichosanthin (GLQ223)

This is a protein-based, botanically derived drug. It has demonstrated in in vitro studies to selectively kill chronically infected macrophage cells, which may act as a reservoir for HIV. It has also been shown to block HIV expression in acutely infected T cells and chronically infected macrophages without harming uninfected cells. Administration of GLQ223 in patients with AIDS was safe and clinically well tolerated and was associated with measurable increases in markers of immunological activity. The drug is now in phase III trials at several centers including San Francisco General Hospital.

Gene Therapy

Gene therapy for many chronic diseases, including HIV infection, is clearly a new frontier in science. If the scientific and technical hurdles can be overcome, gene therapies to combat HIV infection could emerge as important treatment options. If scientists are able to reconstitute damaged immune systems, protecting new immune cells from HIV infection will be essential. Gene therapy via intracellular immunization with anti-HIV genes is a prime candidate for this task.

The basis of gene therapy against HIV derives from the fact that in HIV infection the virus makes use of the host cell genes to replicate itself. The model of gene treatment for HIV is to create in the laboratory a gene, that is defective for HIV replication but does not affect host cell function; to attach the gene to viral DNA, that does not replicate itself, in humans; to "infect" (transduce) donor lymphocytes and macrophages or hematopoietic stem cells, (from patients or from uninfected transplant-compatible donors) and then infuse these resistant cells into HIV-infected patients. In the ideal case, the newly-infused HIV-resistant cells would gradually replace infected cells and prolong the healthy state, and HIV would eventually run out of suceptible host cells to infect.

Currently, the main goals of research into gene therapy for HIV are to define efficient methods of in vivo gene transfer into cells, identify the anti-HIV genes that confer optimal resistance to HIV infection in vitro, and combine gene therapy for HIV with immune reconstitution. Even if gene therapy proves to be of only modest benefit in treating HIV infection, the scientific knowledge gained from this research is likely to have broad applications in other areas of investigation and therapeutic development (Hardy et al., 1994). Currently at least three possible strategies for gene therapy exist.

One strategy involves inserting a gene into white blood cells that would cause them to produce multiple copies of CD4 to bind HIV in the cells' local environment. A second strategy involves inserting a gene into white blood cells that would interfere with the virus's ability to reproduce.

In a third strategy, researchers are attempting to insert a "suicide gene" into white blood cells, which would remain dormant until the cells were infected by HIV. The gene would then direct the cells to begin producing a powerful toxin, such as diphtheria toxin, which would destroy both the cells and the viruses within them.

An aggressive strategy for AIDS gene therapy now being developed is that of Flossie Wong-Staal from the University of California, San Diego. Her group has built gene therapy vectors to deliver a **ribozyme** gene into HIV-infected cells. The ribozyme gene will produce a ribozyme that will seek out and cut the HIV genome in two (Barinaga, 1993). Additional information on molecular targets for gene transfer therapy for HIV infection is presented by Gary Buchschacher (1993).

In other gene therapy experiments, the biotech company, Viagene of San Diego California, made their first attempt to treat AIDS patients with gene therapy (Ziegner et al., 1995). The treatment was tested on four HIV-infected patients. Fibroblasts were removed from the patients' arms and genetically altered to manufacture gp160, a protein that is part of the virus's protective shell. The engineered fibroblasts were irradiated to make them stop dividing (though they survive and continue producing gp160 for a few weeks), and then put back into the patient. This study is an initial attempt to activate cytotoxic T cell activity in HIV-infected patients using a gene therapy immunization approach. The treatment appears to be well tolerated by these patients without any apparent adverse clinical events. It also appears to be capable of generating/ augmenting cytotoxic T cell activity in asymptomatic HIV-infected individuals. These patients will be receiving additional future treatments with continued follow-up in an effort to gain additional understanding of the potential impact of cytotoxic T cell activity in the HIV disease process.

Antisense RNA Used to Treat HIV Infections

Cells use messenger RNA to transmit the genetic code from a gene to a ribosome, a workbench where the cell assembles proteins using RNA as a "blueprint."

What happens when an antisense compound meets its natural opposite? The nucleotides of the messenger RNA and the antisense molecule stick together much as two pieces of Velcro do. (They complementary base pair.) The result: no protein. If the drug engineer has identified the correct illness-producing protein. The production of that protein can be blocked. This should lead to a reduction of illness. Thus, antisense HIV RNA can hybridize to the HIV mRNA strand, stopping the production of viral (HIV) proteins The use of antisense RNA to regulate gene expression or the production of HIV proteins derives from the observation that in prokaryotes and eukaryotes, naturally transcribed antisense RNA species regulate gene expression by hybridizing to their complementary mRNAs. Experi-mentally, exogenous antisense RNA has been introduced into cells and shown to inhibit cellular gene expression (Boyd et al., 1991; Cohen et al., 1994). Antisense RNA would also produce non-functional protein—such protein if made may cause cell death before HIVs are replicated.

HYPERTHERMIA TREATMENT

In early 1990, a 33-year-old Atlanta waiter captured the attention of the nation with his televised claim that doctors had rid his body of the AIDS virus by heating his blood. An official account of the experiment has yet to be published, and was turned down by the *Journal of the American Medical Association* on the basis that it is only a single case report.

BOX 7.5

WILLIAM "SKIP" BLUETTE: MAY 18, 1946–JULY 17, 1988

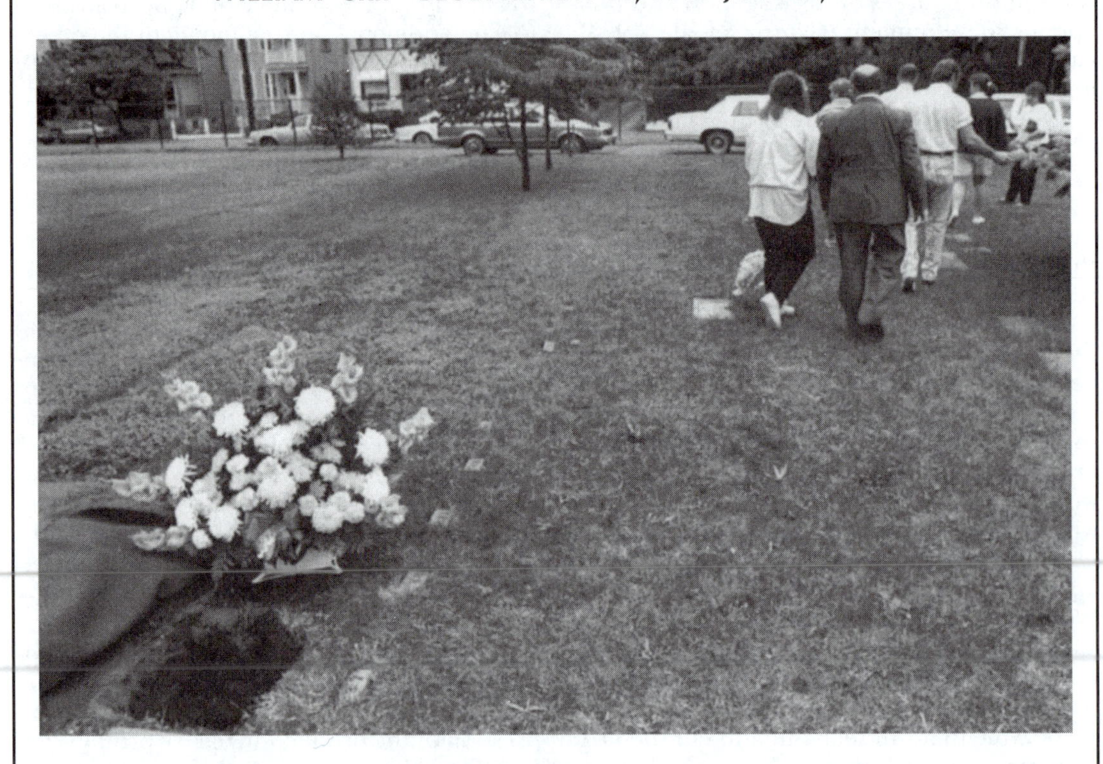

FIGURE 7-11 Free of Pain—One With the Universe–William 'Skip' Bluette. On July 20, 1988 Skip's body was cremated. There was a memorial service. On July 21, Skip's ashes were buried in Evergreen Cemetery. (*By permission of Mara Lavitt and* The New Haven Register)

William Logan, a heart surgeon, and his research partner Kenneth Alonso, a pathologist, claim that a 2-hour hyperthermia session, in which the patient's blood was heated to 108°F outside his body, cooled, and returned to his body, reduced the concentration of AIDS virus and virtually eradicated the purplish patches of Kaposi's sarcoma on his body. This team later reported that it treated a second patient who showed a 50% reduction in Kaposi's sarcoma lesions. In August of 1990, an AIDS patient died while undergoing hyperthermia treatment in Mexico City. Alonso was present during the treatment and said the patient died because his illness was much more severe than they had thought. The cost of the treatment was $36,000 per hypothermia session (Associated Press Release, August 16, 1990). In January of 1995, the FDA approved Biocontrol Technology's expanded study of heating the blood of AIDS patients. The studies are based on HIV being heat sensitive.

It should be mentioned that hypothermia as a medical therapy has been used historically. In 1927, Austrian psychiatrist Julius Wagner-Jauregg received the Nobel Prize in Physiology and Medicine for providing a novel treatment in relieving general paralysis brought on by syphilis. He transfused blood from malarial patients into syphilitic patients. The high fever caused by the ensuing malaria cured the paralysis. The use of hypothermia in cancer patients has been tried over the years with some success in relieving symptoms but it has never been known to result in a cure.

MACROBIOTICS AND AIDS

Macrobiotics is the study of life prolongation through the use of a restricted or balanced diet to promote health and prevent disease. Few today would disagree with the concept that a balanced diet leads to better health. But the question is: Can altering the diet prevent HIV infection and extend or save the lives of HIV/AIDS patients? This is a very difficult question to answer. There are so many variables to any diet and the body's response to it may be as different as there are different people. The problem is establishing meaningful controls in order to determine exactly what a given component of a given diet does in the human body.

With respect to HIV infection and AIDS, it is believed that if one eats only quality foods properly prepared and in certain combinations, the foods will stimulate the immune system and prolong life. The belief is that if a macrobiotic diet were properly adhered to, many, if not most, drug therapies would be unnecessary. Even if diet could provide a pathway to perfect health, it should be pointed out that many AIDS patients are too weak to eat or their mouths are too sore; they have difficulty swallowing, suffer from nausea and vomiting, and are anorexic.

The theory of macrobiotics is presented in the publication *MACROMUSE*. The claims for macrobiotics regarding the prevention and cure of disease often sound too good to be true. This does not mean that diet is unimportant; clearly it is, but at this time there is insufficient knowledge about diet manipulation to cure AIDS or any of the other sexually transmitted diseases.

TASK FORCE ON NUTRITION SUPPORT IN AIDS

In June of 1988, a task force was established to study the implications of nutrition in AIDS patients. The task force was set up in recognition that the course of AIDS is often complicated by profound weight loss, multiple nutrient deficiencies, and, particularly, protein calorie malnutrition (PCM) (Colman et al., 1987; Jansen, 1988). Throughout the progression of AIDS, the patient's nutritional status is challenged by the manifestation of symptoms such as malabsorption, diarrhea, oral/esophageal problems, nausea/vomiting, and infection. The expression of AIDS produces a different combination of symptoms in each individual. As with any chronic disease, the severe malnutrition that accompanies AIDS might decrease longevity and increase morbidity. In addition, the quality of life for people with AIDS is severely compromised when their primary disease is accompanied by major nutritional complications.

Nutritional intervention should begin as soon as an HIV-positive diagnosis is made.

SUMMARY

Therapies available at this time do not prevent HIV infection or the progression from infection to AIDS. Successful treatment of primary HIV infection requires the interruption of the viral replication cycle. This can occur at any of several sites. Binding of the virus to the cell surface receptor (CD4) can be blocked with the cholesterol-stripping agent AL-721 or the pseudomembrane receptor, or soluble CD4 receptors.

Currently, there are no known agents that block viral uncoating, but several agents are effective in inhibiting the reverse transcriptase enzyme. These include zidovudine (ZDV), dideoxyinosine (ddI), and dideoxycytosine (ddC).

Multimillions of dollars are being spent on anything that even remotely looks promising as an anti-HIV or AIDS drug or therapy. Beginning 1995, 250 different drugs, immunomodulators, and vaccines were in use or in development in the United States. It has been evident from the constant protests by AIDS activist groups that they are displeased with the amount of money available for research, the progress made, and the limited availability of experimental drugs. The FDA believes it is doing all that is possible to help move untried or untested drugs to HIV/AIDS patients. The FDA accomplished this by eliminating the need for phase III studies for drugs that might help terminally ill patients.

A problem exists in helping HIV/AIDS patients who become pregnant. How can HIV infection of the fetus be blocked? Studies on the administration of zidovudine in the second and third trimesters of pregnancy are in progress.

A second problem is the appearance of zidovudine and other nucleoside-resistant mutants. Although it was expected, it occurred before alternative drugs were available. In addition to using antiviral drugs, investigators are trying out immunomodulators, which regenerate or revitalize a failing immune system.

In a recent scientific advance, the three-dimensional structure of the HIV protease enzyme was discovered. This should allow for the production of a designer drug that will inhibit the enzyme and stop HIV reproduction. Research is in progress.

DISCLAIMER

This chapter is designed to present information about certain aspects of HIV/AIDS therapy. This chapter does *not* provide medical advice. Consult your health care providers for medical advice before undertaking any treatment discussed herein.

SOME AIDS THERAPY INFORMATION HOTLINES

For HIV/AIDS treatment information, call:

The American Foundation for AIDS Research: 800-39AMFAR (392-6237)

AIDS Treatment Data Network: 212-268-4196

AIDS Treatment News: 800-TREAT 1-2 (873-2812)

For information about AIDS/HIV clinical trials conducted by National Institutes of Health and Food and Drug Administration-approved efficacy trials, call:

AIDS Clinical Trials Information Service (ACTIS): 800-TRIALS-A (874-2572)

For more information about HIV infection, call:

Drug Abuse Hotline: 800-662-HELP (4357)

Pediatric and Pregnancy AIDS Hotline; 212-430-3333

National Hemophilia Foundation: 212-219-8180

Hemophilia and AIDS/HIV Network for Dissemination of Information (HANDI): 800-42-HANDI (424-2634)

National Pediatric HIV Resource Center: 800-362-0071

National Association of People with AIDS: 202-898-0414

Teens Teaching AIDS Prevention Program (TTAPP) National Hotline: 800-234-TEEN (8336)

General information:

English 800-342-AIDS (2437)

Spanish: 800-344-7432

TDD Service for the Deaf: 800-243-7889

General information for health care providers:

HIV Telephone Consultation Service: 800-933-3413

To locate a physician, call your local or state Medical Society

Note: This is not an all-inclusive list. For other sources of information, contact your state HIV hotline. State HIV hotline numbers are located at the end of the "Introduction."

REVIEW QUESTIONS

(*Answers to the Review Questions are on page 479.*)

1. What would be the ideal medical solution for the general population in the fight against HIV?
2. What are the only FDA-approved drugs for antiviral therapy?
3. The FDA has the most rigorous drug approval system in the world. What phase of the system has been changed to bring drugs to the terminally ill more rapidly?

4. Which side of the nonvalidated therapies dispute do you favor? Write an opinion and indicate why. Discuss aspects of ZDV therapy: for example, severe side effects and financial costs. Include data on both adult and pediatric AIDS patients.
5. How does ZDV select for drug-resistant mutants?
6. What single immunomodulator has been found to be safe in human trials and has lowered the number of free HIVs in the bloodstream?
7. Why are scientists so keen on discovering the three-dimensional structure of HIV gene products?
8. Is it possible that macrobiotics can prevent HIV infection?

REFERENCES

ABOULKER, JEAN-PIERRE, et al. (1993). Preliminary analysis of the Concorde trial. *Lancet*, 341:889–890.

AIDS Newslink. (1992 Winter). The twin epidemics of substance use and HIV. 3:4–50.

ANDERSON, R.M., et al. (1991). Potential of community-wide chemotherapy or immunotherapy to control the spread of HIV-1. *Nature*, 350:356–359.

BARINAGA, MARCIA. (1993). Ribozymes: Killing the messenger. *Science*, 262:1512–1514.

BLUNDELL, TOM, et al. (1989). Retroviral proteinases. *Nature*, 337:596–597.

BOYD, MARK T., et al. (1991). Antisense RNA to treat HIV infections. *AIDS*, 5:225–226.

BREO, DENNIS. (1991). Tired of taking the blame, AIDS drug regulatory Ellen Cooper quits. *JAMA*, 265:1027–1028.

BREO, DENNIS. (1993). The US race to 'cure' AIDS–at '4' on a scale of 10, says Dr. Fauc i. *JAMA*, 269:2898–2900.

BUCHSCHACHER, GARY. (1993). Molecular targets of gene transfer therapy for HIV infection. *JAMA*, 269:2880–2886.

CHOW, YUNG-KANG, et al. (1993). Use of evolutionary limitations of HIV-1 multidrug resistance to optimize therapy. *Nature*, 361:650–654.

COHEN, JACK, et al. (1994). The new genetic medicines. *Sci. Am.*, 271:76–82.

COLMAN, N., et al. (1987). Nutritional factors in Epidemic Kaposi's Sarcoma. *Semin. Oncol.*, 14:54.

COTTON, DEBORAH J. (1993). Disappointing Assessment of current antiretrovirals. *AIDS Clin. Care*, 5:51–58.

CRAIN, ELLEN F. (1991). Assessing fever in HIV-infected children. *Emerg. Med.*, 23:137–146.

CROMBLEHOLME, WILLIAM R. (1990). Women's issues are key topic at AIDS conference. *Fam. Pract. News*, 20:26.

DANAR, DAVID A., et al. (1991). Gene therapy for AIDS due. *Med. Tribune*, 32:1,8.

DYDA, FRED, et al. (1994). Crystal structure of the catalytic domain of HIV integrase: Similarity to other polynucleotidyl transferases. *Science*, 266:1981–2006.

ERICKSON, JOHN, et al. (1990). Design, activity, and 2.8 angstrom crystal structure of a C_2 symmetric inhibitor complexed to HIV protease. *Science*, 249:527–533.

EZZELL, CAROL. (1989). AIDS: Closer to becoming a treatable disease. *Nature*, 340:581.

FAUCI, ANTHONY S. (1988). The human immunodeficiency virus: Infectivity and mechanisms of pathogenesis. *Science*, 239:617–621.

FISCHL, MARGARET A. (1994). Combination antiretroviral therapy for HIV infection. *Hosp. Pract.*, 29:43–48.

FREEDMAN, BENJAMIN, et al. (1989). Nonvalidated therapies and HIV disease. *Hastings Center Rep.*, 19:14–20.

GOLDSCHMIDT, RONALD, et al. (1995). Antiretroviral strategies revisited. *J. Am. Board Fam. Pract.*, 8:62–69.

HAMILTON J.D., et al. (1992). A controlled trial of early versus late treatment with zidovudine in symptomatic human immunodeficiency virus infection: results of the Veterans Affairs Cooperative Study. *N. Engl. J. Med.*, 326:437–443.

HARDY, LESLIE M, et al. (1994). Gene therapy for HIV Infection. *JAMA*, 272:423.

HO, DAVID, et al. (1994). Characterization of HIV Variants with Increased Resistance to a C_2-Symmetric Protease Inhibitor. *Virology*, 68:2016–2020.

HO, DAVID, et al. (1995). Rapid turnover of plasma virions and CD4 lymphocytes in HIV infection. *Nature*, 313:123–126.

HODGIN, DEANNA. (1991). AIDS: Desperate Victims—Dangerous drugs. *Insight*, 7:10–17.

JACOBSON L.P., et al. (1993). Changes in survival after acquired immunodeficiency syndrome (AIDS), 1994–1991. *Am. J. Epidemiol.*, 138:952–964.

JANSEN, DOUGLAS D. (1988). Nutrition and the AIDS patient. *Minnesota Pharmacist*, Issue 6, 42:6–9.

KAHN, JAMES. (1991). Clinical Issues in Using Didanosine (ddI). *AIDS Clin. Care*, 3:89–96.

KRIM, MATHILDE. (1986). A chance at life for AIDS sufferers. *New York Times*, August 8:A–27.

LAND, S., et al. (1992). Incidence of ZDV-resistant HIV isolated from patients before, during and after therapy. *J. Infect. Dis.*, 166:1139–1142.

LARDER, BRENDAN A., et al. (1989). HIV with reduced sensitivity to zidovudine (AZT) isolated during prolonged therapy. *Science,* 243:1731–1734.

LARDER, BRENDAN A., et al. (1991). Zidovudine resistance predicted by direct detection of mutations in DNA from HIV-infected lymphocytes. *AIDS,* 5:137–144.

LUNDGREN J.D., et al. (1994). Comparison of long-term prognosis of patients with AIDS treated and not treated with zidovudine. *JAMA,* 271:1088–1092.

MARX, JEAN. (1989). New hope on the AIDS vaccine front. *Science,* 244:1254–1256.

MATTHES, E., et al. (1987). Inhibition of HIV associated reverse transcriptase by sugar-modified derivates of thymidine 5′ phosphate in comparison to cellular DNA polymerases α. *Biochem. Biophys. Res. Commun.,* 148:78–85.

MAY, ROBERT M. (1993). Resisting resistance. *Nature,* 361:593–594.

MCKINNEY, R.E., et al. (1991). A Multicenter trial of oral zidovudine in children with advanced human immunodeficiency virus disease. *N. Engl. J. Med.,* 324:1018–1025.

MCLEAN, ANGELA R., et al. (1991). Population dynamics of HIV within an individual after treatment with zidovudine. *AIDS,* 5:485–489.

MCLEOD, GAVIN, et al. (1992). Nucleoside analogs: Combination therapy. *Hosp. Pract. Suppl. 2,* 27:14–25.

MERLUZZI, VINCENT J., et al. (1990). Inhibition of HIV-1 replication by a nonnucleoside reverse transcriptase inhibitor. *Science,* 250:1411–1413.

Morbidity and Mortality Weekly Report. (1990). Public Health Service statement on management of occupational exposure to HIV, including considerations regarding zidovudine postexposure use. 39:1–14.

Morbidity and Mortality Weekly Report. (1994a). Zidovudine for the prevention of HIV Transmission from Mother to infant. 43:285–287.

Morbidity and Mortality Weekly Report. (1994b). Recommendations of the U. S. Public Health Service Task Force on the Use of Zidovudine to Reduce Perinatal Transmission of Human Immunodeficiency virus. 43:1–15.

NATIONAL INSTITUTES OF HEALTH CONFERENCE. (1990). Intravenous immunoglobulin: Prevention and treatment of Disease. *JAMA,* 264:3189–3193.

NAVIA, MANUEL A., et al. (1989). Three-dimensional structure of aspartyl protease from human immunodeficiency virus HIV-1. *Nature,* 337:615–620.

NOZYCE, MOLLY, et al. (1994). A 12-month study of the effects of oral zidovudine on neurodevelopmental functioning in a cohort of virtically HIV-infected inner-city children. *AIDS,* 8:635–639.

PAUWELS, RUDI, et al. (1990). Potent and selective inhibition of HIV-1 replication *in vitro* by a novel series of TIBO derivatives. *Nature,* 343:470–474.

PHAIR, JOHN P. (1994). Effectiveness of zidovudine in treatment of Advanced HIV Infection. *JAMA,* 271:1121–1122.

PHARMACEUTICAL MANUFACTURING ASSOCIATION. (1990). *New Medicines in Development for Children.* Fall:1–12.

PHARMACEUTICAL MANUFACTURING ASSOCIATION. (1991). *In Development—AIDS Medicines—Drugs and Vaccines.* Oct.:1–11.

PIZZO, PHILLIP A., et al. (1988). Effect of continuous intravenous infusion of zidovudine (AZT) in children with symptomatic HIV infection. *N. Engl. J. Med.,* 319:889–896.

PIZZO, PHILLIP A., et al. (1990). Pediatric AIDS: Problems within problems. *J. Infect. Dis.,* 161:316–325.

RICHMAN, DOUGLAS D. (1993). Playing chess with reverse transcriptase. *Nature,* 361:588–589.

ST. CLAIR, M.H., et al. (1991). Resistance to ddI and sensitivity to AZT induced by a mutation in HIV-1 reverse transcriptase. *Science,* 253:1557–1559.

SKOWRON, GAIL. (1992). Nucleoside analogs: Monotherapy. *Hosp. Pract. Suppl. 2,* 27:5–13.

TASK FORCE ON NUTRITION SUPPORT IN AIDS. (1989). Guidelines for nutrition support in AIDS. *Nutrition,* 5:39–46.

VOLBERDING PAUL A, et al. (1994). The Duration of Zidovudine Benefit in persons with Asymptomatic HIV Infection. *JAMA,* 272:437–442.

VELLA, STEFANO. (1994). Update on a proteinase inhibitor. *AIDS.* 8(suppl. 3):S25–S29.

WEBER, IRENE, et al. (1989). Molecular modeling of the HIV-1 protease and its substrate binding site. *Science,* 243:928–931.

ZIEGNER, ULRIKE, et al. (1995). Cytotoxic T-lymphocyte induction in asymptomatic HIV-infected patients immunized with retrovector-transduced autologous fibroblasts expressing HIV-111B ENV/Rev proteins. *AIDS,* 9:43–50.

CHAPTER

8

Epidemiology and Transmission of the Human Immunodeficiency Virus

Chapter Concepts

- In 1985, HIV-2 was isolated in West Africa.
- Transmission of HIV into the United States may have been via Haiti.
- Lifestyle is associated with HIV transmission.
- HIV is not casually transmitted.
- HIV is not transmitted to humans by insects or other animals.
- HIV transmission is being reported from 160 countries and among all age and ethnic groups.
- The major route of HIV transmission involves an exchange of body fluids.
- The body fluids involved in HIV transmission are exchanged during sexual activities, injection drug use, blood transfusions, use of blood products and during pre- and postnatal events.
- Highest frequency of HIV transmission in the United States is among homosexual and bisexual males and among injection drug users.
- Highest frequency of HIV transmission in Africa is among heterosexuals.
- Prenatal HIV transmission generally occurs after the 12th to 16th week of gestation, most often during childbirth.

When a population becomes infected with a contagious disease, an epidemic results. *Epidemic* is derived from Greek and means "in one place among the people." To understand how an infectious disease can spread or remain established in a population, investigators must consider the relationship between an infectious disease agent and its host population. The study of diseases in populations is an area of medicine known as *epidemiology*.

We learned from earlier epidemics, the danger of complacency. Complacency about HIV infection is especially dangerous because the infection remains hidden for a long time. Because many infected people remain symptom-free for years, it is hard to be sure just who is infected with the virus. The more sexual partners you have, the greater your chances of encountering one who is infected and subsequently becoming infected yourself.

With regard to HIV infection, it is not who you are but your behavior that counts. **The transmission of HIV can be prevented. HIV is relatively hard to contract and can be avoided.** HIV is a communicable disease in a limited sense. A communicable disease is one in which the causative agent passes from one person to another. The modes of transmission for communicable diseases include: direct contact with body fluids, contact with inanimate objects, and contact with vectors, including flies, mosquitoes, or other insects capable of spreading disease. HIV is communicable only in the first of the three modes, that is, through direct contact with certain body fluids. HIV is transmitted in human body fluids by **three** major routes: (1) sexual intercourse through vaginal, rectal, or penile tissues; (2) direct injection with HIV-contaminated drugs, needles, syringes, blood or blood products; and (3) from HIV-infected mother to fetus in utero or through intrapartum inoculation from mother to infant.

Epidemiological data suggest that sexual transmission, in general, is relatively inefficient, in that exposure often does not produce infection. HIV is transmitted more efficiently through intravenous than through sexual routes. However, worldwide the predominant mode of transmission of HIV is through exposure of mucosal surfaces to infected sexual fluids (semen, cervical/vaginal, rectal) and during birth.

HIV is not communicable through contact with inanimate objects or through vectors. Thus people do not "catch" HIV in the same way that they "catch" the cold or a flu virus. Unlike colds and flu viruses, HIV **is not**, according to the CDC, spread by tears, sweat, coughing or sneezing. The virus **is not** transmitted via an infected person's clothes, phone or toilet seat. HIV **is not** passed on by eating utensils, drinking glasses, or other objects that HIV-infected people have used that are free of blood.

HIV **is not** transmitted through daily contact with infected people, whether at work, home, or school. Insects do not transmit the virus. Kissing is also considered very low risk: There has never been a documented case to prove that HIV is transmitted by kissing. However, Paul Holmstrom and colleagues (1992) report that salivary antibodies are detected regularly in HIV seropositive subjects. This suggests that immunoreactivity of these antibodies with HIV may be responsible for the negative results of HIV cultivation or antigen detection in the saliva. The route of HIV into saliva is not fully understood. Both salivary glands and salivary leukocytes have been shown to harbor HIV. Gingival fluid, which is a transudate of serum, has been regarded as the main source of salivary HIV antibodies and infectious HIV.

In its 1990 supplemental guidelines for cardiopulmonary resuscitation (CPR) training and rescue, the Emergency Cardiac Care Committee of the American Heart Association (AHA) noted that there is an extremely small theoretical risk of HIV or hepatitis B virus (HBV) transmission via cardiopulmonary resuscitation (CPR). No known case of seroconversion for HIV or HBV has occurred in these circumstances.

MUST WE STOP HIV TRANSMISSION NOW?

We are standing at a moment in the AIDS epidemic when we have what may be our last opportunity to stem a major new wave of HIV infection: of heterosexuals and in particular minorities in the urban areas, and of gay men and drug users in the smaller cities and suburban and rural areas where infection is currently of less intensity. Stephen Joseph, Commissioner of Health of New York City from 1986 to 1990, states that 10% to 15% of reproductive age men and women in poor minority neighborhoods will be infected. This of course will lead to the birth of a steady stream of HIV-infected infants and the orphaning of a steady stream of older uninfected children as mothers and fathers die of AIDS. To get a sense of the magnitude of the AIDS orphan problem, consider the following: New York City will have 10,000 to 20,000 of these children by the late 1990s (Josephs, 1993).

Education and advocacy for risk reduction remain important tools for preventing HIV infection, but, alone, they will never accomplish the objective of slowing the speed and extent of the virus's spread. This can only be achieved by combining educational and early interven-

POINT OF VIEW 8.1

HIV/AIDS CAN BE STOPPED NOW!

Some HIV/AIDS experts now believe that the AIDS epidemic in America can be all but stamped out, without a vaccine or wonder drug. The strategy would involve concentrating on prevention of risky behavior that is particularly prevalent in 25 to 30 neighborhoods nationwide, in such cities as New York, Miami, Los Angeles, San Francisco, Houston, Newark, and Camden, New Jersey. Among the measures on which public health officials want to concentrate in those neighborhoods are some that many conservatives oppose, including free distribution of clean hypodermic needles, many more drug treatment programs, and explicit sex education adapted to the language and mores of affected neighborhoods. For example, a medical anthropologist at Montefiore Medical Center in the Bronx told of a recent examination that revealed that a patient had been engaging in anal sex. But when the doctor asked him if he had ever had sex with another man, he repeatedly said no. Finally, at the end of the interview, the doctor asked him, "Has another man's penis ever touched your anus?" The man replied, "Oh yeah, all the time." This man practiced anal sex as a trade, for a living; he was homeless. Sex, for him, he said, was something you did with a woman.

Once the controversial idea of stopping HIV/AIDS was proposed, persons of various disciplines immediately began voicing their support or opposition to the idea that the HIV/AIDS epidemic in the United States can be stopped NOW! The following are items of interest both pro and con. After reading both points of view, formulate your own.

PRO:

As Stephen Joseph writes in his book, *Dragon Within the Gates: The Once and Future AIDS Epidemic,* an epidemic requires not only a microbe but also an appropriate social context. HIV/AIDS has found both contexts in the United States: the artistic, cultural, and fashion enterprises and large numbers of gay men. In the late 1980s came the great epidemiological shift away from gay white males and toward minority heterosexuals and needle-sharing injection drug users and their sexual partners. AIDS, like lung cancer, coronary artery disease, and motor vehicle accidents, is a characteristic 20th century epidemic: It is closely related to current behavior—related, in fact, to voluntary, conscious, and intimate behavior, involving sex and drugs. And much of the high-risk behavior is highly concentrated in a few small areas. Because AIDS in America has been associated with stigmatized and illegal behavior, and has been concentrated among marginalized groups—homosexuals and inner-city poor—that feel vulnerable to oppression, there has been a concerted effort to "democratize" the disease. The politically correct message is that everyone is vulnerable—"AIDS does not discriminate." And there has been resistance to targeting the risky behavior of particular groups, groups that tend to be concentrated in given geographical areas of the United States.

Gina Kolata (*New York Times,* March 7, 1993) quotes Don Des Jarlais (day-zhar-lay), a drug-abuse specialist and AIDS researcher at Beth Israel Medical Center in New York, "We could stamp AIDS out. I think that's a realistic goal."

Other experts from a variety of disciplines are also arguing that AIDS can be stopped. They cite two reasons: the pattern of AIDS's spread and the success of programs that have focused tightly on affected groups and neighborhoods.

Their view of the disease's pattern of spread has emerged from a recent analysis by a committee of the National Research Council that suggests AIDS is devastating a handful of neighborhoods while leaving most of the nation relatively unscathed.

In its report, "The Social Impact of AIDS," released in February 1993, the council said the epidemic was "settling into spatially and socially isolated groups and possibly becoming endemic in them." As a result, the committee wrote, "many geographic areas and strata of the population are virtually untouched by the epidemic and probably never will be," while "certain confined areas and populations have been devastated."

The second reason for a new approach is that data now emerging, mostly from abroad, show it is possible to reverse the course of an AIDS epidemic or even to prevent one if efforts are intense and narrowly focused. Such efforts have succeeded even among supposedly recalcitrant populations like injection drug users.

Australia, for example, has managed to control the rate of new infection in the last 5 years by targeting high-risk groups. And Tacoma, Washington has kept its HIV infection rates among injection drug users negligible while rates in New York and other cities have soared to between 50% and 80%. To this end, Allan Brandt of Harvard University states, "If we want to really deal with the epidemic, we have to go where the epidemic is."

Until recently, health officials in Russia performed some 24 million HIV tests a year on pregnant women, hospital patients, soldiers, and just about anyone else. The result: Between 1990 and the end of 1993, 338 people tested positive. It's a similar story throughout much of the former eastern bloc. Out of almost 100,000 AIDS cases so far reported across Europe, only 3.4% are from the continent's eastern half, and some countries—including Azerbaijan, Kazakhstan, Tajikistan, and Albania—have yet to diagnose their first AIDS case. The AIDS virus was not rapidly spread under communism.

A big question facing these countries now is whether the virus can continue to be kept at bay in the wake of the social liberalization and increase in foreign travel that are following the collapse of the old, repressive regimes. The guarded answer from officials at the World Health Organization (WHO) is: Yes, at least in theory. They calculate that the epidemic in eastern Europe and the former Soviet Union is lagging 5 years behind that in the West—just enough time, they argue, to mount an effective anti-HIV effort. Eastern Europe is one of the few parts of the world where it may be posible to stop the virus in its tracks. "These countries have a good chance," says Johannes Hallauer, European coordinator for WHO's Global Program on AIDS, "because it is early enough to prevent a big spread of the virus" (Balter, 1993).

Albert Jonsen, an ethics professor at the University of Washington and the chairman of the National Research Council's Committee on AIDS believes that epidemics throughout history have behaved in a pattern similar to that of HIV/AIDS. "The thing that leaps out at you is the way that almost every historical epidemic was socially-culturally determined." People were not felled indiscriminately.

A second feature of epidemics is that they require a concentration of cases to sustain the disease. In the case of AIDS, if you are going to have sexual transmission outside of infected communities, you need a fairly high rate of contact. The disease can and does break out of the tight communities where it festers, but it cannot sustain itself there.

In concluding the PRO discussion,Jeff Stryker and Ronald Bayer (1933), both members of NRC, believe that if the people of the United States come to believe that AIDS no longer threatens every hamlet and every citizen, political support for AIDS prevention and research might be eroded. Those who agree with this idea believe that focusing on "the universality of risk among all people" helps meet the need of the truly vulnerable (Stryker et al., 1993). Stryker and Bayer believe the time is ripe for new leadership in the fight against AIDS.

The rethinking they propose involves asking some hard questions. Does current AIDS prevention policy in the United States suffer because of a scattershot approach divorced from epidemiological reality? Would a more targeted approach place those outside the current epicenters of HIV infection at risk?Would such an approach to prevention foster stigmatization, possibly weakening the delicate political alliance that currently supports HIV prevention and research.

CON: The Opposing Force

The contention that AIDS is sustained by a small number of epicenters is unrealistic. The opposing force counters that it is, in fact, very unwise to focus prevention efforts on a relatively small number of neighborhoods at the expense of those with fewer AIDS cases. They emphasize that everyone needs help and should be assured of receiving it. June Osborn, chairwoman of the National Commission of AIDS, states that, "AIDS sustains itself awfully well. As soon as the virus is present, as it now is everywhere, risk-taking behavior becomes significant."

Osborn takes issue with the very notion of targeting a few areas: "It is much too broad a brush to say, 'Focus your money in some areas, and everyone else can forget it.' Nobody can forget it. The AIDS epidemic is very rapidly spreading throughout smaller and smaller communities each year." Still others warn that the strategy of focusing on a few target areas could threaten and offend the very groups it is meant to help. There is a real concern among many people that public discussions of HIV and AIDS as a problem among minorities will further stigmatize them without necessarily leading to an allocation of resources to help correct the problem.

Osborn and colleague David Rogers (1993) state that the NRC report "subtly encouraged the virus spread through all segments of society " and feel it is a "cruel influence" and "painful setback [for] responsible public policy."

Another point of view is that if this idea had been tried early on it might have worked—if one could possibly have gotten around the charges of racial discrimination. But it is too late, the horse is out of the barn.

Class Discussion:

What do you think? Is it too late? Has the horse left the barn? Can the barn still be locked up? Can charges of discrimination be justly filed if large sums of money and medical personnel were assigned to those areas with the largest concentration of AIDS cases while the lower incidence areas were left to a lower level of support?

tion efforts with specific measures guiding those resources to the people who need them most: those who are already infected and to their sex and drug partners.

By the end of 1995, there will be over 500,000 AIDS cases in the United States. Figure 8-1 breaks this number down according to means of HIV infection that is, sexual behavior, drug use, medical exigencies, and undetermined causes. Figure 8-2 gives a breakdown by transmission category for those AIDS adult/adolescent cases reported only for 1993. There were 80,473 reported AIDS cases for 1994.

EPIDEMIOLOGY OF HIV INFECTION

The first scientific evidence of human HIV infection came from the detection of HIV antibodies in preserved serum samples collected in Central Africa in 1959. The first AIDS cases appeared there in the 1960s. By the mid-1970s HIV was being spread throughout the rest of the world. The earliest places to experience the arrival of HIV were Central Europe and Haiti. Transmission into the United States may have been by tourists who had vacationed in the area of Port-au-Prince, Haiti (Swenson, 1988).

On entry into the United States the virus first spread among the homosexual populations of large cities such as New York and San Francisco. The first *recorded* AIDS cases in the United States occurred in 1979 in New York. The first CDC *reported* AIDS cases were in New York, Los Angeles, and San Francisco in 1981 (Figure 8-3). In both cases, the diagnosis of AIDS was based on clinical descriptions. Retrospectively, antibody to the AIDS virus was detected in the stored tissue of a 25-year-old British sailor from Manchester who died mys-

FIGURE 8-1 AIDS Cases by Route of Transmission. By the end of 1994, there were about 442,000 AIDS cases in the United States. This diagram gives the percentage of adults and adolescents in each group. Groupings are according to sexual preference, drug use, medical conditions, and others not associated with any of these. (*Courtesy of CDC,* Atlanta)

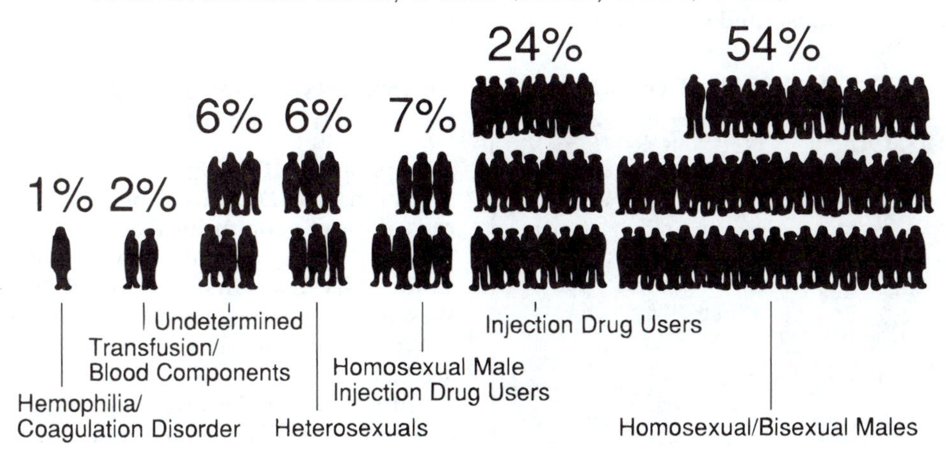

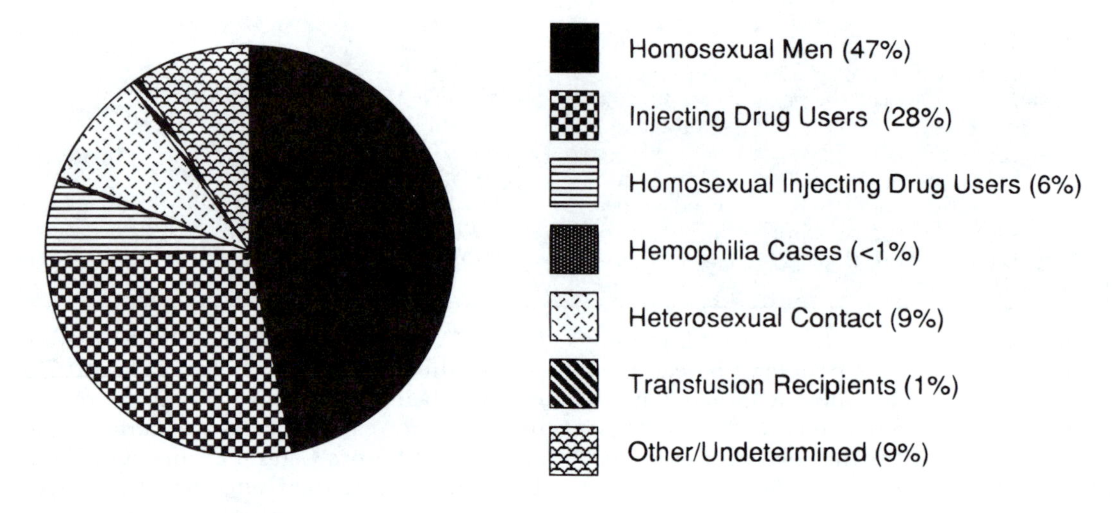

FIGURE 8-2 Adult/Adolescent AIDS Cases by Transmission Category Reported for 1993, United States. Reported for 1994, 80,473. (Pediatric cases for 1993, 959; for 1994, 1,017)

teriously in 1959 (Corbitt et al., 1990). The first case in the United States was identified from a frozen blood sample that was taken from a 15-year-old male in St. Louis, Missouri, who died of AIDS in 1969. He was also infected with chlamydia, herpes, cytomegalovirus, and Epstein-Barr viruses. At his death, his body was severely wasted and he demonstrated Kaposi's sarcoma (Garry et al., 1988). How he contracted the virus is unknown.

According to the CDC AIDS definition (Table 1-2), at least one case of AIDS occurred in New York City in 1952 and another in 1959. Both males demonstrated opportunistic infections and *Pneumocystis carinii* pneumonia, today a hallmark of HIV infection. This early evidence of AIDS suggests that the virus might have been in both the United States and Africa at about the same time (Katner et al., 1987). If HIV has been present for decades as suggested, its failure to spread may reflect a recent HIV mutation, a major change in social behaviors conducive to HIV transmission, or both. For example, the sexual revolution and the widespread use of birth control pills, which began in the 1960s, and the subsequent decrease in the use of condoms may be involved with the transmission of HIV.

POINT OF INFORMATION 8.1

CONSEQUENCES OF IGNORING HIV

You may be offended by the description of how HIV is transmitted. You may feel invulnerable to HIV infection. You may think that given time, HIV infection and AIDS will "go away." You may choose to ignore that it exists. **But ignoring HIV may kill you.** The cost of ignorance about any of the STDs is always high, but with AIDS the cost is a disfiguring, painful death.

TRANSMISSION OF TWO STRAINS OF HIV (HIV-1/HIV-2)

The spread of HIV-1 is global. The clinical presentation of AIDS caused by HIV-1 is similar regardless of geographical area.

HIV-2 is a genetically similar but distinct strain. HIV-2 was first discovered 1n 1985 in West Africa. It is believed to have been present in West Africa as early as the 1960s (Marlink et al., 1994).

Information is lacking concerning clinical outcomes of HIV-2-infected individuals. From

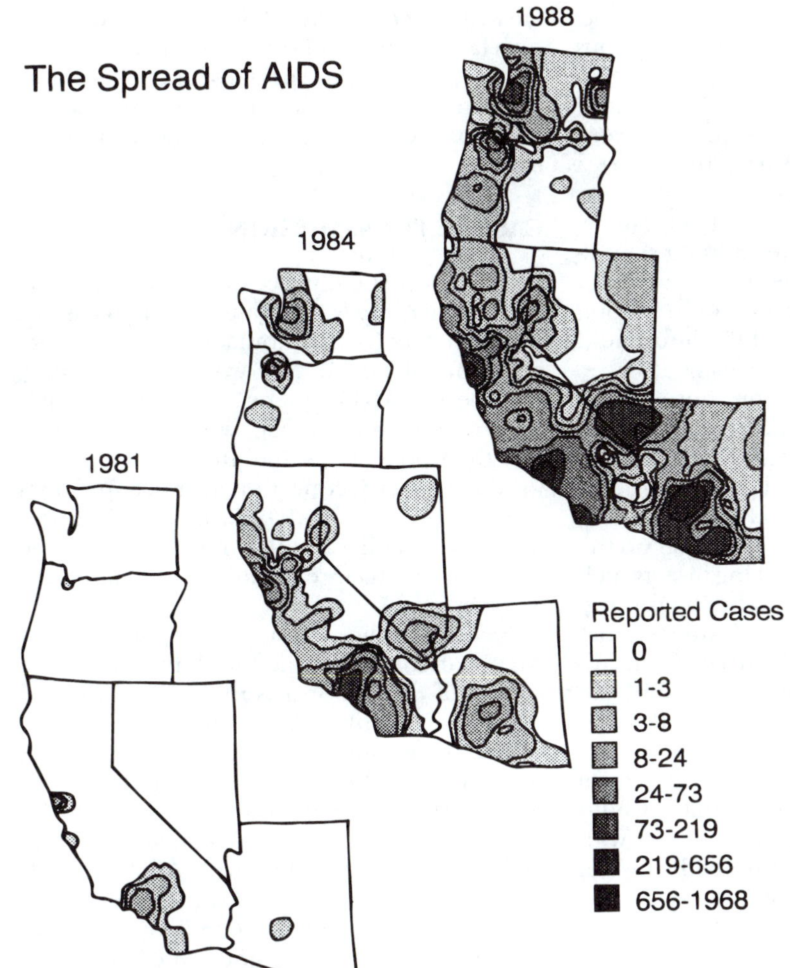

FIGURE 8-3 The Spread of HIV/AIDS on the West Coast. The three separate maps show the rapid spread of AIDS along the Pacific Coast from 1981 through 1988. The maps depict a movement from urban centers into the suburbs and surrounding rural areas. The AIDS epidemic in the West first appeared in Los Angeles and San Francisco, followed by Las Vegas and Phoenix. By 1983, Seattle and Portland encountered the epidemic. The number of AIDS cases continues to increase as HIV infection continues to spread. (*Courtesy of Peter Gould and colleagues, Pennsylvania State University*)

1985 to 1993, a prospective clinical study was conducted in women with HIV-1 and HIV-2 infection to determine and compare rates of disease development. HIV-1-infected women had a 67% probability of AIDS-free survival 5 years after seroconversion in contrast with 100% for HIV-2-infected women. The HIV-2 infected had significantly fewer HIV-related diseases then the HIV-1 infected. The rate of developing abnormal T4 lymphocyte counts with HIV-2 infection was also significantly reduced. These data demonstrate that HIV-2 has a reduced virulence compared to HIV-1 (Marlink et al., 1994).

What appears certain is that HIV-2, like HIV-1, will spread worldwide. HIV-2 has already spread from West Africa to other parts of Africa, Europe, and the Americas. In 1988, HIV-2 infection was discovered in a woman in New Jersey. Both HIV-1 and HIV-2 are transmitted or acquired through the same kinds of exposure.

(Because over 95% of global AIDS cases are caused by the transmission of HIV-1, only data that pertain to HIV-1 (HIV) will be presented unless otherwise stated.)

IS HIV TRANSMITTED BY INSECTS?

In spite of convincing evidence of the ways in which HIV can be transmitted, it remains difficult for the general public to believe that a virus that spreads so rapidly is not either highly contagious or transmitted by an environmental agent. After all, there are many viral and bacterial diseases that are either highly contagious or transmitted by insects. The question was asked: Is this virus being transmitted by insects?

Necessary data to resolve the question were available. Epidemiological data from Africa and the United States suggested that AIDS was not transmitted by insect bites. If it were, many more cases would be expected among school-age children and elderly people, groups that are proportionally underrepresented among AIDS patients. In one study of the household contacts of AIDS patients in Kinshasa, Zaire, where insect bites are common, not a single child over the age of 1 year had been infected with the AIDS virus, while more than 60% of spouses had become infected.

In 1987, the Office of Technology Assessment (OTA) published a detailed paper on the question of whether blood-sucking insects such as biting flies, mosquitoes, and bedbugs transmit HIV (Miike, 1987). The conclusion was that the conditions necessary for successful transmission of HIV through insect bites and the probability of their occurring rule out the possibility of insect transmission as a significant factor in the spread of AIDS. Also, a Central Intelligence Agency report stated that it would take 2,800 bites by a mosquito infected with HIV "to deliver a sufficient virus load (dose of HIV) to pose even a theoretical threat."

EXPOSURE TO HIV AND SUBSEQUENT INFECTION

Early on, it was believed that certain aspects of one's lifestyle and medical status predetermined the risk of HIV infection upon HIV exposure. For example, if the HIV-exposed individual had some previous sexually transmitted disease or an open sore, used drugs, or had an already weakened immune system, he or she would be more susceptible to HIV infection. Such conditions are called **cofactors**. There is, at the moment, considerable argument as to whether cofactors are essential to HIV infection. (See Chapter 4 for a discussion on cofactors.)

TRANSMISSION OF HIV

If most HIV-exposed people can become HIV-infected, can most infected people *transmit* HIV to others? This is a difficult question to answer. Infection with HIV appears to depend on a large number of variables that involve the donor, recipient, and portal of entry. The most important variables are mode of transmission, viral dose, and the genetic resistance of the recipient.

CASUAL TRANSMISSION

There is overwhelming evidence that *HIV is not transmitted casually*. Assurances that HIV is not spread through casual contact are based on observation of health care workers and family members of AIDS patients. These individuals have much closer contact with AIDS patients and their body fluids than the average person would in a social, educational, or occupational setting. Thus, if the AIDS virus could be transmitted through casual contact, it would be found in much larger numbers of health care workers.

Several studies of the family members of AIDS patients have failed to demonstrate the spread of the AIDS virus through household contact. The only cases in which family members have become infected involved the sexual partners of AIDS patients or children born to mothers who were already infected with the virus. Even individuals who bathed, diapered, or slept in the same bed with AIDS patients have not become infected. In one study, 7% of the family members shared toothbrushes with the infected person and none became infected.

Perhaps the best evidence against casual HIV transmission comes from studies of household members living with blood-transfused AIDS patients (Peterman et al., 1988). Transfusion infection cases are unique because their dates of infection are known retrospectively. Prior to the onset of AIDS symptoms, the families were unaware that they were living with HIV-infected individuals. Family life was not altered in any way, yet family members remained uninfected. In some cases, the transfusion patients were hemophiliacs who received weekly or monthly injections of blood products and became HIV-infected. From the combined studies of these households, only the sexual partners of infected hemophiliacs became infected. In some cases, the sexual partners of hemophiliacs remained HIV free after 3 to 5 years of unprotected sexual intercourse.

HIV TRANSMISSION IN HOUSEHOLD SETTINGS

Although contact with Blood and other body substances can occur in households, transmission of HIV is rare in this setting. Through mid-1995, at least eight reports have described household transmission of HIV not associated with sexual contact, injection drug use, or breast feeding (Table 8-1). Of these eight reports, five were associated with documented or probable blood contact. In one report, HIV infection was diagnosed in a boy after his younger brother had died as the result of AIDS; however, a specific mechanism of transmission was not determined.

Home Nursing Exposure

Three reports involved home nursing care of terminally ill persons with AIDS in which a blood exposure might have occurred but was not documented; in these reports, skin contact with body secretions and excretions occured.

In another reported case in the United States, a mother apparently became infected with HIV as a result of extensive, unprotected exposure to her infected child's blood, body secretions, and excretions. The child, who underwent numerous surgical procedures to correct a congenital intestinal abnormality, had become infected through multiple blood transfusions. The mother did not wear gloves when performing procedures such as drawing blood, removing intravenous lines, emptying ostomy bags, changing diapers, and changing surgical dressings. On numerous occasions her hands became contaminated with blood, feces, saliva, and nasal secretions. Although she reported no accidental needlesticks or open wounds on her hands, she often failed to wash her hands immediately after such exposures.

In a similar case, a woman in England developed AIDS after caring for a man who died of AIDS. Again, the care involved frequent contact with body secretions and excretions. The woman reported that she had some small cuts and eczema on her hands during the time that she cared for the man.

HOME CARE PREVENTION

Persons who provide home nursing care for HIV-infected patients should employ precautions to reduce exposures to blood and other body fluids. In particular, needles and sharp objects contaminated with blood should be handled with care. Needles should not be recapped by hand or removed from syringes. Needles and sharp objects should be disposed of in puncture-proof containers, and the containers should be kept out of reach of children and visitors. Bandages should be used to cover cuts, sores, or breaks on exposed skin of persons with HIV infections and of persons providing care. In addition, persons who provide such care should wear gloves when there is a possibility of direct contact with HIV-infected blood or other body fluids, secretions, or excretions. Because urine and feces may contain a variety of pathogens, including HIV, persons providing nursing care to HIV-infected persons should wear gloves during contact with these substances. In addition, even when gloves are worn, hands should be washed after contact with blood and other body fluids, secretions, or excretions.

Because of the social, economic, and medical benefits of home care, the number of persons with AIDS who receive health care outside of hospitals is increasing. Persons infected with HIV and persons providing home care for those who are HIV-infected should be fully educated and trained regarding appropriate infection control techniques. In addition, health care providers should be aware of the potential for HIV transmission in the home and should provide training and education in infection control for HIV-infected persons and those who live or provide care to them in the home. Such training should be an intergral and ongoing part of the health care plan for every person with HIV infection.

The findings of the investigations described in Table 8-1 indicate the transmission of HIV as the result of contact with blood or other

TABLE 8-1 Reported Cases of HIV Infection in Which Transmission Not Associated with Sexual Contact, Injection-Drug Use, or Breast Feeding Occurred from an HIV-Infected Person to a Person Residing in the Same Household or Providing Home Care

Case-Patient	Source-Patient	Activity During Which Transmission May Have Occured	Type of Exposure	Body Substance Through Which Transmission May Have Occured	HIV DNA Sequence Match	Comment
Mother	Child	Home nursing	Cutaneous	Blood/ stool	ND[1]	Mother provided extensive care without gloves (e.g., drawing blood, removing intravenous catheters, and emptying and changing ostomy bags).
Child	Child	Home intravenous therapy for hemophilia	Possible intravenous percutaneous[2]	Blood	Y	Mother administered intravenous therapy to both children in succession and placed used needles in bag within reach of case-patient.
Child	Child	Living in same household	Cutaneous[2]	Blood	Y	Source-patient had frequent bleeding; case-patient had excoriated rash.
Adolescent	Adolescent	living in same household	Cutaneous/ percutaneous	Blood	Y	Case-patient and source-patient shared a razor; each cut himself while shaving with the razor and bled as a result. Both have hemophilia.
Child	Mother	Living in same household	Cutaneous	Blood/ exudate	Y	Source-patient had drained skin lesions; source-patient picked at case-patient's scabs.
Child	Child	Living in same household	Bite[2]	Not specified	ND	Source-patient bit case-patient, skin was not broken, and there was no bleeding. Details of home care not reported.
Adult	Adult	Home nursing	Cutaneous	Body secretions and excretions, including urine and saliva	ND	Case-patient wore no gloves while caring for source-patient; case-patient had eczema and small cuts on her hands.
Mother	Adult son	Home nursing	Cutaneous	Body secretions and excretions, including urine and feces	ND	Case-patient usually wore gloves.

[1]Not done.

[2]No definite exposure documented.

(Source: *MMWR*,1994a)

body secretions or excretions from an HIV-infected person in the household.

Additional infection control recommendations are contained in a recently updated brochure published by CDC, *Caring for Someone with AIDS: Information for Friends, Relatives, Household Members, and Others Who Care for a Person with AIDS at Home.* This brochure is available free in English or Spanish from the CDC National AIDS Clearinghouse, P.O. Box 6003,

Rockville, MD 20849–6003; Telephone (800) 458–5231 or (301) 217–0023. (*MMWR* 1994)

Living in the Same Household

In December 1993, investigators found two cases in which HIV was transmitted from one child and one adolescent to others but not by the usual routes.

One case involved two New Jersey boys, whose ages were given only as between 2 and 5. The other involved two teenage brothers who are hemophiliacs. The investigators found no evidence for the usual modes of transmission—sexual intercourse or contaminated needles. Thus they believe that the most probable route of transmission in both cases was the contact of one child's blood with the blood of another child through a nosebleed or shared razor blade.

In the New Jersey case, the older, infected child had frequent nosebleeds, and the younger child had dermatitis, a condition that can break the surface of the skin.

The brothers with hemophilia shared a razor on one occasion. They told investigators that they did not know who used the razor first. Each had his own injection equipment to deliver the drug needed to prevent uncontrolled bleeding.

In August of 1994,There was a single report of HIV being transmitted during a bloody fight (Ippolito et al., 1994). Two brothers had a severe fight. Brother (1) had been diagnosed with AIDS. Brother (2) beat (1) until blood from (1) flowed freely from both sides of his face. Brother (2) reported that blood from (1) came into contact with his mucosal surfaces of his eyes and lips. Brother (2) developed mononucleosis symptons and tested positive 30 days after the fight. Brother(2) denied contact with needles used by his brother, or sharing of razors, toothbrushes, manicure scissors, or a common sexual partner. Tests for other blood-borne and sexually transmitted diseases were negative. HIV isolated from both brothers showed the same pattern of mutations associated with resistance to zidovudine (AZT) even though only brother (1) had taken the drug.

Since transmission in such a manner has rarely, if ever, been documented, these cases are of special interest to scientists. But these two cases are not cause for alarm and are not cause for changing CDC recommended guidelines for allowing HIV-infected children to attend schools.

The exposures in these nine cases are not typical of the household or social contact most people would have with an HIV-infected or AIDS patient. Nevertheless, they underline the need for observance of commonsense sanitary precautions when caring for an AIDS patient.

NONCASUAL TRANSMISSION

The routes of HIV transmission were established *before* the virus was identified. The appearance of AIDS in the United States occurred first in specific groups of people: homosexual men and injection drug users. The transmission of the disease within the two groups appeared to be closely associated with sexual behavior and the sharing of IV needles. By 1982, hemophiliacs receiving blood products, as well as the newborns of injection drug users, began demonstrating AIDS. By 1983, heterosexual female partners of AIDS patients demonstrated AIDS. Fourteen years of continued surveillance of the general population has failed to reveal other categories of people contracting HIV/AIDS (Table 8-2). It became apparent that the infectious agent was being transmitted within specific groups of people, who by their behavior were at increased risk for acquiring and transmitting it (Table 8-3). Clearly, an exchange of body fluids was involved in the transmission of the disease.

With the announcement that a new virus had been discovered, further research showed that this virus was present in most body fluids. Thus, even before there was a test to detect this virus, the public was told that it was transmitted through body fluids exchanged during intimate sexual contact, contaminated hypodermic needles, contaminated blood or blood products, and from mother to fetus. In addition it was concluded that the widespread dissemination of the virus was most likely the result of multiple or repeated viral exposure because the data from transfusion-infected individuals indicated that they did not necessar-

TABLE 8-2 HIV Transmission and Infection

TRANSMISSION ROUTES

Blood Inoculation

- Transfusion of HIV-infected blood and blood products
- Needle sharing among injection drug users
- Needlesticks, open cuts, and mucous membrane exposure in health care workers
- Use of HIV-contaminated skin-piercing instruments (ears, acupuncture, tattoos)
- Injection with unsterilized syringe and needle (mostly in Africa)

Sexual Contact: Exchange of semen, vaginal fluids, or blood

- Homosexual, between men
- Lesbian, between women
- Heterosexual, from men to women and women to men
- Bisexual men

Perinatal

- Intrauterine
- Peripartum (during birth)
- Breast feeding

(Adapted from Friedland et al., 1987)

TABLE 8-3 Adult/Adolescent AIDS Cases by Sex and Exposure Categories, through December 1994, United States

Male Exposure Category (88.5%)	Total No.	
1. Men who have sex with men	237,035	(62)
2. Injecting drug use	80,286	(21)
3. Men who have sex with men and inject drugs	30,585	(8)
4. Hemophilia/coagulation disorder	3,823	(1)
5. Heterosexual contact:	7,646	(2)
a. Sex with injecting drug user	3,823	
b. Sex with person with hemophilia	25	
c. Sex with transfusion recipient with HIV infection	128	
d. Sex with HIV-infected person, risk not specified	3,670	
6. Receipt of blood transfusion, blood components, or tissue	3,823	(1)
7. Other/undetermined	19,116	(5)
Total male AIDS cases	382,314	(100)
Female Exposure Category (11.5%)		
1. Injecting drug use	24,906	(49)
2. Hemophilia/coagulation disorder	76	(0)
3. Heterosexual contact:	17,714	(35)
a. Sex with injecting drug user	10,097	
b. Sex with bisexual male	1,594	
c. Sex with person with hemophilia	178	
d. Sex with transfusion recipient with HIV infection	354	
e. Sex with HIV-infected person, risk not specified	5,491	
4. Receipt of blood transfusion, blood components, or tissue	3,050	(6)
5. Other/undetermined	5,082	(10)
Total female AIDS cases	50,828	(100)
Total cases	441,982	

ily infect their sexual partners. In other words, it was concluded early on and later confirmed that this viral infection did not occur as easily as other blood-borne viral diseases such as hepatitis B, or viral and bacterial sexually transmitted diseases. Table 8-4 lists the means of HIV transmission worldwide.

Mobility and the Spread of HIV/AIDS

Mobility is an important epidemiological factor in the spread of communicable diseases. This becomes particularly obvious when a new disease enters the scene. In the early stage of the HIV/AIDS epidemic, for example, the route of the virus could be associated with mobility.

The first HIV-infected people in some Latin American and European countries reported a history of foreign travel. In some African countries, spread of the virus could be traced along international roads. Today, increasing numbers of HIV infection have been observed to be associated with the relaxation of travel restrictions in Central and Eastern Europe.

Few countries are unaffected by HIV/ AIDS. This has made it clear that restrictive measures such as refusal of entry to people living with HIV/AIDS and compulsory testing of mobile populations are inappropriate and ineffective measures to stop spread of the virus. In times of increasing international interdependency, it is an illusion to think that the disease can be stopped at any border.

Who Is Mobile?— Mobility is a feature that can be observed in all societies and at all times. It may be characterized as leading to two types of new residence. One is that in which people become more or less settled in their place of destination, establishing a home and eventually integrating, at least somewhat, into the society they have entered. In the other case,

TABLE 8-4 How HIV is Transmitted Worldwide, 1995

Exposure	Efficiency, %	% of Total
Blood transfusion	>90	5
Perinatal	20–40	10
Sexual intercourse	0.1–1.0	75
Injection drug use	0.5–1.0	10
Needle-type exposure	<0.5	<0.1

(Source: WHO/Global Programme on AIDS)

people only temporarily settle in a place, knowing and/or hoping that they will only reside in the new place for a strictly limited period of time. Three such mobile groups are: migrant workers, travelers, and refugees.

Migrant workers are an example of mobile people who often attain a more settled new existence. They constitute a significant mobile population as many national economies depend on manpower provided by foreigners. However, it should be noted that "migrants" do not constitute a homogeneous group. Some go abroad with the intention of making their new home a permanent one, while others may maintain two homes. The latter situation is seen, for instance, with seasonal migrants who travel to a particular destination at a certain time each year, thereafter returning to their place of origin.

Travelers, a multifaceted group, represent mobile people who do not permanently settle in another place. They can be distinguished according to their motives for travel (business or leisure), their destinations (long distance, East-West travel), the social context of their trips (travel alone, with a partner, or in a group), and their length of stay (overnight stops, as is the case for truckers, or several weeks for businessmen, fishermen, or traders).

Refugees, who move to flee war zones or escape from political, economic, or ecological crises, are an example of people who do not intend to resettle elsewhere permanently. Their place of refuge may be a refugee camp or it may constantly change, as in the case of displaced persons who move from one region to another. (See related information in Point of Information 8.2).

HIV Patterns in Different Countries

HIV infection is a global pandemic. Within the global community, three general patterns of HIV transmission have been identified by the World Health Organization and the U.S. Communicable Disease Center: Patterns I, II, and III.

Pattern I transmission occurs in industrialized parts of the world such as the United States, Canada, Western Europe, Australia, and New Zealand, and some Latin American countries such as Brazil, Mexico, and Puerto Rico. HIV was introduced to these countries in the late 1970s. The principal modes of transmission are through homosexual sex, bisexual sex, prostitution, injection drug use, and sex with a drug user. The ratio of male to female AIDS cases is 10:1 to 15:1. However, if the number of gay AIDS cases is subtracted, the male-to-female ratio is about 3:1. Hetero-sexual transmission and perinatal infection account for a small but gradually increasing number of cases. IDUs account for a significant number of AIDS cases in Italy, Spain, and Puerto Rico. Transfusion-associated disease is steadily declining due to effective screening of donated blood.

Pattern II transmission occurs in developing countries in Africa, the Caribbean (Haiti and the Dominican Republic), and parts of South America. Here, HIV was introduced in the early to mid-1970s and has been predominantly spread by heterosexual intercourse. The male to female ratio is about 1:1. Homosexual transmission is believed to be rare. Transmission by IDUs is infrequent due to lack of money and drug availability. Transfusion-associated infection is still significant due to lack of resources required to screen donated blood.

Early in 1994, the World Health Organization stopped using the term "Pattern II" to describe regional differences in transmission because this is no longer a useful way to describe all countries where heterosexual contact is a major mode of HIV transmission. Adult/adolescent heterosexual contact cases formerly classified under "Born in Pattern II country" and "Sex with person born in Pattern II country " are now tabulated under the category "Risk not reported or identified."

POINT OF INFORMATION 8.2

AIDS AND IMMIGRATION

Time magazine reported (February 1993) the results of a telephone poll of 1,000 American adults. The question was: Should the United States allow foreigners who have the AIDS virus to enter [the USA]? Twenty-two percent said yes, 71% said no.

In 1992, the National Commission on AIDS urged the Clinton Administration to scrap the continued prohibition against HIV-infected foreigners. International visitors are questioned by the Immigration and Naturalization Service, and those who admit to testing HIV-positive can be denied visas. An exemption for travelers attending international conferences or business meetings was added in 1990.

Under current regulations, there is a list of communicable diseases—including AIDS, syphilis, gonorrhea, leprosy, and tuberculosis—that are grounds for barring entry into the United States. A Clinton proposal (1993) is to remove all of them except active tuberculosis, which unlike the others can spread through the air. The National Commission on AIDS estimates that as a result between 300 and 600 people with AIDS or infected with HIV might immigrate into the country every year.

Clinton's plan to lift the current ban is supported by most of the medical community, including officials at the Public Health Service, the Centers for Disease Control and Prevention, and the National Academy of Sciences. "AIDS is not transmitted by casual contact, so we don't have a public health concern with Clinton's proposal," says Dr. Charles Mahan, Florida's state health officer. "The argument has been that it's expensive to take care of these patients, but we let in chronic kidney and cancer patients, whose treatment can be even more costly."

Meanwhile, in an interim order in March of 1993, U.S. District Court Judge Sterling Johnson, Jr., ordered the government to immediately move all HIV-infected Haitian refugees in detention at the U.S. naval base at Guantanamo Bay in Cuba. This order moved 158 HIV-positive Haitian immigrants into South Florida and the New York area on humanitarian grounds—medical care at Guantanamo was inadequate to treat HIV-positive persons. By the end of 1993, the U.S. Senate voted 76 to 23 to bar HIV-infected foreigners from permanent immigration into the United States.

Class Discussion:

Is the case for barring HIV-positive persons from establishing permanent residence in the United States based on scientific fact, political fear, or both/neither?

Pediatric perinatal transmission cases in which the child's mother was formerly classified under "Born in Pattern II country" and "Sex with person born in Pattern II country" are now tabulated under the exposure category "Mother with/at risk for HIV infection: Has HIV infection, risk not specified." This change in reporting heterosexual contact is reflected in the data presented in Table 8.3.

Pattern III transmission occurs in countries of Eastern Europe, the Middle East, North Africa, Asia, and the Pacific. In Thailand and India, HIV infection is rapidly increasing, and most cases have been associated with sexual or IDU contact with foreigners. Imported contaminated blood has also been a significant problem in some countries. (See Chapter 11, "Prevalence of HIV Infection and AIDS outside the United States.")

Number of HIVs Required for Infection

Robert Coombs and colleagues (1989) calculated the dose of HIV necessary to cause an HIV infection. They reported that one "infective dose" of 1,000 HIV particles is necessary to establish HIV infection in human tissue culture cells. To establish HIV infection in the body, it was reasoned that it would take 10 to 15 infective doses. Their study indicated that a pint of blood from an AIDS patient contains 1.8 million infective doses, or about 2 billion HIV particles per pint of blood, or about 4.2 million HIV particles per milliliter.

Placing these numbers in perspective, in cases of hepatitis B there may be 100 million to 1 billion hepatitis viruses in *just 1 mL* of blood (25 to 250 times more virus/mL than

BOX 8.1

RELATIVE DOSE: THE SWIMMING POOL ANALOGY

An analogy on the number of viruses it would take to cause an infection can be made by diluting the number of viruses in 1 mL of blood in a swimming pool full of water.

Basically the analogy goes like this: If 1 mL of blood carrying the hepatitis B virus were dropped into 24,000 gallons of water and mixed well, and if 1 mL of that solution were injected into a susceptible individual, that individual would develop hepatitis B. He or she might not develop jaundice, gray stools, chocolate urine, or other clinical conditions, but would develop serological markers indicating hepatitis B infection.

In contrast, if 1 mL of blood from an AIDS patient were dropped into a quart of water and 1 mL of that solution were injected into a susceptible individual, there is only a 1 in 10 chance that the individual would develop HIV antibody indicating HIV infection (Cottone et al., 1990). The implication here is that HIV is not easy to acquire.

for HIV). A pint of blood contains 473 mL. Yet only one in three people who stick themselves with a needle contaminated with blood from a hepatitis B patient becomes infected.

The epidemiology of HIV infection is similar to that of HBV infection, and much that has been learned over the last 15 years about the risk of acquiring hepatitis B in the health care workplace can be applied to understanding the risk of HIV transmission in similar settings. Both viruses are transmitted in the same manner.

Current evidence indicates that despite the epidemiological similarities of HBV and HIV infection, the risk of HBV transmission in health care settings far exceeds that of HIV transmission. The risk of HIV transmission from a needlestick (including "probable " cases) is less than 0.5%. By contrast, the risk of hepatitis B infection from a needlestick has been estimated at 6% to 30%, or anywhere from 12 to 60 times more likely than for HIV. Approximately 12,000 health care workers in the United States develop symptomatic hepatitis B annually. About 1,000 of them become carriers, and approximately 250 die of cirrhosis, fulminant hepatitis, or primary liver carcinoma. A health care worker's risk of dying of hepatitis B after 15 years on the job is about 27 in 10,000; the annual risk of dying in a car crash is 2.4 in 10,000 (Sadovsky, 1989).

Body Fluid Transmission

HIV has been isolated from blood, semen, saliva, serum, urine, tears, breast milk, vaginal secretions, lung fluid, and cerebrospinal fluid (Friedland et al., 1987). HIV has not been found in sweat. Because HIV has been identified in these fluids does not, however, mean they are important in transmission. Jay Levy and colleagues (1989) isolated HIV from 10 cell-free body fluids and from the cells found in five of them (Table 8-5). The results indicated that except for cerebrospinal fluid, large quantities of cell-free HIV are not present in any of the nine other body fluids tested.

TABLE 8-5 HIV in Body Fluids and in Cells within Body Fluids

	Estimated Number of HIV[a]
Cell-free fluid	
Plasma	10–50
Serum	10–50
Tears	<1
Ear secretions	5–10
Saliva	<1
Urine	<1
Vaginal/cervical	<1
Semen	10-50
Sweat	0
Breast milk	<1
Cerebrospinal fluid	10–1,000
Infected cells (T4 and macrophages)	
PBMC	0.001–0.1
Saliva	<0.01
Bronchial fluid	not detected
Vaginal/cervical fluid	present but not quantitated
Semen[b]	0.01–5

[a]Cell-free fluid is expressed in infectious particles per milliliter; infected cells, in percentage of infected cells observed.

[b]HIV has been detected in cell-free seminal fluid and in nonspermatazoal mononuclear cells and in the DNA of sperm from some HIV-infected men (Meriman et al., 1991; Bagasra et al., 1994).

(Source: Adapted from Levy, 1989)

The low levels of HIV in cell-free body fluids and within the cells of these fluids does not mean that HIV cannot be transmitted via these fluids or cells—it can, but the dose (number of viruses) is so small that the risk of infection is minimal, thus the low number of health care workers contracting HIV infection after touching, being splashed by, or needlesticking themselves with blood containing HIV. Particularly interesting is the finding that there is no detectable HIV in bronchial fluid and almost none in saliva (there has always been a great fear that HIV could be transmitted by kissing), breast milk, urine, and tears.

HIV is found in greatest numbers (100 to 10,000 infectious units per milliliter, mL) *within the T4, macrophage, and monocytes of blood, vaginal fluids, and semen*; yet these fluids carry relatively low levels of cell-free HIV. Laboratory findings, along with overwhelming empirical observations, support the scientific conclusion that the major route of HIV transmission is through human blood and sexual activities involving exchange of semen and vaginal fluids. Semen carries significantly larger numbers of HIV than vaginal fluid. It appears that of all body fluids, these three contain the largest number of infected lymphocytes (Figure 8-4), which provide the largest HIV concentration in a given area at a given time.

Cell-to-Cell Transmission

According to classic models of viral infection, which draw heavily from research on bacteriophage (viruses that attack bacteria), the process of infection starts with adherence of free virus to host cells. This view has dominated the thinking about mechanisms of infection by HIV. Researchers have only recently appreciated that cells can have a direct role in transmission of HIV.

FIGURE 8-4 Electron Micrograph of an HIV-Infected T4 Lymphocyte. The T4 cell has produced a large number of HIVs that are located over the entire lymphocyte. The photograph shows part of the convoluted surface of the lymphocyte magnified 20,000 times. (*Courtesy of The National Biological Standards Board, South Mimms, U.K. and David Hockley*)

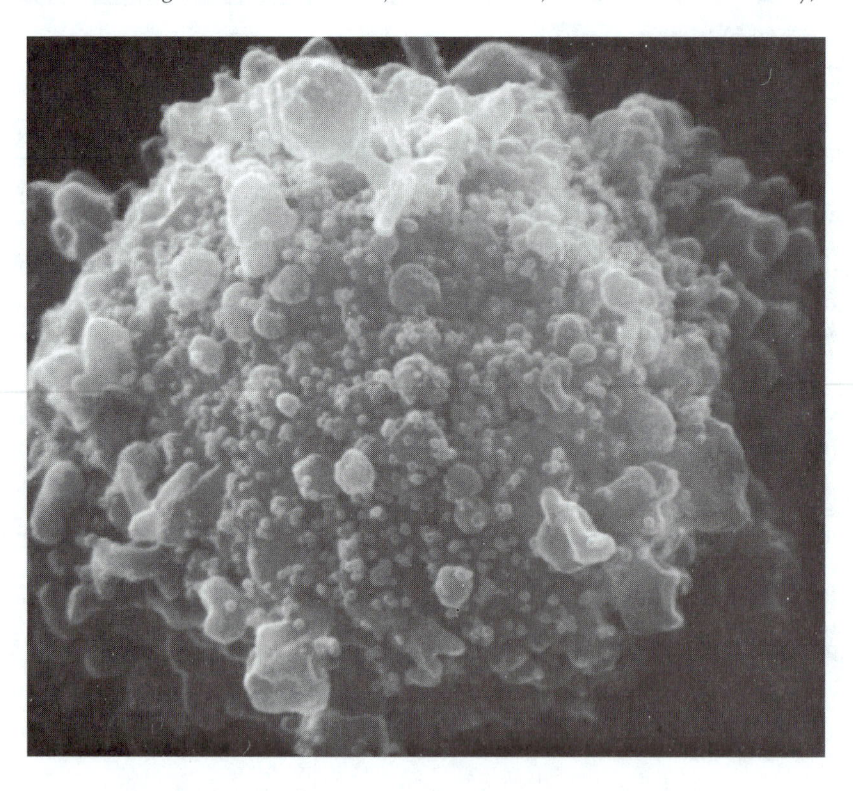

There is overwhelming evidence that HIV infection can be initiated by cell-associated HIV in the blood and body fluids. Current data support the idea of direct transfer of HIV from one cell to another by syncytia formation and by cell-to-cell transmission without syncytia formation. Cell-to-cell HIV transfer could hypothetically take place either between host and donor cells within the host or between a donor HIV-secreting mononuclear cell and intact host epithelium of the genital, digestive or urinary tract, or the placenta. Different mechanisms of cell-mediated transmission are illustrated in Figure 8-5.

Presence of HIV-Infected Cells in Body Fluids

Blood— Cell-to-cell transmission assumes that HIV-infected cells are present in the body fluid of the infected donor individual Also, the infected donor cells must produce virus, although theoretically a latently infected cell could produce virus if it were activated after it entered the recipient host. Recent observations indicate that both latent and HIV-producing cells are present throughout the course of infection, but latent cells are far more common. Although virus is primarily confined to lymphatic organs, considerable numbers of HIV-infected cells can also be detected in the blood. Thus it is probable that HIV-infected people harbor substantial numbers of HIV-infected mononuclear cells from soon after the initial infection to the terminal stage of the disease.

Semen— Semen from healthy men typically contains many leukocytes, including T4 cells. But the number and type of all mononuclear cells in the semen of a healthy man differs considerably from day to day.

If T4 cells (lymphocytes and macrophages) are the vectors of HIV, then reducing their numbers in semen could decrease the chances of infection. Lymphocytes and macrophages can originate from the testes, epididymis, seminal vesicles, or prostate and inflammation of the genital tract results in an increased number of these cells in semen. Very litttle information is available on the relative percentages of mononuclear cells that orginate from the

FIGURE 8-5 Schemes of Four Possible Mechanisms of Cell-Mediated Transmission of HIV. (1) An HIV-secreting donor mononuclear cell (MC) releases virus that infects nearby host cells; (2) an HIV-infected donor MC fuses with a host cell; (3)and (4)adhesion-based cell-to-cell transmission without syncytia. Cell-to-cell transfer of virus could hypothetically take place either between cells within the body of the host (3) or between a donor HIV-secreting MC and a host epithelial cell at the portal of entry (4). (*Source:* Phillips, 1994.)

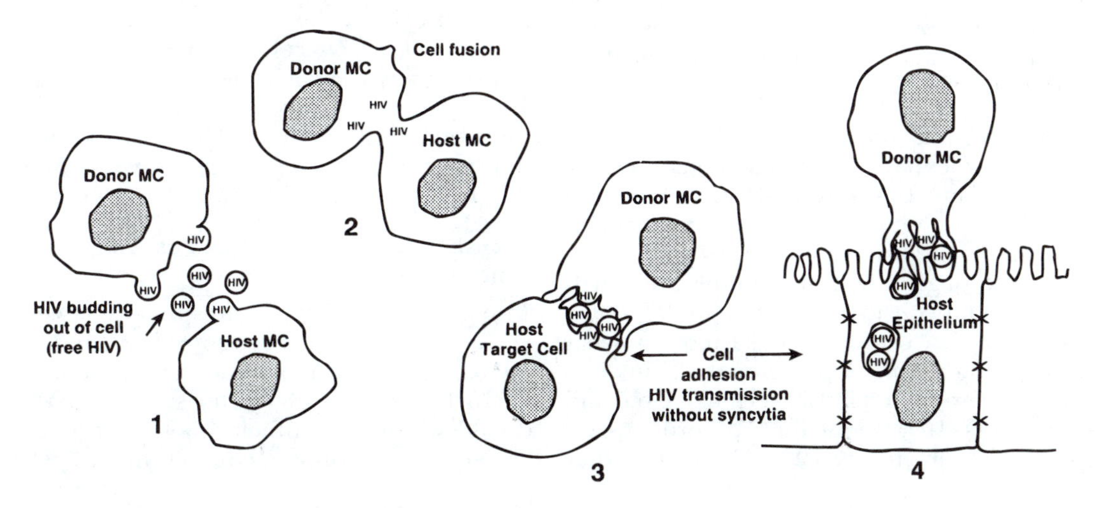

POINT OF INFORMATION 8.3

DANGER OF HIV INFECTION VIA ARTIFICIAL INSEMINATION

By mid-1994, five women were reported to the CDC to have been HIV-infected through the use of donor sperm to initiate pregnancy. About 80,000 women each year are artificially inseminated with donor sperm. But 14 years into the AIDS epidemic, the increasingly popular fertility business remains largely unregulated and unmonitored, even though it traffics in semen,long known to be one of the two main HIV transmission routes.

Only a few states (New York, California, Ohio, Illinois, and Michigan) require HIV testing of semen donors. **There are no federal regulations.**

Medical and public health experts agree that artificial insemination is an HIV risk that somehow fell through the cracks of public education and health regulations. They insist, however, that the risk is low.

Lack of federal and state regulations means you must protect yourself! (1) Stay away from private physicians unless you know the doctors are using only certified sperm banks to get their products (2) Review a doctor's or clinic's testing and record-keeping procedures and demand to see donor medical records, which can be shared even if the donor's identity is protected (3) Accept only frozen donor semen that has been HIV-tested twice at 3- to 6-month intervals.

different organs of the male reproductive tract, what factors control their numbers, or what function(s) these lymphocytes and macrophages perform in semen. It has been suggested that vasectomy could reduce the infectivity of HIV-infected men because it would eliminate mononuclear cells or cell-free virus in semen originating from the testes and epididymis. Although vasectomy has been reported to reduce the number of white blood cells in semen, HIV-infected mononuclear cells have been detected in semen from seropositive vasectomized men. Further studies are necessary to determine the efficacy of vasectomy for AIDS prevention.

In summary, semen from HIV-infected men can contain both cell-free and cell-associated virus. From the available evidence, as in blood, it is not yet possible to determine to what extent cell-free and cell-associated virus mediate HIV infectivity (Phillips, 1994).

Saliva— Several large-scale epidemiological studies have failed to demonstrate HIV transmission to household members and health care workers by casual contact, suggesting that transmission by saliva is uncommon. Although saliva from healthy individuals may contain considerable numbers of leukocytes, very few of these are T4 mononuclear cells. Using the DNA polymerase chain reaction test (presented in Chapter 12), Goto and co-workers (1991) found that HIV provirus was present in saliva from all 20 AIDS patients they examined. However, half of the patients required multiple analyses to demonstrate that proviral sequences were present. It should also be noted that AIDS patients frequently have oral lesions that result in blood in the oral cavity. Thus, it is possible that both cell-free virus and HIV-infected mononuclear cells in saliva from AIDS patients could originate from blood (Phillips, 1994). A recent report suggests that a secretory protease inhibitor in saliva attaches to the surface of lymphocytes blocking HIV infection.

Milk— Several studies have shown that HIV can be transmitted by breast-feeding. Van de Perre and co-workers (1993) found that infection of babies via breast milk was most strongly correlated with the presence of HIV-infected cells in the milk, suggesting that infection might be cell-mediated. However, infection was also correlated with low levels of antibodies to HIV, suggesting that infection was initiated by cell-free virus. Thus this study does not present stronge evidence in favor of infection by cell-associated versus cell-free virus.

Transmission by Cell-to-Cell Fusion: Syncytia Formation

The idea that a virus could spread from one cell to another was recognized in the mid-1950s. Induction of syncytium formation (Figure 3-8) is a characteristic effect produced when HIV-infected cells expressing surface gp120 come in contact with T4 cells.

Theoretically, cell-to-cell transmission mediated by syncytium formation could take place when HIV-infected mononuclear cells enter the host and fuse with host T4 target cells. Although the importance of gp120-T4-induced syncytium formation in vivo has been questioned, this phenomenon has been investigated in detail in other virus systems.

Hironori Sato and co-workers (1992) have suggested how syncytium formation may mediate HIV infection and spread. These workers compared the kinetics of infection of T4 cells following either the addition of HIV-infected H9 cells or cell-free virus obtained from H9-infected cell culture fluids. The synthesis of new viral protein or unintegrated DNA began within hours of addition of the infected cells. However, with cell-free virus, new viral protein and DNA were not detected until 2 or 3 days after addition of the culture supernatant. Examination of the cultures by light microscopy revealed that addition of HIV-infected cells, but not free virus, resulted in numerous small syncytia 1 hour after infection, large syncytia by 2 to 4 hours, and giant syncytia, containing hundreds of nuclei, by 8 hours. Although the amount of the virus produced by HIV-secreting T4 cells may not be comparable to that of free virus in culture medium because T4 cells are a continuous source of virus, Sato and co-workers' conclusion that cell-mediated infection was much more efficient than infection by cell-free virus appears justified in view of the striking difference in kinetics of virus production (Phillips, 1994).

Transmission by Cell-to-Cell Adhesion

Mononuclear Cell to Mononuclear Cell—Spread of HIV from one cell to another across a confined space between donor and host cells without the involvement of syncytia may have consequences very different from syncytium formation (Figure 8-6). Unlike the infected syncytial cells, which contain surface major histocompatibility compex (HLA) antigens of the

FIGURE 8-6 HIV Infection of Epithelial Cells. An HIV (*arrow*) budding from an infected cervix-derived epithelial cell (above) appears to be entering an adjacent cell (below) by a coated pit. (aoriginal magnification ×65,000.) (reprinted with permission of David M. Phillips, The Population Council.))

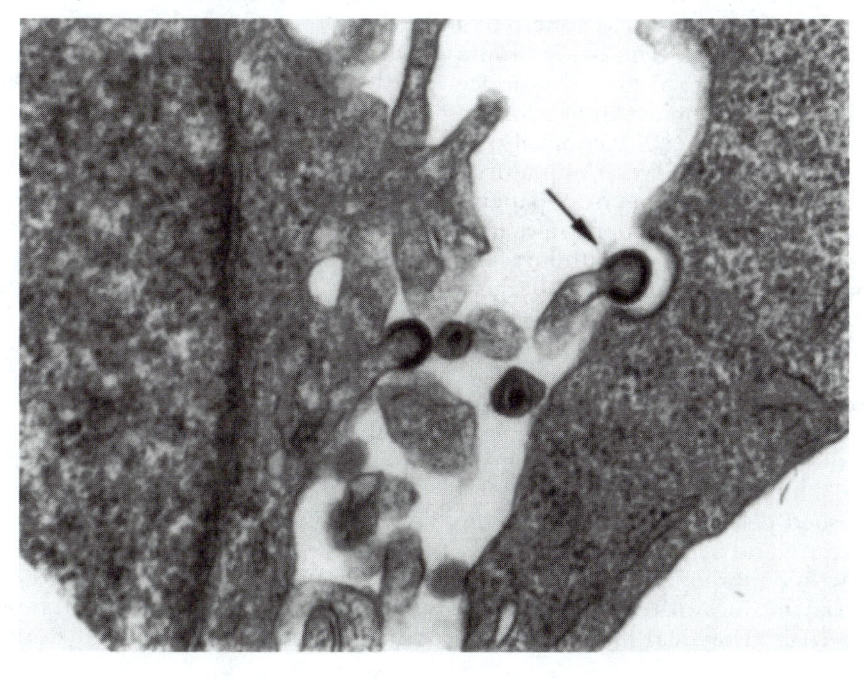

donor cell, the host cell infected by cell-to-cell adhesion would not necessarily be recognized as a foreign cell by the host's immune system. In addition, unlike a syncytium, the infected cell might be able to divide and spread the virus to many recipient cells.

Cell-to-cell spread of HIV without syncytium formation has only recently been addressed. Theoretically, the transmission of virus from one mononuclear cell to another, without syncytium formation, involves a three-step process. First the donor and recipient cells adhere. Following adherence, the donor cell sheds virus into the space between the two cells. Finally, viruses are taken up by the recipient cell. Secretion of HIV, direction of secretion, and uptake could be influenced by cytokines produced by the adherent donor and/or recipient cell. In contrast to syncytium formation, which can be easily visualized by light microscopic examination of living cells, adherence-mediated infection has been difficult to document both in vitro and in vivo. However, such cell-to-cell interactions are probable, and the results of in vitro experiments suggest that cell-to-cell transmission of HIV can occur without syncytium formation.

A critical consideration in cell-to-cell transmission without fusion is whether it is possible for a cell that is secreting virus to adhere to a T4 cell without fusing to it. The answer would depend on the amount of gp120 on the surface of the HIV-infected cell and the amount of surface CD4 on the recipient cell. It could also be dependent on virus strain. Several laboratories have shown that viruses isolated from patients soon after infection tend to be nonsyncytial. It is possible that virus that spread without forming syncytia are more transmissible because they use a cell-to cell mechanism to infect that does not involve syncytia (Phillips et al., 1994).

Cell Transmission of HIV to Epithelial Cells— To examine the possibility that HIV could directly infect epithelia at the portal of entry, David Phillips and co-workers (1994) grew established cell lines derived from the gut, genital tract, and placenta, potential sites of HIV entry. Initially they attempted to infect these epithelial cell lines with culture fluid containing free HIV. They had limited success. However, when they added HIV-infected T4 cells or monocyte cell lines to the epithelia, they were able to detect infection.

HIV-infected cells were much more efficient in infecting epithelical cells than free virus because the mononuclear cells continued to adhere to the epithelia even after the cultures were washed vigorously. In the scanning electron microscope they observed many cells attached to the epithelium. These cells frequently display pear shapes and ruffles disposed away from the epithelium (Figure 8-7 a and b).

Summary— Although most HIV/AIDS scientists have used the term "cell-to-cell transmission" almost synonymously with syncytium formation, contact-mediated transmission without syncytia merits further consideration. Theoretical and experimental evidence suggests that contact-mediated transmission by adherence can occur and that mononuclear cell-to-epithelial infection may be an important entry mechanism for HIV.

There continues to be some concern over the presence of HIV in saliva because of the exchange of saliva during "deep" kissing, the saliva residue left on eating utensils, and saliva on instruments handled by health care workers, especially in dentistry. Results of studies on hundreds of dental workers, many of whom have cared for AIDS patients, have shown no evidence of HIV infection (Friedland et al., 1987). Also, in a recent CDC study, none of 48 health care workers became infected after parenteral (IV) or mucous membrane exposure to the saliva of HIV-infected patients (Curran et al., 1988). A recent study by Philip Fox, (1991) National Institute of Dental Research, showed that saliva from three healthy men stopped HIV infection of lymphocytes in vitro. Additional studies by D.W. Archibald and colleagues (1990) and Pourtois and colleagues (1991) also showed that human saliva contains factors that inhibit HIV infectivity. Robert Woolley (1989) attempted to calculate the amount of hemoglobin that might be transferred during passionate kissing, and concluded that kissing *does not* pose a serious health threat. Further saliva inhibition tests are in progress.

Spitzer and colleagues (1989) reported that a male became HIV-infected during unpro-

A

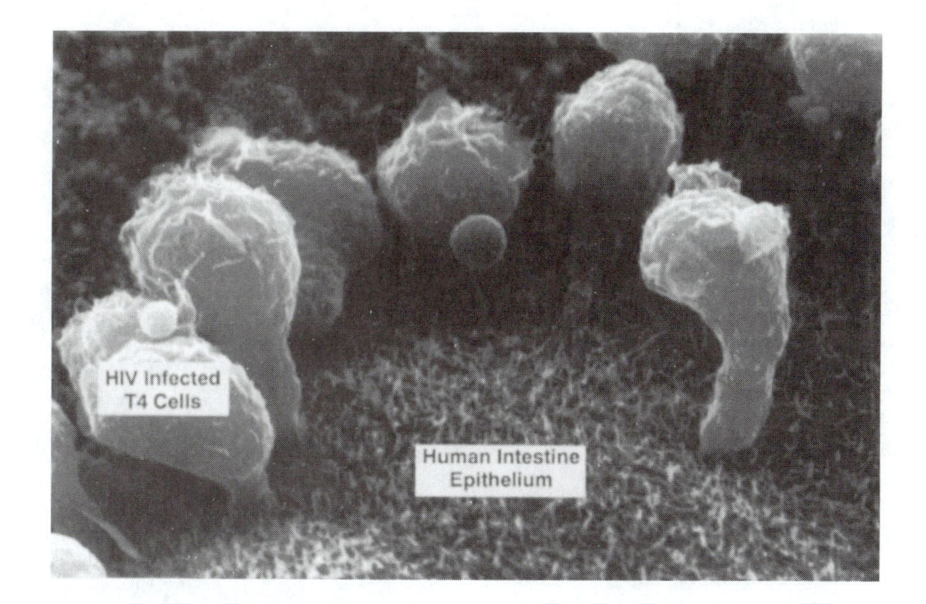

B

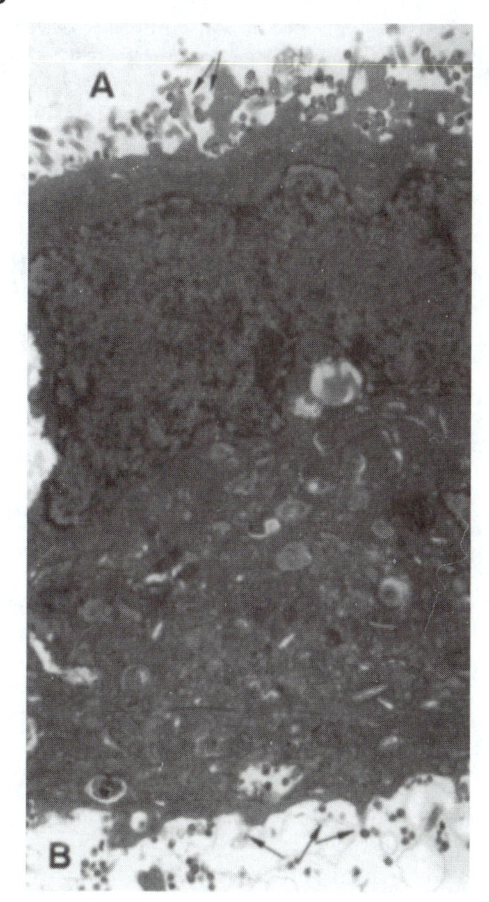

Figure 8-7 HIV Tisue Adherence and Infectivity. A) Scanning electron micrograph of HIV-infected T cells(MOLT-4/HIV-1_{IIIB}) adhering to an epithelium derived fromthe human intestine (1407). Following adherence T cells tend to become pear-shaped.(Original magnification × 4,500.) B) HIV-infected cervix-derived epitheial cell. The epithelium has been cut perpendicular to the filter. Budding HIV (*arrows*) are observed on both the apical (*A*) and basal (*B*) surfaces. (Original magnification × 17,000.) (Reprinted with permission of David M. Phillips, The Population Council).

POINT OF INFORMATION 8.4

DISTRIBUTION OF HIV-CONTAMINATED BLOOD: FRANCE, GERMANY, THE UNITED STATES, AND OTHER COUNTRIES

Near the end he could not bring himself to visit his youngest brother, to see him dying of AIDS. He too was dying of AIDS. Their deaths would close out a family of four HIV-infected hemophiliac brothers, all diagnosed with AIDS. The first died at age 24, the second committed suicide at age 33, the last two brothers died in 1993. The four brothers became HIV-infected about 1985 from using HIV-contaminated blood-clotting factor.

FRANCE

The French National Center of Blood Transfusions (CNTS) knowingly distributed HIV-contaminated blood products to hemophiliacs in 1985. The scandal, which broke in 1991, prompted the center's director to resign and an official government investigation.

In the confidential minutes of a 1985 CNTS meeting, agency officials concluded that 100% of the concentrated blood-clotting factors used to treat French hemophiliacs were contaminated with HIV. The agency, which has a monopoly on blood for transfusions, kept its secret and ignored a 1984 recommendation from the U.S. Centers for Disease Control and Prevention that blood products be heated in order to kill the deadly virus (Dorfman, 1991).

In July 1985, the CNTS decided to heat all blood products and to institute national testing of donated blood. But for the next 3 months, the agency continued to sell the HIV-contaminated blood products to hemophiliacs without warning them of the risk. That policy, which was approved by the Ministry of Health and the French Association of Hemophiliacs, was reportedly intended to ward off a blood shortage.

Whatever the reasons, the secrecy and delay produced catastrophic results. Nearly half of France's 3,000 hemophiliacs were infected with HIV; subsequently 256 have died. Bowing to public and media pressure, the French government will provide compensation for some 7,000 French citizens who have been infected with HIV through blood products and transfusions (Aldhous, 1991).

The Unfolding Tragedy

Ann Marie Casteret, a 43-year-old French physician, gave up her career in medicine to expose this tragedy. She wrote a series of articles that appeared in the spring of 1991. They were entitled *L'Evenement du Jeudi* (The Event that Happens on Thursday). This national tragedy has two parts:

1. *The Intentional Delay in the Use of an American Blood Test for HIV.* For almost 6 months, the French public authorities blocked the use of an American test for detecting antibodies to HIV. This allowed time for Pasteur Diagnostics of The Pasteur Institute to produce its own HIV test. This gave Pasteur Diagnostics the *first* domestic license. The French government owns half of the Pasteur enterprise.
2. *The Intentional Use of HIV-Contaminated Blood Products.* The National Center for Blood Transfusions in Paris decided to use up its stocks of blood products worth $10 million even though it had been told that "probably all" of the pooled plasma from Parisian donors was HIV-contaminated. Administrators of the Center decided not to tell the physicians who run the 163 transfusion centers about the HIV risk.

On October 23, 1992, the French courts found the three health administrators guilty of the distribution of HIV-contaminated blood. Michel Garretta, the former director of France's blood bank had moved to Boston, Massachusetts. In October 1992, he returned to France, was fined $100,000, stripped of his license to practice medicine, and is serving a 4-year sentence. Co-defendant Jean-Pierre Allain received a 4-year sentence with 2 years suspended. Both were ordered to pay $1.8 million in compensation to victims and their families. Jean Roux was given a 4-year suspended sentence. Technically, the convictions are for fraud in the field of consumer protection; those convicted are held to have "sold, or allowed to be sold," products that were not what their consumers had a right to expect.

French Ministers to Face Poisoning Charges

Formal charges of "collusion in poisoning" were made in October 1994 against Laurent Fabius, the former Socialist prime minister, and four of his colleagues—Edmond Hervé, then deputy health minister, and Georgina Dufoix, then minister of social affairs, Francois Gros, scientific advisor to Fabius, and Claude Weisselberg, physician and advisor to Fabius—over their role in France's HIV-contaminated blood scandal in the mid 1980s.The charge carries a maximum sentence of 30 years in prison. In Addition to these three men, the charge of collusion to poison were also be brought against Jean-Pierre Allain (just released from prison) and Michel Garretta (still in prison) (Butler, 1994a,1994b).

GERMANY

The German blood scandal began with two questions. The first question was how to explain several unexpected cases of HIV infection. And the second question, associated with the first, was how could 7,000 units of blood have been screened for HIV using 2,500 HIV blood testing kits (it takes one kit/unit of blood screened). The search for the answers led investigators to a blood supply company called UB Plasma in the city of Koblenz. The investigators concluded that either the firm had failed to test thousands of units, or it had "pooled" units from multiple donors before conducting the test, an illegal practice that reduces the chances of detecting HIV contamination.

Investigators discovered that after UB Plasma began running into financial trouble in 1991, technicians were told to pool units to save money on the $2 test kits. Åfter German kit manufacturers stopped deliveries (UB Plasma failed to pay its bills) technicians switched to an unauthorized and less reliable test. There was also evidence that the firm may have distributed blood that was not screened at all.

Because of the extent of blood banking violations, German authorities closed UB Plasma. They arrested the manager and three employees on charges of fraud and "negligent bodily harm." Batches of company blood were distributed to at least 88 hospitals and four companies in Germany and abroad. UB Plasma records show shipments went to Austria, Greece, and Saudi Arabia, as well as to intermediary companies that may have sent the products to France, the Netherlands, Britain, Portugal, Sweden, Italy, and Switzerland. In November of 1993, the German Health Minister recommended that anyone who received blood or blood products from the early 1980s on should be HIV tested. According to the German press, the Health Minister's recommendation started a panic that caused thousands of individuals to cancel routine and in some cases urgent surgery. In 1987, a UB Plasma employee reported that the company distributed questionable blood products, and that for-profit blood collection companies were buying blood from unscreened donors and, in addition, were pooling blood for HIV testing. This information has led to charges that health officials covered up the fact that they knew HIV-infected blood was being distributed. The current health minister disbanded the German Federal Health Bureau. And the Director of Pharmaceuticals was relieved of his duties relating to the control of blood and blood products. In stark contrast to the HIV blood scandals in France and the United States, German investigators attribute the distribution of HIV-contaminated blood and blood products to incompetence rather than company greed—UB Plasma did not attempt to distribute known HIV-positive blood until current stocks were used up!

The question for the reader is whether incompetence is a crime and, if so, what kind of crime and what should be the punishment?

To help in your private thoughts and class deliberations, one may refer to the traditions of professions. For example, are not engineers who give faulty advice in the construction of a bridge, a building, or a plane held accountable if afterwards the construction fails because of their incompetent advice? And more recently, accountants who were found to have incompetently audited the accounts of companies for which they were responsible were held liable in lawsuits from those injured in the process. And haven't certain automobile manufacturers who supplied dangerous or defective products been sued for damages done to those who acquired them? Then should those who allow contaminated blood onto the market expect to be exempt from whatever penalties are prescribed for incompetence and carelessness?

THE UNITED STATES

In late 1993, a class action suit was filed on behalf of 9,000 hemophiliacs who became infected with HIV after using HIV-contaminated blood products, called Blood Factor 8, which is essential for proper blood clot formation following an injury. In the case of severe hemophilia, many persons spontaneously bleed into their joints. Blood Factor 8 is sometimes referred to as Anti-Hemolytic Factor or AHF. Hemophiliacs are now dying of AIDS at the rate of one a day.

The suit charges that five manufacturers of AHF and the National Hemophilia Foundation continued to pursue aggressive advertising and marketing of AHF while downplaying the risk of viral infection.

By the mid-1970's, the dangers of viral infection from blood products was well known and methods had been provided for blood viral inactivation. Such methods were patented and available by 1977. In 1981, Donald Francis, an epidemiologist then with the CDC, and Max Essex, a retrovirologist at Harvard Cancer Biology Laboratory, were convinced that AIDS, then referred to as Gay Related Immune Deficiency or GRID, was caused by an infectious agent, most likely a virus. But others thought GRID was related to the gay male lifestyle. The disease was spreading rapidly among gay males through sexual contact. But the evidence continued to mount that the disease, or agent causing the disease, was being transmitted by blood. And in that same year, the president of an AHF-producing company stated the agent was in the blood supply. He said he thought it was a 100% fatal retrovirus. At this time, a major part of blood stocks came from paid donors, mostly from poor neighborhoods. To offset taking in contaminated blood, this single company began questioning donors face-to-face: Are you homosexual? In the first 2 weeks of new guideline operations, 308 donors said yes and their blood was not taken. Another 500 refused to answer and left.

The FDA's Blood Products Advisory Committee (then) and other blood banks across the United States said that gays should not be prevented from donating blood and they should not be questioned. Yet the evidence for blood transfusion-associated AIDS related to the blood and plasma of gay men was known and information shared, but the blood bankers chose to ignore it. The head of the American Association of Blood Banks (AABB) led a revolt against the concept of transfusion-associated AIDS. The blood banking industry generates more than a billion dollars a year. Withdrawal of blood products at this time would have required dumping more than $100 million in AHF currently in the pipeline, and would have drastically reduced company profits until the newer products became available. The AABB and the American Red Cross issued a joint statement that "Direct or indirect questions about a donor's sexual preferences are inappropriate." Clearly, they kept open the door to high behavioral risk blood donors. The FDA went along with the joint statement and against the CDC recommendations for screening blood donors.

Interestingly, while the head of AABB was stating publicly that there was no proof that the agent causing AIDS was in the blood supply, he had written a confidential report to the AABB board stating that there is an increased probability that AIDS may be spread by blood! He stated, "I believe the most we can do in this situation is buy time. There is little doubt in my mind that additional transfusion-related cases and additional cases in patients with hemophilia will surface."

According to Milton Musin, former medical research director of Cutter Laboratories, by the end of 1983 he knew that the hemophiliacs clotting factor could transmit AIDS. And virtually all lots of the concentrate were contaminated with the AIDS virus. "You'll never convince me that profit margins and fear of the product liability and fear of losing a very lucrative business did not drive the CEOs and leaders of these companies."

By mid-1983, the U.S. government was fully aware that there was a substantial problem of AIDS in the blood supply and they invited participants from all the blood industries as well as academicians to come to a meeting to present their ideas and findings. A surrogate test to reduce the likelihood of AIDS in the blood supply was explained. And, many tests were described, but the test that seemed to make the most sense economically was the antibody to the hepatitis B core (a component of the hepatitis B virus).

The night before that meeting, officials from the four major clotting factor producers held a meeting in a suburban Washington hotel room. A memo describes how, at that meeting, the companies agreed to propose a task force to study the question of testing as a **delaying tactic.**

The following morning the study proposal was adopted by the FDA. Several different surrogate tests were to be considered and evaluated by the task force subcommittee. This committee didn't issue a report for 6 or 8 months and ultimately majority and minority reports were issued, with the majority favoring no testing and the minority favoring the institution of the hepatitis B core. So the ultimate outcome of that meeting was nothing—no testing.

Finally there was a breakthrough. In 1985, the FDA announced a blood test. "This test adds a major dimension of protection to our present safeguards. Its use will keep our blood supply safe and indeed make them even safer."

The HIV antibody test, called the ELISA test, would help make the blood supply, in large part, safe. But it came at a cost to the blood banks. Technicians had to be hired and trained. Donors had to be checked and every new unit of blood tested and logged. **But, astonishingly, the blood banks were not required to go back to the inventories on their shelves.** In hindsight, the current head of the AABB says that was a mistake.

But perhaps the worst was yet to be learned. While the AABB was stalling testing, it convinced the FDA to reduce the number of blood bank inspections at the very time HIV was entering the blood system of the country.

It wasn't until 1988 that the blood banks began recalling HIV-positive blood. FDA reports were discovered that told of errors and accidents. Between 1985 and 1987 thousands of units of potentially contaminated blood had been released and officially recalled. But recalling blood that was released for transfusion is a bit misleading because, depending on when and how you are trying to recall it, the chances of being able to get it all back are almost zero. Once it is released, it is used. Potentially contaminated blood had been used, most of it quickly, in emergency rooms. The FDA now had no choice but to take action. In September 1988, the FDA and the Red Cross entered into what is known as a voluntary agreement to comply with all FDA regulations. From now on there would be yearly inspections! But that did not work. The Red Cross kept poor records at local blood banks and the FDA constantly had to threaten license revocations.

Finally, in 1993, FDA commissioner, Dr. David Kessler, went to federal court and obtained an injunction against the Red Cross for failure to fulfill its promise under the 1988 voluntary agreement.

> We filed a complaint for injunctive relief in the district court and we obtained a consent decree in May of this year (1993) to put the American Red Cross under court supervision.
>
> The injunction that applies to the American Red Cross, applies to all facilities throughout the country, all American Red Cross blood banking facilities, both in the field and at headquarters. It doesn't apply to any one blood banking facility over another. All facilities are covered by the injunciton.

It is now estimated that as many as 30,000 Americans were infected with AIDS through blood. It is a tragedy that has exposed critical weaknesses in the rules and practices in blood banking. It's also a story of missed opportunities, vested interests, and lax regulations stretching back more than a decade when a mysterious virus entered America's bloodstream. In November 1993, Donna Shalala, Secretary of Health and Human Services, asked for a high-level investigation of how thousands of American hemophiliacs became HIV-infected from contaminated blood products.

Question: Do you feel this saga of delayed and controlled misuse of blood in the United States is equal to or greater than the French and/or German scandals? Explain. (Class discussion)

USE OF HIV-CONTAMINATED BLOOD OR BLOOD PRODUCTS IN OTHER COUNTRIES

Canada and Nova Scotia

A flood of lawsuits is expected to follow the decision to award more than half a million Canadian dollars to the HIV-infected wife of a man who died of AIDS after receiving a transfusion of HIV-contaminated blood. The outcome of this case was announced on the eve of a deadline set by all except one of Canada's provinces and territories for acceptance of a compensation package by more than a thousand recipients of HIV-infected blood. To obtain the money, victims had to sign wavers promising not to sue Ottawa, the provinces or territories, hospitals, the Red Cross, and pharmaceutcal and insurance companies. Compensation was set at C$515,000 per case or per person plus interest and legal fees.

The Canadian compensation is less generous than the province of Nova Scotia, which, as well as making annual payments of C$30,000 to the HIV-infected, pays for expensive AIDS drugs, as well as funeral costs and post-secondary education for their children (Spurgeon, 1994).

Switzerland

In mid-1994, the former head of the Swiss Red Cross Central Laboratory in Bern was charged with causing "grievous bodily harm" by allowing HIV-tainted blood-clotting factors to be distributed to Swiss hemophiliacs in 1985 and 1986.

The Swiss case resembles the French scandal. In both cases, a national lab continued to distribute blood products that were known to be potentially infected with HIV. France stopped using such products in October 1985, but in Switzerland they were marketed until April 1986.

The suspect Swiss factors were made with blood collected some months before July, 1985, when

HIV testing became routine. The trial is likely to center on his failure to stop production of the factors in July, 1985, when the New York Blood Center identified one HIV-positive sample among 3,375 units of donated Swiss blood. But the Swiss Red Cross insists that no alternative supplies were available: "If these products would not have gone out, the hemophiliacs would have bled to death." (Holden, 1994)

Japan

In July of 1993, 92 Japanese hemophiliacs filed suit against the Japanese government and blood product manufacturers. They are seeking compensation for failure to protect them from blood products contaminated with HIV. Blood product manufacturers continued to advertise untreated blood products in Japan without warning until late-1985; Japanese hemophiliacs used them into 1986. They are seeking one million dollars each in compensation.

Donald Francis, who testified for the hemophiliacs, said that by early 1983, the danger posed to U.S. blood supplies by AIDS was "absolutely black and white," after six cases of AIDS in five adults and one baby had been traced to transfusions of blood from donors who subsequently developed AIDS. Yet, during 1983–1985, Japan dramatically increased its imports of untreated U.S. blood products and, as a result, about 2,000 of Japan's 4,000 hemophiliacs were infected with HIV. Francis said the tragedy could have been avoided. This court case will take years to resolve in Japan (Swinbanks, 1993, 1994).

OTHER BLOOD SCANDALS IN BRIEF

In Columbia, a drug-addicted bisexual who knew he had AIDS sold his blood 12 times to a laboratory. Twelve patients received the blood between 1989 and 1990 and went on to infect a further 200 people through sexual contact.

In Romania during the Communist era, HIV-contaminated blood infected 2,376 children.

Developing countries at the moment must rely on paid donors, who may include gay and bisexual men, prostitutes, and drug addicts needing money. Countries like India, Pakistan, and Russia have an open paid donor system.

Parts of Africa and Latin America use family replacement donors—a scheme that allows paid donors to pose as relatives of the patient. Paying unquestioned donors without HIV screening their blood is an invitation for the transmission of HIV. But developing countries do not have the capital nor sufficient trained personnel to do anything else at the moment.

tected fellatio with an HIV-infected prostitute. A second similar case has also been reported. The mechanism of transmission, saliva, in these cases may be suspected, but it is not conclusive!

The precise risk of oral sex is difficult to assess because most couples engage in other sexual practices. However, Rozenbaum and colleagues (1988) and Monzon and colleagues (1987) reported that this was a probable route of HIV transmission (see discussion under ORO-GENITAL SEX in this chapter). Regardless, special precautions for dentistry are recommended by the CDC. A small number of hepatitis B viral infections have been documented in dental workers (*MMWR*, 1988b; 1991a).

Dentist with AIDS Infects Patient During Tooth Extraction?

In July of 1990, the CDC reported on the possible transmission of HIV from a dentist with AIDS to a female patient (*MMWR*, 1990a). This case, like no other before it, sent chills through many. But why this case? Because the vast majority of people go to dentists! They don't inject drugs and are not gay. This case, however, is difficult to resolve. For example, 2 years had elapsed from the time of the dental work to when the patient, Kimberly Bergalis (Figure 8-8), was diagnosed HIV-positive. Both patient and dentist, David J. Acer of Stuart, Florida, were uncertain of exactly what happened. Some of the pertinent factors in this case are (1) review of dental records and radiographs suggest that the two tooth extractions were uncomplicated; (2) interviews with Bergalis and the dentist did not identify other risk factors for HIV infection (Bergalis, age 22, stated over national TV in 1990 that she was still a virgin;) This point was disputed on June 19, 1994, during the TV program *60 Minutes* (with Mike Wallace) as well as the CDC's ge-

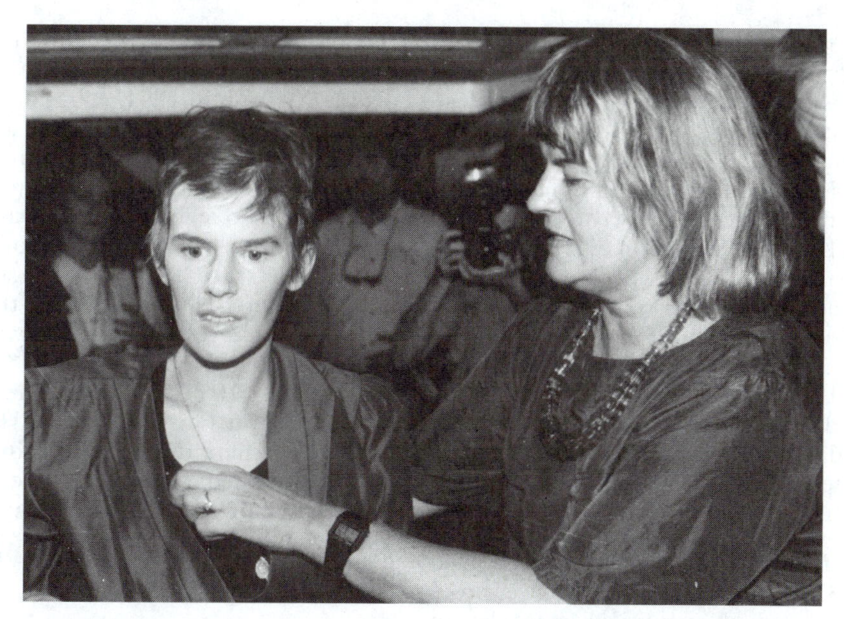

FIGURE 8-8 Kimberly Bergalis, Age 23. Bergalis is being comforted by her mother after their train trip from their home in Florida to Washington, D.C. She made the trip to testify before a congressional committee on September 26, 1991. Bergalis favored mandatory HIV testing for health care personnel. She died December 8, 1991. (*Photograph courtesy of AP/Wide World Photos*)

netic match between Dr. Acer's HIV and his patient's strain of HIV. Yes, she did engage in sexual foreplay, but not intercourse. Yes, she was infected with the human papilloma virus, which can be sexually transmitted, but this is not at all uncommon in immune-suppressed AIDS patients with no history of sexual intercourse; (3) nucleotide sequence data indicated a high degree of similarity between the HIV strains infecting her and the dentist; and (4) the time between the dental procedure and the development of AIDS was short (24 months), and Bergalis developed oral candidiasis 17 months after infection. Only 1% of infected homosexual/ bisexual men and 5% of infected transfusion recipients develop AIDS within 2 years of infection.

David Acer, a bisexual, was diagnosed with symptomatic HIV infection in 1986 and with AIDS in 1987. He died on September 3, 1990. Since then, 1,100 patients of his were contacted for HIV testing. In January of 1991, the test results of 591 of these patients revealed that five others were HIV-positive: a 68-year-old retired school teacher, a middle-aged father of two, a 37-year-old carnival worker, an unemployed drifter, and a 19-year-old student. As with Bergalis, infection in these patients may have come from some other source. All six patients denied having sexual contact with the dentist or with one another (*MMWR*, 1991a). If an absolute case can be made that Acer transmitted the virus to Bergalis, this will be the *first documented case of a health care professional infecting a patient.* Bergalis is reported to have settled her first claim for $1 million from Acer's malpractice insurance company. She settled a second claim against his estate for an undisclosed sum.

Bergalis died of AIDS on December 8, 1991. She was 23 years old and weighed 48 pounds. In January 1993 a life-size bronze statue of Kimberly Bergalis was unveiled at the high school she attended. Her dying wish was that what happened to her should never happen to anyone else. To this end, weak and near death, she traveled by train to testify before the United States Congress urging mandatory testing for all health care workers. The 'Bergalis Bill' never got out of committee, the CDC and Congress rejected the call for mandatory testing of health care workers. On April 6, 1991, Ms. Bergalis wrote a two-page unmailed letter to the Florida State Department of Health and Rehabilitative Services. She wrote "Whom do I blame? I blame Dr. Acer and every single one of you bastards. Anyone who knew Dr. Acer was infected and had AIDS and stood by not doing a damn thing about it. You are all just as guilty as he was."

In July, 1991, a guest on the *Sally Jessy Raphael Show* stated in front of Mr. and Mrs. Bergalis, that their daughter Kimberly, knowing she was HIV-infected, went to another dentist and did not tell him that she was infected.

Acer's Dental Practice— Staff reported that by 1987 all surgical instruments were routinely autoclaved. Nonsurgical heat-tolerant instruments (e.g., dental mirrors) were autoclaved when practice conditions, such as time and instrument supply, allowed, or were immersed in a liquid germicide for varying lengths of time. Tests of the autoclave in October, 1990, demonstrated that it was functioning properly (*MMWR*, 1991a).

There is no shortage of ideas as to how Acer might have infected his patients. For example, he could have used the same dental instruments on himself or his sexual partners that he used on his patients without sterilizing them. Or he could have had HIV in his sweat which could have dropped into his patients' oral cavities. However, the polymerase chain reaction (the latest in DNA detection technology) was used to detect the presence of HIV in the natural sweat from 40 HIV-infected people. All 40 tested HIV-negative. It appears that by the available methodology of detection HIV is *not* present in the sweat of HIV-positive people.

The actual route of HIV transmission in the Acer–Bergalis case will most likely never be known. There have been suggestions that the dentist did not wish to die alone and chose certain people to infect. It was suggested that he may have attempted to infect still others, but was unsuccessful. A friend of the dentist said that he believed that Acer intentionally infected his patients to call attention to the HIV/AIDS problem in the United States. Acer felt that mainstream America was ignoring the problem. In mid-1994, Continental Broadcasting Systems (CBS), during an interview with Lionel Resnick, chief of retrovirology research at Mt. Sinai Medical Center in Miami, said that, based on his research, David Acer was not the source of HIV infection for the six persons. He said the CDC "vastly overstated the reliability of the DNA tests." But, to the contrary, the CDC believes it has *understated* its case based on the evidence!

A recent CDC estimate put the theoretical risk of HIV transmission from an HIV-infected dentist to patient during a procedure with potential blood exposure at 1 chance in 263,158 to 1 chance in 2,631,579 (Friedland, 1991).

Point for Discussion: Is this last point, one of revenge against society, reasonable?

(Read: Denis Breo (1993). The dental AIDS cases—murder or an unsolved mystery? *JAMA*, 270:2732–2734.)

Summary— The CDC states that based on the following considerations, their investigation strongly suggests that at least three patients of Acer's were infected with HIV during dental care: (1) the three patients had no other confirmed exposure to HIV; (2) they all had invasive procedures performed by an HIV-infected dentist; and (3) DNA sequence analyses of the HIV strains from these three patients indicated a high degree of similarity to each other and to the strain that had infected the dentist—a finding consistent with previous instances in which cases have been linked epidemiologically. In addition, these strains are distinct from the HIV strain from another of Acer's patients who had a known behavioral risk for HIV infection, and from the strains of the eight HIV-infected people residing in the same geographic area and from the 21 other North American HIV isolates.

As of January, 1995, four of the six patients believed to have been infected by Acer have progressed to AIDS and have died: Kimberly Bergalis, Richard Driskill, John Yecs, and Barbara Webb. To date, the six people have received $10 million from Acer's insurance company.

See Point of Information 8.5.

POINT OF INFORMATION 8.5

EFFECTIVENESS OF SCREENING HEALTH CARE WORKERS FOR HIV IN THE UNITED STATES

There is considerable public concern regarding the potential transmission of the human immunodeficiency virus (HIV) from health care worker to patient. This risk is manifest in the results of a 1991 *Newsweek* poll, which found that 90% of Americans favor testing health care workers for HIV and revealing the results to patients. The same poll indicated that 49% of the public believed health care workers should be forbidden to practice if they are HIV-positive, and the majority indicated they would no longer seek treatment from an infected practitioner.

In contrast to this perceived risk, the CDC has estimated the theoretical probability of this type of transmission to be between 0.000024 and 0.0000024. Daniels (1992) points out that the risk of being infected by an HIV-positive surgeon is roughly 10% of the chance of being struck by lightning, 25% as probable as being killed by a bee, and half as likely as being hit by a falling aircraft. Part of the basis of the public's concern is that, in contrast to the other risks mentioned, transmission of HIV from a health care worker to a patient is potentially avoidable. Still, the CDC has recommended against mandatory screening because the low risk does not warrant the anticipated cost associated with testing.

William Chavey and co-workers (1994) examined a screening protocol that included a sequence of antibody tests (enzyme-linked immunoabsorbent assay and the Western blot) and culture for HIV. The incremental cost-effectiveness of applying this protocol as opposed to the status quo for the prevention of transmission of HIV from health care worker to patient was evaluated. The incremental cost-effectiveness ratio was then compared with that of other interventions. Their study showed that the expected annual cost of screening for a large hospital would be $244,382 to prevent 0.02663 transmission. The incremental cost-effectiveness ratio was $9,177,615 per transmission prevented. (*Question:* Is it worth over $9 million to prevent the transmission of HIV to one person? *Discussion.*) The conclusion reached was that screening health care workers for prevention of potential HIV transmission to patients is an expensive use of health care resources.

The results of another cost-effectiveness study of HIV testing of just physicians and dentists in the United States by Kathryn Phillips and coworkers (1994) showed that, although one-time mandatory testing of surgeons and dentists with mandatory restriction of those found to be HIV-positive is more cost-effective than other policies, the cost-effectiveness varies tremendously under different scenarios. Results were highly sensitive to several data inputs, especially HIV seroprevalence of surgeons and dentists and transmission risk. For example, under a medium seroprevalence and transmission risk scenario, mandatory testing of all surgeons might avert 25 infections at a total cost of $27.9 million or $1,115,000 per infection averted and an incremental cost of $291,000 compared with current testing; however, the incremental cost-effectiveness per patient infection averted ranges from $29,807,000 under a low-risk scenario to a savings of $81,000 under a high-risk scenario.

Sexual Transmission

Sexual transmission of HIV occurs when infected blood, semen, or vaginal secretions from an infected person enter the bloodstream of a partner.This can happen during anal, vaginal, or oral penetration, in descending order of risk. Unprotected anal sex by a male or female is perhaps the most dangerous, since the rectal wall is very thin. Masturbation without a partner and abstinence are totally safe. In general, a person's risk of acquiring HIV infection through sexual contact depends on (1) the number of different partners, (2) the likelihood (prevalence) of HIV infection in these partners, and (3) the probability of virus transmission during sexual contact with an infected partner. Virus transmission, in turn, may be affected by biological factors, such as concurrent STD infections in either partner. If there is a genital ulcer caused by syphilis or chancroid or herpes, the risk of getting HIV increases 10- to 20-fold. If there is gonorrhea or chlamydial infection, which are more common, the risk increases probably 3- to 4-fold. Behavioral factors, such as type of sex practice and use of condoms, or varying levels of infectivity in the source partner related to clinical stage of disease also increase the risk of HIV transmission/infection. Based on these factors, the risk for HIV infection is highest for a regular partner of an HIV-infected person practicing unsafe sex. Persons who have sex partners with risk factors for HIV infection or who themselves have multiple partners from urban settings with high rates of injection drug and "crack" cocaine use, prostitution, and other STDs are also at increased risk.

Personal Choice–Personal Risks

About 90% of the HIV infections that occur within the heterosexual non-injection drug use population occur through one or more sexual activities. Some 90% of the HIV infections that occur among gay males occur through anal intercourse (Kingsley et al., 1990). In any sexual activity, HIV is transmitted via a body fluid. Transmission may occur between men, from men to women, or women to men.

Female-to-female transmission has been reported in one case and suggested in another (Curran et al., 1988). As with the other sexually transmitted diseases, HIV transmission among lesbians is very low. However, CDC investigators warn that vaginal secretions and menstrual blood are potential sources of HIV in an infected female. A review of the 9,717 AIDS cases in American women over the last decade found 79 women classified as lesbian and 103 as bisexual. The vast majority of women acquired the virus through injection drug use (Chu et al., 1990). The Women's AIDS Network (1988) of San Francisco states in their publication *Lesbians and AIDS* that if there is a possibility that either woman is carrying the virus, she should not allow her menstrual blood, vaginal secretions, urine, feces, or breast milk to enter her partner's body through the mouth, rectum, vagina, or broken skin.

BOX 8.2

VASECTOMY LOWERS BUT DOES NOT ELIMINATE HIV TRANSMISSION RISK DURING UNSAFE SEX

Vasectomized men infected with HIV have less of the virus in their ejaculate than do men who have not had the sterilization procedure, according to a study released at the recent American Urological Association meeting.

But HIV-positive men who have had a vasectomy still can transmit the virus during unprotected sex. Thus men must still use a condom to prevent HIV transmission.

Unlike sperm, which is entirely absent in vasectomized men, small numbers of lymphocytes still are present in the ejaculate of men who have had the procedure. Therefore, a vasectomy cannot be viewed as a way to prevent transmission of HIV completely (Pudney et al., 1991).

Heterosexual HIV Transmission

Heterosexual HIV transmission means that the virus was transmitted during heterosexual sexual activities. As such, the proportion of HIV infection and AIDS cases among the heterosexual population in the United States is now increasing at a greater rate than the proportion of HIV infections and AIDS cases among homosexuals or IDUs (Friedland et al., 1987). Persons at highest risk for heterosexually transmitted HIV infection include adolescents and adults with multiple sex partners, those with sexually transmitted diseases (STDs), and heterosexually active persons residing in areas with a high prevalence of HIV infection among IDUs. In 1985, fewer than 2% of AIDS cases were from the heterosexual population; by 1989, 5% were from the heterosexual population. For the year 1993, 9% of cases were from the heterosexual population. The large increase is a reflection of the new AIDS definition of 1993. But overall, the incidence of heterosexual AIDS cases remains between 6% and 7% of the total number of reported AIDS cases in the United States.

Studies in Africa, Haiti, and other Caribbean and Third World countries indicate that HIV transmission is most prevalent among the heterosexual population. The male-to-female ratio in Africa is 1:1. In late 1991, the World Health Organization stated that 75% of worldwide HIV transmission occurred heterosexually. By the year 2000, up to 90% will occur heterosexually. Homosexuality and injection

POINT OF INFORMATION 8.6

HIV INFECTION AMONG WOMEN

Alarming News for Women (*World News Tonight* ABC, September 7, 1993). Until now, AIDS has been perceived to be a disease primarily afflicting homosexual men and injection drug users. **In nine U.S. cities, AIDS has become the leading cause of death in women of childbearing age. For the first time, in 1992, the number of women infected with HIV through heterosexual transmission approximated those women infected via virus-contaminated needles.** In 1993, the number of women infected via heterosexual transmission surpassed those infected via injection drug use. Officials at the World Health Organization estimate that four million women will die of AIDS by the year 2000, many of them Americans. The Federal Centers for Disease Control plans to expand the focus of future public health messages to include women.

There are six million women ages 18 to 40 in the United States who are unmarried and having sexual relationships. Those most at risk for HIV infection are (1) those who have multiple sexual partners (defined as having more than four different partners/year), and (2) those women who **do not** insist on the use of a condom.

Antonia Novello, past Surgeon General of the United States, who called AIDS "a family disease" in a talk at the Harvard School of Public Health in October, 1993, said that currently 12% (of 51,000 through 1994, about 15,000 were heterosexually infected) of AIDS patients in this country are women, but by the year 2000, more women than men will have AIDS. She also noted that the incidence of heterosexual transmission is much higher in African-American and Hispanic communities.

Most of what we know about the natural history of AIDS comes from studies in men. "Researchers now need to identify opportunistic infections in women. For example, studies have shown a high prevalence of HIV infection among women with pelvic inflammatory disease (PID)." Novello cautioned physicians who see women with cervical dysplasia, pelvic inflammatory disease, or monilia, which does not respond to the usual therapy, to consider the possibility that they may be dealing with gynecological manifestations of HIV infection.

The nation's top five cities with a female population of 100,000 or more that have the highest incidence of AIDS among women are as follows:

Rate/100,000 Women (1993)

City	White	Black (non-Hispanic)
(1) New York, NY	41.5	90.9
(2) West Palm Beach, FL	38.1	295.4
(3) Ft. Lauderdale, FL	34.1	199.5
(4) Newark, NJ	29.6	105.5
(5) Miami, FL	29.1	125.2

Clearly, in all five cities, HIV disease and AIDS affects black, non-Hispanic women disproportionately.

Three of the nation's cities with the highest incidence of AIDS in women are located in Florida within a 70 mile radius of each other (West Palm Beach, Ft. Lauderdale, and Miami). This area is an epicenter of HIV infection in women. Florida has 10% of the nation's AIDS cases. Nationally, 12% of AIDS cases are women. In Florida's Palm Beach County the rate is 24%; in Broward and Dade Counties, 18%. Nationally, about 6% of AIDS cases are due to heterosexual contact, as opposed to 32% in Palm Beach County, 19% in Broward, and 20% in Dade. Throughout Florida, the prevalence of AIDS cases is 18%. The epidemiologist for the state of Florida stated that what is happening in Florida is happening in the inner cities nationwide. What may distinguish the AIDS epidemic in women is that it hinges on the low self-esteem and lack of personal power experienced by women in many walks of life.

Most of Florida's women with AIDS are poor and receive their medical care through the public health system. Among women in South Florida, HIV transmission is associated with crack cocaine. Pam Whittington, director of the Boynton Community Life Center, a family support facility in southern Palm Beach County, said, "If you have 10 women on crack, probably eight of them are HIV-infected." Injection drugs are a top risk factor for women throughout the United States.

Crack cocaine is cheap and readily available. Its use contributes to anonymous, high-risk sex with multiple partners. Those who can not afford crack exchange sex for it. In isolated communities of crack users, there is a high degree of sharing sex partners, many of whom are HIV-positive.

Perhaps more overwhelming from the viewpoint of education and prevention are risk factors rooted in the region's cultural mix from Latin America, South America, and the Caribbean islands.

The Role of Culture

South Florida is a melting pot of Haitians, Nicaraguans, Panamanians, Cubans, and many other nationalities. Each year thousands of people immigrate and migrate to South Florida with their own cultures, and in those cultures it is taboo to even talk about sex.

A South Florida physician said that among some foreign groups "Machismo rules; homosexuality and bisexuality are akin to heinous crimes. You will never see open admissions. These men are difficult to identify, for outreach purposes, because there is no meeting place. Their cultures also teach that only passive partners are homosexual, so men view themselves as heterosexual as long as they are the active partner during intercourse."

Women are endangered by having sex with husbands or lovers who may have been infected through homosexual contacts. Even if a woman suspects her partner has been with a man, her male-dominated culture prevents her from suggesting condom use. Their greatest risk factor is denial.

Many of South Florida's diverse cultures also believe that only prostitutes use condoms. A woman who raises the issue risks domestic violence or emotional and financial abandonment. At the same time, it is perfectly acceptable for their men to frequent prostitutes, many of whom have come to this country illegally and put themselves at high risk for infection merely to survive.

Another source of risk stems from island religious practices over which ministers hold extreme authority. When a male minister has sex with a male congregation member, it is viewed as a worshiper's union with his god, not a sexual act.

The Bisexual HIV Threat to Women

About 11% of women's AIDS cases occurred from having sexual intercourse with a bisexual male. Approximately 87% of women who were wives of bisexual men did not know it during the time of their marriage. There are about 10 million bisexual men in the United States.

drug use occurs in Africa but the incidence is reported to be very low. The high frequency of AIDS cases in Third World countries is thought to be due to poor hygiene, lack of medicine and medical facilities, a population that demonstrates a large variety of sexually transmitted diseases and other chronic infections, unsanitary disposal of contaminated materials, lack of refrigeration, and the reuse of hypodermic syringes and needles due to supply shortages.

Transmission from men to women in Nairobi has been shown to be facilitated by common genital ulcers, the use of oral contraceptives rather than condoms, and the presence of chlamydia, a type of bacterium. Chlamydia infection probably increases the inflammatory response in the vaginal walls and increases the likelihood of having lymphocytes there that can attach to the virus and allow transmission. The damage that sexually transmitted ulcerative diseases cause to genital skin and mucous membranes is believed to facilitate HIV transmission. Prevention and early treatment of STDs could slow HIV transmission in the United States and in other countries.

Vaginal and Anal Intercourse— Among routes of HIV transmission, there is overwhelming evidence that HIV can be transmitted via anal and vaginal intercourse. In vaginal intercourse, male-to-female transmission is much more efficient than the reverse. This is believed to be due to (1) a consistently higher concentration of HIV in semen than in vaginal secretions, and (2) abrasions in the vaginal mucosa. Such abrasions in the tissue allow HIV to enter the vascular system in larger numbers than would occur otherwise, and perhaps at a single entry point.

The same reasoning explains why the receptive rather than the insertive homosexual partner is more likely to become HIV-infected

BOX 8.3

HIV/AIDS ROULETTE

Case I: The Woman Executive

I am a successful executive woman. A year ago I applied for life insurance. I was required to take an HIV antibody test. It came back positive.

I am not a prostitute or promiscuous. I am not and have never been an injection drug user. I am not a member of a minority group, indigent nor homeless, and I have not slept with a bisexual male (?).

I don't fit any of the stereotypes that people have designated for those infected with HIV. I got HIV from a man I love and have been seeing for 5 years. He is not homosexual or bisexual. He has never used injection drugs. He had no idea he was carrying the virus. He believes he may have been infected about 6 years ago by a woman with whom he had a brief, meaningless relationship. For that one indiscretion we will both pay the ultimate price.

Case II: The HIV-Infected Male

In February of 1994, a 21-year-old man walked into a sexually transmitted disease clinic and told the doctor he had "the clap," or gonorrhea. But he carried HIV.

When a counselor inquired about his sex partners, he told them about several, including a 12-year-old girl. The girl had gone elsewhere to be treated for gonorrhea and tested positive for HIV.

The man admitted to sleeping with 27 women, including 13 teenagers. Ten of the partners couldn't be found. Of the 27 others, 12 tested positive for HIV.

The man has since died, and the clinic has not been able to track all of his sexual partners.

There is a real message to be found in these two cases: People with HIV are much more dangerous to a community than someone with AIDS. Those with AIDS are symptomatic. They are losing weight. They are sick. They have little or no sexual appetite. Those with HIV are healthy and vigorous. That's where the sexual roulette begins.

during anal intercourse. It appears that the membranous linings of the rectum are more easily torn than are those of the vagina. In addition, recent studies indicate the presence of receptors for HIV in rectal mucosal tissue. A recent report by Richard Naftalin (1992) states that human semen contains at least two components, collagenase and spermine, that cause the breakdown of the membrane that supports the colonic epithelial cell layer of the rectal and colon mucosa. This leads to the loss of mucosal barrier function allowing substances to penetrate the rectal and colon mucosa.

Homosexual Anal Intercourse— Today about 60% of homosexual men in San Francisco are infected, probably the highest density of infection anywhere in the developed world. "It colors everything we do out here," says a gay activist, "the gay community, to a large extent, is about addressing AIDS. It has to be, because it's literally a war: your entire community is under siege."

When AIDS struck, it struck hard. In a single year, 1982, 21% of the uninfected gay male population became infected, and for some reason not yet known, many of those infected early, died early. "Soon everyone, and I mean everyone, had a friend who was dying" (Science in California, 1993).

It appears that of all sexual activities, **anal intercourse** is the most efficient way to transmit HIV (DeVincenzi et al., 1989). Information collected from cross-sectional and longitudinal (cohort) studies has clearly implicated receptive anal intercourse as the major mode of acquiring HIV infection. The proportion of new HIV infections among gay males attributable to this single sexual practice is about 90%.

Major risk factors identified with regard to HIV transmission among gay males include anal intercourse (both receptive and insertive), active oral-anal contact, number of partners, and length of homosexual lifestyle (Kingsley et al., 1990).

Heterosexual Anal Intercourse— A number of sexuality oriented surveys of the heterosexual population indicate that between one in five and one in 10 heterosexual couples have tried or regularly practice anal intercourse. Bolling (1989) reported that 70% to 80% of women may have tried anal intercourse and that 10% to 25% of these women enjoyed anal sex on a regular basis. He also reported that 58% of women with multiple sex partners participated in anal sex. James Segars (1989) reported that the highest rates of anal sex occur among teenagers who use drugs and older married couples who are broadening their sexual experiences.

Although it may increase the risk of HIV infection, it must be emphasized that anal intercourse is not necessary for HIV transmission among heterosexuals. In fact, most HIV-infected heterosexuals say that they have never practiced anal intercourse.

Risk of HIV Infection; Number of Sexual Encounters— The risk of HIV infection to a susceptible person after one or more sexual encounters is very difficult to determine. In some cases, people claim to have become infected after a single sexual encounter. Four of eight women developed an HIV infection after being artificially inseminated with what turned out to be HIV-infected donor sperm (Stewart et al., 1985). Other sexually transmitted diseases such as syphilis, gonorrhea, herpes, and hepatitis, carry a significant risk for infection after a single encounter. This risk increases with repeated exposure (Peterman et al., 1986).

In some reported transfusion-associated HIV infections, the female partners of infected males remained HIV-negative after 5 or more years of unprotected sexual intercourse. Television star Michael Glaser said that he had normal sexual relations with his wife for 5 years prior to her being diagnosed as HIV-infected. He was not HIV-infected. She received HIV during a blood transfusion, but was not diagnosed until after their first-born child was diagnosed with HIV. In other studies of heterosexual HIV transmission, many couples had unprotected sexual intercourse over prolonged periods of time with no more than 50% of the partners becoming HIV-infected. There are many instances of heterosexuals and homosexuals who remained HIV-negative after having repeated sexual intercourse with HIV-infected partners.

The fact that not all who are repeatedly exposed become infected suggests that biological factors may play as large a role in HIV infection as behavioral factors. For biological reasons, some people may be more efficient transmitters of HIV; while others are more susceptible to HIV infection, that is, require a smaller HIV infective dose.

Number of Sexual Partners and Types of Activity— One relatively large risk factor for HIV infection in both homosexuals and heterosexuals is believed to be the number of sexual partners. The greater the number of sexual partners, the greater the probability of HIV infection. However, the amount of protection one actually obtains from limiting one's number of partners depends mainly on who those partners are. Having one partner who is in a high-risk group may be more dangerous than having many partners who are not. An example of this is seen in prostitutes, who may be more likely to be infected by their regular injection drug using partners than by customers, who are not in a high-risk group. The risk status of a person who remains faithful to a single sexual partner depends on that partner's behavior: if the partner becomes infected, often without knowing it, the monogamous individual is likely to become infected (Cohen et al., 1989).

Sexual Activities— In addition to a high-risk partner or a number of sexual partners, the types of sexual activities that occur are also significant (Table 8-6). Any sexual activity that produces skin, anal, or vaginal membrane abrasions prior to or during intercourse increases the risk of infection.

OROGENITAL SEX. Orogenital sex may be a greater risk factor for AIDS than previously thought. Of 82 HIV-infected gay men in three San Francisco area studies, 14 (17%) gave orogenital sex as their only high-risk behavior (AIDS Research, 1990). A case was reported of a heterosexual male becoming HIV-infected after receiving oral sex (fellatio) from a prostitute who was HIV-infected (Fischl et al., 1987). Ireneus Keet and colleagues (1992) reported on several studies on the risk of HIV

BOX 8.4

SPORTS AND HIV/AIDS: EARVIN "MAGIC" JOHNSON AND OTHER ATHLETES

HIV-Infected Athletes and Competition

The question regarding whether HIV-infected athletes should be allowed to compete has two facets:

1. Should these athletes be banned from competition to avoid the risk of spreading HIV infection?
2. Does the exercise that is demanded in competition accelerate progression of HIV disease?

As yet, there is no hard, fast, scientifically supported answer to either question. However, through mid-1995, there has not been a single reported case of HIV transmission in any sporting event worldwide!

Magic Johnson: Age 32; Professional Basketball Player, Los Angeles Lakers, HIV-Positive

On November 7, 1991, Magic Johnson (Figure 8-9) appeared at a nationally televised press conference and said, "Because of the HIV virus I have obtained, I will have to announce my retirement from the Lakers today." He admitted having been "naive" about AIDS and added, "Here I am saying **it can happen to anybody,** even me, Magic Johnson." He also assured the world that his wife, Cookie Kelly, 2 months pregnant, had tested negative for the virus. As he spoke, Johnson promised to battle the disease and "become a spokesman" for it. New York AIDS activist Rodger McFarlane said, "If you tried to come up with the perfect person to carry the message of AIDS awareness to the people it ought to reach, you couldn't do better than Magic Johnson."

The National AIDS Hotline lit up with 40,000 phone calls on the day of Johnson's announcement, instead of the usual 3,800. At the Centers for Disease Control and Prevention in Atlanta, AIDS-related calls, which usually average 200 per hour, jumped to 10,000 in a single hour. And shares of Carter-Wallace, Inc., the maker of Trojan condoms, were up $3 on Johnson's announcement that he would become a spokesperson for safer sex. Following Johnson's HIV infection announcement, STD/HIV sexual risk behaviors of persons of an STD clinic in a Maryland suburb of Washington, D.C. were studied. Information was gathered during the 14 weeks prior to his announcement and for 14 weeks after his announcement. The same 283 people were interviewed before and after Johnson's announcement. The mean age was 25 years, 85% had a high school diploma, 60% were males, and 73% of the males were black. Johnson's announcement appeared to lower the number of one night stands for persons between ages 16 to 48, but it had no effect on the use of condoms. Persons between 25 and 48 reduced their number of sexual partners but those between the ages of 16 and 24 did not (Boekeloo et al., 1993). Prior to Magic's announcement, the black community lacked a focal point for action: no leader of national stature had claimed a prominent space from which to ad-

FIGURE 8-9 Earvin "Magic" Johnson, National Basketball Association Basketball Star. The photograph was taken on November 7, 1991 as he announced that he is HIV-positive and that because of the infection, he retired from the Los Angeles Lakers team. He was 32 years old at this time and at the peak of his basketball career. His wish is to become a spokesperson for the struggle against HIV/AIDS.

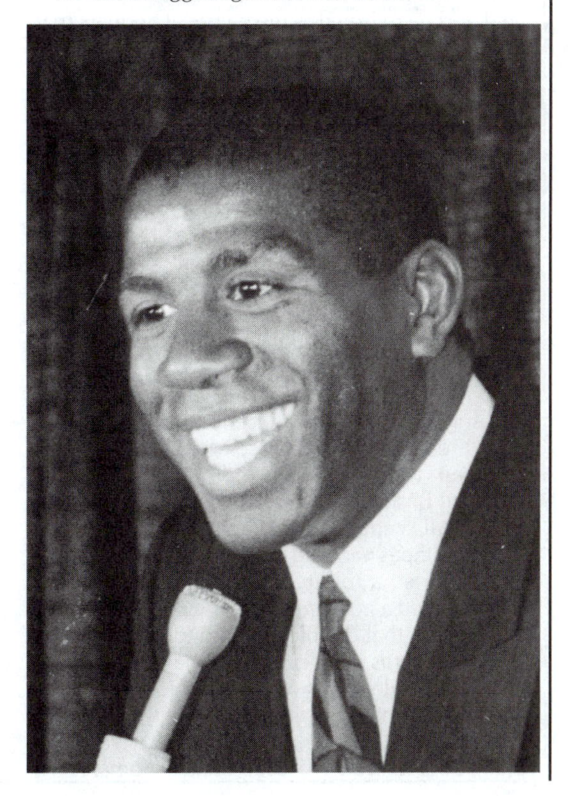

dress HIV disease. Few black politicians, entertainers, civil rights leaders, or sports figures had tackled the issue of AIDS either through public service announcements, television talk shows, radio addresses, church pulpits, theaters, or school auditoriums. Magic's announcement—at least for a time—changed that.

Some Events Since Magic's Announced Retirement

June 4, 1992—Earvin the III is born *without* antibody to HIV. (As of June 15, 1995 Magic is age 35. His wife age 35 and baby age 3 are HIV-negative.)

Sept. 27, 1992—Announces he will return to the Lakers and play limited schedule in the upcoming 1992–1993 NBA season.

Nov. 2, 1992—Announces his retirement in a statement issued by the Lakers. The reason for this retirement given by Magic was that his presence on the court struck fear among his fellow players—controversies over player safety surrounded his return to the game. During a pre-season game, Magic's forearm was scraped. He was immediately taken out and treated. His wound was covered and he returned to the game. It appears that this single event caused a great deal of concern to Magic and to other players. According to an interview with Magic, it was the most important single event in determining his retirement.

Nov. 5, 1992—Announces that a woman has filed a $2 million lawsuit in Michigan federal court claiming he gave her the AIDS virus in June, 1990. Johnson, through his lawyers, told ABC's *Prime Time Live* TV he had sex with the woman, but said he doesn't know if he got the virus from her, or if she got it from him, or neither.

Also in 1992, he published his book *My Life* in which he reveals his many sexual exploits.

In March, 1994 he became head coach of the Los Angeles Lakers for a brief period.

In the three seasons since Magic Johnson announced he had contracted the AIDS virus, National Basketball Association players have attended AIDS education seminars, listened to safe sex audiotapes narrated by Spike Lee and Arsenio Hall, phoned a toll-free hotline for counseling, and received a novel gift from the player's union: a key chain that doubles as a condom holder.

But in words and deeds NBA players continue to send mixed signals on whether Johnson's announcement has had any impact on their behavior—and whether they are heeding the warnings of the doctors who visit their locker rooms.

Other Sports, Other Athletes

Basketball players are not the only athletes whose behavior may place them at risk for HIV infection. John Elson (1991) wrote a revealing article for *Time* magazine just after Magic Johnson revealed his HIV status. Elson tells of groupies that follow athletes in all sports. They are usually college-age or older. Mainly they seek money, attention, and the glamor of associating with celebrated and highly visible "hard bodies." According to a 31-year-old who has had affairs with athletes in two sports, "For women, many of whom don't have meaningful work, the only way to identify themselves is to say whom they have slept with. A woman who sleeps around is called a whore. But a woman who has slept with Magic Johnson is a woman who has slept with Magic Johnson. It's almost as if it gives her legitimacy."

Baseball players call them "Annies." To riders on the rodeo circuit, they are "buckle bunnies." To most other athletes, they are "wannabes" or just "the girls." They can be found hanging out anywhere they might catch an off-duty sports hero's eye and fancy, or in the lobbies of hotels where teams on the road check in. To the athletes who care to indulge them—and many do—these readily available groupies offer pro sport's ultimate perk: free and easy recreational sex, no questions asked. Recently, an HIV-infected female stated publicly that she had had sex with at least 50 Canadian ice hockey players. She could not recall their names. The sex may be free, but now there is a price for the lifestyle—HIV/AIDS.

Concerns over the transmission of HIV are shared throughout sports, particularly those sports that cause blood-letting injuries—football, hockey, and boxing. In football Jerry Smith, a former Washington Redskin, died of AIDS in 1986; no others are known at this time. In boxing, Esteban DeJesus, WBC lightweight champion, died of AIDS in 1989. Three other boxers are known to be HIV-positive. In professional ice skating, the Calgary Herald reported that, by 1992, at least 40 top United States and Canadian male skaters and coaches have died from AIDS (among them, Rob McCall, Brian Pockar, Dennis Coi, and Shawn McGill). In February, 1995, Greg Louganis, the greatest diver in Olympic history, announced that he has AIDS.

An informal poll of 20 NFL Pro Bowl football players in February of 1992 showed that 10 of the 20 believed HIV-positive athletes should be banned from competition.

TABLE 8-6 Sexual Activity According to Degree of Risk for Transmitting HIV

Risk	Activity
Lowest risk	1. Abstinence
	2. Masturbating alone
	3. Hugging/massage/dry kissing
	4. Masturbating with another person but not touching one another
	5. Deep wet kissing
	6. Mutual masturbation with only external touching
	7. Mutual masturbation with internal touching using finger cots or condoms
	8. Frottage (rubbing a person for sexual pleasure)
	9. Intercourse between the thighs
	10. Mutual masturbation with orgasm *on,* not *in* partner
	11. Use of sex toys (dildos) with condoms, or that are not shared by partners and that have been properly sterilized between uses
	12. Cunnilingus
	13. Fellatio without a condom, but never putting the head of the penis inside mouth
	14. Fellatio to orgasm with a condom
	15. Fellatio without a condom putting the head of the penis inside the mouth and withdrawing prior to ejaculation
	16. Fellatio without a condom with ejaculation in mouth
	17. Vaginal intercourse with a condom correctly used and spermicidal foam that kills HIV and withdrawing prior to orgasm
	18. Anal intercourse with a condom correctly used with a lubricant that contains spermicide that kills HIV and withdrawing prior to ejaculation
	19. Vaginal intercourse with internal ejaculation with a condom correctly used and with spermicidal foam that kills HIV
	20. Vaginal intercourse with internal ejaculation with a condom correctly used but no spermicidal foam
	21. Anal intercourse with internal ejaculation with a condom correctly used with spermicide that kills HIV
	22. Brachiovaginal activities (fisting)
	23. Brachioproctic activities (anal fisting)
	24. Use of sex toys by more than one partner without a condom and that have not been sterilized between uses
	25. Vaginal intercourse using spermicidal foam but without a condom and withdrawing prior to ejaculation
	26. Vaginal intercourse without spermicidal foam and without a condom and withdrawing prior to ejaculation
	27. Anal intercourse with a condom and withdrawing prior to ejaculation
	28. Vaginal intercourse with internal ejaculation without a condom but with spermicidal foam
	29. Vaginal intercourse with internal ejaculation without a condom and without any other form of barrier contraception
Highest risk	30. Anal intercourse with internal ejaculation without a condom

(Source: Shernoff, 1988

transmission among gay males. They concluded that the orogenital route of HIV transmission is difficult to assess. Information on questionnaires was frequently contradicted in follow up interviews. For example, of 20 men who denied having receptive anal intercourse, 11 later changed their statements. However, Keet and colleagues concluded that there is sufficient evidence to conclude that orogenital HIV transmission does occur.

Madalene Heng and colleagues (1994) reported that HIV-infected patients with oral herpes simplex lesions are at risk of transmitting HIV to others through oral sex. They tested keratinocytes (live skin cells) from the oral lesions of six men with AIDS and oral herpes infection (HSV-1), and compared those biopsies from six men with HSV-1 but not HIV.

The tissue from the HIV/herpes patients was infected with both viruses, and the number of virus in that tissue was much higher than the number found in samples from the other men—736 particles per skin cell compared to 31 and 0 in the other two groups.

This shows that HIV is capable of infecting epidermal cells when herpes virus is present. Epidermal keratinocytes were thought to be resistant to HIV infection because they lack the CD4 receptor molecule.

Data from this study is similar to that from a previous study of brain cells of people infected with both HIV and cytomegalovirus. The brain tissue also lacks CD4 receptors, yet HIV was able to invade the cells and replicate.

The researchers speculated that the association of HIV envelope proteins with HSV-1 proteins may allow HIV to infect cells without the aid of CD4 molecules.

Prostitution (Sex Worker). There is little if any evidence that prostitutes in pattern I countries play a large role in heterosexual HIV transmission (Cohen et al., 1989).

An unfortunate consequence of the attention prostitutes or sex workers have attracted in relation to AIDS in the United States and other countries, is that they tend to be seen as responsible for the spread of HIV — an attitude reflected in descriptions of prostitutes as reservoirs of infection or high-frequency transmitters. But, the sex worker is only the most "visible" side of a transaction that involves two people: for every sex worker who is HIV-positive there is, somewhere, the partner from whom she or he contracted HIV. Given the fact that the chance of contracting HIV during a single act of unprotected six is not high, infection in a sex worker is likely to mean that she or he has been repeatedly exposed to HIV by clients who did not or would not wear condoms. Thus the more useful way of reading the statistics of HIV infection in prostitutes or sex workers is to view them as an indication of how strong a foothold the epidemic has gotten within a community.

Risk Estimates for HIV Infection During Sexual Intercourse in the Heterosexual Population— Norman Hearst and Stephen Hulley of the University of California, San Francisco calculated that the odds of heterosexual HIV transmission range from one in 500 for a single act of sexual intercourse with an HIV-infected partner when no condom is used to one in five billion if a condom is used and the sexual partner is HIV-negative **at the time**.

Table 8-7 presents estimates of the risk of HIV infection from a single heterosexual encounter and after 5 years of frequent heterosexual contact for various types of partners. Risk depends on the following: (1) the probability that the sexual partner carries the virus; (2) the probability of infection given a single sexual exposure to an infected partner; and (3) the reduction in risk by using condoms and spermicides.

The most striking feature of the table is the large variation in the risk of HIV infection under different circumstances. The most important cause of this variation is risk status of sexual partners (Figure 8-10). Choosing a partner who is not in a high-risk group provides almost 5,000-fold protection compared with choosing a partner in the highest-risk category.

Condoms are estimated to provide about 1,250-fold protection. A negative HIV antibody test provides about 2,500-fold protection.

The implication of this analysis is clear: **Choose sex partners carefully and use condoms**.

In a study by Nancy Padian and colleagues (1991), only 1% of HIV-positive women passed HIV by sexual contact to their male partners. In contrast, one of every five uninfected female partners of HIV-infected men acquired the virus through sex. Overall, the study revealed that women are 17.5 times more likely to become HIV-infected from an infected male than men are to contract the disease from an infected female. The ratio of 18:1 came from a limited study (379 heterosexual couples) and as such may underestimate the relative frequency of female-to-male HIV transmission. But, Padian's findings support recent Centers for Disease Control and Prevention figures showing that 90% of the more than 33,000 adults who became HIV-positive through heterosexual contact were women.

Injection Drug Users and HIV Transmission

The hypodermic syringe and needle play an essential role in medical therapy; they also play a role in HIV transmission. Injection drug use

TABLE 8-7 Risk of HIV Infection for Heterosexual Intercourse in the United States

Risk Category of Partner	Estimated Risk of Infection: 1 Sexual Encounter	Estimated Risk of Infection: 500 Sexual Encounters
HIV SEROSTATUS UNKNOWN		
Not in any high-risk group		
Using condoms	1 in 50,000,000	1 in 110,000
Not using condoms	1 in 5,000,000	1 in 16,000
High-risk groups[a]		
Using condoms	1 in 100,000 to 1 in 10,000	1 in 210 to 1 in 21
Not using condoms	1 in 10,000 to 1 in 1,000	1 in 32 to 1 in 3
HIV SERONEGATIVE		
No history of high-risk behavior[b]		
Using condoms	1 in 5,000,000,000	1 in 11,000,000
Not using condoms	1 in 500,000,000	1 in 1,600,000
Continuing high-risk behavior[b]		
Using condoms	1 in 500,000	1 in 1,100
Not using condoms	1 in 50,000	1 in 160
HIV SEROPOSITIVE		
Using condoms	1 in 5000	1 in 11
Not using condoms	1 in 500	2 in 3

[a]High-risk groups with prevalences of HIV infection at the higher end of the range given include homosexual or bisexual men, injection drug users from major metropolitan areas, and hemophiliacs. Groups with prevalences at the lower end of the range include homosexual or bisexual men and injection drug users from other parts of the country, female prostitutes, heterosexuals from countries where heterosexual spread of HIV is common (including Haiti and central Africa), and recipients of multiple blood transfusions between 1983 and 1985 from areas with a high prevalence of HIV infection.

[b]High-risk behavior consists of sexual intercourse or needle sharing with a member of one of the high-risk groups.

(Source: Adapted from Hearst and Hulley, 1988.

(IDU) is the second highest risk behavior in the United States and Europe, accounting for about 30% of AIDS cases in 1989. In 1990, IDUs made up about 50% of *all* new AIDS cases in the United States. About two-thirds of the females and about half of the heterosexual males who were diagnosed with AIDS had a sex partner who was an IDU (*MMWR,* 1991b). State surveillance reports for New York indicate that 60% of IDUs are HIV-infected; in New Jersey, 80% are HIV-infected. Because 70% to 80% of IDUs have sex with non drug users, IDUs are a major source of heterosexual and perinatal HIV infection in the United States and Europe. HIV is also spreading rapidly among IDUs in developing countries such as Brazil, Argentina, and Thailand (Des Jarlais et al., 1989).

Ninety percent of injection drug users in the United States are heterosexuals. Thirty percent are women, of whom 90% are in their child-bearing years. From 1988 through 1990, female IDUs made up 52% of all AIDS cases in women. In 1991, of 5,457 female AIDS cases, 70% became HIV-infected due to drugs. Forty-nine percent of these women were IDU; 21% were infected by sexual intercourse with men who were IDUs. During this same period, 735 new cases of AIDS in children occurred—56% were from IDU mothers and 18% were from

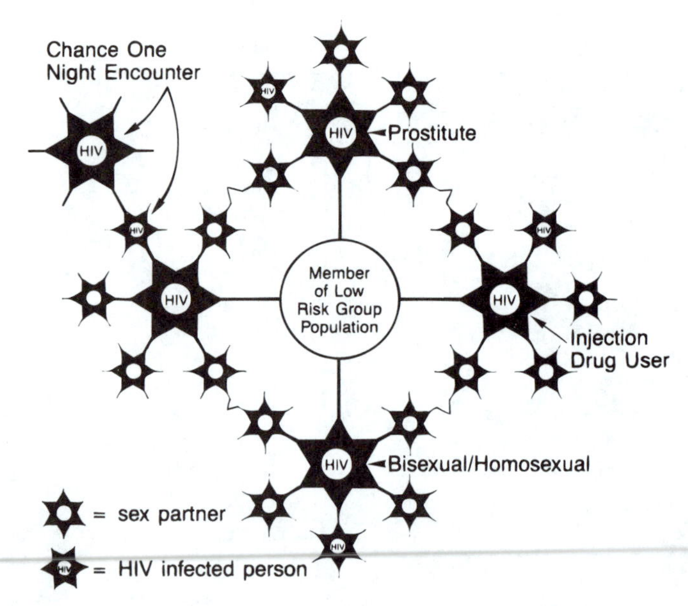

FIGURE 8-10 Risk Transmission of HIV. Sexual transmission can occur among homosexuals or heterosexuals. Prostitutes can be either male or female. The diagram shows possible bridges for transmission of HIV from high-risk groups into low-risk groups. To be safe, *you* must not become part of the chain. Be sure your sexual partner is free of HIV.

mothers whose sex partners were IDUs (*MMWR*, 1992). These drug users and the sexual partners of male drug users represent the largest part of the estimated 100,000 HIV-infected women of child-bearing age. Thus, there is a direct correlation between HIV perinatal transmission and pediatric AIDS cases and injection drug use. In addition, 30% to 50% of female injection drug users have engaged in prostitution, and as such represent the largest pool of HIV-infected heterosexuals in the United States and Europe (Drucker, 1986). The use of alcohol (Avins, 1994) and the use of other noninjection drugs such as crack cocaine are believed to play an increasing role in HIV transmission among heterosexuals.

More than 60% of reported adult *heterosexual* AIDS cases are associated with people who have a history of injection drug use. Twenty-eight percent of *all* AIDS cases in the United States occur in IDUs; 21% of these cases occur where IDU is the only risk factor. Of pediatric AIDS cases, 90% occur perinatally. Of these, over 64% are associated with IDU by either the mother or her sexual partner (HIV/AIDS Surveillance Report, 1994).

The prevalence of HIV infection in IDUs varies widely with geography. Data from more than 18,000 people tested in nearly 90 surveys consistently show high rates in eastern towns and cities with close proximity to New York City and northern New Jersey. Eighty-two percent of AIDS cases among all *reported* IDUs have been in New York City. It should be noted that most of the surveys were conducted in drug treatment facilities for heroin abuse. Since only 10% to 20% of the estimated 1,100,000 IDUs are currently in treatment, geographical conclusions based on the surveys may be misleading. More data are needed on HIV prevalence among injection drug users not currently in treatment.

BOX 8.5

PLACING THE RISK OF DEATH DUE TO HIV INFECTION AND AIDS IN PERSPECTIVE IN RELATION TO DEATHS CAUSED BY OTHER DISEASES, ACCIDENTS, AND MURDERS

Before reading this section it might be useful to keep in mind that the line between **risk** and **blame** is very thin. Too often risk figures are used to place or fix blame. Risk figures are used to transmit fact but may give misleading impressions. And misleading impressions can have enormous impact on public policy. Thus the need to place HIV disease in perspective.

In 1986, 1.6 million people in the United States died from six major chronic diseases: cardiovascular, cerebrovascular, lung, liver, diabetes, and various cancers. These six diseases accounted for 75% of all deaths. An additional 8% of deaths were caused by infectious diseases and 7% were caused by accidents, suicides, and homicides. AIDS was responsible for 0.5% of the total number of deaths. In 1994, 538,000 people died from cancer; about 37,000 died from AIDS. In this same year, there were 1,208,000 new cancer cases, there were about 60,000 new AIDS cases (about 5% of new cancer cases).

An estimated 48 million Americans over age 18 smoke about 24 billion packages of cigarettes each year (*MMWR*, 1994c).

Tobacco use in various forms was associated with the deaths of over 400,000 people in 1991, 1992, 1993, 1994, and most likely will continue at this rate through 1995, at an annual cost to the work force of at least $52 billion. Former Surgeon General C. Everett Koop said in early 1989 that smoking was the single most preventable cause of death known. It kills more people than HIV/AIDS, cocaine, heroin, alcohol, fire, automobile accidents, homicide, and suicide combined (Will, 1991). One in six deaths is caused by smoking and smoking-related deaths continue in spite of a 28-year-old warning concerning the risks of smoking. Worldwide, mid-1992, it was reported that about 3 million people a year die due to the Brown Plague, smoking-related diseases (Peto, 1992). In 1993, some 160,000 deaths resulted from various forms of cancer due to tobacco used (Munzer, 1994).

In the United States in 1988, 32,000 people died from AIDS—yet 32,000 people died from tobacco-related diseases every 32 days. Also in 1988, there were 1.5 million heart attacks resulting in 550,000 deaths; and 1,800,000 people were involved in automoble accidents resulting in 48,700 deaths. In that year, between 30,000 and 40,000 people committed suicide and about 30,000 were killed in shootings. In 1 week in 1989, from May 1 to May 7, 464 people were shot to death. The victims ranged in age from 2 to 87. They were white, black, Hispanic, and Asian and represented 42 of the 50 states. Over 30,000 others shared this same fate in 1989.

From 1981 to 1990, about a quarter of a million people died because of drunken drivers on American highways. In this same time period about 70,000 people died from AIDS.

According to UNICEF, about 39,000 children under age 5 die **each day** in Latin America, Asia, and Africa. They die of starvation, lack of medicine, poor sanitary conditions, and such. Far more children and adults are dying each day from famine than from AIDS. In these countries, HIV infection is not a major concern—their next meal is.

HIV/AIDS is real, it is here, but it is **preventable**. The odds of heterosexual HIV infection after a single penile–vaginal encounter with a low-risk partner when a condom is used are about 1 in 50 million. Without the condom it is about 1 in 5 million. The long-range risk of death from smoking is about 1 in 200; motorcycling, about 1 in 1,000; automobile driving, about 1 in 6,000; canoeing, 1 in 100,000; and having a legal abortion before 9 weeks, 1 in 400,000.

In short, there are many more ways to die than from HIV/AIDS. Worldwide hunger leads the list. AIDS, like so many other diseases, is preventable. Whether you become HIV-infected depends on you.

Other Means of HIV Transmission

Other means of HIV infection have been documented. There has been a reported case of HIV transmission via acupuncture. It is believed that HIV-infected body fluids contaminated the acupuncture needles (Vittecoq et al., 1989). The CDC reported that a woman became HIV-positive after being artificially inseminated with semen from her HIV-infected husband

BOX 8.6

HIV TRANSMISSION: PREPARATION AND USE OF INJECTION DRUGS

Group use of drug paraphernalia and the type of substance used are factors in transmission of HIV from person to person.

Drugs in powdered form are usually placed in a bottle cap, or "cooker," an item often found on streets or in garbage cans. Water is added and heated to dissolve the powder into a solution.

The solution is withdrawn by needle through a "cotton," or a filter through which the drug solution is drawn into the syringe. Cotton swabs, lint from clothing, cigarette filters, and a variety of other materials are used.

The needle then punctures a vein wherever there is one that can be used. Blood is drawn up into the syringe to mix with the drug solution and the blood–solution mixture is injected into the vein (Figure 7-8). If the vein is missed, the drug injected subcutaneously (under the skin) hurts and may cause an abscess. Small quantities of a drug may be injected repeatedly—each time blood is drawn up into the syringe.

The "works," as the syringe and needle are referred to, become contaminated with the user's blood. The "works " and the "cookers " are shared and the amount of sharing depends on the number of users present. Everyone after the first user in the "shooting gallery" line receives potentially HIV-infected lymphocytes from all those with HIV infection who used the equipment before them.

It should be noted that in the injection drug culture, the sharing of needles is a sign of comradery, a sign of mutual trust. An unwillingness to share needles may cause others in the group to become suspicious of possible police connections.

Drug paraphernalia are commonly rented in shooting galleries by users who lack the equipment. A set of "works" is usually rented out until the needle is too dull to penetrate the skin. By then the needle has been sharpened often on whatever was available to give it a penetrating edge. Thus, not only is HIV transmitted among those in a "shooting gallery" but other bacteria and viruses that contaminate their surroundings are also shared.

The world of injection drug use is "designed" to transmit infectious agents. However, *it is not the drug that is responsible for HIV transmission, rather it is the infected blood shared by each of the users of an HIV contaminated "works."* The practice of sharing "works" appears to be equally common among homosexual and heterosexual drug users. Thus it provides a common link between the homosexual and heterosexual population placing both at risk for HIV infection.

Cocaine vs. Heroin— The use of injected cocaine is rising as is exposure to HIV in cocaine IDUs. One major difference between cocaine and heroin abuse is that IV cocaine abusers are binge users or repeat injectors, while the heroin abuser falls asleep after one injection. Studies in New York and San Francisco show that IV cocaine abusers are the more likely to test HIV-positive.

FIGURE 8-11 An Injection Drug User. Note that the arm is tied to force veins to fill with blood making them easier to reach. A candle is used to heat the drug into a solution. This is referred to as "cooking" the drug.

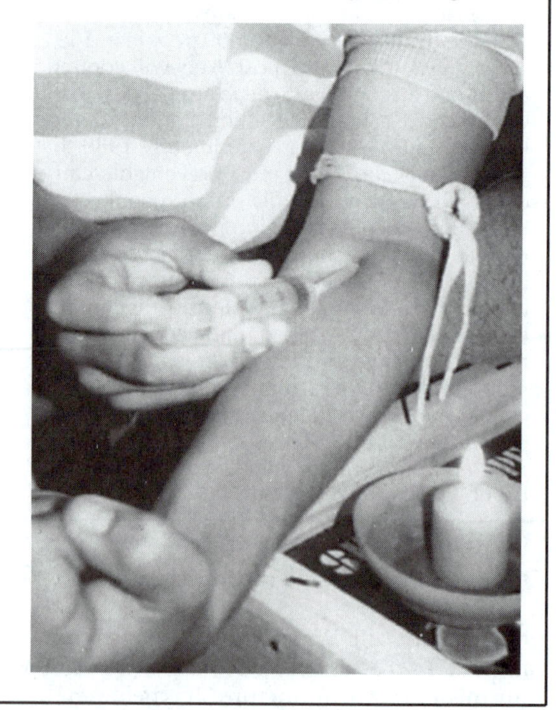

BOX 8.7

SEXUAL ABUSE OF CHILDREN RESULTS IN HIV INFECTION: THREE CASES

Childhood sexual abuse is a common problem that is present in all social and economic groups. Approximately one-half of children who are sexually abused are between 6 and 12 years old, and 30% to 46% have been sexually abused on more than one occasion. Most investigators report a female-to-male ratio of 8:1 or 9:1. These reports, however, come from medical centers and may not reflect the true ratio, because sexual abuse of boys is more often reported only to the police and less likely to be assessed by physicians.

Ninety-eight percent of perpetrators of childhood sexual abuse are male, one of the few common characteristics of pedophiles. No classic profile of a pedophile exists. Little evidence supports the identification of a potential pedophile on the basis of race, religion, income, social class, intelligence, occupation, or education. Forty percent of abusers are family members, and an additional 40% are known to the family. Only 20% of pedophiles are unknown to the child.

Sexually Transmitted Disease

Sexually transmitted diseases (STDs) are infrequently encountered in childhood victims of sexual abuse. However, most authorities agree that nonsexual transmission of STDs is rare in children older than 2 years. Routine cultures for STDs are positive in 5% to 12% of sexually abused children. The epithelium and relatively alkaline pH of the prepubertal vagina inhibit the growth of many sexually transmitted organisms (Gibbons, (1994).

Case I

A woman called from an AIDS organization, asking for someone who could speak to a girl who was HIV-infected at the age of 12. The girl is not a hemophiliac and her father is the only other HIV-infected member of her family. When asked if she had considered sexual abuse as a means of transmission, the wife responded. "The family doesn't talk about that."

Case II

When I was 13 years old, my mother's boyfriend, who was also a drug supplier, raped me. He infected me with HIV. I was robbed of my teen years and my life. I live knowing I will die soon—yet I have not begun to live.

Case III

On March 10, 1994, the headline of a local paper read, "Abused Girl with AIDS Dies." This headline says so much yet says so little with regard to this case.

When this physically and mentally tormented young girl came to live with her foster parents in 1992 she was sad, easily frightened, and withdrawn. She had been badly abused sexually. At least a dozen men sexually abused this child. Just one was arrested and given a 10-year sentence.

She was 10 years old and couldn't read or write. She had never heard of Jesus or celebrated Christmas. She also had AIDS. She was close to death.

With the loving care of her foster parents and medications, she rebounded and lived another 2 years. She died at age 11.

The local Department of Health and Rehabilitative Services (HRS) began receiving reports involving this girl in September 1986, when she was 3. At 6, she was treated for herpes and gonorrhea. Her vaginal warts were so enlarged the cervix was not visible. Her collection of sexually transmitted diseases caused such pain that the physician had to render her unconscious to examine her vagina. She was placed on medicine for the virus, for her ears, eyes, tongue, throat, sinus, vagina, itching (which was so intense she would scrape until she bled). She suffered from severe neuropathy in her hands and feet (due to ddI), had Pneumocystis pneumonia, herpes zoster infection, diarrhea, etc. She had four close encounters with death during the 2 years she was with her foster parents.

Although at least two reports were confirmed, HRS didn't permanently remove her from her home until March, 1992.

The foster mother said people were so frightened of her that some physicians "examined" her from across the room—**"they would not touch her!"**

The girl's foster father said their goal was to give her a safe and normal childhood for the time she had left.

She was tutored at home. She went to Disney World. They took her to California to meet Roseanne Arnold. Every occasion was celebrated to the max because she had never had a party.

She had never heard of God or Jesus, so her foster parents had her baptized. When she went up to the altar for her first communion, she put the wafer in her mouth and said in a loud voice. "Oh, that tastes nasty." And everybody broke up.

With regard to Christmas, she told her foster parents, "Santa Claus never found me." Her foster father said he explained that Santa sends parents a bill and if it's not paid, children don't get presents. "And, I told her, 'I have already sent a check to Santa, so you've got to come home.' And she said, 'Oh, boy!'" That Christmas she had seven Christmas trees and 267 gifts. "Most of them were from garage sales, but it didn't make any difference," he said. "She was thankful for anything."

With regard to dying, there were many conversations about God and heaven. She told her foster mother she wanted a God who laughed. And she hoped heaven was like Disney World. She had told her foster mother once that she was afraid to die because she didn't know how to get to heaven. "I told her, 'You'll go to sleep and you won't feel a thing, and when you wake up God will be holding your hand instead of mommy.' And that's exactly how it happened. I believe she said to God, 'This is it. Take me.' And he did."

During the 2 years of making a home for this child, the foster parents lost friends. Even relatives stopped coming to visit. But these people said they would gladly do it over again!

HIV is now the fifth leading cause of death in children under age 15 (Oleske, 1994).

(*MMWR*, 1990b). Unlicensed and unregulated tattoo establishments may present an unrecognized risk for HIV infection to patrons. If the operator does not use new needles or needles which have been autoclaved (steam sterilized), the possibility exists that infection with HIV or a number of other blood-borne pathogens may take place. In addition, single-service or individual containers of dye or ink should be used for each client.

Human Bites— According to police reports, a Florida woman with a history of arrests for prostitution and who has tested HIV-positive, bit a 93-year-old man on his arm, head, and leg while robbing him. The bits required stitches. The man initially tested HIV-negative but a test several months later was HIV-positive. A complete investigation into his personal life ruled out previous HIV infection.

Sexual Abuse— The subject of sexual abuse, in all its forms, of children by adults or adult on adult is beyond the scope of this text. However, each time there is a date-rape or any other type of rape there is the chance that the rapist may be HIV-positive. One in five adult women has been the victim of a completed rape at some time in her life (Koss et al., 1991). Although 61% of the women stated that physicians should routinely ask about these experiences, only 4% had been asked by their physicians (Walker et al., 1993). Without a complete sexual history that includes questions about rape and so forth, the proper care and medication can be delayed until the onset of HIV disease or AIDS.

Through the end of 1993, there have been at least a dozen cases of purposeful HIV infection of males by HIV-infected females or vice versa. This too should be looked on as a form of sexual abuse—one partner is being sexually deceived by the other. In some of these cases the jury found the HIV-positive persons who kept this knowledge from their sexual partner guilty of attempted murder (see Chapter 16 for individual legal cases).

Transplants— On any given day, about 20,000 Americans are waiting for a transplant. There is a small but present risk of receiving HIV along with the transplant tissue. A CDC report revealed that a bone transplant recipient became HIV-infected from an HIV-infected donor. HIV transmission has also occurred in the transplantation of kidneys, liver, heart, pancreas, and skin (*MMWR*, 1988a). In May of 1991, the CDC reported on 56 transplant patients who received organs and tissues from an HIV-infected donor in 1985. A transplantation service company supplied tissues to 30 hospitals in 16 states. All tissues came from a single young male who was shot to death during a robbery. He twice tested HIV-negative before his heart, kidneys, liver, pancreas, cornea, and other tissues were removed for transplant. By mid-1991, three recipients of these tissues had died of AIDS and six others were HIV-positive. As of mid-1991, 32 other recipients had been located, 11 of whom tested HIV-negative. The others had not yet been tested.

In May of 1994, the CDC published guidelines for preventing HIV transmission through transplantation of human tissue (*MMWR*, 1994b).

Nosocomial

Nosocomial (nos-o-ko-mi-al) refers to hospital-acquired infections. A chain of nosocomial HIV transmission has occurred in southern Russia and among children in Romanian orphanages. Instances of nosocomial HIV transmission have also been reported from industrialized countries such as the United States, where transmission occurred from patient to patient. While nosocomial transmission accounts for a very small fraction of HIV transmission, nosocomial HIV transmission in any country at this time is unacceptable, and underscores deficiencies in present medical practices (Heymann et al., 1994).

Influence of Sexually Transmitted Diseases on HIV Transmission and Vice Versa

Sexual intercourse occurs more than 100 million times daily around the world. Results: 910,000 conceptions and over 600,000 cases of sexually transmitted disease. In the United States over 12 million new cases of sexually transmitted diseases occur each year (World Health Organization study as reported in *The New York Times*).

Because HIV can be sexually transmitted, the association between HIV and other sexually transmitted diseases can be in part attributed to the shared risk of exposure and shared modes of transmission. If sexually transmitted diseases are biological cofactors of HIV infection and dissemination, one would expect a time-sequence (temporal) relationship. In-deed, HIV infection and other sexually transmitted diseases may be acquired in sequence, but because of the delay between HIV infection and development of antibodies, STD detection and HIV seroconversion may occur in reverse order.

For the purpose of understanding which STDs best promote HIV transmission, the sexually transmitted diseases can be divided into genital ulcer and genital nonulcerative diseases.

Genital Ulcer Disease (GUD)— Signs of genital ulcer disease appear as open sores on the penis, vagina, other genital areas and at times elsewhere on the body. The most widespread genital ulcer STDs are syphilis, genital herpes, and chancroid.

TABLE 8-8 Bidirectional Interaction between HIV and Sexually Transmitted Genital Ulcer Disease

Types of Biological Transactions	Epidemiological Observation
GUD Increases HIV Prevalence	
Type I interaction: *Transmission*	
GUD increases susceptibility to HIV	Increased incidence of HIV in people with GUD
GUD increases infectiousness of HIV	Increased transmission of HIV with co-exposure to GUD and HIV
HIV Increases GUD Prevalence	
Type II interaction: *Virulence*	
HIV immune disease increases virulence of GUD pathogens	Increased incidence and prevalence of GUD in HIV-infected patients Decreased effectiveness of GUD therapy

Two categories of interaction between sexually transmitted genital ulcer disease (GUD) and HIV are relevant to transmission and to disease. Facilitated transmission (type I interaction), in which GUD operates to increase the prevalence of HIV, and enhanced virulence (type II interaction), in which HIV operates to increase the prevalence of GUD, may amplify the prevalence of each in a network of sexual contacts, such as a "core group" of prostitutes and clients, forming an efficient reservoir of high-frequency HIV and sexually transmitted disease transmitters.

(Source: Adapted from Cameron et al., 1990)

William Cameron and colleagues (1990) reported on the bidirectional biological interactions between HIV and STDs, especially the genital ulcerative STDs. Bidirectional interaction between HIV and STDs occurs with respect to both transmission and virulence (Table 8-8). HIV transmission is a consequence of both infectivity and susceptibility, both of which can be increased by genital ulcer disease. Virulence, the capacity of a pathogen to produce disease, is a consequence of both pathogen and host factors. Thus, HIV infection and associated immune deficiency disease may account for the increased prevalence of genital ulcer disease; and this in turn may further amplify HIV transmission in a network of social contacts.

Evidence that genital ulcer disease may increase the risk of acquiring HIV has been reported from at least one STD clinic in the United States (Quinn et al., 1988). Since 1986, the incidence of primary and secondary syphilis in the United States has been increasing, especially among minority heterosexuals in urban areas. Between 1986 and 1988, cases of primary and secondary syphilis increased 98%, chancroid cases increased 105%, and herpes simplex increased 78%. In one study at the STD clinic at Kings County Hospital in Brooklyn, the number of GUD cases more than tripled from 1986 to 1988 and by the first half of 1989, 35% of STD clinic visits were for GUDs (Chirgwin et al., 1991).

Nonulcerative Disease— The nonulcerative STDs include gonorrhea, chlamydial, and trichomonal infections, and genital warts. In most populations, these are much more common than genital ulcer diseases. None causes the noticeable open sores that occur in the ulcer diseases but they do cause microscopic breaks in affected tissue, and are associated with HIV transmission (Laga et al., 1993). The most common symptoms are warty growths on the genitals, discharge from the penis or vagina, and painful urination.

Collectively, worldwide there are over 250 million cases a year of just seven major STDs: syphilis, herpes, and chancroid, which cause ulcers; and trichomoniasis, chlamydia, warts, and gonorrhea, which do not (Figure 8-12).

HIV infection and other sexually transmitted diseases (STDs) share the same risk factors. The major difference between HIV/AIDS and the other STDs is the degree of cell and tissue destruction and the mortality of HIV/AIDS.

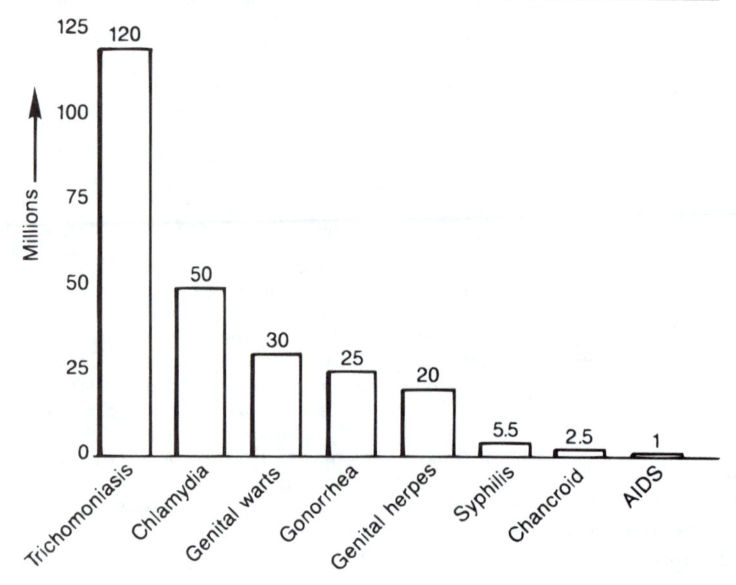

FIGURE 8-12 Global Incidence of Eight Sexually Transmitted Diseases.

HIV is transmitted most often during sexual contact with an infected partner. There is abundant evidence that if a sexual partner has an active STD, especially one that causes an ulcer, he or she is at greater risk of becoming HIV-infected (Laga, 1991).

The types of blood cells, lymphocytes, or macrophages most likely to become infected if exposed to HIV tend to collect in the genital tract of people with STDs. This makes an STD-infected person both more likely to transmit HIV and more vulnerable to it (Laga, 1991). The relationship of STDs to HIV can be seen in Figure 8-13.

Pediatric Transmission

Children can acquire HIV from their mothers in several ways. A pregnant HIV-infected woman can transmit the virus to her fetus in utero (during gestation) as the virus crosses over from the mother into the fetal bloodstream (Jovaisas et al., 1985; St. Louis et al., 1993). At least 50% of newborn infections occur during delivery by ingesting blood or other infected maternal fluids (Scott et al., 1985; Boyer et al., 1994; Kuhn, et al., 1994). If breast fed, the newborn may also become infected from breast milk (Zigler et al., 1985;

FIGURE 8-13 Bidirectional Interaction Between STDs and HIV. Medical studies support a complex bidirectional interaction between HIV and other sexually transmitted diseases with respect to transmission and virulence. In a group of sexually active, frequently HIV-exposed people with multiple sex partners (e.g., urban prostitutes), a subgroup of efficient, high-frequency HIV transmitters may occur. The epidemiology of HIV dissemination through sexual intercourse may in part be related to regional and demographic differences in the nature and size of sexually active groups and on the patterns of sexual mixing between high-risk groups and low-risk groups in the general population.

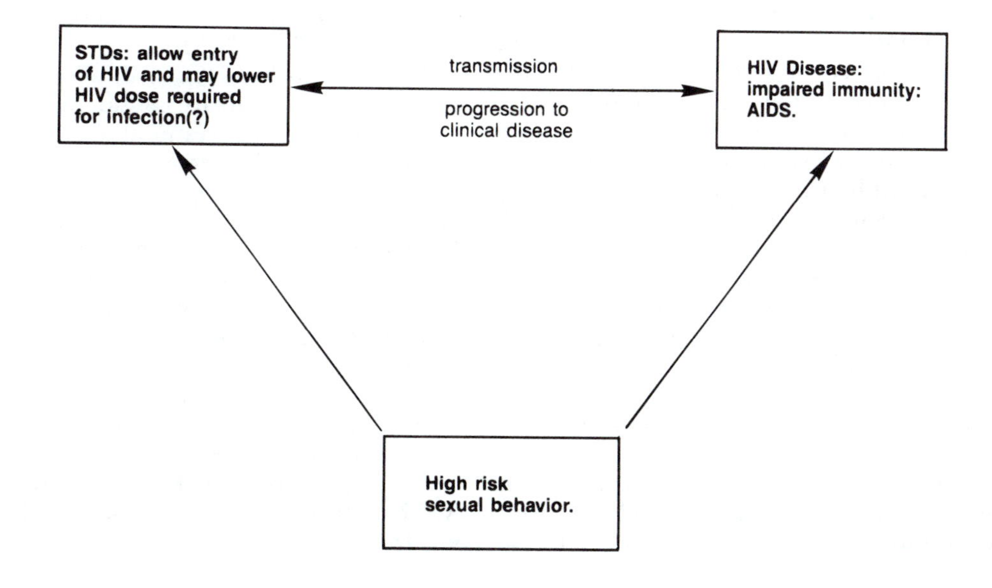

deMartino et al., 1992; Van DePerre et al., 1993). In case reports, three women who contracted HIV by blood transfusions *immediately after birth* subsequently infected their newborns via breast feeding (Curran et al., 1988). Other studies suggest that the risk of HIV transmission through breast feeding is increased if the mother becomes HIV-infected during lactation (Hu et al., 1992).

The relative efficiency of these three routes of infection is unknown. However, the data on mothers' milk add to the urgency of learning more about mucosal transmission, because the most likely explanation for HIV transmission through breast feeding is that the virus penetrates the mucosal lining of the mouth or gastrointestinal tract of infants. If this occurs in newborns, then what of older children, adolescents, and adults? Does the mucosal lining change with development and become HIV-resistant?

HIV-Infected Babies— One major problem in perinatal transmission is how to determine which babies are truly HIV-infected as opposed to just carrying the mother's HIV antibodies (which would produce a false-positive test). HIV transmission can occur during pregnancy (in utero), as well as at the time of delivery (**intrapartum**) and through breast milk. HIV transmission is more likely if virus can be cultured from the mother's blood, or if she has later stage HIV disease, or if her CD4 (T4) counts are low; and is more likely to occur in the first born than in the second born of twins. A baby automatically acquires the mother's antibodies and may carry them for 2 or more years. Usually by 18 months of age, most of the mother's antibodies will be gone. The babies may then begin to show signs of clinical AIDS-related illness. But, even at 18 months, a child cannot be unequivocally diagnosed. The most commonly used HIV antibody test is not sufficiently accurate until the child is at least 2 years old. A new antibody test in development shows promise in recognizing newborn infection by examining the type of HIV antibodies the infected mother is producing.

Although the rate of perinatal and breast milk HIV transmission is unknown, evidence from 1986 through mid-1995 indicates that over 90% of pediatric AIDS cases acquired the virus in utero from an HIV-infected mother after the first trimester (12th through 16th weeks) (Marion et al., 1986; DeRossi et al., 1992; Backe et al., 1993). In 1990, researchers concluded that a fetus can become infected as early as the 8th week of gestation (Lewis et al., 1990). HIV has been isolated from a 20-week-old fetus after elective abortion by an HIV-positive female and from a 28-week-old newborn delivered by Caesarean section from a female who was diagnosed with AIDS (Selwyn, 1986).

Reports on the probability of a fetus becoming HIV-infected when the mother carries the virus vary widely. The most often quoted estimate is from 30% to 50%. However, the results of four in-depth follow-up studies on the frequency of HIV transmission by infected mothers to their fetuses gives a range of incidences of from 7% to 65%.

There is little documented information on maternal factors that influence vertical transmission. As with other congenital infections, only one of a pair of twins may be HIV-infected (Newell et al., 1990). A mother's clinical status during pregnancy and the duration of her infection (stage of disease) may be important, but evidence remains circumstantial (St. Louis et al., 1993). Studies to determine mother-to-fetus transmission relative to stage of disease are in progress. One reason that all fetuses of HIV-infected mothers are not HIV-infected during gestation may be because the mothers' antibodies have a high affinity for HIV.

According to the CDC classification, children under 13 years of age are considered pediatric AIDS cases. They make up about 1.3% of all AIDS cases in the United States. Through mid-1995, about 5% of reported pediatric male AIDS cases occurred due to blood transfusions, 4% received HIV-contaminated blood factor VIII used in treating hemophiliacs, and in 1%, the cause was undetermined (Table 8-9).

The prognosis for AIDS children is not good; some 53% of the pediatric AIDS cases reported to the CDC have died. Half of them died within 9 months after diagnosis. At least two children infected from birth lived beyond age 12; a New York girl lived to age 12 and 7 months and a New Jersey boy lived to age 13.

TABLE 8-9 Causes of Pediatric AIDS in the United States Estimates through July 1995

Pediatric[a] Exposure Category	Totals	(%)
Hemophilia/coagulation disorder	239	(4)
Mother with/at risk for HIV infection:	5,611	(90)
a. Injecting drug use	2,413	
b. Sex with injecting drug user	1,185	
c. Sex with bisexual male	92	
d. Sex with person with hemophilia	27	
e. Sex with transfusion recipient with HIV infection	24	
f. Sex with HIV-infected person, risk not specified	437	
g. Receipt of blood tissue transfusion, blood components, or tissue	121	
h. Has HIV infection, risk not specified	1,556	
Receipt of blood transfusion, blood components, or tissue	317	(5)
Undetermined	67	(1)
Total pediatric AIDS cases (Total AIDS Cases July 1995, 476,500)	6,234	(100)

[a]CDC classification: Pediatric cases means AIDS cases in children less than 13 years old.

(Adapted CDC *HIV/AIDS Surveillance Mid-Year Report*, 1994)

The largest number of pediatric AIDS cases through mid-1995 were in New York, Florida, and New Jersey, in that order. The highest incidence of all pediatric cases occurs in minority populations. By mid 1995, there were about 6,500 pediatric AIDS cases in the United States. Blacks and Hispanics make up 12% and 6% of the United States population, respectively, yet make up 55% and 20%, respectively, of all pediatric AIDS cases. Thus 75% of pediatric AIDS cases occur within two minority populations.

Recent studies demonstrate that HIV seropositivity has reached alarming levels among child-bearing women in some major cities. For example, a New York Health Department study conducted in November 1987 indicated that one out of every 61 babies

CASE IN POINT 8.1

WHEN THE WONDERFUL NEWS "YOU'RE PREGNANT" BECOMES A TRAGEDY

First Case: Amy Sloan

In 1982, AIDS was a homosexual disease. Amy Sloan became HIV-infected from a blood transfusion. She received the blood because of ulcerative colitis (ulcers in the colon). In 1985, 3 years after her transfusion, and 2 days *after* she learned she was pregnant, Amy was told she had AIDS. She was 24 years old.

By 1985, the general public was being educated to the devastating effects of AIDS; the virus had been named and it was known that blood transfusions were a major route of HIV transmission. Amy Sloan had become pregnant not knowing that she was carrying the AIDS virus. Amy delivered an uninfected son in 1986. She died in January 1987.

Second Case: Elizabeth and Paul Michael Glaser

On March 13, 1990, Elizabeth and Paul Michael Glaser, former star of *Starsky and Hutch*, testified before the House Budget Committee's Human Resource Task Force arguing for increased funding for pediatric AIDS research, education, and treatment.

Elizabeth Glaser was infected with HIV in 1981, after she was given a blood transfusion while giving birth to daughter Ariel. At that time, AIDS did not have a name, and the reporting of cases was just beginning. No one knew about the risk of contracting the virus through transfusions. Elizabeth breast-fed Ariel, unknowingly passing the virus to her daughter. Three years later, Paul and Elizabeth had a son, Jake, who later also tested positive for HIV. Paul is the only one in the family not infected.

Elizabeth testified that she watched her daughter suffer from symptoms that did not seem to affect adults. She watched her daughter's central nervous system atrophy as she became, at age 6, unable to walk, talk, or even sit up.

Ariel Glaser died in 1988, just after her 7th birthday. Elizabeth Glaser died on December 4, 1994. Son Jake, age 8, remains asymptomatic.

born in New York City was born to a woman infected with HIV. Approximately 100,000 women of child-bearing age are estimated to be infected with HIV. The majority of these women do not know they are infected; they are identified as infected only after their children are diagnosed as having an HIV infection or AIDS. It is not uncommon for HIV-infected women to go through several pregnancies before expressing HIV disease.

Mother-to-fetus infection could be avoided by avoiding pregnancy, but this is possible only in cases where the female is aware of her infection and takes measures to prevent pregnancy (e.g., birth control or tubal ligation). In many cases, pregnancy has occurred before the mother knew she was carrying the virus. In other cases, the mother has become infected after she has become pregnant.

HIV Infection in Older People

Stuart Lichtman and colleagues (1991) reported on 26 patients, aged 60 and over, who were HIV-positive. Twenty were male. Collectively, 58% of the 26 had become HIV-infected via blood transfusions. Other causes were homosexual behavior (19%), heterosexual transmission (15%), injection drug use (4%), and unknown (4%). The means of transmission for one-half of the female patients (three out of six) was heterosexual sex.

HIV Transmission in the Workplace

The idea of contracting HIV from a fellow employee generates fear in many employees regardless of their jobs. It is believed that most people in the United States have been exposed to information on the routes of HIV transmission and on how to practice safer sex. But remote possibilities remain worrisome to many in the job force. Many still believe that HIV can be transmitted casually via handshakes, coffee cups, and food handling.

It is the anxiety of uncertainty that engenders suspicion about the possibility of HIV infection in the workplace—an anxiety that HIV/AIDS scientists could be wrong about the routes of HIV transmission. As Judith Wilson Ross states, "We have spent our lives in a culture in which infectious disease does not represent a significant threat. And thus we had consigned living in fear of life-threatening contagious diseases to the pages of history books." But today, HIV/AIDS forces us to reexamine our faith in the certainty of science. We want to believe, we want to accept—but the fear of death prevents complete surrender to education.

Business Responds to AIDS Education

On December 1, 1992, CDC initiated a new long-term, primary program for HIV/AIDS education. This program, "Business Responds to AIDS" (BRTA), encourages business executives, managers, and labor leaders to undertake comprehensive workplace HIV education that includes developing written HIV policies; providing employee education; supporting education efforts for employees' families; developing manager, labor leader, and supervisor training about companies' HIV policies and education programs; and providing corporate support and encouraging employees to provide volunteer support for community HIV-prevention activities. BRTA will help CDC in increasing public understanding of, involvement in, and support for HIV prevention.

To assist business and labor in initiating their own HIV-education programs, the CDC National AIDS Clearinghouse has established the BRTA Resource Service. The BRTA Resource Service has available the BRTA manager's kit, which includes materials for policy development, education program development and additional resources. The manager's kit (cost: $25 per kit) can be obtained from the Business Responds to AIDS Resource Service, P.O. Box 6003, Rockville, MD 20849-6003.

PUBLIC CONFIDENCE: ACCEPTANCE OF CURRENT DOGMA ON ROUTES OF HIV TRANSMISSION

Although no new routes of HIV transmission have surfaced over the last 14 years of this pandemic, many people still do not believe "that's all there is." People still make the arguments that: (1) scientists do not yet know enough about this disease to be certain there are no other routes of transmission; and (2) scientists know other routes exist but are either too frightened to tell the truth, or are under political pressure not to do so for fear of creating a public panic. Many thousands of people in the United States firmly believe that in a few years they will look back and say "I told you so": You can get HIV from HIV-infected people if they breathe on you or if you touch their sweat and so on.

*Question: How do you get everyone to believe what medical and research scientists say? **Should we get everyone to believe scientific dogma?***

National Aids Resourses

Aids Action Council	1-202-547-3101
Coalition for Leadership on AIDS	1-202-628-4160
Gay Men's Health Crisis	1-212-807-6655
Mothers of AIDS Patients	1-619-234-3432
National AIDS Information Clearinghouse	1-301-762-5111
National AIDS Network	1-202-546-2424
National Association of Persons with AIDS	1-202-483-7979
Project Inform (Alternative AIDS Info.)	1-800-822-7422
Public Health Service Hotline	1-800-342-2437
Centers for Disease Control and Prevention Technical Information	1-404-639-2077
American Red Cross, National AIDS Education	1-202-639-3223
Guide to Socal Security and SSI Disability Benefits for People with HIV Infection	1-800-772-1213

(You can write or call for this Social Security brochure: Social Security Administration, Public Information Distribution Center, P.O. Box 17743, Baltimore, Maryland 21235.

SUMMARY

The World Health Organization began keeping records of AIDS cases in 1980. By the end of 1994, there were over 5 million AIDS cases reported from 160 countries and territories. About 16% of these cases occurred in the United States. It has been reported that the first cases of AIDS entered the United States via homosexual men who had vacationed in Haiti in the late 1970s. However, there is evidence of AIDS cases in the United States as early as 1952. While testing West Africans for HIV infection, a second strain of HIV was discovered: HIV-2. Both are transmitted in the same manner and both cause AIDS. However, HIV-2 appears to be less pathogenic than HIV-1.

There are two major variables involved in successful HIV transmission and infection. First is the individual's genetic resistance or susceptibility and second is the route of transmission. Not all modes of HIV exposure are equally apt to cause infection, even in the most susceptible individual. There have been a number of studies and empirical observations that demonstrate that HIV *is not casually acquired.* HIV is difficult to acquire even by means of the recognized routes of transmission.

HIV is transmitted mainly via sexual activities involving the exchange of semen and vaginal fluids, through the exchange of blood and blood products, and from mother to child both prenatally and postnatally (breast milk). Besides a few cases of breast milk transmission, no other body fluids have as yet been implicated in HIV infection.

The current belief is that anal receptive homosexuals have a higher risk than heterosexuals (in the United States) of acquiring HIV because the membrane or mucosal lining of the rectum is more easily torn during anal intercourse. This allows a more direct route for larger numbers of HIVs to enter the vascular system.

Others at high risk for acquiring and transmitting HIV are injection drug users. They infect each other when they share drug paraphernalia. Changes in sexual and injection drug use behavior can virtually stop HIV transmission among these people.

REVIEW QUESTIONS

(Answers to the Review Questions are on page 480.)

1. True or False: Africa makes up the largest percentage of **reported** AIDS cases worldwide. Explain.

2. What evidence is there that HIV may have evolved in the United States and Africa at the same time?

3. Are HIV-1 and HIV-2 related? Explain.

4. True or False: HIV-1 and HIV-2 are transmitted differently and therefore are located in geographically distinct regions of the world. Explain.

5. True or False: HIV is not believed to be casually transmitted. Explain.

6. Name the routes of HIV transmission.

7. True or False: Deep kissing wherein saliva is exchanged is a direct route for efficient HIV transmission. Explain.

8. True or False: Insects that bite or suck have been claimed to be associated with HIV transmission. Explain.

9. True or False: Among heterosexuals, HIV transmission from male to female and from female to male are equally efficient. Explain.

10. True or False: If a person has unprotected intercourse with an HIV-infected partner he or she will become HIV-infected. Explain.

11. What is the percentage of risk that a developing fetus with an HIV-positive mother will be born HIV-positive?

12. Despite the warnings, groups that continue to engage in high-risk sexual activity include:
 a) high school students
 b) black women
 c) injection drug users
 d) all of the above

13. True or False: Prior to 1985, use of blood component therapy put the hemophiliac at risk for contracting HIV.

14. True or False: Relapse to risky sexual behavior can be an important source of new HIV infection in the homosexual community.

15. True or False: The body fluids shown most likely to transmit HIV are blood, semen, vaginal secretions, and breast milk.

16. True or False: Participation in risk behaviors and not identification with particular groups puts an individual at risk of acquiring HIV infection.

17. True or False: Unprotected receptive anal intercourse is the sexual activity with the greatest risk of HIV transmission.

18. True or False: Women who are HIV-infected always transmit the virus to their fetus during pregnancy or delivery.

19. True or False: A person infected with HIV can transmit the virus from the first occurrence of antigemia throughout the rest of his/her life.

20. True or False: Women constitute the fastest growing segment of the population with HIV infection.

21. True or False: The majority of HIV-infected women whose source of infection is known became infected through vaginal intercourse.

22. True or False: HIV infection in children is now a leading cause of death in children between the ages of 1 and 4.

23. True or False: Sexual contact is the major route of HIV transmission among blacks.

REFERENCES

AIDS Research. (1990). Roundup: Oral sex. *Med. Asp. Human Sexuality,* 24:52.

Aldhous, Peter. (1991). France will compensate. *Nature,* 353:425.

Archibald, D.W., et al. (1990). *In vitro* inhibition of HIV-1 infectivity by human salivas. *AIDS Res. Human Viruses,* 6:1425–1431.

Avins, Andrew., et al. (1994). HIV infection and risk behaviors among heterosexuals in alcohol treatment programs. *JAMA* 271:515–518.

Backe, E., et al. (1993). Fetal organs infected by HIV-1. *AIDS,* 7:896–897.

Bagasra, Omar, et al. (1994). Detection of HIV proviral DNA in sperm from HIV-infected men. *AIDS,* 8:1669–1674.

Boekeloo, B., et al. (1993). Sexual risk behaviors of STD clinic patients before and after Earvin 'Magic' Johnson's HIV-infection Announcement—Maryland 1991–1992. *MMWR,* 42:45–48.

Bolling, David R. (1989). Anal intercourse between women and bisexual men. *Med. Asp. Human Sexuality,* 23:34.

Boyer, Pamela J., et al. (1994). Factors predictive of maternal-fetal transmission of HIV. *JAMA,* 271:1925–1930.

Breo, Dennis L. (1991). The two major scandals in France's AIDSGATE. *JAMA* 266:3477– 3482.

BUTLER, DECLAN. (1994a). Allain freed to face new changes. *Nature,* 370:404.

BUTLER, DECLAN. (1994b) Blood scandal raises spectre of Dreyfus case. *Nature,* 371:548.

CAMERON, WILLIAM D., et al. (1990). Sexual transmission of HIV and the epidemiology of other STDs. *AIDS,* 4:S99–S103.

CDC (Centers for Disease Control and Prevention). (1990). *HIV/AIDS Surveillance Report,* Oct.: 1–18.

CHIRGWIN, KEITH, et al. (1991). HIV infection, genital ulcer disease, and crack cocaine use among patients attending a clinic for sexually transmitted diseases. *Am. J. Public Health,* 81:1576–1579.

CHU, S.Y., et al. (1990). Epidemiology of reported cases of AIDS in lesbians, United States 1980–89. *Am. J. Public Health,* 80:1380.

COHEN, J.B., et al. (1989). Heterosexual transmission of HIV. *Immunol. Ser.,* 44:135–137.

COOMBS, ROBERT W., et al. (1989). Plasma viremia in HIV infection. *N. Engl. J. Med.,* 321:1526.

CORBITT, G., et al. (1990). HIV infection in manchester, 1959 *Lancet,* 336:51.

COTTONE, JAMES A., et al. (1990). The Kimberly Bergalis case: An analysis of the data suggesting the possible transmission of HIV infection from a dentist to his patient. *Phys. Assoc. AIDS Care,* 2:267–270.

CURRAN, JAMES W., et al. (1988). Epidemiology of HIV infection and AIDS in the United States. *Science,* 239:610–616.

DANIELS, NORMAN. (1992). HIV-infected Professionals, patient rights, and the switching dilemma. *JAMA,* 267:1368–1371.

DEMARTINO, MAURIZIO, et al. (1992). HIV-1 transmission through breast-milk: Appraisal of risk according to duration of feeding. *AIDS,* 6:991–997.

DEROSSI, ANITA, et al. (1992). Vertical transmission of HIV: Lack of detectable virus in peripheral blood cells of infected children at birth. *AIDS,* 6:1117–1120.

DES JARLAIS, DON C., et al. (1989). AIDS and IV drug use. *Science,* 245:578.

DEVINCENZI, I., et al. (1989). Risk factors for male to female transmission of HIV. *Br. Med. J.,* 298:411–415.

DORFMAN, ANDREA. (1991). Bad blood in France. *Time,* 138:48.

DRUCKER, E. (1986). AIDS and addiction in New York City. *Am. J. Drug Alcohol Abuse,* 12:165–181.

ELSON, JOHN. (1991). The dangerous world of wannabes. *Time,* 138:77–80.

Emergency Cardiac Care Committee, American Heart Association. (1990). Risk of infection during CPR training and rescue: Supplemental guidelines. *JAMA,* 262:2714–2715.

FISCHL, M.A., et al. (1987). Evaluation of heterosexual partners, children and household contacts of adults with AIDS. *JAMA,* 257:640–644.

FOX, PHILIP. (1991). Saliva and salivary gland alterations in HIV infection. *J. Am. Dental Assoc.* 122:46–48.

FRIEDLAND, GERALD H., et al. (1987). Transmission of the human immunodeficiency virus. *N. Engl. J. Med.,* 317:1125–1135.

FRIEDLAND, GERALD H. (1991). HIV transmission from health care workers. *AIDS Clin. Care,* 3:29–30.

GARRY, ROBERT F., et al. (1988). Documentation of an AIDS virus infection in the United States in 1968. *JAMA,* 260:2085–2087.

GIBBONS, MARY. (1994). Childhood sexual abuse. *Am. Fam. Phys.,* 49:125–136.

GOTO, Y., et al. (1991). Detection of proviral sequences in saliva of patients infected with human immunodeficiency virus type 1. *AIDS Res. Hum. Retroviruses,* 7:343–347.

HEARST, NORMAN, AND HULLEY, STEPHEN B. (1988). Preventing the heterosexual spread of AIDS: Are we giving our patients the best advice? *JAMA,* 259:2428.

HENG, MADALENE, et al. (1994). Co-Infection and synergy of human immunodeficiency virus-I and herpes simplex virus-I. *Lancet,* 343:255–258.

HEYMANN, DAVID, et al. (1994). The laboratory, epidemiology, nosocomial infection and HIV. *AIDS,* 8:705–706.

HIV/AIDS Surveillance Report (1994 Draft copy). Center for Disease Control and Prevention, Atlanta GA, March 29, 1994.

HOLDEN, CONSTANCE. (1994). Switzerland has its own blood scandal. *Science,* 264:1254.

HOLMSTROM, PAUL, et al. (1992). HIV antigen detected in gingival fluid. *AIDS,* 6:738–739.

HU, DALE J., et al. (1992). HIV infection and breastfeeding: Policy implications through a decision analysis model. *AIDS,* 6:1505–1513.

IPPILITO, GIUSEPPE, et al. (1994). Transmission of zidorudine-resistant HIV during a bloody fight. *JAMA,* 272:433–434.

JOSEPH, STEPHEN C. (1993). Dragon within the gates: The once and future AIDS epidemic. *Med. Doctor,* 37:92–104.

JOVAISAS, E., et al. (1985). LAV/HTLV III in 20-week fetus. *Lancet,* 2:1129.

KATNER, H.P., et al. (1987). Evidence for a Euro-American origin of human immunodeficiency virus. *J. Natl. Med. Assoc.,* 79:1068–1072.

KEET, IRENEUS, et al. (1992). Orogenital sex and the transmission of HIV among homosexual men. *AIDS,* 6:223–226.

KINGSLEY, L.A., et al. (1990). Sexual transmission efficiency of hepatitis B virus and human immunodeficiency virus among homosexual men. *JAMA,* 264:230–234.

KOSS, M.P., et al. (1991). Deleterious effects of criminal victimization on women's health and medical utilization. *Arch. Intern. Med.,* 151: 342–347.

KUHN, LOUISE, et al. (1994). Maternal-infant HIV transmission and circumstances of delivery. *Am. J. Public Health,* 84:1110–1115.

LAGA, MARIE. (1991). HIV infection and sexually transmitted diseases. *Sexually Transmitted Dis. Bull.,* 10:3–10.

LAGA, MARIE, et al. (1993). Non-ulcerative STDs as risk factors for HIV transmission in women: Results from a cohort study. *AIDS,* 7:95–102

LEVY, JAY A. (1989). Human immunodeficiency viruses and the pathogenesis of AIDS. *JAMA,* 261:2997-3006.

LEWIS, S.H., et al. (1990). HIV-1 introphoblastic villous Hofbauer cells and haematological precursors in eight-week fetuses. *Lancet,* 335:565.

LICHTMAN, STUART M., et al. (1991). Greater attention urged for HIV in older patients. *Infect. Dis. Update,* 2:5.

MARION, R.W., et al. (1986). Human T cell lymphotropic virus type III embryopathy: A new dysmorphic syndrome associated with intrauterine HTLV III infection. *Am. J. Dis. Child,* 140:638–640.

MARLINK, RICHARD, et al. (1994). Reduced rate of disease development after HIV infection as compared to HIV-1.*Science,* 265:1587–1590.

MERIMAN, J.H., et al. (1991). Detection of HIV DNA and RNA in semen by the polymerase chain reaction. *J. Infect. Dis.,* 164:769–772.

MIIKE, LAWRENCE. (1987). Do insects transmit AIDS? *Office of Technological Assessment,* Sept. 1:43.

MONZON, O.T., et al. (1987). Female to female transmission of HIV. *Lancet,* 2:40–41.

Morbidity and Mortality Weekly Report. (1988a). Update: Universal precautions for prevention of transmission of human immunodeficiency virus, hepatitis B virus, and other bloodborne pathogens in health-care settings. 37:377–382,387–388.

Morbidity and Mortality Weekly Report. (1988b). Transmission of HIV through bone transplantation: Case report and public health recommendations. 37:597–599.

Morbidity and Mortality Weekly Report. (1990a). Possible transmission of HIV to a patient during an invasive dental procedure. 39:489–493.

Morbidity and Mortality Weekly Report. (1990b). HIV infection and artificial insemination with processed semen. 39:249–256.

Morbidity and Mortality Weekly Report. (1991a). Update: Transmission of HIV infection during an invasive dental procedure—Florida. 40:21–27,33.

Morbidity and Mortality Weekly Report. (1991b). Drug use and sexual behaviors among sex partners of injecting-drug users—U.S. 40:855–860.

Morbidity and Mortality Weekly Report. (1992). Childbearing and contraceptive-use plans among women at high risk for HIV infection—Selected U.S. sites, 1989–1991. 41:135–144.

Morbidity and Morality Weekley Report. (1994a). Human immunodeficiency virus transmission in household settings—United States. 43:347, 353–357.

Morbidity and Morality Weekley Report. (1994b), Guidelines for preventing transmission of HIV through transplantation of human tissue and organs. 43:1–15.

Morbidity and Morality Weekley Report. (1994c) Medical-care expenditures attributable to cigarette smoking—United States, 1993. 43:469–472.

MUNZER, ALFRED. (1994). The threat of secondhand smoke. *Menopause Management,* 3:14–17.

NAFTALIN, RICHARD J. (1992). Anal sex and AIDS. *Nature,* 360:10.

NEWELL, MARIE-LOUISE, et al. (1990). HIV-1 infection in pregnancy: Implications for women and children. *AIDS,* 4:S111–S117.

OLESKE, JAMES M. (1994).The many needs of HIV-infected children. *Hosp Pract.* 29:81–87.

PADIAN, NANCY S., et al. (1991). Female to male transmission of HIV. *JAMA,* 266:1664–1667.

PETERMAN, THOMAS A., et al. (1986). Sexual transmission of human immunodeficiency virus. *JAMA,* 256:2222–2226.

PETERMAN, THOMAS A.,et al. (1988). Risk of human immunodeficiency virus transmission from heterosexual adults with transfusion-associated infections. *JAMA,* 259:55–58.

PETO, RICHARD. (1992). Statistics of chronic disease control. *Nature,* 356:557–558.

PHILLIPS, DAVID. (1994). The roll of cell-to-cell transmission in HIV infection. *AIDS,* 8:719–731.

PHILLIPS, KATHRYN, et al. (1994). The cost effectiveness of HIV testing of physicians and dentists in the United States. *JAMA,* 271:851–858.

POURTOIS, M., et al. (1991). Saliva can contribute in quick inhibition of HIV infectivity. *AIDS,* 5:598–599.

PUDNEY, J., et al. (1991). White blood cells and HIV in semen from vasectomized seropositive men. *Lancet,* 338:573.

QUINN, THOMAS C., et al. (1988). HIV infection among patients attending clinics for sexually transmitted diseases. *N. Engl. J. Med.,* 318: 197–203.

ROGERS, DAVID, et al. (1993). AIDS policy: Two divisive issues. *JAMA,* 270:494–495.

ROZENBAUM, W. et al. (1988). HIV transmission by oral sex. *Lancet,* 1:1395.

SADOVSKY, RICHARD. (1989). HIV-infected patients: A primary care challenge. *Am. Fam. Pract.,* 40:121–128.

SATO, HIRONORI, et al. (1992). Cell to cell spread of HIV occurs within minutes and may not involve the participation of virus particles. *Virology,* 186:712–724.

Science in California. (1993). AIDS: I want a new drug. *Nature,* 362:396.

SCOTT, G.B., et al. (1985). Mothers of infants with the acquired immunodeficiency syndrome: Evidence for both symptomatic and asymptomatic carriers. *JAMA,* 253:363–366.

SEGARS, JAMES H. (1989). Heterosexual anal sex. *Med. Asp. Human Sexuality,* 23:6.

SELWYN, PETER A. (1986). AIDS: What is now known. *Hosp. Pract.,* 21:127–164.

SHERNOFF, MICHAEL. (1988). Integrating safer-sex counseling into social work practice. *Social Casework: J. Contemp. Social Work,* 69:334–339.

SPITZER, P.G., et al. (1989). Transmission of HIV infection from a woman to a man by oral sex. *N. Engl. J. Med.,* 320:251.

SPURGEON, DAVID. (1994). Canadian AIDS suit raises hope for HIV-blood victims. *Nature,* 368–281.

ST. LOUIS, MICHAEL E., et al. (1993). Risk for perinatal HIV transmission according to maternal immunologic, virologic and placental factors. *JAMA,* 269:2853–2860.

STEWART, G.J., et al. (1985). Transmission of human T cell lymphotropic virus type III by artificial insemination by donor. *Lancet,* 1:581–584.

STRYKER, JEFF, et al. (1993). AIDS policy: Two divisive issues. *JAMA,* 270:2436–2437.

SWENSON, ROBERT M. (1988). Plagues, History and AIDS. *Am. Scholar,* 57:183–200.

SWINBANKS, DAVID. (1993). American witnesses: Testify in Japan about AIDS risks. *Nature,* 364:181.

VAN DE PERRE, PHILIPPE, et al. (1993). Infective and anti-infective properties of breast milk from HIV-infected women. *Lancet,* 341:914–918.

VITTECOQ, D., et al. (1989). Acute HIV infection after acupuncture treatments. *N. Engl. J. Med.,* 320:250–251.

WALKER, EDWARD A., et al. (1993). The prevalence rate of sexual trauma in a primary care clinic. *J. Am. Board Fam. Pract.,* 6:465–471.

WILL, GEORGE F. (1991). Foolish choices still jeopardize public health. *Private Pract.,* 24:46–48.

Women's AIDS Network. (1988). Lesbians and AIDS: What's the connection? *San Francisco AIDS Foundation,* 333 Valencia St., 4th Floor, P.O. Box 6182, San Francisco, CA 94101-6182.

WOOLLEY, ROBERT J. (1989). The biologic possibility of HIV transmission during passionate kissing. *JAMA,* 262:2230.

ZIGLER, J.B., et al. (1985). Postnatal transmission of AIDS-associated retrovirus from mother to infant. *Lancet,* 1:896–897.

CHAPTER

9

Preventing the Transmission of HIV

CHAPTER CONCEPTS

- HIV transmission can be prevented; the responsibility rests with the individual.
- No new routes of HIV transmission have been found after 15 years.
- Safer sex essentially means using condoms and not having intercourse with an HIV-infected person.
- New female condom (vaginal pouch) was FDA approved in 1993.
- Oil based lubricants must not be used with condoms.
- Free syringe and needle exchange programs may help lower the incidence of HIV transmission.
- Blood bank screening to detect HIV antibodies began in 1985.
- Vaccines are made from whole or parts of dead microorganisms, inactivated viruses, or attenuated viruses and microorganisms.
- Experimental subunit vaccines are prepared using recombinant DNA techniques.
- Animal models are being prepared for vaccine trial studies.
- A moral problem exists in attempting to get human volunteers for AIDS vaccine testing.
- Universal precautions and blood and body substance isolation are techniques to help health care workers prevent infection.
- Under universal precautions certain body fluids from all patients are to be considered potentially infectious.
- Partner notification is a means of notifying at risk partners of HIV-infected individuals.

PREVENTION OF INFECTIOUS DISEASES

The first responsibility in an epidemic is the protection of the uninfected.
Stephen C. Joseph

Infectious agents have persisted over the centuries through transmission from an infected person to an uninfected one. To combat these infections, prevention programs have attempted to interrupt the chain of transmission. While some methods focus on stopping transmission from person-to-person contact by using vaccines or prophylactic therapy, other methods focus on stopping the transmission that occurs through environmental contamination by sanitary improvements.

With regard to HIV infection, there is no available vaccine against the virus, but effective methods for preventing it do exist. The leading preventative is education: teaching people how to adjust their behavior to reduce or eliminate HIV exposure. Because the vast majority of HIV infections are transmitted through consensual acts between adolescents and adults, the individual has a choice as to whether to risk infection or not.

Despite widely supported educational efforts at both institutional and street levels, a large number of gay males, drug abusers, and heterosexuals, continue to participate in *unsafe* sexual practices. Unsafe sex is defined as having sex without using a condom. This allows the exchange of potentially infectious body fluids such as blood, semen, and vaginal secretions. Unsafe sex most often occurs with injection drug users, and bartering sex for drugs with multiple partners. The sharp increase in the use of crack cocaine and its connection to trading sex for drugs has led to a dramatic rise in almost all of the sexually transmitted diseases. **The idea of *Safer* sexual practices began in the early 1980s and now refers almost exclusively to the use of a latex condom with or without a spermicide.**

Among the severely addicted, concerns about personal safety and survival are secondary to drug procurement and use. Thus their range of acceptable unsafe behaviors leads to random sex and sex without condoms. These behaviors are in part responsible for the increased incidence of HIV and other sexually transmitted diseases (Weinstein et al., 1990). **Eliminating all unsafe sex is not a reasonable goal. Preventing all future HIV infections is impossible, but striving for anything less is unacceptable.**

AIDS prevention is, in a sense, more powerful than, say, cancer prevention. Preventing one HIV infection now will not simply prevent one death from AIDS, as preventing one incurable cancer would prevent one cancer death. Preventing an HIV infection now will help break the chain of transmission, averting the risk that the infected person will unknowingly pass the virus on to others who in turn might infect a still wider circle of people.

PREVENTING THE TRANSMISSION OF HIV

HIV/AIDS: The News Is Mostly Bad

We are now 15 years into an epidemic that has touched—directly or indirectly—virtually every person on the planet. We know so much about the virus, yet despite our knowledge, our only option is to *prevent* the initial infection. Prevention is foremost because there are *no* truly effective viral therapies, *no* vaccines, and *no* cure. As we face this realization, alarming statistics continue to emerge about the spread of HIV infection.

HIV disease/AIDS is the leading cause of death among young men and women in eastern coastal states, where injection drug use is most prevalent. In San Francisco, estimates suggest that at least 50% of homosexual African-American men are infected with HIV. Unsafe sexual practices that could lead to HIV transmission are common among adolescents and young adults, as evidenced by the epidemic of other sexually transmitted diseases in this population. And tens of millions of persons in developing countries will become HIV-infected and most likely die. Entire generations are threatened with extinction in these countries.

The social, cultural, and economic factors that have led to the HIV pandemic seem overwhelming. How can a drug user be convinced to use clean needles to prevent an infection that may kill him in 10 years, when he faces an immediate struggle in a violent environment every day? How can condom use be promoted in countries with inadequate resources to provide even basic immunizations? Why should young women on the streets of New Delhi or Bangkok who depend on the sex industry for daily survival care about safer sex when it might lead to rejection by their customers and an end to their livelihood?

Hopelessness threatens reason. But there is reason to believe that education may reduce the number of new HIV infections. In San Francisco, gay men organized grassroots efforts to educate themselves about HIV transmission, and the results are impressive: less than 1% of the gay male population was infected with HIV after 1985, compared to 10% to 20% in the preceding years. People **can** change their behavior when educated about the risks of transmission (Clement, 1993).

But, if these successes were known in the mid-1980s, why the continued delay in educating the general population, especially sexually active adolescents? Most likely because early efforts to describe the HIV epidemic focused on risk groups rather than the **behaviors** associated with HIV transmission. The epidemic was and still is described with labels—the gay, bisexual, injection drug user, hemophiliac, and heterosexual—rather than in terms of the human behaviors that lead to HIV infection. (It would be analogous to say that only alcoholics engage in drunk driving.) Labeling has resulted in an "us versus them" mentality providing an emotional safety net for the general population.

The continued lack of a coordinated federal program to address the HIV pandemic has allowed this false safety net to remain in place. The former AIDS "Czar" Kristine Gebbie (Figure 9-1) and the former Surgeon General (Joycelyn Elders) placed prevention and education at the top of their list of priorities in fighting this epidemic.

The importance of prevention is especially clear as one comes to understand the state of the art in HIV/AIDS therapy. Regardless of

FIGURE 9-1 Kristine Gebbee as the newly appointed "AIDS Czar" for the United States. She is giving her acceptance speech, June 1993. She resigned August 2, 1994. Congressman Stewart B. McKinney of Connecticut died of AIDS on May 8, 1987. His AIDS quilt panel can be seen in this photograph.

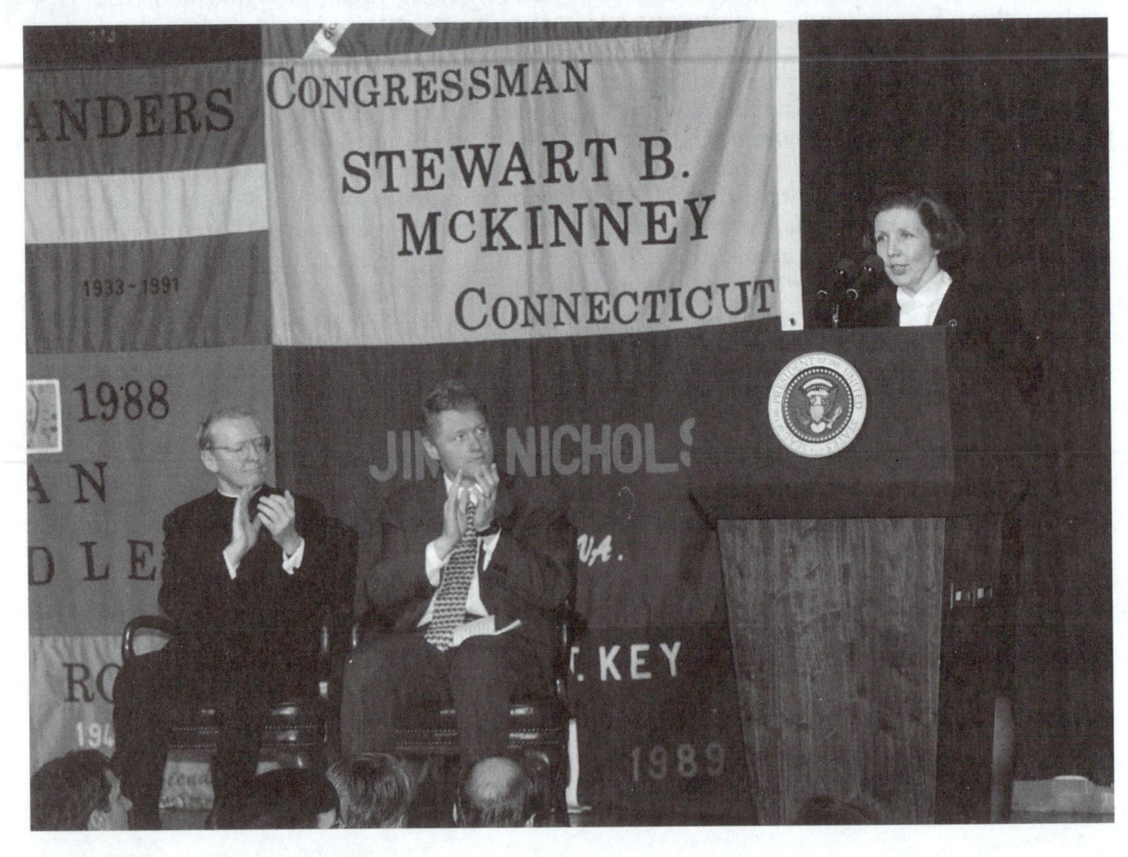

what can be medically done for patients with HIV disease, there is no cure. Thus officials from the Centers for Disease Control and Prevention (CDC), the World Health Organization (WHO), and the American Health Organization (AHO) have placed the responsibility of prevention in the hands of the educators, which include health care professionals, parents, and teachers.

Grim Reality

Steven Findlay (1991) wrote that burying those who have died from AIDS has become almost routine. With about 290,000 AIDS deaths expected by the end of 1995, most Americans are indeed becoming accustomed to HIV/ AIDS related deaths. But how many will die, say, by the year 2000? Will a cure or preventive and therapeutic vaccines be produced? Will our health care system become swamped and ineffective? The best guess by scientists is that neither an effective vaccine nor cure will be found by the end of this century. By the year 2000 it is projected that over 12 million people will have died of AIDS, over 1 million of them in the United States. San Francisco may lose 4% of its population; New York 3%; Central Africa 15%. To avoid the realization of these projections, people of the world must work on HIV/AIDS *prevention*.

Based on over 14 years of intensive epidemiological surveys, scientific research, and empirical observations, it is reasonable to conclude that HIV is not a highly contagious disease. HIV transmission occurs mainly through various sexual activities, HIV-contaminated blood or blood products, prenatal events, and in a few cases postnatally through breast milk. Since 1981, no new route of HIV transmission has been discovered. The virus is fragile and, with time, self-destructs outside the human body. The most recent data show that HIV remains active for up to 5 days in dried blood, although the number of virus particles (titer) drops dramatically. However, it is dangerous to assume that there are no infectious viruses remaining in the dried blood or body fluids from an HIV/AIDS patient. In cell-free tissue culture medium, the virus retains activity for up to 14 days at room temperature (Sattar et al., 1991). The bottom line is that, although HIV is more resistant to the environment than originally believed, it is relatively easy to inactivate. Chemical agents used to destroy or inactivate the virus are listed in Table 9-1.

It appears that HIV transmission can be prevented by individual action but it will require change in social behaviors. The absolutely best way to protect against all sexually transmitted diseases is ***sexual abstinence***. The next best way is a mutually monogamous sexual relationship. Following these two options is the use of a barrier method during sexual activities—male and female condoms or rubber dams.

Table 9-2 provides a number of recommen-

TABLE 9-1 Agents Effective Against Human Immunodeficiency Virus

Agents (freshly prepared)	Recommended Concentration
Sodium hypochlorite (household bleach)[a]	Full strength **(no dilution)**
Chloramine-T	2%
Sodium oxychlorosene	4 mg/mL
Sodium hydroxide	30 mm
Glutaraldehyde	2%
Formalin	4%
Paraformaldehyde	1%
Hydrogen peroxide	6%
Propiolactone dilution	1:400
Nonoxynol-9	1%
Ethyl alcohol	70%
Isopropyl alcohol	30%–50%
Lysol	0.5%–1%
NP-40 detergent[b]	1%
Chlorhexidine gluconate/ethanol mix	4/25%
Chlorhexidine gluconate/isopropyl mix	0.5%/70%
Tincture of iodine/isopropyl	1/30%–70%
Betadine	0.5%
Quarternary ammonium chloride	0.1%–1%
Acetone/alcohol mix	1:1
pH of 1 or 13	
Heat[c] 56°C for 10 minutes	

[a]In 1993, the CDC and Public Health Association recommended that household bleach (e.g., Clorox) be used at full strength.

[b]To be used at 1% solution at room temperature for 2 to 10 minutes.

[c]Dried HIV is ineffective at room temperature after 3 or more days. HIV at high concentration in liquid at room temperature remained ineffective for over 1 week.

Isopropanol (35%), ethanol (50%), Lysol (0.5%), hydrogen peroxide (0.3%), paraformaldehyde (0.5%), and detergent NP-40 (1%) effectively inactivate HIV when incubated at room temperature for 2 to 10 minutes.

(Adapted from Tierno, 1988)

TABLE 9-2 Guidelines for Prevention of HIV Infection

I. For the General Public:

1. Sexual abstinence
2. Have a mutual monogamous relationship with an HIV-negative partner (the greater the number of sexual partners, the greater the risk of meeting someone who is HIV-infected).
3. If the sex partner is other than a monogamous partner, use a condom.
4. Do not frequent prostitutes—too many have been found to be HIV-infected and are still 'working' the streets.
5. Do not have sex with people who you know are HIV-infected or are from a high-risk group. If you do, prevent contact with their body fluids. (Use a condom and a spermicide from start to finish.)
6. Avoid sexual practices that may result in the tearing of body tissues (e.g., penile–anal intercourse).
7. Avoid oral–penile sex unless a condom[a] is used to cover the penis.
8. If you use injection drugs, use sterile or bleach cleaned needles and syringes and *never* share them.
9. Exercise caution regarding procedures such as acupuncture, tattooing, ear piercing, and so on, in which needles or other unsterile instruments may be used repeatedly to pierce the skin and/or mucous membranes. Such procedures are safe if proper sterilization methods are employed or disposable needles are used. Ask what precautions are being taken before undergoing such procedures.
10. If you are planning to undergo artificial insemination, insist on frozen sperm obtained from a laboratory that tests all donors for infection with the AIDS virus. Donors should be tested twice before the sperm is used—once at the time of donation and again 6 months later.
11. If you know that you will be having surgery in the near future and you are able to do so, consider donating blood for your own use. This will eliminate the small but real risk of HIV infection through a blood transfusion. It will also eliminate the more substantial risk of contracting other transfusion blood-borne diseases, such as hepatitis B.
12. Don't share toothbrushes, razors, or other implements that could become contaminated with blood with anyone who is HIV-infected, demonstrates HIV disease, or has AIDS.

II. For Health Care Workers:

1. *All* sharp instruments should be considered as potentially infective and be handled with extraordinary care to prevent accidental injuries.
2. Sharp items should be placed into puncture-resistant containers located as close as practical to the area in which they are used. To prevent needlestick injuries, needles should not be recapped, purposefully bent, broken, removed from disposable syringes, or otherwise manipulated.
3. Gloves, gowns, masks, and eye-coverings should be worn when performing procedures involving extensive contact with blood or potentially infective body fluids. Hands should be washed thoroughly and immediately if they accidentally become contaminated with blood. When a patient requires a vaginal or rectal examination, gloves must always be worn. If a specimen is obtained during an examination, the nurse or individual who assists and processes the specimen must always wear gloves. Blood should be drawn from all patients—regardless of HIV status—only while wearing gloves.
4. To minimize the need for emergency mouth-to-mouth resuscitation, mouthpieces, resuscitation bags, or other ventilation devices should be strategically located and available for use where the need for resuscitation is predictable.

III. People at Risk of HIV Infection:

1. See recommendations for general public.
2. Consider taking the HIV antibody screening test.
3. Protect your partner from body fluids during sexual intercourse.
4. Do not donate any body tissues.
5. If female, have an HIV test before becoming pregnant.
6. If you are an injection drug user, seek professional help in terminating the drug habit.
7. If you cannot get off drugs, do not share drug equipment.

IV. People Who Are HIV-Positive:

The prevention of transmission of HIV by an HIV-infected person is probably lifelong, and patients must avoid infecting others. HIV seropositive persons must understand that the virus can be transmitted by intimate sexual contact, transfusion of infected blood, and sharing needles among injection drug users. They should refrain from donating blood, plasma, sperm, body organs, or other tissues. HIV-infected people should:

(continued)

TABLE 9-2 *Continued*

1. Seek continued counseling and medical examinations.
2. Do not exchange body fluids with your sex partner.
3. Notify your former and current sex partners, encourage them to be tested.
4. If an injection drug user, do not share drug equipment and enroll in a drug treatment program.
5. Do not share razors, toothbrushes, and other items that may contain traces of blood.
6. Do not donate any body tissues.
7. Clean any body fluids spilled with undiluted household bleach.
8. If female, avoid pregnancy.
9. Inform health care workers on a need-to-know basis.

V. Practice of Safer Sex:

Safer sex is body massage, hugging, mutual masturbation, and closed mouth kissing. HIV seropositive patients must protect their sexual partners from coming into contact with infected blood or bodily secretions. Although consistent use of latex condoms with spermicide containing nonoxynol-9 can decrease the chance of HIV transmission, condoms do break. If engaging in sexual intercourse with an HIV-positive person use two condoms. But even this is no guarantee. (also see 1 through 6 under "For the General Public" in this table.)

[a]Tests show that HIV can sometimes pass through a latex condom. Experts believe that natural-skin condoms are more porous than latex and therefore offer less effective protection. Never use oil-based products such as Vaseline, Crisco, or baby oil with a latex condom, because they make the latex porous and nullify the protection the condom provides against the virus. The use of condoms containing a spermicide is recommended.

dations for preventing the spread of HIV. These recommendations place the responsibility for avoiding HIV infection on both adults and adolescents. **Lifestyles must be reviewed, choices made, and risky behavior stopped**. The public health service and the CDC have established guidelines that, if followed, will prevent HIV transmission while still allowing individuals to be somewhat flexible in their personal behaviors (*MMWR*, 1989a).

Quarantine

With few exceptions, proposals to quarantine all individuals with HIV infection have virtually no public support in the United States. Given the civil liberties implications of quarantine, its potential cost, and the realization that alternative, less repressive strategies can be effective in limiting the spread of HIV infection, quarantine proposals have been dismissed. Despite claims that AIDS is similar to other diseases for which quarantine has been used, public health officials have insisted on distinguishing between behaviorally transmitted infections and those that are airborne. AIDS is not tuberculosis. The CDC and Public Health Association believe that strategies less repressive than quarantine are more effective, for example, effective education and counseling. But many people believe that less repressive strategies are inadequate.

In the first 10 years of the epidemic 25 states enacted revised public health statutes providing for conditions under which individuals who engaged in behaviors that could spread disease could be restricted or quarantined (Table 9.3) (Bayer et al., 1993). In 19 of these states, statutes criminalizing HIV transmission-related behavior were also enacted. Framed broadly to cover public health threats, such legislative action was clearly inspired by the AIDS epidemic. Note that neither California nor New York, states that together account for close to 40% of AIDS cases in the United States, enacted criminal laws or revised public health statutes to cover the sexual transmission of HIV. Despite the extended and often acrimonious debate over the use of the power to quarantine in the context of AIDS, little is known about how such powers have been used in states where they have been granted to public health officials. Through mid-1995, the official policy of the United States for HIV prevention remained education, counseling, voluntary testing and partner notification, drug abuse treatment, and needle exchange programs. To date, the power to quarantine has rarely been used in the United States. In fact, only one country, Cuba, officially used the power of quarantine to stem the spread of HIV. Data to date indicate that the use of quarantine of HIV-infected and AIDS persons in

TABLE 9-3 State Quarantine Policies on Individuals Whose Behavior Poses a Risk of HIV Transmission

State	Quarantine Authorized 1981–1992	State	Quarantine Authorized 1981–1992	State	Quarantine Authorized 1981–1992
AL	-	KY	-	NY	-
AK	-	LA	-	OH	-
AZ	+[a]	MA	-	OK	+[a]
AR	-	ME	+	OR	+
CA	-	MD	+[a]	PA	-
CO	+[a]	MI	+[a]	RI	-
CT	+	MN	+	SC	+[a]
DC	-	MO	+[a]	SD	-
DE	-	MS	-	TN	+[a]
FL	+[a]	MT	+[a]	TX	+[a]
GA	+[a]	NC	-	UT	-
HI	-	ND	+[a]	VA	+[a]
ID	-	NE	-	VT	-
IL	+[a]	NH	-	WA	+[a]
IN	+[a]	NJ	-	WI	-
IO	-	NM	-	WV	+
KS	+[a]	NV	+[a]	WY	+

Source: Quarantine data are from Intergovernmental Health Policy Project publications and files.
[a]Criminal penalties for HIV transmission-related behavior also available.
(Adapted from Bayer et al., 1993)

Cuba had been very effective. Cuba had 13 sanatoriums holding some 900 persons of which about 180 have AIDS. Cuba stopped the quarantine of HIV infected persons in mid-1994.

BARRIERS TO HIV INFECTION

The two most effective barriers to HIV infection and other sexually transmitted diseases are (1) abstinence, which can be achieved by saying *NO* emphatically and consistently; and (2) forming a no-cheating relationship with one individual, preferably for life. These solutions to the danger of HIV infection may not be "cool," but they definitely work. These two completely safe approaches are endorsed by the Surgeon General as the *preferred* methods. For those who do not practice abstinence or have multiple sex partners, barrier methods are necessary to prevent HIV infection/transmission.

The barrier methods used to prevent HIV infection are the same methods used to prevent other sexually transmitted diseases (STDs) and often pregnancy. They include latex condoms, plastic condoms (new in 1995), and latex dams, and diaphragms, used in conjunction with a spermicide. Barrier dams are thin sheets of latex or similar material used in oral–vaginal and oral–anal sex. Spermicides are chemicals that kill sperm. These same chemicals have also been shown to kill bacteria and inactivate viruses that cause STDs (Bolch et al., 1973; Singh, 1982; Amortegui et al., 1984; Hicks et al., 1985). Spermicides are commercially available in foams, creams, jellies, suppositories, and sponges. Use of these products may provide protection against the transmission of STDs, but the only recommended barrier protection against HIV infection is a **condom with a spermicide.** National Condom Week is the week of February 14–21.

Condoms are classified as medical devices. Every condom made in the U.S. is tested for defects and must meet strict quality control guidelines enforced by the federal Food and Drug Administration (FDA).

Condoms are intended to provide a physical barrier that prevents contact between vaginal, anal, penile, and oral lesions and secretions and ejaculate.

At least 50 brands of condoms are manufactured in the United States. They are pro-

POINT OF INFORMATION 9.1

CLARIFYING THE ISSUES OVER CONDOM USE

Two major issues surface in the debate over advocating condom use in the prevention of HIV infection: One concerns the concept of efficacy, the condoms ability to stop the virus from passing through, and the other, the fear that making condoms available will encourage early sexual activity among adolescents and extramarital sex among adults.

Efficacy (do they work)

All condoms are not 100% impermeable; they are not all of the same quality. Investigators using different testing methods have reported that latex condoms are effective physical barriers to high concentrations of *Chlamydia trachomatis, Neisseria gonorrhoeae,* the herpes and hepatitis viruses, cytomegalovirus, and HIV (Judson, 1989). But for maximum effectiveness condoms must be properly and consistently used from start to finish (Table 9-4).

To be effective, a condom must be worn on the penis during the entire time that the sex organ is in contact with the partner's genital area, anus, or mouth. Care must be taken that the condom is on before vaginal, anal, or oral penetration, and that it does not slip off. If properly used, the condom provides protection against most of the STDs that occur within the vagina, on the glans penis, within the urethra or along the penile shaft.

Because the condom covers only the head and shaft of the penis, it does not provide protection for the pubic or thigh areas, which may come in contact with body secretions during sexual activity.

Margret Fischel reported in 1987 that 17% of women whose husbands were HIV-positive became HIV-infected while using condoms properly and consistently.

Susan Weller (1993) reported on the use of condoms as a barrier to HIV transmission. She analyzed the data from 11 studies involving 593 partners of HIV-infected people. The resulting data showed that condoms are only 69% effective in preventing HIV transmission in heterosexual couples. These data surprise people because earlier contraceptive research indicated that condoms are about 90% effective in preventing pregnancy. Thus many people assume condoms prevent HIV transmission with the same degree of effectiveness. However, transmission studies by Weller do not show that to be true. Weller states that condom effectiveness in blocking HIV transmission may be as low as 46% or as high as 82%!

TABLE 9-4 Proper Placement of a Condom[a] on the Penis

1. Open the packaged condom with care; avoid making small fingernail tears or breaks in the condom.
2. Place a drop of a water based lubricant inside the condom tip before placing it on the head of the penis. Be sure none of the lubricant rolls down the penis shaft as it may cause the condom to slide off during intercourse.
3. Hold about a half an inch of the condom tip between your thumb and finger—this is to allow space for semen after ejaculation. Then place the condom against the glans penis (if uncircumcised, pull the foreskin back).
4. Unroll the condom down the penis shaft to the base of the penis. Squeeze out any air as you roll the condom toward the base.
5. After ejaculation, hold the condom at the base and withdraw the penis while it is still firm.
6. Carefully take the condom off by gently rolling and pulling so as not to leak semen.
7. Discard the condom into the trash.
8. Wash your hands after the procedure.
9. Never use the same condom twice.
10. Condoms should not be stored in extremely hot or cold environments.

[a]Males should practice putting on and removing a condom prior to engaging in sexual intercourse.

Isabelle deVincenzi (1994) reported on HIV transmission among heterosexual sexual couples in which one partner was known to be HIV-positive. Study participants were advised to use condoms during intercourse, and among the 124 (or 48%) of couples who followed that advice consistently, no seronegative partner became HIV infected during roughly 24 months of follow-up. However, despite knowledge about HIV transmission, more than 50% of the couples failed to use condoms consistently. Twelve of the seronegative individuals in that group became HIV-positive during the study.

The importance of compliance is illuminated by an analogy with pregnancy prevention programs. Although typical pregnancy rates for couples who use condoms are as high as 10% to 15%, rates are estimated to be as low as 2% for couples who use condoms correctly and consistently.

A mathematical model predicts that consistent condom use could prevent nearly half of the sexually transmitted HIV infections in persons with one sexual partner and over half of HIV infections in persons with multiple partners. A reduction of this magnitude could help interrupt the propagation of the epidemic. Therefore, promoting more widespread understanding of condom efficacy or effectiveness, and advocating their consistent use by those who choose to be sexually active, is crucial to protecting people from HIV infection and to slowing the spread of the HIV and sexually transmitted disease epidemic.

Do Condoms Encourage Sexual Activity?

Many persons assert that those who promote condom use to prevent HIV infection appear to be condoning sexual intercourse outside of marriage among adolescents as well as among adults. Recent data from Switzerland suggest that a public education campaign promoting condom use can be effective without increasing the proportion of adolescents who are sexually active. A 3-year, 10-month study showed condom use among persons aged 17 to 30 years increased from 8% to 52%. By contrast the proportion of adolescents (aged 16 to 19 years) who had sexual intercourse did not increase over that same period. A report from Deborah Sellers and colleagues (1994) also concluded that the promotion and distribution of condoms did not increase sexual activity among adolescents. The study involved 586 adolescents who were 14 to 20 years of age.

The AIDS epidemic has brought new dimensions of complexity and urgency to the debate over adolescent sexual activity. Some have urged abstinence as the only solution; while others champion condom use as the most practical public health approach. Thus a clear message about condoms may have been obscured by controversy over providing condoms for adolescents in schools while at the same time trying to discourage these same young people from initiating sexual activity.

There must be a common ground: People should be able to agree that premature initiation of sexual activity carries health risks. Therefore, young people must be encouraged to postpone sexual activity. Parents, clergy, and educators must strive for a climate supportive of young people who are not having sex. Let them know it is a very positive and intelligent decision, and so help to create a new health-oriented social norm for adolescents and teenagers about sexuality.

The message that those who initiate or continue sexual activity must reduce their risk through correct and consistent condom use needs to be delivered as strongly and persuasively as the message, "Don't do it." Protection of the individual and the public health will depend on our ability to combine these messages effectively (Roper et al., 1993).

ANECDOTE

Presenting facts without understanding won't work! Here is a simple story to emphasize the point: A minister following his custom, paid a monthly call on two spinster sisters. While he was standing in their parlor, holding his cup of tea, engaged in their usual chit chat, he was startled by something that caught his eye. There on the piano was a condom! 'Ladies, in all the years we've known each other I have never intruded into your private lives, and never felt the need to. But now I am forced to ask what is that thing doing there?' 'One of the ladies replied, 'Oh, that's a wonderful thing, pastor, and they really work!' 'The minister was agitated: I'm not talking about their value or effectiveness. I just want to know what that thing is doing on your piano?'

'Well, my sister and I were watching television. We heard this lovely man, the Surgeon General of the whole United States. He said that if you put one of those on your organ, you'll never get sick. Well, as you know we don't have an organ, but we bought one and put it on the piano, and we haven't had a day's sickness since!'

duced to fit every fancy. There are colored condoms—pink, yellow, and gold; flavored condoms; and condoms that are perfumed, ribbed, stippled, and phosphorescent (glow in the dark). This assortment of condoms exposes the user and his partner not only to rubber but also to a variety of different chemicals—some that can cause allergic skin reactions (contact dermatitis). One to two percent of people are sensitive to latex rubber and demonstrate contact dermatitis.

Condoms are also called rubbers, prophylactics, bags, skins, raincoats, sheaths, and French letters. They can be lubricated or not, have reservoir tips or not, and can contain spermicide—the choice is yours.

Over the years we have been told to use condoms to prevent STDs and pregnancy. Today we are told that an additional use of the condom is to save lives.

History of Condoms

It has been reported that early Egyptian men used animal membranes as a sheath to cover their penises (Barber, 1990). Animal intestines were flushed clean with water, sewn shut at one end and cut to the length of the erect penis. In 1504, Gabriel Fallopius designed a medicated linen sheath that was pulled on over the penis. A Japanese novel written in the 10th century refers to the uncomfortable use of a tortoise shell or horn to cover the penis.

It is interesting to note that condoms were used far more often throughout history as protection against STDs than as contraceptives. For example, an 18th century writer recommended that men protect themselves against disease by placing a linen sheath over the penis during intercourse.

The term condom came into common usage in the 1700s. It has been suggested that the name came from Dr. Condom, who designed a penile sheath for King Charles II of England. According to accounts, in the early 1700s, condoms were sold and even exported from a London shop whose proprietress laundered and "recycled" them in a back room (Barber, 1990). Condoms became more widely available after 1854 when the method for making rubber was invented by Charles Goodyear (as in Goodyear tires). The latex condom was first manufactured in the 1930s.

Condoms have been available in the United States for over 130 years, but have never been as openly accepted as they are now. Their sale for contraceptive use was outlawed by many state legislatures beginning in 1868 and by Congress in 1873. Although most of these laws were eventually repealed, condom packages and dispensers until only a few years ago continued to bear the label "*Sold only for the prevention of disease,*" even though they were being used mainly for the prevention of pregnancy.

After the advent of nonbarrier methods of contraception during the 1960s (mainly the use of the birth control pill) there was an ensuing epidemic increase in most sexually transmitted infections including HIV. Condoms once again are being marketed for the prevention of disease (Judson, 1989).

In 1979, only 8% of respondents to a *Consumer Reports* survey on condoms said they used condoms for the prevention of STDs. However, in *Consumer Reports'* 1989 study, 26% said they used condoms to prevent STDs, especially HIV infection (Figure 9-2, A and B).

Safer Sex, the Choice of Condom

Although a variety of preventative behaviors have been recommended (Table 9-2), the responsibility of *safer sex,* with a condom, is a personal choice. If one decides to use a condom, then the choice is what kind, and whether or not to use a spermicide.

The Male Condom— The American- made condom most often sold is made of latex, is about 8 inches long, and in general, one size fits all (Figure 9-3). About 500 million condoms were sold in the United States in 1992. Over five billion are sold annually worldwide (Grimes, 1992).

Intact latex condoms provide a continuous mechanical barrier to HIV, herpes virus (HSV), hepatitis B virus (HBV), *Chlamydia trachomatis,* and *Neisseria gonorrhoeae.* A recent laboratory study indicated that latex condoms are the most effective mechanical barrier to fluid containing HIV-sized particles (0.1 μm in diameter) available.

Three prospective studies in developed countries indicated that condoms are unlikely to break or slip during proper use. Reported breakage rates in the studies were 2% or less for vaginal or anal intercourse (*MMWR,* 1993a).

There is another kind of condom made from lamb's intestine. It is commonly called a "skin." It is believed that it may allow viruses to slip through and is **not recommended** for use. Animal-derived condoms are used mainly because they allow greater passage of body heat, provide better tactile sensation, and can be reused.

Choice— The best choice for preventing STDs and pregnancy is condoms that are made of latex and contain a *spermicide.* The spermi-

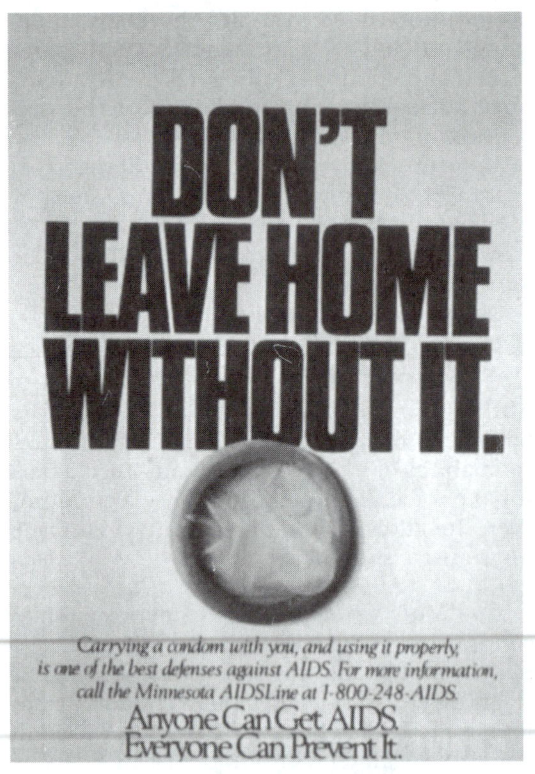

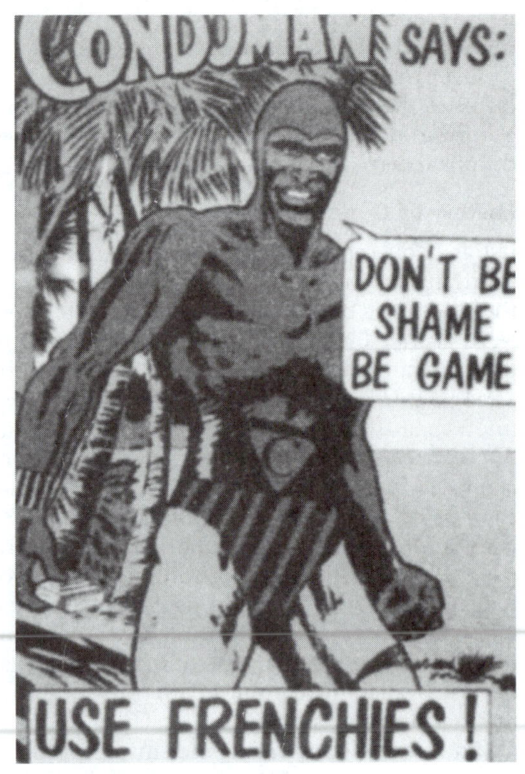

FIGURE 9-2 Advertisements for Condoms. **A,** A common theme centered around the use of a condom to protect against sexually transmitted diseases. **B,** A specific type of condom in a comic book style advertisement.

cide is added protection in case the condom ruptures or spills as it is taken off. During in vitro studies, condoms were artificially ruptured in a medium containing nonoxynol-9 or N-9 (*p*-diisobutylphenoxypolyethoxethanol). On examination, no virus capable of reproduction was found. Tests done without the spermicide resulted in viruses capable of reproducing (Connell, 1989). It must be mentioned, however, that there is no evidence that N-9 has any effect on HIVs that are carried within lymphocyte cells in the semen.

Nonoxynol-9— Evidence from the mid-1970s has lent support to the prophylactic use of N-9 as a spermicide against sexually transmitted diseases (Bird, 1991). There are reports, however, that some males and females are sensitive to it. N-9 has been shown to variably inactivate *Neisseria gonorrhoeae, Tri-chomonas vaginalis, Ureaplasma urealyticum, Treponema pallidum, Candida albicans,* herpes and hepatitis B viruses, and cytomegalovirus and HIV. There is some question about its effectiveness against *Chlamydia trachomatis,* and it has been reported to be ineffective against the genital wart virus (Stone et al., 1986; Rosenberg et al., 1992). More recently, concern has been raised that N-9 may serve to digest nonspecific protective mucosal coatings and induce the increased presence of lymphocytes and bleeding, which by itself might promote HIV and other viral and bacterial infections (Fisher, 1991).

Condom Advertising on American Television— On January 4, 1994, condoms danced into America's living rooms as part of the most explicit HIV prevention campaign the nation has even seen. Previously, condoms were rarely seen or even mentioned on American television. But the Centers for Disease Control and Prevention (CDC) launched a series of radio and

POINT OF VIEW 9.1

SHOULD CONDOMS BE DISTRIBUTED IN SCHOOLS?

The pro and con of this question was debated in the *New Haven Register*, New Haven, Connecticut, August 4, 1993. It could well be any large city school district in the United States.

PRO:

New Haven has the greatest number of cases of HIV in Connecticut. Nationally for adults aged 25 to 44, AIDS is the second leading cause of death in men, and sixth in women; in New Haven it has become the No. 1 cause of death for both young men and women.

The New Haven Board of Education, amid much controversy, approved a plan intended to protect public school students from infection with HIV. The program calls for an array of efforts to minimize the risk of contracting HIV.

It is first a plan to educated teens, parents, and teachers about AIDS risk reduction. It is a plan to expand peer education where teens teach other teens about behaviors which placed them them at risk.

Proponents of the program include parents, students, health care professionals and AIDS activists. Testimony presented by members of the health care community came from a cross-section of federal, state and community organizations. Underlying the emotional testimony of every advocate for the plan was the fact that young men and women in the community are dying each day, and the spread of AIDS will continue unchecked without efforts at prevention.

The Superintendent of Schools conceded that sometimes the school system does intervene on behalf of the city's children on issues that in a better world, would preferably be left to parents in the home. He cited the school breakfast program, and providing clothing and shelter to needy students as examples of the school system's addressing social and health needs which for some children would otherwise go unmet. The reality that New Haven youth were succumbing to a fatal illness underscored the need for intervention.

If one thing is clear from the three weeks of public testimony, it is that greater efforts to educate the community about AIDS are needed. Right now the best approach to preventing AIDS lies in behavior modification, a necessary but less-than-perfect strategy. Michael H. Merson discussed the different mechanisms for promoting safer behavior, ranging from repeated educational messages about AIDS to spermicides with antiviral capacity that can help empower women worldwide. The need for more effective education must not be ignored. Currently, condoms can be an effective, prophylactic vaccine. Therefore, in order to protect our teenagers, a major component of our AIDS strategy should be an intelligent program of sex education in the schools.

The current options for treating AIDS are limited at best, and there is little hope on the horizon for any imminent breakthroughs in treatment. The only significant efforts which can be taken in our community at this time to combat the epidemic are through prevention.

Abstinence will still be stressed as the only foolproof way to prevent sexual transmission of HIV. However, for those teens who, despite our best wishes, continue to engage in sex, *condoms will only be made available by health care providers in the school-based clinics, along with counseling about the risks of HIV and other sexually transmitted diseases.*

CON:

It won't work. Instead of solving problems—AIDS, teenage pregnancy—in-school condom distribution makes them worse. It does so by encouraging children and teenagers to engage in the precocious and promiscuous sexual activity that causes the problems in the first place.

The case for condoms is, of course, perfectly clear: nothing else will help so let's give this a try—maybe a few kids will be saved from the worst consequences of their behavior.

Maybe. But many more won't. The failure rate of condoms has been documented time and again. Where sexual promiscuity is accepted as the behavioral norm—sanctioned and encouraged, be it noted, by schools—this is the functional equivalent of Russian roulette played several times a week. The odds are stacked against the kids. This is not something responsible adults should do.

What should be done? The answer is obvious. Sexual abstinence is the only 100 percent effective way to prevent the disastrous consequences of teenage sex.

To be sure, abstinence is not a popular prescription in a sex-saturated, feel-good culture, but it has a great advantage—It works!

People constantly abstain—from drugs, from drink, from sugar, from fats, from countless other habits or negative inclinations or appetites. The idea that young people can't responsibly resist AIDS, teen pregnancy, or other self-injury, if given the right reasons with the right emphasis, is not convincing.

The principle to be taught is not self-indulgence, but self-control.

Another principle of great importance is that of parental right and duty. Parents have the primary responsibility to make decisions about the education and ethical formation of their children especially when the children are still very young.

Many parents wish to exercise this right and fulfill this duty, yet find themselves opposed and frustrated by circumstances in society beyond their control. It is grossly unfair to such parents, struggling against hostile and destructive cultural currents to fulfill their obligations to their children, to throw the weight of the schools into the balance against them.

But, it will be objected, some parents shirk their duty; some families have been weakened to the point of collapse. No doubt that is true. The answer, however, doesn't lie in bypassing parents and families, but in drawing them into the educational program so that they will be constructively involved in their children's lives and decisions.

Of course this will be difficult, but the difficulty is not an argument for giving up. Instead of undermining parental authority and family structures, education policy and practice need to seek creative ways of reinforcing and strengthening them.

As a society, we have gone very far down the road of tolerating and encouraging precocious sexual activity on the part of our young people—so far that some people now suppose there is no turning back. Nonsense. We can turn back when we decide, as a community and a society, to do so.

The grave threats to health and well being now menacing our children make it imperative that we do. Forget the condoms. For a change, let's really help the kids.

Class discussion: Are you Pro or Con on this issue?

television public service announcements (PSAs) targeting sexually active young adults, a group at high risk for HIV infection.

One of the television ads, entitled *Automatic*, features a condom making its way from the top drawer of a dresser across the room and into bed with a couple about to make love. The voice-over says, "It would be nice if latex condoms were automatics. But since they're not, using them should be. Simply because a latex condom, used consistently and correctly, will prevent the spread of HIV." Another, entitled *Turned Down*, features a man and woman kissing, when the woman asks the man, "Did you bring it?" When he says he **forgot it**, she replies, "Then **forget it**," and turns on the light. There is also a pair of abstinence ads, in which condom use is not mentioned. The ads feature a man and woman talking. She says, "There is a time for us to be lovers. We will wait until that time comes."

Language that was once forbidden on TV has now become routine. Will it prevent HIV infection? Will it save lives?

The advertising campaign was hailed as a milestone, marking a high point of visibility for the condom on network television and introducing a new level of explicitness to the Centers for Disease Control and Prevention's public pronouncements about AIDS prevention.

In the 4 months following the advertising campaign's January debut, supermarkets, drug stores, and mass-merchandise outlets sold 137.6 million condoms—virtually the same as in the year-earlier period. Some established condom brands even experienced a sales drop in the wake of the CDC campaign. Trojan brand, by far the category leader, saw unit sales slip 3% in the 4 month period. Sales of the Sheik and Ramses brands were off 4% and 25%, respectively. A behavioral epidomologist at the University of California believes that there has already been a condom "saturation effect." People who want to use condoms are already using them.

Class Discussion: What is your opinion on condom advertising?

Buying Condoms— Women are taking a more active role in buying condoms. In 1985, women bought about 10% of the condoms sold. In 1989, they purchased 40% to 50%. According to surveys, most women buying condoms are single, and their concern is about HIV infection rather than pregnancy.

BOX 9.1

CONDOMS: A LIFE OR DEATH ISSUE

Adults

Some males argue that they want to feel the *real you,* others argue that they don't make condoms *large* enough, while others say they are an inconvenience and putting one on takes away the pleasure of the moment. But not to use a condom or insist on the use of a condom *invites* infection. And if it's an HIV infection, the invitation will, most likely, lead to death.

There are many men and women who want to practice safer sex and are willing to use a condom. The problem is, many do not carry condoms with them 100% of the time. If they happen to have a condom available, they might be thought of as promiscuous. If they do not have a condom, they may not get the chance to have sex, especially if their potential partner is `safe sex' conscious. In other words, to demand one's sexual partner to use a condom may be taken as an accusation, while an offer to use a condom may be viewed as a confession.This is a kind of "Catch-22" scenario—damned if they do and damned if they do not.

Teenagers

Although information alone does not keep young people from having sex, becoming infected with HIV, or getting pregnant, accurate information about the consequences of unsafe sex may strengthen a youth's resolve not to have sex or not to have it without protection. Knowing that many of their peers do not have sex also helps youth understand they have the option to abstain.

In order for information to influence decisions, teenagers must understand that the information is about them.

According to data from the CDC's national school-based Youth Risk Behavior Survey, at least half of all high school students have had sexual intercourse. By the age of 17, 72% were sexually active. The survey, based on a questionnaire given to 12,272 students at 137 schools in the United States, revealed that 48% said they used a condom the last time they had sex, but that figure dropped to 19% for couples using birth control pills to prevent pregnancy.

That suggests students understand the importance of using birth control but do not understand the value of condoms in preventing HIV infection.

In another study, the CDC found that 88% to 98% of teenagers in homeless shelters, medical clinics, and correctional institutions were sexually active.

Note: In attempting to promote condom use among sexually active teenagers, be truthful. Promoting condoms as an erotic gadget for sex does not work. They are not fools. They will become angry with whomever told them this, when they find themselves clumsily fiddling with a condom the first time around. Tell them to practice their skills. They've already learned many things in life that were more complicated than putting on a condom. Millions of people do it every day—men and women—because they are smart, want to stay healthy, and have healthy children, and because they care for one another.

Many condoms are purchased from vending machines. The FDA recommends the following guidelines when purchasing condoms from a vending machine:

1. Is the condom made of latex?
2. Is the condom labeled for disease prevention?
3. Is the spermicide (if any) outdated?
4. Is the machine exposed to extreme temperatures or direct sunlight?

In mid-1992, the first drive-up "Condom Hut" opened in Cranston, Rhode Island. With each purchase the customer receives a brochure on safer sex.

Free Condoms— In the south of France, the regional tourism authority announced, in 1991, that condoms would be placed alongside soap and shampoo in all hotel rooms and would be supplied free to all people using campsites in the area. Some 8 million tourists visit the south of France every summer—the region has the highest incidence of HIV/AIDS in the country.

Condoms are now being dispensed without charge in most college and university and public health clinics, and an increasing number of high school health offices in the United States. Some cities in Canada have been providing access to free condoms in high schools since 1984. By the end of 1992, 260,000 students at 120 schools across the United States were provided with safer sex education and free condoms. In mid-1992, the New York City Board

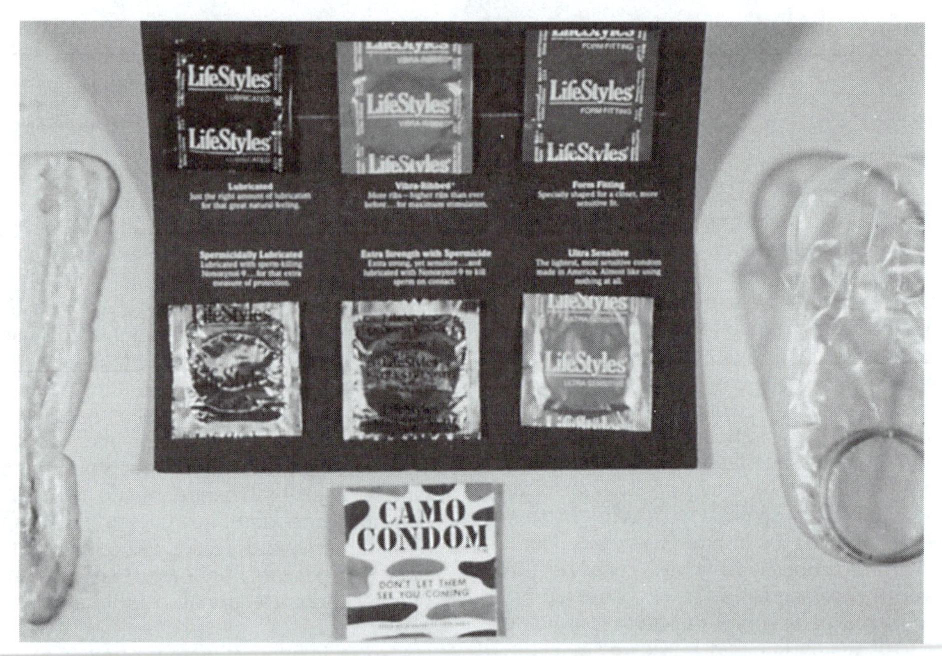

FIGURE 9-3 A Collection of Condoms. The condom is sealed in an aluminum foil package, sometimes along with a spermicide. On the left side is an unfolded or unrolled male condom; on the right side is a vaginal pouch (female condom) (see Figure 9-4).

of Education agreed to adopt an AIDS curriculum for elementary schools that introduces the use of condoms in the *fourth grade.* The board also agreed to a voluntary program to make free condoms available to teenagers at school. In December 1993, a New York appeals court handed HIV/AIDS and sex educators a stunning defeat when it struck down the New York City public school system's voluntary program to make condoms available to teens at school. At issue is a recommendation by the Chancellor of the New York City Board of Education to make condoms available on request in high schools as part of an expanded HIV-AIDS prevention curriculum. Under the plan, students who asked for condoms could do so **without parental permission** but were required to receive counseling on how to use them.

New York City teenagers account for 1 in every 5 cases (20%) of the reported adolescent AIDS in the United States. Supporters of the program called it a necessary response to a public health emergency. Parents challenging the condom distribution program argued that it violated their due process rights in raising their children.

The New York appellate court wrote that condom distribution in public schools was a "health service," rather than health education, and absent a parental opt-out provision, violated public health and common laws. Under law, medical or health services cannot be provided to minors without informed consent. "Supplying condoms to students upon request has absolutely nothing to do with education, but rather is a health service occurring after the education phase has ceased."

Regardless of educational programs on safer sex and condom usage, recent studies indicate that teenagers still refuse to use condoms. **What they know is not equal to what they do!** Based on their findings, the researchers said information-oriented school- and community-based AIDS prevention programs will not succeed in getting adolescents to use condoms, because there is no association between knowledge and preventive behavior.

Condom Availability in Developing Nations

Access to condoms in developing nations, although crucial, is poor even though over **1 billion** condoms are distributed in developing nations each year. The World Health Organization spends some $70 million a year for condoms distributed in 14 countries. But, it would cost $460 million to provide just Africa with an adequate condom program. The United Kingdom, in 1992, purchased 66 million condoms for Zimbabwe but the country needs at least 120 million condoms per year. And it must be recognized that a number of cultures in developing nations prohibit the use of condoms.

Condom Quality

Some have touted condoms as a bulletproof vest for preventing HIV infection. This is simplistic and inaccurate because condoms may break or be used improperly. Condoms have been shown to *reduce* significantly but not *eliminate* the transmission of HIV. Condom use is a form of *safer* sex but *not* absolutely safe sex. The March 1989 issue of *Consumer Reports* did a rather extensive study on the quality of different brands of condoms. The reader survey revealed that one in eight people who used condoms had two condoms break in one year of sexual activity; one in four said one condom had broken. Calculated from its data, about one in 140 condoms broke, with condom breakage occurring more often during some sexual activities than others. For example, the breakage rate during anal sex was calculated at one in 105 compared to one in 165 for vaginal sex. One in 10 heterosexual men admitted to engaging in anal sex using condoms (*Consumer Reports*, 1989).

In 1987, FDA inspectors began making spot checks for condom quality. They fill the condom with 10 ounces (about 300 mL) of water to check for leaks. If leaks are found in more than four per 1,000 condoms, that entire batch is destroyed. Over the first 15 months of spot inspections, one lot in 10 was rejected. Import condoms failed twice as often—one lot in five.

The Female Condom (Vaginal Pouch)— The female condom was FDA approved in May of 1993, and has become available to the general public. Before giving the Reality condom final approval, the FDA asked that two caveats be put into the labeling. First, the agency required a statement on the package label that male condoms are still the best protection against disease, and second, that the label compare the effectiveness of female condoms with that of other barrier methods of birth control. According to the FDA, in a study of 150 women who used the female condom for 6 months, 26% became pregnant. The manufacturer contends that the pregnancy rate was 21%—and only because many women did not use the condom every time they had sex. With "perfect use," company officials say, the rate is 5%, in contrast to 2% for male condoms. Both conditions were met to the FDA's satisfaction. Gaston Farr and co-workers (1994) concluded that the female condom provided contraceptive efficacy in the same range as other barrier methods, particularly when used consistently and correctly, and has the added advantage of helping protect against sexually transmitted diseases.

The female condom is now called the vaginal pouch. It is 17 cm long and it consists of a 15-cm polyurethane sheath with rings at each end (Figure 9-4). The closed end fits into the vagina like a diaphragm. The outer portion is designed to cover the base of the penis and a large portion of the female perineum (the area of tissue between the anus and the beginning of the vaginal opening) to provide a greater surface barrier against microorganisms. Studies of acceptability, contraceptive effectiveness, and STD prevention are currently underway. Potential advantages of this product are: (1) it provides women with the opportunity to protect themselves from pregnancy and STDs; (2) it provides a broader coverage of the labia and base of the penis than a male condom; and (3) its polyurethane membrane is stronger than latex.

At least three versions of the female vaginal pouch are currently undergoing testing and awaiting Food and Drug Administration approval—one developed by a Wisconsin company, another by a father and son doctor team in California, and a third by a Wyoming physician. The Wisconsin version has recently been named *Reality*. The cost for the Reality condom is about $2.50 each. The female condom has been sold in Switzerland since 1992 and in France and Britain since mid-1993.

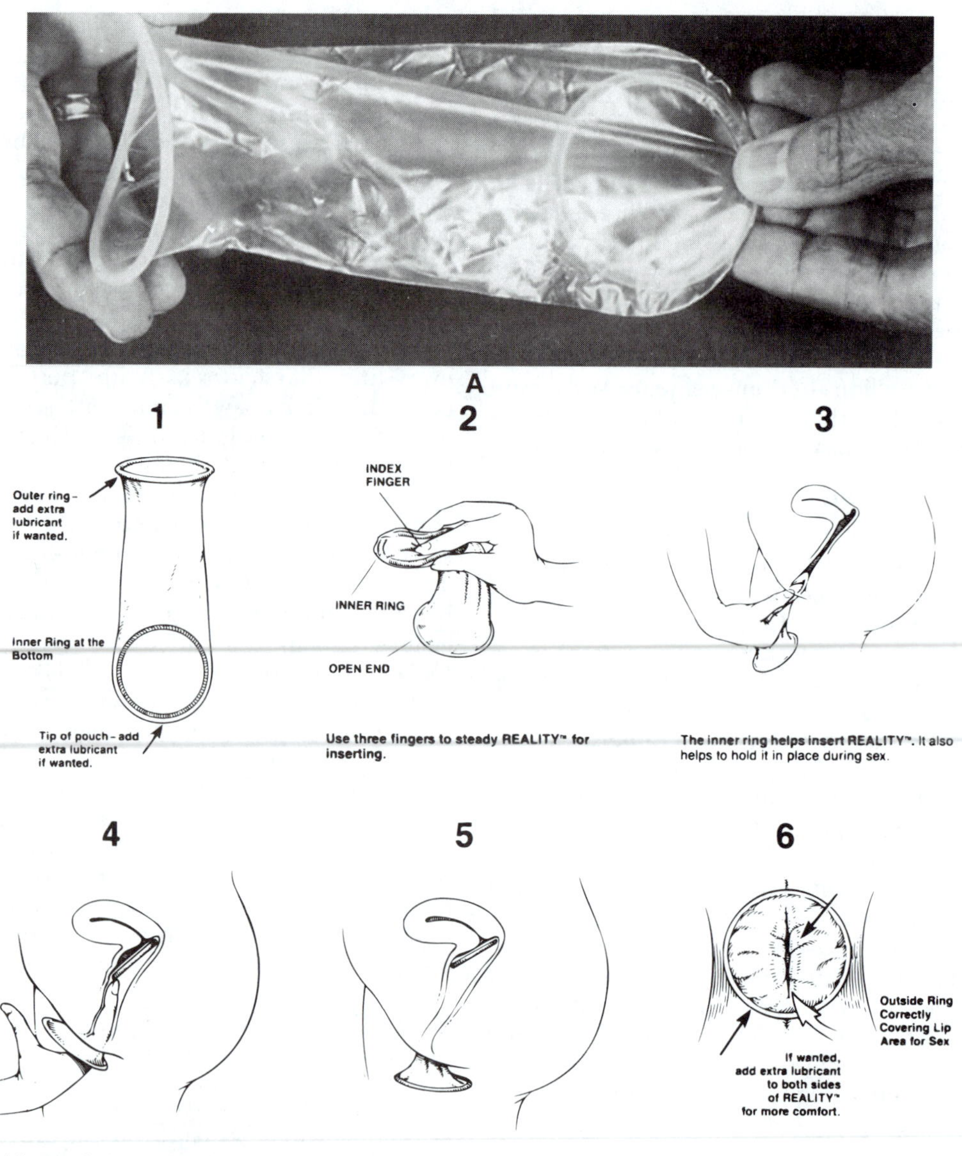

FIGURE 9-4 **A,** The Vaginal Pouch. **B,** The 7-inch female condom or vaginal pouch is made of lightweight, lubricated polyurethane and has two flexible rings (1), one at either end. It is twice the thickness of the male latex condom. The inner ring (2) is used to help insert the device and fits behind the pubic bone. The outer ring remains outside the body. Unlike the diaphragm, the vaginal condom protects against the transmission of HIV, which can penetrate the vaginal tissues. The pouch can be inserted anytime from several hours to minutes prior to intercourse. The vaginal pouch is inserted like a diaphragm and removed after sex. FDA approved in May, 1993. (*Courtesy of Wisconsin Pharmacal Co.*)

POINT OF INFORMATION 9.2

QUESTIONS AND ANSWERS ABOUT THE FEMALE CONDOM

1. **Does one have to be fitted for use of a female condom?** The female condom is offered in one size and is available without prescription. Unlike using a diaphragm, the female condom covers not only the cervix but also the vagina, thereby containing the man's ejaculate.
2. **Should a lubricant be used with the female condom?** A lubricant is recommended for use with the female condom to increase comfort and ease the entry and withdrawal of the penis. The female condom is prelubricated on the inside with a silicone-based, nonspermicidal lubricant. Additional water-based lubrication is included. The lubricant can be placed either inside the female condom or on the penis.
3. **Can oil-based lubricants be used with the female condom?** The female condom is made of polyurethane which is not reported to be damaged by oil-based lubricants.
4. **Can a spermicide be used with the female condom?** Use of a spermicide has not been reported to damage the female condom. It is recommended that a spermicide containing nonoxynol-9 be used with the female condom for additional protection against HIV in the event of displacement, breakage, or leakage.
5. **How far in advance of sexual intercourse can the female condom be inserted?** The female condom may be inserted up to 8 hours before sexual intercourse. Most women insert it 2 to 20 minutes before engaging in vaginal intercourse.
6. **Can the female condom be reused?** No. A new female condom must be used for each act of vaginal intercourse. After intercourse, the condom must be removed before the women stands, to ensure that semen remains inside the pouch.
7. **Should a female condom and a male condom be used at the same time?** The female condom and male condom can be used at the same time but it is not recommended because the condoms may not stay in place due to friction between the latex in the male condom and the polyurethane in the female condom.
8. **Does Medicaid cover the female condom?** Currently Medicaid does not cover this device, as it does the male condom, spermicide, and other barriers. However, Medicaid coverage is expected in 1995. (*Information provided by the New York State Department of Health AIDS Institute Division of HIV Prevention,* Info Bulletin, *Jan. 1994, Number Five.)*

The symbolic importance of the female condom should not be understated: it is the *first* woman-controlled barrier method officially recognized as a means for the prevention of sexually transmitted disease. The female condom allows women to be able to deal with the twin anxieties—AIDS and unwanted pregnancy—with a method that is under their own control.

The Wyoming pouch is folded into the crotch of a latex G-string. The three products all perform in essentially the same way. They are disposable, contain protective sheaths of rubber or plastic, and are worn on the inside of a woman instead of on the outside of a man.

Condom Variant

A variant of the traditional condom is under review by the FDA. It is called a microcondom. It is a smaller version of the standard condom. It is only a glans cap which covers the tip of the penis.

Condom Lubricants

It has been demonstrated that petroleum or vegetable oil based lubricants should not be used with latex condoms. Nick White and colleagues (1988) have reported that these lubricants weaken latex condoms. Latex condoms exposed to mineral oil for 60 seconds demonstrated a 90% decrease in strength (Anderson, 1993). There are a number of water based lubricants that do not adversely affect latex condoms; these should be the lubricants of choice (Table 9.5).

World Health Organization Searches for Alternative Barrier Protection

It takes two people to have sex, but only one to slow the spread of sexually transmitted diseases and AIDS. A man can use condoms, but a woman's choices are limited. The most glaring gap in AIDS prevention is the lack of a method a woman can use when she suspects her partner may have a sexually transmitted disease or HIV infection and she cannot compel him to use a condom.

The risks of AIDS and other sexually transmitted diseases are stacked against women. Sexually transmitted diseases present fewer symptoms but cause more long-term damage in women than in men; sexualy transmitted diseases and HIV pass more easily from men to women than vice versa, so even though the average man has more sexual partners than most women, women acquire HIV at an earlier mean age than men; and women can pass sexually acquired infections and HIV to the next generation during pregnancy, delivery, or breast feeding. HIV and other sexually transmitted diseases spread most rapidly where women are most disadvantaged: among prostitutes it is those who charge least who are most likely to get infected. The female condom is a welcome new choice for women that should slow HIV transmission, but it cannot be used without the man's knowledge.

TABLE 9-5 Water-Based[a] and Oil-Based[b] Lubricants Often Used with Latex Condoms

Lubricants Recommended	Lubricants Not Recommended
Aqualube	Petroleum jellies
Astroglide	Mineral oils
Cornhuskers Lotion	Vegetable oils
Forplay	Baby oil
H-R Jelly	Massage oil
K-Y Brand Jelly	Lard
RePair	Cold creams
Probe	Hair oils
Today Personal Lube	Hand lotions containing vegetable oils
Contraceptives with nonoxynol 9:	Shaft
Delfen Foam	Elbow Grease
Koromex Foam	Natural Lube
Koromex Jelly	
Ramses Jelly	

[a]Water-based lubricants can be used with latex condoms.

[b]Oil-based lubricants will chemically weaken latex, causing it to break.

The above lists are not exhaustive of all available lubricants used by consumers.

Source: The STD Education Unit of the San Francisco Department of Public Health

Chemical methods that can be controlled by women are likely to have a powerful effect on the spread of HIV for several reasons. They could be distributed rapidly and cheaply by well understood social marketing techniques. They have the potential to slow HIV transmission directly and to reduce other sexually transmitted diseases that are cofactors in transmission.

In the United States, HIV-infected women are among the most rapidly growing groups affected by the disease. Globally, the largest number of cases are the result of heterosexual transmission. From a public health perspective, a modest reduction in HIV transmission brought about by a vaginal microbicide made available today might save as many lives as a more effective method (e.g., a vaccine) made available in 10 years' time, when there might be 5 or 10 times as many infected people (Potts, 1994).

In November of 1993, the WHO began a strategy to identify a safe and effective substance that can be inserted into the vagina in a foam, gel, sponge, or other form to kill HIV or prevent it from infecting cells in the body. Researchers hope that it can be used by a woman without her partner's knowledge. WHO scientists believe that if there is one thing which truly can make a difference to the epidemic, it is a vaginal microbicide.

In developing a vaginal microbicide, scientists must be sure that the substance is safe, does not kill microbes naturally present in the vagina that benefit female hygiene, and does not impair a woman's ability to conceive. Any microbicide will have to be tested to determine whether it damages spermatozoa, which could result in birth defects. Currently 10 substances are being explored as potential microbicides.

The earliest expected success is some years off. However, even if an early vaginal microbicide proves to be far less that 100% effective, it still can make a major impact on the AIDS epidemic. The prevalence of HIV infection in some populations, particularly in the developing countries, is so high that even something that was 50% effective would be a great advance.

PREVENTION OF INJECTION DRUG USE/HIV TRANSMISSION: THE TWIN EPIDEMICS

Syringes and needles used to inject drugs or steroids, or to tattoo the body, or to pierce the ears, should never be shared. If an individual is going to assume the risk of HIV transmission through needle sharing, the risk can be reduced by sterilizing the needle, and the syringe, if one is used, in undiluted chlorine bleach. The needle and syringe should be flushed through twice with bleach and rinsed thoroughly with water.

Both injection drug use (IDU) and HIV infection are on the increase. They are twin epidemics in the United States and Europe because the virus is readily transmitted by the use of injection drugs; and then from infected drug users to their noninfected sexual partners. Stopping injection drug-associated HIV transmission in theory is easy—just avoid drugs. But, that is a difficult proposition for most of the over 1 million IDUs in the United States. IDUs will remain a major HIV connection to the homosexual, heterosexual, and pediatric populations (Figure 9.5).

What can be done and what is being done to prevent HIV transmission by this population? Available drug rehabilitation programs are far too few. Even if there were a sufficient number, there are always the hard core IDUs who will not enter a program.

A massive education program on how to clean drug equipment and **not sharing** such equipment has for the most part failed. IDUs have an economic motive to share equipment (Mandell et al., 1994). In addition, it takes time and effort to clean the syringe and needle and it takes time to find and purchase cleansing chemicals (detergents or bleach). The most important drawback may be that IDUs have little interest in health care or changing their behaviors. In addition, there is always the problem of legality. IDU is illegal throughout the United States. IDUs know this and fear incarceration without the possibility of a "fix." A "Catch-22" situation also exists for

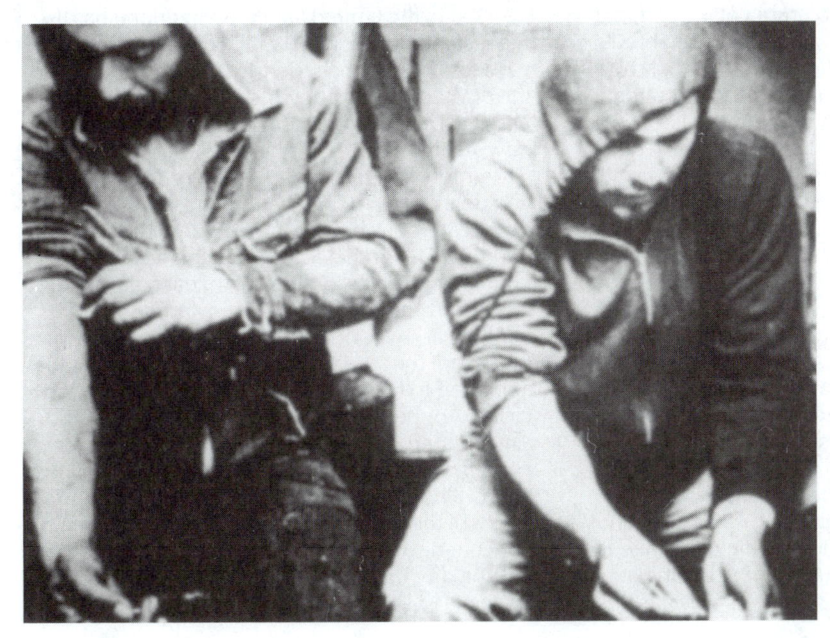

FIGURE 9-5 Injection Drug Users. Note that the person on the left is injecting the drug while the person on the right is preparing his injection. He is drawing up the "cooked" drug, most likely cocaine or heroin, into the syringe.

BOX 9.2

THE CONTROVERSY: PROVIDING STERILE SYRINGES AND NEEDLES TO INJECTION DRUG USERS (IDUs)

Providing sterile syringes and needles to injection drug users is controversial. *Pro forces* believe that it is impossible to eliminate injection drug use. Providing IDUs with free sterile equipment is an attempt at slowing the spread of HIV among drug users and their sexual partners, subsequently reducing the number of people in the general population that will become infected. In support of the Pro forces, the CDC reviewed the 37 needle-exchange programs operating in the United States in 1993 (In 1994 there were 41) and others in Canada and Europe. The most important conclusion is that needle exchanges are preventing HIV infections in drug users, their sex partners, and their children. That finding was based, in part, on evidence collected in Tacoma and Seattle, Washington and in New Haven, Connecticut where there was a 33% reduction in the rate of new infections among needle-exchange clients. In another key finding, they found no evidence that *distributing needles leads to an increase in drug use.*

Con forces feel that to provide free sterile equipment is to condone drug addiction and perhaps promote injection drug use among those who would not otherwise participate. A side issue of course is the fact that it is illegal to sell needles and syringes (NSs) over the counter in 10 of the 50 states and the District of Columbia. Statutes in 44 states and the District of Columbia place criminal penalties on the possession and distribution of NSs (drug paraphernalia laws) (*MMWR*, 1993b). Laws restricting these sales were intended to discourage drug use, but instead they have most likely increased the number of addicts sharing works, thereby helping to spread HIV (Fisher, 1990).

There is a *third force* of people who take the middle ground. They advocate providing free bleach to IDUs to clean their drug equipment. People from many AIDS-action groups in metropolitan areas are involved in the free bleach dispensing program. With each bottle of bleach is a set of directions. But as many IDUs can not read, they are given verbal instructions, though some are too "spaced out" to listen or too uncomfortable to care. Third force people have to understand that needle exchanges and distribution of bleach kits have to be accessible privately, off the street and out of sight, as well as publicly. Use of a public, streetcorner needle exchange is a statement to the entire community that the person exchanging a needle is an IDU. This has potentially very different consequences for women than for men. Women who have children have good reason to try to conceal their addiction as they risk losing custody or contact with their children if the state finds out they are actively using drugs—and if they are using a public needle exchange the child welfare bureaucracy is more likely to find out than if they are not getting needles in public. Perhaps needle exchanges should provide some type of informal child care so that a mother doesn't have to literally exchange needles in front of her children. Addiction among women is often taken as a statement of sexual availability.

A *fourth force* suggests that drugs be legalized so that they can be used openly, thereby reducing the threat of HIV transmission through illegal "shooting galleries." Discussion of the fourth force's position is beyond the scope of this text. However, a quasi-fourth force situation did exist in Zurich, Switzerland until 1992.

Zurich gained notoriety for its vast amounts of gold but in 1988 it gained a new image—that of an open Needle Park. The city of 250,000 people experimented in setting aside a park where cocaine and heroin addicts could openly buy, sell, and use injection drugs. The park attracted up to 4,000 drug users/day.

Next to the United States, Switzerland has the highest incidence of HIV/AIDS in the developed world. The city has tried to stop the spread of the disease among addicts sharing contaminated needles by isolating them and giving them free new needles. A cart laboratory has been converted for this purpose. For every used needle an addict turns in, he or she will get a free, sterile one. About half of the young people in the park are HIV-infected. All of them are slowly killing themselves. At the end of each day, some 7,000 dirty needles have been turned in. The needle park was not run to prevent drug use but to prevent the spread of HIV/AIDS. The program appeared to be working. The incidence of AIDS cases dropped from 50% to 5% (*Time*, 1992). An example of the people in the park are Reno, age 28, and Sophie, age 24. She has not only tested HIV-positive, she is suffering the first stages of the disease. For both of them their main concern now is not AIDS but getting the $400 or $500 a day they need to support their drug addiction.

There are no figures on how many of these addicts in the park die from AIDS. Many just drift away. It is known that more than 250 died in 1991 from addiction alone. And the rate of addiction is increasing, the population of the park is increasing, and the number overdosing is increasing. The medical staff tries to help, and the addicts, many of whom have lost hope for themselves, try to help each other. One man tries to keep the other who has overdosed upright and moving, trying to stop death. The fight is for life. A social worker volunteer says she has watched life and death in Needle Park for 4 years. She feels that death may be the best alternative. She does not make that statement lightly. Her own 22-year-old son has been in the park for almost 5 years—one who lives from fix to fix, one of the players in the drama that is played out each day in one of the world's financial capitals. But in early 1992, the park was closed because the park became a magnet for professional dealers, especially Lebanese, Yugoslav, and Turkish gangs that overran small dealers in a violent price war. Some of the park's inhabitants clustered around the central train station, others headed off in search of methadone. Others went back to the alleys and shelters from which they came. With sales suddenly back underground, addicts complained that the price of heroin had doubled overnight to $214 a gram (454 grams/pound = $97,156). Health workers said efforts to prevent the spread of HIV/ AIDS will now be much more difficult.

those who want to help make injection drug use safer: **many governmental agencies and law enforcement officers interpret the intention of making drug use safer as advocating drug use.** As a result, many proponents of safe drug use have avoided becoming involved in the issue.

Free Syringe-Needle Exchange Programs Begin in the United States

Tacoma, Washington— The nation's first "needle" exchange (syringes and needles) program began in August 1988. It began as a one-man program. Dave Purchase, a 20-year drug counselor, bought supplies out of pocket and between August 1988 and April 1989, he traded out over 19,000 needle packages. The following conversation between Purchase and an IDU offers a sense of what happens daily at the Tacoma needle exchange site:

> Many of the 40 or so clients to use the needle exchange one day last month were regulars. They knew the drill. If they dropped five syringes into the red box marked *BIOHAZARD*, they got five clean ones in return (Figure 9-6). Soon two new clients appear. One leans close to Purchase and quietly asks for a syringe. They have none to trade.
>
> "You've got to give me one to get one," Purchase says loudly. "It's an absolute rule."
>
> "But he's going by this girl's," says the spokesman, leaning closer. "She don't know nothin' about these. I didn't know nothin' about it either."
>
> "It pisses me off that I can't do it. But this is an exchange program. I can't do it. I'm under too much pressure to shut this place down. Go down to Bimbo's, man, and get the ones they

FIGURE 9-6 Needle and Syringe Exchange. The injection drug user drops the used syringe and needle into the collection box. For each deposit, the user receives a new syringe and needle. The use of clean equipment prevents the spread of HIV. (Through mid-1995, federal money could not be used for needle exchange programs.)

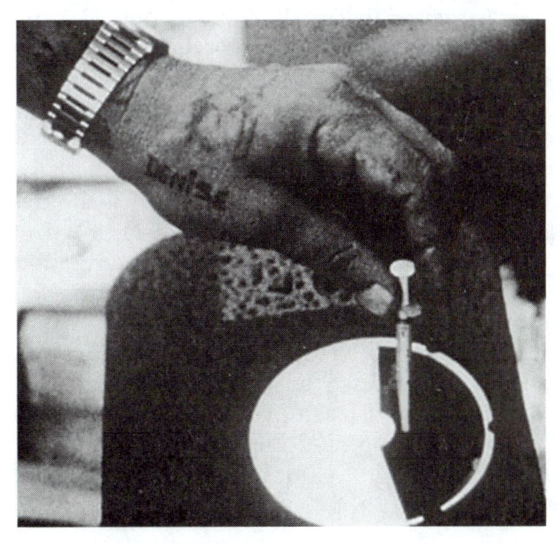

throw away," Purchase advises. "I don't care where you get it, just get me one."

They leave in the direction of Bimbo's, a nearby restaurant, across the street from which junkies often shoot up, but they never come back (Perrone, 1989).

New York City— In November 1988, after many delays, New York City began its needle exchange program. The program was canceled in early 1990—the reason: because over 50% of NYC's 240,000 IDUs are HIV-infected, the program offered too little too late to have an impact. IDUs make up about 38% to 40% of NYC AIDS cases. In late 1991, New York City commissioners recommended reestablishing a needle exchange program to the mayor.

New Haven, Connecticut— The 2-year-old program has demonstrated that needle exchange dramatically slows the rate of infection without encouraging new injection drug use. Some indicators even suggest that the program has been responsible for a decrease in both crime and the amount of drugs used illegally. The city's police chief claims that crime actually dropped 20% over the past 2 years, perhaps because of the improved relationship between city workers and the community. Meanwhile, referrals to drug treatment centers increased. These results have enabled policymakers elsewhere to call for needle exchange programs. Edward Kaplan of Yale University reported at the Eighth International AIDS Conference that the New Haven needle program cut the rate of new HIV infections by 33% to 50%. His data come from comparing the number of HIV-contaminated needles found on the streets versus those turned in at needle exchange points.

The mayor of Washington has called for needle exchange for addicts, as well as the distribution of free condoms in city schools and jails. Rhode Island, New Hampshire, and Connecticut will probably soon take the even more dramatic step of decriminalizing the possession of hypodermics. Movements are underway in New Jersey, California, and Massachusetts to remove legal barriers and begin officially sanctioned needle programs. Even in the U.S. Congress, Charles Rangel, who has led the opposition to needle exchange on the ground that it threatens blacks, has asked the General Accounting Office to reevaluate the effects of such programs.

The most important catalyst for this change has been the experiment conducted in New Haven (Thompson, 1992; *Time,* 1992).

Hawaii— In 1990, Hawaii became the first state to legalize a statewide syringe-needle exchange program. The state legislature felt it was necessary to stem the rate of HIV infection in women and newborns. The results of this program will have an impact on decisions to be made in other states. In Hawaii, a drug user comes in, drops a dirty needle into a plastic bucket, and receives a fresh sterile syringe and needle in exchange. No name is given, no questions are asked. Under the 2-year pilot project, an addict can swap a used needle for a new one supplied by the nonprofit Life Foundation up to 5 times a day 5 days a week.

Needle Exchange Programs in Other Countries

Needle exchange program results from England, Austria, the Netherlands, Sweden, and Scotland, presented at the Fourth International AIDS Conference (1988) suggest that the European programs attracted IDUs who had no previous contact with drug treatment programs; and that IDUs were drawn from clean needle programs into treatment programs, thus the decrease in drug use. There was no indication in these studies of an increase in injection drug use in cities with exchange programs. Where HIV testing had been done, the rate of HIV infection showed a marked decline after the introduction of the exchange program. Furthermore, self-reported instances of needle sharing and sexual intercourse without condoms, to the extent that they are reliable, also showed a downward trend (Raymond, 1988; Hagen, 1991).

Some of the countries with active needle sharing programs are:

Canada— In 1989, Montreal, Toronto, and Vancouver began syringe-needle exchange programs.

England— In 1992, over 2 million syringes and needles were exchanged in 120 programs. Needles and syringes can be legally purchased throughout England. Free distribution and exchange remains a relatively nonpolitical and noncontroversial issue (Stimson et al., 1989). Overall, the programs in England indicate that although changes in IDUs' behavior are slight, they are encouraging and may be important in reducing the spread of HIV (Hart et al., 1991). One problem found in England, the United States, and elsewhere is that these exchange programs attract IDUs who are at *lower risk* for HIV infection while *high-risk* IDUs are less likely to participate.

Netherlands— Needle exchange programs are available in 40 municipalities. Data from these programs suggest that the staff operating the needle exchange centers should be multilingual and the centers should be operational 24 hours a day.

Australia— As of March 1990, five states and one territory had needle exchange programs. The remaining state and one jurisdiction may have since joined the program. An evaluation concluded that a substantial number of IDUs have made appropriate changes in their behavior to support the continuation of these programs (Wodak, 1990).

An assessment of Sydney's program in 1989 suggested that some 9 to 12 million needles and syringes a year would have to be distributed to meet the need for sterile equipment. By 1994 the program was distributing around 3 million syringes, and some exchanges in the suburbs of Sydney as well as in the city center were seeing attendances rise by 1,000 clients per month from late 1992.

Italy— Only a few limited exchange programs have been reported. However, between 1983 and 1988, the sale of syringes and needles, which is legal, increased by 50%.

Advocates for and against safe drug use activities present forceful arguments. The major problem is that HIV infection is now increasing rapidly among the IDU population. The proportion of AIDS cases involving adult/adolescent males with a history of homosexual/bisexual activity as the only risk factor decreased from 70% in 1987 to 56% in 1991. But in the same time period, the proportion of AIDS cases in adult/adolescent males with a history of IDU as the only risk factor increased from 14% to 20%. In adult/adolescent single risk female AIDS cases the proportion of IDUs was 49% in 1987 and 49% in 1991. The proportion of AIDS cases in children whose mothers had sexual intercourse with IDUs rose from 11% before 1985 to 21% through 1991 (*MMWR*, 1989b; 1992a).

BLOOD AND BLOOD PRODUCT TRANSMISSION

Blood Donors

There is **no risk** in the United States or in other *developed nations* of contracting HIV by donating blood. Blood centers use a new, sterile needle for *each* donation, yet a 1993 survey revealed that 25% of those polled believed that they could become HIV-infected by donating blood. In Third World nations, it is important to make certain that a new, sterile needle is used before donating blood.

About 8 million people have been donating some 13 million units of blood annually in the United States. Blood can carry HIV in a cell-free state or HIV may be carried within cells of the blood. The amount of virus taken in (dose) and a person's biological susceptibility determines whether infection will occur after HIV exposure. A large dose of HIV received via blood transfusion almost universally results in HIV infection. A small dose of HIV-contaminated blood, such as the blood received by a needlestick seldom results in infection (Francis et al., 1987). The mean volume of blood injected by a needlestick has been calculated to be 1.4 μL (1.4 millionths of a liter). It is difficult to determine exactly how large a viral dose is necessary to cause infection because it is difficult to quantitate virus in humans. However, it is known that infection is more likely to occur if blood is donated close to the time the HIV-infected donor becomes symptomatic. Becoming symptomatic may mean that HIV is being less rapidly neutralized within the body. Through mid-1995, 2% of HIV-infected adults and 12% of HIV-infected children in the United States are believed to have become infected via blood transfusions or by the use of contaminated blood products. The majority of HIV infections occurred prior to the initiation of the blood screening program. To date *only* whole blood, blood cellular components, plasma, and blood clotting factors have been involved in transmitting HIV.

Blood Collection and Blood Screening for HIV

Regardless of whether blood comes from volunteer donors or is purchased, it is now screened for HIV antibodies. If the test indicates that the blood carries antibodies to HIV, it is treated to destroy the HIV and then discarded. Current blood screening procedures have reduced the number of blood transfusion-associated HIV infections.

Blood Screening for HIV— In March of 1983, the major United States blood banking organizations instituted procedures to reduce the likelihood of HIV transmission through blood transfusions. People with signs or symptoms suggestive of HIV disease/AIDS, sexually active homosexual and bisexual men with multiple partners, recent Haitian immigrants to the United States, past or present IDUs, men and women who have engaged in prostitution since 1977 or have patronized a prostitute within the past 6 months, and sexual partners of individuals at increased risk of HIV infection were asked to refrain from donating blood.

In March of 1985, the FDA approved the ELISA test for use in commercial blood banks, plasma centers, and public health clinics to screen blood for antibodies to HIV. This test did not and still does not diagnose AIDS. It merely indicates whether or not a blood donor has been infected with HIV.

All blood that tests positive for antibody to the HIV virus is rejected. This test, in conjunction with current measures to exclude blood donations by members of behavioral high-risk groups, has substantially reduced the chance of transmitting HIV through blood transfusion (ELISA and other test procedures are presented in Chapter 12). The risk of becoming HIV-infected from a blood transfusion has dropped by more than 99% from 1983 to 1991.

BOX 9.3

EXAMPLE OF BLOOD SUPPLY HIV PREVENTION

Testimonial: I'm 56 and have donated over 90 pints of blood. After my last donation, I received a letter that read, in part: "Unfortunately, we can no longer accept you as a donor because there was something in your blood detected in our HIV antibody screening test. . . . However, we did additional testing by a more specific method and the final result was negative for antibody to HIV. . . . It is our policy, based on current federal and state guidelines, not to accept blood donors whose blood has been found to be falsely positive for anti-HIV." (State of California)

Explanation: The first screening test his blood bank used was probably the ELISA test, a quick, relatively cheap screening method that occasionally yields false-positive results (see Chapter 12). Blood that tests positive for HIV in the ELISA test is then put through a more specific test called the Western blot (WB). Even though the WB showed no HIV antibodies in his blood, the blood bank's rules required it to reject his blood—on the theoretical but unlikely possibility that the first test could be right and the second one wrong. This person can request a more specific HIV test that is less likely to give a false-positive result. If that test is negative and he wants to resume blood donations, he can check to see if the blood bank has a donor re-entry program. He will have to wait 6 months and then get negative results on both the ELISA and Western blot tests before being allowed to donate.

Blood Transfusions Worldwide— Ten years after the industrialized world began to screen all blood used in transfusions for HIV, as many as 1 in 10 seropositives in developing countries are still being infected through this route.

A combination of the lack of screening with high levels of infected donors turns transfusion into a form of Russian roulette. A survey carried out by WHO in 1990, for example, showed that centres in Kinshasa, Zaïre, screened fewer than a quarter of blood units for HIV, even though about 5% of donors were HIV-infected. Ending 1994, blood transfusions accounted for 5% to 10% of HIV infections world wide (Butler, 1994).

Problems that Contribute to Transfusion-Associated HIV Infection—

1. Lack of coordination among international agencies (e.g., how to obtain HIV tests, who will supply, who will administer, and so on).
2. Lack of trained staff to use supplies and equipment.
3. Lack of refrigeration to keep supplies.
4. Lack of facilities for testing and counseling.
5. Failure to take local culture into account.

Blood Safety— From 1985 through the end of 1994, over 112 million blood or plasma donations had been screened for HIV antibody in the United States. By excluding those who test HIV-positive and by asking people from high-risk behavior groups not to donate blood, the incidence of HIV transmission from the current blood supply is relatively low. And with faster and more accurate testing procedures now in use, the risk is becoming even lower. **However, the probability or risk of receiving HIV-contaminated blood will never be zero.** The reason a small risk still exists is because some people infected with HIV may donate blood during what is known as the "window period." During that period, a person may be infected with the AIDS virus, but the test can not yet detect the infection. And, the test is not 100% accurate.

In 1991, the CDC estimated the risk of receiving HIV-infected blood at 1 in 39,000 to 1 in 250,000. That is, for every 39,000 to 250,000 units of whole blood used in transfusions, one patient will receive HIV-infected blood. On average, a blood transfusion requires five or more units of whole blood (Pines, 1993). A recent study of 12,000 heart patients who received blood transfusions found the risk to be 1 in 60,000 units (*Wellness Letter*, 1993).

Playing the Odds. For comparison, the odds of dying in a highway accident are 1 in 5,960 in a lifetime of driving. The CDC calculates that, *at worst*, with a risk factor of 1 HIV infection in 39,000 transfusions, there will be about 540 new HIV infections per year. (Eighteen million units of blood transfused each year means that three one thousandths of one percent (.00003%) of the 18 million units of blood are infected or 540 units.) By contrast, the CDC estimates that 10 times the number (5,400) will become infected with hepatitis C, which can be fatal.

BOX 9.4

BLOOD TRANSFUSIONS: A GIFT OF LIFE OR THE CARRIER OF DEATH?

In 1987, a grief-stricken mother wrote an open letter to her neighbors thanking them for their compassion when her oldest son, a hemophiliac, died of AIDS. In 1989, this mother was to experience the loss of her second son to AIDS. He was also a hemophiliac. Her letter was to thank her community for caring for one of its members as a family cares for its child. It was an example of compassion to a nation demonstrating mixed emotions about those with AIDS.

In contrast, vandals burned down the home of Clifford and Cynthia Ray of Arcadia, Florida in 1987. Their three young boys, all hemophiliacs, acquired HIV from blood products used to stop life-threatening bleeding episodes. They also developed AIDS. Unlike the first family's experience, the Rays lost their friends, became the targets of hate mail, received threats of physical violence, were recipients of verbal abuse, and their children were not permitted to attend school. The Desoto County School Board, after threat of lawsuit, offered to let the boys attend class in a portable trailer in isolation from other children. Food would be served using disposable plates, cups, and utensils. The playground and library could be used only when other children were in class. Pickets again marched at the school and verbally abused the Ray family. Finally, their home was burned down and the Rays moved to Sarasota, Florida where the boys were enrolled in school without incident.

Blood Supply Shortages— For over 50 years Americans have been giving blood. But today, subtle trends are altering the nation's ability to provide a safe and adequate blood supply.

Because of HIV infection, fewer people can give blood now than gave in 1980. Today donated blood must pass seven laboratory tests that screen for HIV antibody, HTLV I (the virus associated with tropical spastic paraparesis and some forms of leukemia), Non-A Non-B hepatitis, syphilis, hepatitis B and hepatitis C antigens, and HIV-2.

New screening criteria are reducing the donor pool by 10% to 15%. Many former blood donors, some of whom routinely donated several times each year, are no longer eligible. In addition, some states have outlawed paid blood donations.

Blood banks in New York, Miami, Los Angeles, and San Francisco have, at times, had to issue urgent pleas for blood donations. Recent blood shortages have been the most severe in the nation's history and the situation is expected to get much worse. The reasons for the shortages are: (1) the additional transfusions necessary for the ever increasing number of symptomatic HIV and AIDS patients; (2) the restrictions on who may now donate blood; and (3) the loss of a significant percentage of potential blood donors who still believe they can become HIV-infected by donating blood.

Autologous Transfusions— These are transfusions using "*self*" blood. It has been suggested that the two groups that benefit most from autologous blood storage are: expectant mothers facing Caesarean section and certain elective surgical candidates where substantial loss of blood is anticipated. A person's blood is drawn and refrigerated for transfusion back into his or her own body when needed. (Stored whole blood remains usable for a maximum of 42 days.) This is the safest blood available. A healthy person taking iron supplements can donate one unit of blood a week, generally, for up to 6 weeks. In emergency situations, including some surgeries, it may be necessary to receive another person's blood through transfusion. If a transfusion is necessary to sustain life, the risk of contracting HIV from the transfusion is outweighed by the risk of refusing the transfusion and suffering further consequences from the emergency.

INFECTION CONTROL PROCEDURES

With no cure or vaccine for HIV/AIDS, prevention of infection is of paramount importance. With the advent of the HIV/AIDS epidemic, health care workers and others who are occupationally exposed to body fluids, especially blood, are understandably concerned about the risk of contracting HIV disease/AIDS. However, when precautions are observed, the risk is very small, even for those treating HIV/AIDS patients.

Two sets of infection control procedures are in use in hospitals, medical centers, physicians' offices, and units that deal with people in medical emergencies. One is called universal precautions, the other blood and body substance isolation.

Universal Precautions

Universal precautions (Table 9.6) are standard practices that workers observe on the job to protect themselves from infections and injuries. These precautions or safety practices are called "universal" because they are used in all situations even if there seems to be no risk. Universal precautions had their beginnings in 1976 when barrier techniques were first recommended for the prevention of hepatitis B infection. Precautions required the use of protective eyewear, gloves, and gowns, and careful handling of needles and other sharp instruments. In 1977, hepatitis B immune globulin was recommended for those exposed to hepatitis B through needlesticks. In 1982, hepatitis B vaccine became commercially available and recommended for all health care workers exposed to human blood.

In 1983, the CDC published "Guidelines for Isolation Precautions in Hospitals." It contained a section that recommended specific blood and body fluid precautions to be followed when a patient was known or suspected to be infected with blood-borne pathogens. In 1987, the CDC published "Recommendations for Prevention of HIV Transmission in Health-Care Settings." It recommended that blood and body fluid precautions be consistently

TABLE 9-6 Universal Precautions

Definition

Universal precautions (UP) are a set of infection control practices, developed by the Centers for Disease Control and Prevention (CDC), in which health care workers (HCWs) appropriately utilize barrier protection (gloves, gowns, masks, eyewear, etc.) for anticipated contact with blood and certain body fluids of *all* patients.

1. The hands and skin must be carefully washed when contaminated with blood or certain body fluids.
2. Particular care is taken to prevent injuries caused by sharp instruments.
3. Resuscitation devices should be available where the need is predictable.
4. HCWs with exudative lesions or weeping dermatitis should refrain from patient care until the condition resolves.

Blood and Body Fluids to Which UP Apply

Blood is the single most important risk source of HIV, HBV, and other blood-borne pathogens in the occupational setting. Thus prevention of transmission must focus on reducing the risk of exposure to blood and other body fluids or potentially infectious materials containing visible blood.

1. UP should be used when exposure to the following body fluids may be anticipated:
    a. Blood
    b. Semen
    c. Vaginal secretions
    d. Cerebrospinal fluid (CSF)
    e. Amniotic fluid
    f. Synovial fluid
    g. Pleural fluid
    h. Peritoneal fluid
    i. Pericardial fluid
    j. Any other body fluid containing visible blood (but not feces, urine, saliva, sputum, tears, nasal secretions, or sweat, unless they contain visible blood).
2. Note: Blood, semen, and vaginal secretions have been shown to transmit HIV. The others, with the exception of fluids containing visible blood, remain a theoretical risk.

Rationale

1. UP reduce the risk of parenteral, mucous membrane, and skin exposure to blood-borne pathogens such as, but not limited to, HIV and HBV.
2. For several reasons, focusing precautions only on diagnosed cases misses the vast majority of persons who are infected (many of whom are asymptomatic or subclinical) and who may be as infectious as the diagnosed cases. Persons who have seen a physician and have been diagnosed with acute or active disease represent only a small proportion of all persons with infection. Infectivity always precedes the diagnosis, which often is made once symptoms develop.

(Adapted from Mountain-Plains Regional AIDS Education Training Center. *HIV/AIDS Curriculum,* Nov. 1994.)

followed for all patients regardless of their blood-borne infection status. This extension of blood and body fluid precautions to all patients is referred to as *Universal Precautions.*

Under universal precautions, the blood and certain body fluids of all patients are considered potentially infectious for HIV, hepatitis B virus (HBV), and other blood-borne pathogens.

Universal precautions are intended to prevent parenteral (introduction of a substance into the body by injection), mucous membrane, and broken skin exposure of health care workers (HCWs), teachers, or any other person who may become exposed to blood-borne pathogens. In 1987, the CDC also published a report that got the immediate attention of most, if not all, informed health care workers. The report stated that three health care workers who were exposed to the blood of AIDS patients tested positive for HIV. What was so startling was that until that time, needle punctures and cuts were thought to be the only dangers in a clinical setting. These three cases appeared to involve only skin exposure to HIV-contaminated blood. One of the three cases involved a nurse

BOX 9.5

DOES THE PATIENT HAVE HIV? I CAN'T TELL

Treating disease can be difficult. Dealing with the legal system and the politics of disease can be a conundrum.

Recently, a nurse in California brought charges against a patient after the nurse accidentally cut herself with a contaminated scalpel and subsequently learned that the patient had AIDS. The prosecution based its case on the patient's failure to fully disclose information relevant to her care. The defense case centered on the failure of medical personnel to use **universal precautions** for treating all patients regardless of their health history.

I side with the nurse and so did the Los Angeles jury who convicted the patient of fraud for failing to disclose that she had AIDS.

Yes, **universal precautions** are required for all patients regardless of health history, but the practical fact is that different situations in medicine require different levels of attentiveness. Care for a young man with a simple cough will and should differ from care for a young man who has a cough and mentions he has AIDS and has had pneumocystis pneumonia in the past. In an emergency department, activity levels vary from dull and routine to harried and panicked. If medical personnel put on gloves, gowns, and masks and slowed their activities to the safest pace for every patient, regardless of known or suspected risk, gridlock would result.

Medical history is critical to proper patient care. When a patient comes to a hospital and is unable to provide a detailed history, medical records are often enormously helpful in providing proper treatment. Therefore, I was surprised recently when a new directive was tacked to the bulletin board in one of the emergency departments where I work. It said that a patient's HIV status could not be recorded on the emergency department chart. I can document syphilis, cancer, schizophrenia, or violent or suicidal behavior, which are all pertinent to a patient's history. Such documentation may help other healthcare professionals provide proper care or take "more attentive" precautions. But I cannot document HIV status. I asked why and was told that this was an effort to comply with a new part of the state of California's Health and Safety Code.

I understand the rationale for this directive. Not only do those who are HIV-positive live with the threat of a terminal disease, but they are discriminated against in the workplace and by insurance carriers, even while they are healthy. The state code is an effort to prevent paranoid discrimination. But I believe the effort to preserve a patient's privacy may put healthcare workers at greater risk.

AIDS is a terrible disease, and paranoia about it is rampant., But protecting patient privacy by putting blinders on healthcare workers is not good medicine.

(Reprinted, with permission, from Pollack B. (1994). Does the patient have HIV? I can't tell. *Postgrad Med* 96(3):19. Copyright © 1994 McGraw-Hill Inc.)

Class Discussion: Your Assessment of Dr. Pollack's concerns?

whose chapped and ungloved hands were exposed to an AIDS patient's blood.

The second case involved a nurse who broke a vacuum tube during a routine phlebotomy on an outpatient. The blood splashed on her face and into her mouth. A blood splash was also involved in the third case. The worker's ungloved hands and forearms were exposed to HIV-contaminated blood (Ezzell, 1987).

The importance of these three cases of HIV infection is that they informed health care workers in the most dramatic way that they were all *vulnerable.* In addition to hepatitis and other infections, they could now add the most lethal virus of all to their occupational hazards. Perhaps these three cases produced a fear among health care workers out of proportion to the actual risk of their becoming infected. However, the fear of an individual and the actual reason he or she has for it are very difficult to judge. Although calculations show that the risk of HIV infection after exposure to blood from an HIV/AIDS patient is about one in 200, if you are that one, probability is meaningless. Some health care workers have used, and still use, such data to support their decisions to avoid caring for HIV/AIDS patients.

The universal precautions as published by

BOX 9.6

WHAT TO ASK YOUR DOCTOR

Few health care workers will willingly disclose their HIV status, but the chances of your becoming HIV-infected are slim if HCWs follow standard procedures. Here are a few examples of what to look for:

1. Do the doctors and nurses wear gloves when doing invasive exams, such as dental, vaginal, or rectal exams?
2. Do they use a new set of gloves and freshly disinfected instruments with each patient?
3. Do they routinely wash their hands before seeing every patient?
4. Do all health care workers follow universal precautions, wearing masks, protective eyewear, and gowns in addition to gloves when there's a risk of being sprayed with blood or other body fluids?
5. How often does the clinic or hospital make sure its staff is actually following universal precautions?

the CDC currently apply to some 5.3 million health care workers at 620,000 work sites across the United States and another 700,000 Americans who routinely come in contact with blood as part of their job, for example, people in law enforcement, education, fire fighting and rescue, corrections, laboratory research, and the funeral industry.

In July of 1991, the CDC published an additional set of recommendations. These recommendations are also for preventing the transmission of HIV and hepatitis B virus to patients during exposure-prone procedures.

In summary, the concept of universal precautions assumes that *all* blood is infectious, no matter from whom and no matter whether a test is negative, positive, or not done at all. Rigorous adherence to universal precautions is the surest way of preventing accidental transmission of HIV and other blood-borne pathogens.

Blood and Body Substance Isolation (BBSI)

An alternative, and some believe superior, approach to the CDC's universal precautions in areas of high HIV prevalence is the system referred to as body substance precautions or Blood Body Substance Isolation (BBSI) (Gerberding, 1991).

In practice, these precautions are similar to universal precautions, in that prevention of needlestick injury and use of barrier methods of infection control are emphasized. Philosophically, however, the two are quite different. Whereas universal precautions place a clear emphasis on avoidance of blood-borne infection, body substance precautions take a more global view. Body substance isolation (BSI) requires barrier precautions for *all* body substances (including feces, respiratory secretions, urine, emesis, etc.) and moist body surfaces (including mucous membranes and open wounds). BSI is designed as a system to reduce the risk of transmission of all nosocomial pathogens, not just blood-borne pathogens. Gloves are worn for any anticipated or known contact with mucous membranes, or nonintact skin and moist body substances of all patients.

The degree of contact with the blood and body fluids or tissues of each patient is considered to determine the type of precaution (if any) required. Unlike the CDC system in which precautions are based on the premise that all blood is infectious, body substance precautions are procedure-specific, that is, based on the degree of anticipated contact. Users of the BBSI system find that this approach is actually easier to teach and implement than universal precautions, although the end result is much the same: the prevention of HIV infection.

PARTNER NOTIFICATION

Partner notification, formerly called contact tracing, is the practice of **identifying** and **treating** people exposed to certain communicable diseases. The term *partner notification* is used by the CDC and some health care providers because it more comprehensively describes the process by which the physician, other health care workers such as Disease Intervention Specialists (DIS, someone who is specially trained in STD work), and the infected person may provide information to at- risk partners.

There are two very different approaches to informing unsuspecting third parties about their potential exposure to medical risk.

Each approach has its own history, including a unique set of practical problems in its implementation, and provokes its own ethical dilemmas. The first approach, involving the moral **duty to warn**, arose out of the clinical setting in which the physician knew the identity of the person deemed to be at risk. This approach provided a warrant for disclosure to endangered persons without the consent of the patient and could involve revealing the identity of the patient. The second approach—that of contact tracing— emerged from sexually transmitted disease control programs in which the clinician typically did not know the identity of those who might have been exposed. This approach was founded on the voluntary cooperation of the patient in providing the names of contacts. It never involved the disclosure of the identity of the patient. The entire process of notification was kept confidential (Bayer, 1992).

History of Partner Notification

The concept of partner notification was proposed in 1937 by Surgeon General Thomas Parran for the control of syphilis (Parran, 1937). By tracing and treating all known contacts of a syphilitic patient, the chain of transmission could be interrupted. According to George Rutherford (1988), contact tracing has been successfully used in a number of STDs beginning in the 1950s. It is still used in cases of syphilis, endemic gonorrhea, chlamydia, hepatitis B, STD enteric infections, and particularly in cases of antibiotic-resistant gonorrhea.

In 1985, when the HIV antibody was first used in screening the blood supply, notification of blood donors and other HIV-infected individuals and their contacts became possible. The strategy in HIV partner notification is the same as that used for the other STDs: to identify HIV-infected individuals, counsel them, and offer whatever treatment is available. In asymptomatic HIV-infected people only counseling is given. But, symptomatic HIV-infected patients receive counseling and treatment, if available, for their signs and symptoms. Partner notification depends on HIV-positive people to give the names of their partners; but, they may be reluctant to do so if they fear that their own identities will be revealed and their jobs or housing threatened.

Opposition to Partner Notification for HIV Disease

There is currently wide opposition to partner notification on the grounds that: (1) nothing can be done medically for the HIV-positive asymptomatic person, nor can he or she be segregated from the noninfected population; (2) it is not cost effective; (3) there is little evidence that those who are informed of their infection will do anything about changing the high-risk behaviors that got them infected in the first place; (4) the threat of social discrimination undermines the intent of contact tracing; and (5) in 24 states homosexuality is a crime, and HIV-infected homosexuals fear prosecution if they acknowledge same-sex contacts and be responsible for having their sexual partner(s) prosecuted.

By the end of 1985, five states, Colorado, Idaho, South Carolina, North Carolina, and Virginia, had reported data to the CDC from their partner notification programs. The first four states emphasize provider referral as the best method for notifying sexual and needle-sharing partners of HIV-infected individuals. Virginia provides contact tracing services to HIV-infected patients who **request assistance** with notifying their sexual and needle-sharing partners (*MMWR*, 1988). By the end of 1988, 22 states declared a need for contact tracing. All 50 states are now somewhere in the process of establishing the capacity for contact tracing at the request of a patient (Bayer, 1992).

In Support of Partner Notification

The following discussion is from Stephen J. Josephs' article, "The Once and Future AIDS Epidemic," *Medical Doctor*, 37:92—104. Mr. Joseph is the past Commissioner of Health of New York City, 1986–1990.

POINT OF VIEW 9.2

PRO AND CON OF PARTNER NOTIFICATION

CON: HIV testing and contact tracing or partner notification amount to a cruel hoax. A gay representative of Act Up Now from the West Coast said, "There are not enough beds to take care of known AIDS patients. Why identify more?"

PRO: Amitai Etzioni (1993) said that "testing is cruel only in a world where captains of sinking ships do not warn passengers because the captains cannot get off. We must marshall the moral courage to tell those infected with HIV: It is truly tragic that currently we have no way to save your life, but surely you recognize your duty to try to help save the lives of others."

CON: Telling others that you are HIV positive is unnecessary because everybody **should** behave safely **all the time**.

PRO: Collective data indicate that most people will not act safely all the time. Warning people that they are about to enter a highly dangerous situation may help them take special precautions. The moral duty of those already infected is clear. They must not become intimate without prior disclosure. Not to do so is like serving poisoned candy. Not informing previous contacts (or not helping public authorities trace them without disclosing your name) leaves them, unwittingly, to transmit the virus to others.

CON: Testing and partner notification may lead to a person's being deprived of a job, health insurance, housing and privacy, and many other types of discrimination.

PRO: This is true today, but ways must be found to protect civil rights without sacrificing public health. It may seem mean spirited but the fact that an individual may suffer as a result of doing what is right does not make doing so less of an imperative. Recognize that the first victims of nondisclosure are the loved ones of those already infected with HIV, in the case of infected women—their children.

CON: It is not cost effective to trace sexual partners of HIV-infected persons.

PRO: A nonclinic HIV test costs, on average, between \$60 and \$70 (most HIV/AIDS clinic HIV/AIDS tests are free). Etzioni (1993) estimates that if those who were HIV-positive were to transmit the disease to only one less person on average, the suggested tests would pay for themselves much more readily than various surgical operations like coronary bypasses, and so forth. Etzioni states that there are many other excesses and rationalizations being put forth to prevent HIV partner notification programs. But, he says, "If AIDS were any other disease—say, hepatitis B or tuberculosis—we would have no trouble (and indeed we have had none) introducing the necessary preventive measures. Moreover, we should make it clear that doing all you can to prevent the spread of AIDS or any other fatal disease is part and parcel of an unambiguous commandment: Thou shalt not kill."

Whose side do you favor in this discussion? What are your reasons? (class discussion)

The New York City Medical Examiner looked at a large sample of dead persons who were tested postmortem and found to be HIV-positive, but who had no notification in their medical records of having been diagnosed as infected. Over 35% of those persons had a readily identifiable spouse or steady sexual partner. Josephs asks,

How can one justify, on clinical, public health or humanitarian grounds, *not* notifying that surviving partner, who might be the source of the infection in the deceased, or the recipient of infection? Arguments against this procedure border on the absurd; one has to start with the premise that increased medical knowledge is more dangerous than helpful to the individual, and that the rights of the uninfected count for nothing against the rights of the infected.

Josephs states that vigorous contact tracing, under conditions of strict public health confidentiality, is the most important step we can now take to reduce the further progress of the HIV virus, and to protect those who, unsuspecting, are at greatest risk of infection or in greatest need of early medical management.

What is you response to Stepen Joseph's point of view on partner notification?

HIV VACCINE DEVELOPMENT

What the World Needs NOW Is a Vaccine for HIV Disease—Why Isn't There One?

On April 24, 1984, Margaret M. Heckler, who was then Secretary of the Department of Health and Human Services, announced the discovery of the AIDS virus. She predicted an AIDS vaccine within 2 years. Even though the prediction proved wrong, research has remained guided by the idea that finding the virus was the hard part, and vaccines could be made by simply injecting people with crucial viral proteins. Her optimism was most likely based on the success of the polio, measles, and flu vaccines. The approach to combating these diseases was: isolate the virus, develop a vaccine, and prevent the disease!

Vaccines are designed to provoke the immune system into making antibodies against a disease-causing agent. Most are made of killed or attenuated (genetically weakened) viruses and, in the case of some newer vaccines, extracts of viral coat proteins. In some cases, vaccination may result in worsening the disease. The distinction between protective, useless, and dangerous responses is essential for vaccine design.

POINT OF VIEW 9.3

THE GOAL OF DEVELOPING AN HIV VACCINE

The ideal HIV vaccine would eradicate HIV infection. But ideals are seldom realized in biology and this ideal in particular does not seem likely. For all of the infectious agent vaccines that have been marketed, *only smallpox* has been eradicated!

For an infectious agent to be a good candidate for eradication, several conditions must exist. The most important of these are: (1) that only humans are affected, (2) that infection is easily recognized, and (3) that infected persons do not remain asymptomatic for long periods of time. HIV meets only the first of these conditions, and even this is questionable as it may have mutated from closely related monkey viruses. Thus a realistic HIV vaccine goal would be to develop candidate vaccines that demonstrate some percent of efficacy, with fewest side effects, and begin their distribution. Saving some lives is better than a complete loss. Because there are an increasing number of HIV strains evolving, no one vaccine is expected to be effective in everyone.

Large-scale human HIV preventive vaccine trials are scheduled to begin in San Francisco by the end of 1995. Any successful preventive vaccine found during this study would take about 5 years to reach wide scale distribution. Therapeutic vaccines may be further off than that. Studies on pediatric vaccines are in progress.

In 1984, Mrs. Margaret Heckler, then the U.S. Secretary of Health and Human Services, spoke convincingly of the immediate production of an HIV vaccine. Is it surprising that both the scientists and public are disappointed with this work to date?

The ideal HIV vaccine has to be safe, orally administered, single dose, stable, inexpensive, confer permanent life-time immunity, and be effective against all HIV strains. This is an unrealistic expectation, at least in the next 10 to 20 years.

Vaccines that work well are the most cost-effective medical invention known to prevent disease. A vaccine is a suspension of whole microorganisms, or viruses, or a suspension of some structural component or product of them that will elicit an immune response after entering a host. In brief, vaccines mimic the organisms or virus that cause disease, alerting the immune system to be aware of certain viruses or bacteria. Because of this advance warning system, when the real organism or virus invades the body, the immune system marshals a response before the disease has time to develop.

Ideally, the body will make antibodies that bind to and disable the foreign invader (humoral immunity) and trigger white blood cells called T cells to attack cells in the body that have been infected by viruses (cellular immunity). Once the immune system's T cells and B cells, which make antibodies, are activated, some of them turn into **memory cells.** The more memory cells the body forms, the faster its response to a future infection.

Vaccines can trigger these responses in three ways. Some vaccines, such as those against smallpox, measles, and tuberculosis, contain genetically altered or weakened (attenuated) organisms or viruses that are reproduced in the body after being administered but do not generally produce disease. Yet since the virus or bacterium is still alive, there is a small risk of developing the disease.

Whooping cough, cholera, and influenza vaccines are made of inactivated (killed) whole organisms and virus or pieces of them. Because killed organisms and virus do not replicate inside the recipient, the vaccines confer only humoral immunity, which may be short-lived.

Finally, vaccines can be made against toxic products produced by microorganisms. In diseases like tetanus, it is not the bacteria that kill, but the toxins they release into the bloodstream (Christensen, 1994a).

An effective vaccine usually blocks viral entry into a cell. But vaccines are generally not 100% effective. Because HIV, once inside the cell, is capable of integrating itself into the genetic material of infected cells, a vaccine would have to produce a constant state of immune protection, which not only would have to block viral entry to most cells, but also would continue to block newly produced viruses over the lifetime of the infected person. Such complete and constant protection has never before been accomplished. But, perhaps more pertinent explanations for why there is still no HIV vaccine nor is one likely to be available soon are the facts that scientists lack sufficient understanding of HIV infection, the virus rapidly develops mutant strains, and the biology of HIV disease/AIDS is very complex.

Scientists know that the body defends itself against HIV in the early years of infection. But the great mystery has always been why it cannot neutralize HIV completely. One possibility is that the body has trouble seeing all of the variant viruses. Like a Stealth fighter plane, some HIV may have hidden parts that do not show up on the immune system scanner. As a result, the immune system may not produce the right kind of antibody to neutralize all the variant HIVs.

Types of HIV Vaccines

Scientists are attempting to design three types of vaccines: (1) a **preventive** or **prophylactic vaccine** to protect people from becoming HIV-infected, analogous to classic virus vaccines such as those for measles and polio; (2) a **therapeutic vaccine** for those who are already infected with HIV to prevent them from progressing to AIDS (with recent findings that within days of infection massive quantities of HIV has seeded the lymph nodes, a therapeutic vaccine may be too little, too late); and (3) a **perinatal vaccine** for administration to pregnant HIV-infected women to prevent transmission of the virus to the fetus. Stephen Straus and co-workers (1994) reported that researchers have developed a therapeutic vaccine for the herpes virus. The new, therapeutic vaccine reduces the frequency with which genital sores appear in patients infected with the herpesvirus. While it fails to outperform the existing antiherpes drug, acyclovir, it sets the stage for a more effective treatment in the future. Over 25 million people in the United States are infected with the herpes virus, which stays in the body for life.

The ability to influence the frequency of genital herpres outbreaks with this vaccine inspires optimism that similar successes may be possible with other chronic viral diseases, such as AIDS.

Scientists are confronted with a number of perplexing problems (Table 9-7). One is that people infected with HIV develop antibodies that inactivate the virus in clinical laboratory

TABLE 9-7 Problems with Vaccine Development Against HIV

1. HIV integrates its genetic material into cellular DNA.
2. Regulatory genes are responsible for controlled, low-level viral expression.
3. Cells of the immune system serve as both targets of viral infection and vehicles of immune protection.
4. Mimicry between viral envelope proteins and MHC II (HLA) molecules.
5. Rapid rate of HIV mutations.
6. HIV antigens may act as decoys to antibody-producing cells.
7. Viral envelope proteins are poor antigens due to high carbohydrate content.
8. HIV rapidly sheds its viral envelope glycoproteins.
9. Cell-to-cell fusion may result in transmission of HIV RNA without complete assembly of virus particles.
10. Presence of HIV antibody may induce viral latency.
11. Vaccines have not been developed for any lentiviral infections.
12. The need to maintain a constant level of protective immune activation in the face of an immune system suppressor network.

(Adapted from Peter Nara, *Los Alamos Science,* 1989)

tests, yet they become sick and die anyway. Why don't these patients' antibodies work against the virus? Researchers are in the difficult position of trying to design a vaccine without even knowing what kinds of immune responses will protect a person from HIV infection. This uncertainty has prompted some researchers to question whether a protein from HIV or the entire virus should be used to make a vaccine.

Recent reports by David Ho (1995) and Xiping Wei (1995) state that HIV and the immune system engage in a desperate struggle of survival that begins with HIV infection. From early on, a billion or more new viruses are released each day into the bloodstream and a billion or more white blood cells die each day in the battle to keep the infection under control. The body, in the meantime, attempts to replace the billion white blood cells lost each day. The virus wins, in the end, because it has an edge in the fight. This edge is not yet completely understood. But, an important component of that "edge" has to be the ability of HIV to mutate, i.e., to produce immune and drug-resistant variants within the first 2 to 4 weeks after infection.

VACCINE PRODUCTION

To make vaccines, scientists use either **dead microorganisms** and **inactivated viruses** or **attenuated viruses** and **microorganisms**. Attenuated means that viruses and other microorganisms are modified; they are capable of reproducing and invoking the immune response but lack the ability to cause a disease.

Attenuated Viruses

Attenuated viruses in vaccines provide a better immunity than inactivated viruses because attenuated viruses continue to reproduce, thereby acting as a constant source of antigenic stimulus to the immune system. Thus attenuated vaccines appear to provide lifelong immunity *without* requiring periodic boosters. One of the major concerns with using attenuated virus vaccine is the fear that the virus may mutate back to the virulent form. This is why attenuated HIV is not used in government-sponsored experimental vaccine preparations. There is, however, an equally great fear that has not received proper attention; that is, no one knows the long-term consequences of having an attenuated retrovirus (HIV) inside the body for 20 to 50 years. Such viruses inserted into human DNA may turn genes off and on at the wrong time causing cancer and other types of disease.

Inactivated Viruses

To inactivate viruses for use in vaccines, the viruses are treated with formalin or another chemical. There is a danger in using inactivated viruses—they may not all be inactivated. Inactivated virus vaccines have been made against hepatitis B, rabies, influenza, and polio (Salk vaccine). The Salk vaccine, which has not yet been known to cause a single case of polio, *is given by injection* and therefore accounts for less than 1% of polio vaccine doses per year in the United States.

Jonas Salk announced at the Fifth International Conference on AIDS (1989) the development of a new HIV vaccine. He used gamma radiation to destroy the virulence of HIVs and stripped them of their outer envelope. Salk's vaccine was injected into three chimpanzees. After reasonable success in protecting the chimpanzees, Salk asked for and received permission to inject volunteer priests and nuns over age 65 with his vaccine. The project was suspended in 1993, as there were little if any observable beneficial effects of his vaccine, e.g., specific neutralizing antibody to HIV was not found.

ROLE OF GENETIC DIVERSITY IN VACCINE DEVELOPMENT

Genetic diversity, or the production of HIV variants, is a major problem in vaccine development. In 1988, Robert Gallo, a leader in HIV research, reported that *every* HIV isolate has been different. Even sequential HIV isolates from the same patient differ and demonstrate different susceptibilities to a standard neutralizing antibody. The problem can be underscored by a report from Gallo's laboratory that even a *single amino acid* change in the HIV envelope can result in a virus that resists the same neutralization antibodies that had previously neutralized parent HIV. Further, it has been reported that at least 25% of the amino acids in HIV envelope protein are subject to change at any time during the production of HIV.

Subunit Vaccines

Subunit vaccines are made from antigenic fragments of an organism or virus most suitable for evoking a strong immune response. The genetic code for producing particular components, such as proteins found in the HIV envelope, an internal core protein, or the reverse transcriptase enzyme, can be genetically engineered in a bacterium, fungus (yeast) or another virus. These subunits can then be mass produced and used in pure form to make a specific vaccine. Vaccine against hepatitis B is made from a subunit of the hepatitis B virus produced in quantity in yeast.

In the United States, researchers are currently basing their vaccine strategies on the use of proteins found in the envelope of HIV (Goldsmith, 1991).

PROBLEMS IN THE SEARCH FOR HIV VACCINE

This virus poses some unique problems for making a human vaccine. *First,* scientists have not established what immune responses are crucial for protecting the body against HIV infection. Without this information, they cannot tailor the vaccine to produce those particular responses. This question is complicated by the fact that it is too risky to use the entire weakened or inactive HIV, as was done to make vaccines for less deadly viruses such as polio or measles. Most HIV vaccine development is focusing on using parts of the virus to ensure that it cannot replicate when it is introduced into a human host. This strategy applies genetic engineering to synthesize a piece of the virus in hopes that this piece alone will produce an immune response that will prevent HIV infection. So far, scientists have successfully used this approach only once, to develop the hepatitis B vaccine.

Second, HIV undergoes a high rate of mutation as it replicates, and strains from different parts of the world vary by as much as 35% in terms of the proteins that comprise the outer coat of the virus. Even within an infected individual, over a period of years, the virus may change its proteins by as much as 10%. This degree of antigenic drift or variation means that a vaccine made from one strain of HIV may not protect against a different strain. While it may be possible to design a vaccine to protect against multiple strains, all current vaccines are based on single strains. To prove their effectiveness, these vaccines may have to be tested in geographic areas where the prevalent strains are the same as the strain used in the vaccine.

Third, the immune response raised by the vaccine may be protective for only a short period of time. In such cases, booster vaccinations would be required too frequently to be practical. For all of these reasons, scientists think that current HIV vaccine candidates are likely to be, at best, only partly effective: they may protect only a proportion of those who get vaccinated or only for limited periods of time, or only against certain HIV strains (Osmond, 1992).

Fourth, it is possible that the vaccine may make people more susceptible to HIV infection.

Fifth, Jon Cohen, writing for the journal *Science* (1994a) reported on a *Science* survey of an international sample of over 100 of the field's leading researchers, public health officials, and manufacturers. All told, 67 people from 18 countries on six continents reponded. And when it came to describing the obstacles that hinder vaccine development, the respondents—be they from Russia, Indonesia, Egypt, Europe, India, or Brazil—had remarkably similar views. The scientific uknowns are the highest hurdles, they said, but they also stressed that the field lacks the strong leadership and funding to speed progress.

Predictably, money—or rather, lack of it—was one of the most frequently mentioned obstacles. Even though vaccines are among the most cost-effective medical interventions ever devised, they are not big money-markers.

In 1990, AIDS researchers and stock analysts hailed Repligen Corp., A Massachusetts biotechnology firm, as a leader—many said *the* leader—in the race to develop a vaccine against HIV. Not only was Repligen collaborating with top AIDS researchers and publishing impressive scientific papers, the startup had won financial backing from pharmaceutical giant Merck & Co. A 1990 investors' guide from Shearson Lehman Hutton predicted that if human tests of the vaccine went well, Repligen and Merck might ask the U.S. Food and Drug Administration to license it as early as the end of 1994.

Fast forward to July 19, 1994. On that day, Repligen announced that, because of a "lack of available funding," it was axing its HIV vaccine research and development program.

Economics clearly isn't the only factor that is discouraging companies from entering the search for an AIDS vaccine. Another is the fact that the science is very tough. Animal models used to test AIDS vaccines have severe limitations; the genetic diversity of HIV may require an effective vaccine to be based on many viral strains; and no researcher has successfully demonstrated which immune responses correlate with protection from HIV (Cohen, 1994b.)

POINT OF INFORMATION 9.3

PATHOLOGICAL UNIQUENESS OF HIV

There has been much written about the uniqueness of HIV. Perhaps the most singular feature is that it is lethal to humans. A national state of immunity has not yet been documented in humans. Once infected with HIV, there is a high probability of death within 10 to 15 years.

Most human pathological viruses, including HIV, behave in a somewhat similar fashion with one important exception. Other viruses, including all of the other sexually transmitted viruses, enter cells, cause cell lysis, and remain in the body. The body "learns" to live with viral infections, latent periods, and recurrent episodes. But HIV is different: it infects and suppresses an immune system that holds other viral infections in check. Perhaps it is because we survive these other viral infections that there has not been the urgency to learn more about host response to viruses: how viruses actually infect cells, become proviruses, and are activated to reproduce. There is not even a respectable spectrum of antiviral drugs available, mostly because we do not know enough about the viruses.

There are vaccines available for smallpox, polio, measles, mumps, yellow fever, rubella, rabies, and influenza; but, only one vaccine—hepatitis B is available for a sexually transmitted viral disease. And, only one vaccine has ever eradicated a human disease, the smallpox vaccine.

Use of Whole Inactivated HIV: A Vaccine-Induced Enhancement of HIV Infection

Whole inactivated viruses are believed to be unsuitable for vaccine production because: (1) one cannot be 100% certain that every HIV is inactivated, and (2) the envelope surrounding HIV may prevent the production of suitable antibodies. The best reason not to use whole HIV, however, may be the possibility of **vaccine-induced enhancement** of disease. It has been shown by a number of investigators that some HIV antibodies actually help HIV enter host cells, primarily monocyte cells (Koff, 1988). This phenomenon is called **antibody-enhanced infectivity**. Antibodies that enhance HIV infectivity have been identified in the serum of HIV-infected patients and in HIV-infected and immunized animals.

The viral antigens responsible for the enhancement phenomenon must be identified and removed before a vaccine is made; otherwise there would be an increased risk of HIV infection following vaccination (Homsy et al., 1989; Levy, 1989).

BOX 9.7

RETHINKING "STERILIZING IMMUNITY"

Since the AIDS virus was first isolated, HIV/AIDS immunologists have been searching for a vaccine that can completely prevent HIV infection. Vaccine researchers feared that if even a single HIV particle infected a cell, it might ultimately lead to AIDS. So the only safe course was to create a vaccine that blocked infection completely, producing so-called **"Sterilizing Immunity."** The usual means for developing such a vaccine has historically been monkey experiments using SIV, the simian cousin of HIV. But monkey studies with disappointing results forced researchers to rethink this all-or-nothing strategy. Immunologists now point to a phenomenon that, just a few years ago, seemed implausible: the immune system does have some capacity to contain infection with the AIDS virus. Therefore, even a vaccine that fails to deliver sterilizing immunity should still be able to delay or prevent disease. As a result of this new thinking, prevention of symptoms, rather than sterilizing immunity, is being considered as a hallmark of vaccine success.

Staging a trial with a disease as a clinical end point would probably require several years—and tens of thousands of people—to arrive at a statistically meaningful answer. And that makes it tough, since retaining people in a vaccine trial for more than a few years is difficult, and the costs of running multiyear tests is astronomical. A trial with infection as an end point might take as little as 3 years and require fewer than 3,500 people (Cohen, 1993).

The Use of the Tuberculosis Vaccine: It Is Not 100% Effective

In spite of conflicting evidence of its ability to prevent infection, the tuberculosis (TB) vaccine is, surprisingly, the most widely used vaccine in the world. Its rise to prominence began in 1908, when Albert Calmette and Camille Guérin at the Pasteur Institute in Paris developed a weakened strain of a bacterium that causes TB in both cows and humans. They first tested this vaccine in people in 1921; since then, more than 3 billion people have received the BCG (bacille Calmette-Guérin) vaccine.

Although BCG is recommended by the World Health Organization's Expanded Program on Immunization, doubts about its effectiveness remain. Some clinical trials have shown it to protect 80% of those vaccinated; others have found it to offer no protection at all. Numerous theories have been proposed to explain these conflicting results, including the possibility of subtle differences in the BCG vaccines used.

The relatively low incidence of TB in the United States, coupled with uncertainties about the effectiveness of the BCG vaccine, has led the U.S. Public Health Service to recommend TB testing and drug therapy for those infected, rather than vaccination. But TB cases are on the rise, and the spread of the hard-to-treat multidrug-resistant tuberculosis (MDR TB) has encouraged the Centers for Disease Control and Prevention (CDC) to take another look at BCG.

The CDC sponsored a review of 14 prospective trials and 12 case-control studies of the BCG vaccine. After analyzing these studies, it was concluded that the vaccine protected just over half of those inoculated.

It's on the lower end of efficacy for a vaccine, but it still provides protection for some people. BCG is effective and should be considered for use in the United States (Christensen, 1994b).

It can be argued that regardless of whether BCG is 80% or less than 50% effective, it is a better treatment then treating drug-resistant TB with an ineffective drug.

Testing HIV Vaccines

Whether a vaccine will stimulate antibody production and is *safe* can be easily determined. It will not require a long time nor will it require many volunteers. But to gauge a vaccine's *efficacy* will require a large number of volunteers who are free of HIV but in danger of becoming infected with it (members of behavioral high risk groups). To determine a vaccine's efficacy, two large groups of subjects are selected, one that receives the vaccine and one that receives a placebo, to see whether the vaccinated group has a lower rate of HIV infection. In carrying out efficacy trials, the number of participants, the length of the follow-up period, the rate of HIV infection, and the presumed efficacy of the vaccine are related to each other. Because the rate of HIV infection is low, even in "high-risk" populations, researchers estimate they will need to study several thousand participants to determine whether an HIV vaccine is effective. The original polio vaccine trial was completed in a year but required nearly half a million children.

An important variable in determining the parameters of the trial is whether the vaccine is prophylactic or therapeutic. If the vaccine actually prevents infection, the trial will measure the rate at which participants develop HIV antibodies. If, however, the vaccine allows infection but prevents or greatly retards disease progression, the trial will measure the rate at which disease develops and will therefore require many more years of follow-up.

Morality of Testing HIV Vaccines

The greater the number of volunteers who are exposed to HIV, the faster investigators will learn whether the vaccine works. But researchers carrying out the trials have a moral obligation to inform, educate, and counsel the volunteers against high-risk behavior that might expose them to the AIDS virus. Thus researchers will be in the paradoxical position of recommending safer sex guidelines while recognizing that an adequate test of a vaccine will require that some participants ignore those guidelines. There is also the additional problem of creating **vaccine** HIV-positive persons who can not be distinguished from those who are naturally HIV-infected. They, too, will be subjected to adverse social, employment, and other discrimination following a positive antibody test.

Having to use volunteers from high behavioral risk groups, such as gay men, prostitutes, and injection drug users—assuming a sufficient number could be recruited—presents its own set of complications. It will be necessary for investigators to keep track of volunteers for as long as 5 years and to be informed of their drug and sexual practices during this time. This may be extremely difficult, considering that the same volunteers will be engaged in illegal activities.

Partners and spouses of AIDS-infected hemophiliacs are at high risk of acquiring infection and would be excellent as vaccine volunteers, but their limited numbers diminish the prospect of evaluating vaccines in this population. There is the possibility of testing an HIV vaccine overseas—particularly in Africa, which has a significant AIDS problem.

HIV Vaccine Costs

Perhaps the most difficult moral question is the cost of the vaccine. A successful vaccine that sells for a high price will be of little use to poor and uninsured Americans and most people of developing nations, who have no more than a few dollars a year to spend on health care. Nine years have passed since the discovery of a vaccine for hepatitis B, a viral disease that is also spread by sexual contact and the sharing of hypodermic needles. But the product has yet to reach many poor people in the United States and Third World countries largely because it costs more than $120 for a series of three injections. Polio and measles vaccines are relatively cheap but are still not in universal use and they have been available for decades!

HUMAN HIV VACCINE TRIALS

The basic principle behind human vaccine trials has changed little since the 19th century. To test for an HIV/AIDS vaccine, several thousand people at high risk for the disease will be inoculated with the experimental agent, most likely an altered version of HIV or some portion of it. The vaccine should not be dangerous enough to cause the disease, but enough like HIV to confer immunity by triggering the production of antibodies and other virus-fighting components of the immune system. The subjects in the trial will be carefully monitored to see if they have a better rate of avoiding infection than others who were not vaccinated.

In 1994, there were at least 15 candidate HIV Prophylactic vaccines and 10 therapeutic vaccines in phase I or II clinical trials in Europe and North America (Lurie et al., 1994). As of early 1995, no vaccine has been tested in a phase III trial.

In June of 1994 the National Institutes of Health delayed human testing of two of its most promising vaccines until sometime in 1995 because of insufficient efficacy and safety data.

The two candidate vaccines had not been formally tested for efficacy. During phase I and II vaccine studies, 8 of 1,400 volunteers became HIV-positive. Thus NIH concluded that the vaccine was unlikely to be effective enough to make the 4,500-person trial worthwhile. The phase 3 efficacy trial was to involve 9,000 people. Using this large number of people was to show whether the vaccines were more than 60% effective or less than 30% effective. A larger follow-up would be required if their effectiveness was between those levels. (Belshe et al., 1994; Macilwain, 1994). Regardless of the United States decision of not to begin vaccine trials, the world Health Organization, in October, 1994, recommended large-scale trials of HIV vaccines moved forward. One of the first candidate country for the vaccine experiments in Thailand. These trials are set to begin sometime in 1995. Data from these trials will not be available for some 7 years. (HIV vaccines Get Green Light for Third World Trials, 1994; Weniger, 1994).

Liability Is a Major Hurdle in Vaccine Development

Jon Cohen (1992) states that some pharmaceutical and biotechnical companies are very concerned about potential damage suits by injured trial subjects. Some companies have stopped their HIV vaccine development work due to the fear of liability. Given our litigious society, concerns of product liability are slowing the progress in vaccine research.

In 1986, the National Childhood Vaccine Injury Compensation Act was passed by Congress. The act was made necessary because of the large number of liability cases that arose from the vaccines for polio, diphtheria-tetanus-pertussis, and swine flu. This act allowed for the reward of victims *without* punishing the vaccine manufacturers. HIV/ AIDS vaccine manufacturers are *not* covered by this act because this *no fault* program was designed to include *only childhood vaccines.* Vaccine manufacturers are asking Congress for similar adult/adolescent vaccine liability protection. The World Health Organization, which plans to begin efficacy trials in four countries in 1995, is currently analyzing the liability issue and expects to find potential solutions by early 1995.

Vaccine Testing Confidentiality

Confidentiality must be maintained for the duration of the vaccine trials because people immunized with candidate AIDS vaccines who mount effective immune responses will appear positive for HIV antibody. They may be subject to the social stigma and discrimination associated with being truly HIV-positive.

Vaccine-induced seroconversion may lead to difficulties in donating blood, obtaining insurance, traveling internationally, or entering the military. Vaccine-induced antibodies may be long-lived, thus volunteers in AIDS vaccine trials must be given some form of documentation that certifies that their antibody status is due to vaccination and not HIV infection. The National Institute of Allergy and Infectious Disease has recently (1993) provided a tamper-proof identification card to help uninfected participants in vaccine trials. The seroconversion issue may play a major role in recruitment efforts and in the future welfare of vaccine trial participants (Koff, 1988). So the question for anyone is: **Should I enter an HIV vaccine trial when I know safeguards are limited?** I know why I ought to do it...but! (Class discussion)

Is an Effective Vaccine Enough to Stop HIV Disease/AIDS?

Data from the San Francisco Young Mens Health Study, which is an HIV transmission study of young gay men, suggests that it is very unlikely that effective vaccines alone will eradicate HIV in San Francisco. Sally Blower and colleagues (1994) suggest that an effective vaccine could cause a sharp *increase* in new HIV infections because of the false sense of security it may create causing people to take greater risks. Their work suggests that risk behavior change and mass vaccination would have to occur together.

Finally, the question: Have AIDS prevention programs produced long-term behavior change?

Kyung-Hee Choi and colleagues (1994) state unequivocally that current AIDS prevention programs have produced long-term behavior changes. In their study they critically review the scientific literature on AIDS prevention programs in an attempt to determine the extent to which behavioral intervention research has demonstrated the efficacy of methods for reducing risk behaviors. They focused on the three most critical questions in intervention research: (1) have AIDS prevention programs had long-term success in behavior change; (2) what recommendations can be made to program developers; and (3) where should HIV prevention research be heading. They reviewed published abstracts, journal articles, and other reports that formally evaluated intervention programs aimed at changing HIV risk behavior. They selected evaluation research on HIV testing and counseling since August 1991, because Higgins and colleagues (1991) provided critical evaluations of relevant materials presented or published up to July 1991. Intervention studies reviewed were divided by AIDS risk or intervention target groups (gay or bisexual men, IDU, heterosexuals, young adults, and adolescents) and treatment units (individual, group, organization, or community) or implementation settings (clinic, school). Each intervention was summarized in terms of its content, duration, intensity and impact, and was assessed according to methodologic strength (inclusion of comparison groups, subject self-selection, sample attrition, analysis of secular trend). The report by Choi and Coates is recommended reading for those wanting greater detail on the question of whether HIV/AIDS prevention programs are working and what else can be done.

SUMMARY

The key to stopping HIV transmission lies with the behavior of the individual. That behavior, if the experience of the past 14 years can be used as an indicator, has proven to be very difficult to change.

Changing sexual behavior and using a condom is referred to as *safer* sex. The latex condom is the only condom believed to stop the passage of HIV; and a spermicide should be used with the condom. Oil-based lubricants must not be used because they weaken the condom, allowing it to leak or break under stress. Water-based lubricants are available and should be used. There is at least one female condom, called a vaginal pouch, approved by the FDA. It is inserted like a diaphragm. It offers protection to both sexual partners.

Many cases of HIV infection have come from contaminated blood transfusions. A test developed in 1985 to screen all donated blood in the United States has reduced the risk of HIV transfusion infection. But blood bank screening has reduced the size of the blood donor pool. Many hospitals are encouraging people who know they might need an operation to donate their own blood for later use—autologous transfusion.

To date there is no FDA-approved vaccine for pre- or post-HIV infection. Scientists have ruled out the possibility of an attenuated HIV vaccine because HIV may mutate to a virulent form once injected into the body. Inactivated whole virus vaccines are also being held back because there is no 100% guarantee that all HIV used in the vaccine will be inactivated.

Even if a vaccine is developed, will it be effective against all of the HIV mutants in the HIV gene pool? Can the threat of vaccine-induced enhancement of HIV infection be overcome? Will an animal model be developed that will allow investigators to study each step of the HIV infection process so that a proper therapy can be designed? How are vaccine testing agencies going to handle the ethical question of vaccine seroconverting normal subjects to positive antibody status? The social repercussions will be devastating for those who, when tested, test HIV-positive even though they are HIV free.

There are some 5.3 million health care workers in the United States. It is crucial that they adhere to the Universal Protection Guidelines set down by the CDC, as a significant number of them are exposed to the AIDS virus annually. The risk of HIV infection after exposure to HIV-contaminated blood is about 1 in 200.

A few states have implemented HIV-partner notification; many other states are beginning to experiment with HIV-partner notification or contact tracing programs. It is too early to tell just how successful locating and testing high behavioral risk partners will be, or the cost-to-benefit ratio. One thing is certain; if these programs are to be successful, they will have to ensure confidentiality to those who are traced. Partner notification or contact tracing continues to work well for other sexually transmitted diseases.

REVIEW QUESTIONS

(Answers to the Review Questions are on page 480.)

1. Which is the better condom for protection from STDs, one made from lamb intestine or one made from latex rubber? Explain.
2. Which lubricant is best suited for condom use? Explain.
3. Briefly explain safer sex.
4. True or False: If a person has unprotected intercourse with an HIV-infected partner, he or she will become HIV-infected. Explain.
5. Yes or No: If injection drug users (IDUs) were given free equipment—no questions asked—would that stop the transmission of HIV among them? Explain.
6. What is the current risk of being transfused with HIV-contaminated blood in the United States?
7. What do you think should happen in cases where a person who knows he or she is HIV-positive, lies at a donor interview, and donates blood?
8. Why do most scientists wish to avoid using an attenuated HIV vaccine or an inactivated HIV vaccine?
9. What is the advantage of using recombinant HIV subunits in making a vaccine?
10. Explain vaccine-induced enhancement. How does it occur?
11. Why is it necessary to practice strict confidentiality with respect to volunteers for AIDS vaccine tests?
12. What are universal precautions? Who formulated them?
13. True or False: Research continues to show that AIDS prevention messages are effective in causing teens to change their sexual behaviors.
14. True or False: Latex condoms eliminate the risk of HIV transmission.
15. True or False: Partner notification is usually performed by the infected individual or a trained and authorized health department official.
16. True or False: The Centers for Disease Control and Prevention estimates that as many as 1 in 100,000 units of blood in the blood supply may be contaminated with HIV.
17. True or False: The three types of vaccines that scientists are interested in developing are preventive, therapeutic, and perinatal vaccines.
18. True or False: Used disposable needles should be recapped by hand before disposal.
19. True or False: Prompt washing of a needlestick injury with soap and water is sufficient to prevent HIV infection.

REFERENCES

AMORTEGUI, A.J., et al. (1984). The effects of chemical intravaginal contraceptives and betadine on *Ureaplasma urealyticum*. *Contraception,* 30: 35–40.

ANDERSON, FRANK W.J . (1993). Condoms: A technical guide. *Female Patient,* 18:21–26.

BARBER, HUGH R.K. (1990). Condoms (not diamonds) are a Girl's best friend. *Female Patient,* 15:14–16.

BAYER, RONALD et al. (1992). HIV Prevention and the two faces of partner notification. *Am. J. Public Health,* 82:1158–1164.

BAYER, RONALD, et al. (1993). AIDS and the limits of control: Public health orders, quarantine and recalcitrant behavior. *Am. J. Public Health,* 83:1471–1476.

BELSHE, ROBERT, et al.(1994). HIV infection in vaccinated volunteers. *JAMA,* 272:431.

BIRD, KRISTINA D. (1991). The use of spermicide nonoxynol-9 in the prevention of HIV infection. *AIDS,* 5:791–796.

BLOWER, SALLY M., et al. (1994). Prophylactic vaccines, risk behavior change, and the probability of eradicating HIV in San Francisco. *Science,* 265:1451–1454.

BOLCH, O.H., JR, et al. (1973). In vitro effects of Emko on *Neisseria gonorrhoeae* and *Trichomonas vaginalis*. *Am. J. Obstet. Gynecol.,* 115:1145–1148.

BUTLER, DECLAN. (1994). Concern over invisable problems of HIV blood in developing countries. *Nature,* 369:429.

CHRISTENSEN, DAMARIS. (1994a). A shot in time: The technology behind new vaccines. *Science News,* 145:344–345.

CHRISTENSEN, DAMARIS. (1994b) Another look at the TB vaccine. *Science News,* 145:393.

CHOI, KYUNG-HEE, et al. (1994). Prevention of HIV infection. *AIDS,* 8:1371–1389.

CLEMENT, MICHAEL J. (1993). HIV disease: Are we going anywhere? *Patient Care,* 27:13.

COHEN, JON. (1992). Is liability slowing AIDS vaccines? *Science*, 256:168–170.

COHEN, JON. (1993). A NEW GOAL: Preventing disease, not infection. *Science*, 262:1820–1821.

COHEN, JON. (1994a). Bumps on the vaccine road. *Science*, 265:1371–1372.

COHEN JON. (1994b) Are researchers racing toward success, or crawling? *Science*, 265:1373–1374.

CONNELL, ELIZABETH B.(1989). Barrier contraceptives—their time has returned. *Female Patient*, 14:66–75.

Consumer Reports. (1989). Can you rely on condoms? 54:135–141.

DE VINCENZI, ISABELLE. (1994). A longitudinal study of HIV transmission by heterosexual partners. *N. Engl. J. Med.*, 331:341–347.

ETZIONI, AMITAI. (1993). HIV sufferers have a responsibility. *TIME*, 142:100.

EZZELL, CAROL. (1987). Hospital workers have AIDS virus. *Nature*, 227:261.

FARR, GASTON, et al. (1994). Contraceptive efficacy and acceptability of the female condom. *Am. J. Public Health*, 84:1960–1964.

FINDLAY, STEVEN. (1991). AIDS: The second decade. *U.S. News World Rep.*, 110:20–22.

FISHER, ALEXANDER A. (1991). Condom conundrums: Part 1. *Cutis*, 48:359–360.

FISHER, PETER. (1990). A report from the underground. *International Working Group on AIDS and IV Drug Use*, 5:15–17.

FRANCIS, DONALD P., et al. (1987). The prevention of acquired immunodeficiency syndrome in the United States. *JAMA*, 257:1357–1366.

GERBERDING, JULIE LOUISE. (1991). Reducing occupational risk of HIV infection. *Hosp. Pract.*, 26:103–118.

GOLDSMITH, MARSHA F. (1991). AIDS vaccines inch closer to useful existence. *JAMA*, 265: 1356–1357.

GRIMES, DAVID A.(1992). Contraception and the STD epidemic: Contraceptive methods for disease prevention. *The Contraception Report: The Role of Contraceptives in the Prevention of Sexually Transmitted Diseases*, III:1–15.

HAGEN, HOLLY. (1991). Studies support syringe exchange. *FOCUS*, 6:5–6.

HART, GRAHAM J. et al. (1991). Prevalence of HIV, hepatitis B, and associated risk behaviors in clients of a needle exchange in central London. *AIDS*, 5:543–547.

HICKS, D.R., et al. (1985). Inactivation of HTLV/LAV-infected cultures of normal human lymphocytes by nonoxynol-9 in vitro. *Lancet*, 2:1422–1423.

HIGGINS, D.L., et al. (1991). Evidence for the effects of HIV-antibody counseling and testing on risk behaviors. *JAMA*, 266:2419–2429.

HIV vaccines get the green light for third world trials. (1994). *Nature*, 371:644.

HO, DAVID, et al. (1995). Rapid turnover of plasma virons and CD4 lymphocytes in HIV infection. *Nature*, 373:123-126.

HOMSY, JACQUES, et al. (1989). The Fe and not CD4 receptor mediates antibody enhancement of HIV infection in human cells. *Science*, 244: 1357–1359.

JUDSON, FRANKLYN N. (1989). Condoms and spermicides for the prevention of sexually transmitted diseases. *Sexually Transmitted Dis. Bull.*, *9:3–11*.

KOFF, WAYNE C. (1988). Development and testing of AIDS vaccines. *Science*, 241:426–432.

LEVY, JAY A. (1989). Human immunodeficiency viruses and the pathogenesis of AIDS. *JAMA*, 261:2997–3006.

LURIE, PETER, et al. (1994). Ethical behavioral and social aspects of HIV vaccine trials in developing countries. *JAMA*, 271:295–302.

MACILWAIN, COLIN. (1994). U.S. puts larger-scale AIDS vaccine trials on ice as premature. *Nature*, 369:593.

MANDELL, WALLACE, et al. (1994). Correlates of needle sharing among injection drug users. *Am. J. Public Health*, 84:920–923.

Morbidity and Mortality Weekly Report. (1988). Partner notification for preventing human immunodeficiency virus (HIV) infection—Colorado, Idaho, South Carolina, Virginia. 37:393–396; 401–402.

Morbidity and Mortality Weekly Report. (1989a). Guideline for prevention of transmission of HIV and hepatitis B virus to health care workers. 38:3–17.

Morbidity and Mortality Weekly Report. (1989b). AIDS and human immunodeficiency virus infection in the United States: 1988 Update. 38:1–33.

Morbidity and Mortality Weekly Report. (1992a). Childbearing and contraceptive-use plans among women at high-risk for HIV infection—selected U.S. sites, 1989–1991. 41:135–144.

Morbidity and Mortality Weekly Report. (1992b). Sexual behavior among high school students—United States, 1990. 40:885–888.

Morbidity and Mortality Weekly Report. (1993a). Update: Barrier protection against HIV infection and other sexually transmitted diseases. 42:589–591.

Morbidity and Mortality Weekly Report. (1993b). Impact of new legislation on needle and syringe purchases and possession—Connecticut 1992. 42:145–147.

NARA, PETER.(1989). AIDS viruses of animals and man: Non living parasites of the immune system. *Los Alamos Sci.* 18:54-84.

OSMOND, DENNIS. (1992). Ethical and legal issues of vaccine clinical trials. *FOCUS*, 8:1–4.

PARRAN, THOMAS P. (1937). *Shadow on the Land: Syphilis.* New York: Reynal and Hitchcock.

PERRONE, JANICE. (1989). U.S. cities launch new AIDS weapon. *Am. Med. News,* March:68–71.

PINES, MAYA. (1993). Blood: Bearer of life and death. *Howard Hughes Med. Inst.,* 6:17.

POTTS, MALCOLM. (1994). Urgent need for a vaginal microbicide in the prevention of HIV transmission. *Am. J. Public Health,* 84:890–891.

RAYMOND, CHRIS ANNE. (1988). U.S. cities struggle to implement needle exchanges despite apparent success in European cities. *JAMA,* 260:2620–2621.

ROPER, WILLIAM L., et al. (1993). Commentary: Condoms and HIV/STD prevention—clarifying the message. *Am. J. Public Health,* 83:501–503.

ROSENBERG, MICHAEL J., et al. (1992). Commentary: Methods women can use that may prevent STDs including HIV. *Am. J. Public Health,* 82:1473–1478.

RUTHERFORD, GEORGE W. (1988). Contact tracing and the control of human immunodeficiency virus infection. *JAMA,* 259:3609–3670.

SATTAR, SYED A., et al. (1991). Survival and disinfectant inactivation of HIV: A critical review. *Rev. of Infect. Dis.,* 13:430–447.

SELLERS, DEBORAH, et al. (1994). Does the promotion and distribution of condoms increase teen sexual activity? Evidence from an HIV prevention program for Latino youth. *Am. J. Public Health,* 84:1952–1958.

SINGH, B., et al. (1982). Demonstration of a spirocheticidal effect by chemical contraceptives on *Treponema pallidum. Bull. Pan. Am. Health Organ.,* 16:59–64.

STIMSON, GERRY V., et al. (1989). Syringe exchange. *International Working Group on AIDS and IV Drug Use,* 4:15.

STONE, KATHERINE M., et al. (1986). Personal protection against sexually transmitted diseases. *Am. J. Obstet. Gynecol.,* 155:180–88.

STRAUS, STEPHEN, et al. (1994). Placebo-controlled trial of vaccination with recombinant glycoprotein D of herpes simplex virus type 2 for immunotherapy of genital herpes, *Lancet,* 343:1460.

THOMPSON, DICK. (1992). Getting the point in New Haven. *Time,* 139:55–56.

TIERNO, PHILIP M. (1988). AIDS overview: New guidelines for handling specimens. *Am. J. Cont. Ed. Nurs.,* Special Issue:1–14.

Time. (1992). Closed: Needle Park. 139:53.

WEI, XIPING, et al. (1995). Viral dynamics in HIV infection. *Nature,* 373:117–122.

WEINSTEIN, STEPHEN P., et al. (1990). AIDS and cocaine: A deadly combination facing the primary care physician. *J. Fam. Prac.,* 31:253–254.

WELLER, SUSAN. (1993). A meta-analysis of condom effectiveness in reducing sexually transmitted HIV. *Soc. Sci. Med.* 36:1635–1644.

Wellness Letter. (May 1993). AIDS. School of Public Health Publication, 9:1-8.

WENIGER, BRUCE C. (1994).Experience from HIV incedence cohorts in Thailand: Implications for HIV vaccine efficacy trials. *AIDS,* 8:1007–1010.

WHITE, NICK, et al. (1988). Dangers of lubricants used with condoms. *Nature,* 335:19.

WODAK, ALEX. (1990). Australia smashes international needle and syringe exchange record. *International Working Group on AIDS and IV Drug Use,* 5:28–29.

CHAPTER

10

Prevalence of HIV Infection and AIDS Cases in the United States

Chapter Concepts

- AIDS is a new plague.
- People with AIDS can be associated with certain lifestyle risks.
- AIDS can be associated with single or multiple exposures.
- AIDS cases can be separated by sex, age group, race, ethnicity, and sexual preference.
- Risk is strongly tied to social behavior.
- Behavioral risk groups include homosexual and bisexual men, injection drug users (IDUs), hemophiliacs, transfusion patients, the sex partners of these people, and the children of infected mothers.
- IDU and prostitution are strongly associated with HIV infection.
- All military personnel are tested for HIV.
- Two per 1,000 college students are HIV-infected.
- High rates of HIV infection have been found among prisoners.
- The greatest threat to health care workers is needlestick injuries.
- All 50 states and U.S. territories have reported adult/adolescent AIDS cases.
- People do not always tell the truth when completing questionnaires, especially with regard to sexual behavior.

The **prevalence** of a disease refers to the percentage of a population that is affected by it at a given time. For example, the total number of AIDS cases or number of HIV infections reported in the United States, by your state or city to the CDC. The **incidence** means the number of times an event occurs in a given time frame, for example, the number of new AIDS cases each month or new HIV infections each week. Much has been learned about the prevalence of HIV infection, HIV disease, and its terminal stage called AIDS since the 1981 CDC report that awakened the world to this new epidemic.

Although cases of AIDS appear retrospectively to have occurred in the United States as early as 1952, the **AIDS pandemic** is considered to have begun with the initial report early in 1981. Since then, there has been an exponential rise in reported AIDS cases (Table10-1). The exponential rise means that there must be a reservoir of asymptomatic HIV-infected people who *with time* progress to AIDS.

If all the cumulative world AIDS deaths had occurred in a single year, this pandemic would top the list of the worst natural disasters of the 20th century. Natural disasters are often analyzed in terms of global vulnerability to events with a rapid onset such as tropical storms, earthquakes, and volcanic eruptions. The slower onset of the AIDS pandemic, with over 260,000 deaths from early 1981 through mid 1995, sets it apart from natural disasters; but in terms of cost and human suffering, it is no different. Even if only the 30,000 lives lost to AIDS in 1990 or 35,000 to 40,000 deaths per year from 1991 through 1994 are used as reference points, the yearly numbers are still greater than the number of deaths caused by most of the natural disasters recorded in this century. By the end of this century, AIDS will be the third most common cause of death in the United States (HIV Guideline Panel, 1994).

TABLE 10-1 AIDS Cases as a Percentage of Total Population: United States 1982–1995

Year	Total Population[a]	Number of AIDS Cases[b]	Percent with AIDS
1982	231,534	1,500	<0.0005
1983	233,981	2,760	<0.001
1984	236,158	4,445	0.001
1985	238,740	8,249	0.003
1986	241,078	12,932	0.005
1987	243,400	21,070	0.009
1988	245,807	31,001	0.013
1989	248,239	33,722	0.014
1990	248,710	44,757	0.018
1991	252,177	53,176	0.020
1992	254,462	49,106	0.019
1993	257,301	105,990	0.041
1994[c]	260,507	80,473	0.031
1995[c]	262,605	64,000	0.023

[a]United States total resident population in thousands.

[b]Number of AIDS cases reported, by year, to the Centers for Disease Control and Prevention, Atlanta, Georgia, USA. AIDS cases are underreported by 10% to 20%.

[c]1995 data are estimated based on reports adapted from *MMWR*, 1994.

BOX 10.1

THE HIV/AIDS SCENARIO

HIV/AIDS is unstoppable in the short term. Because it takes an HIV infection so long to develop into AIDS, virtually all of the AIDS cases that occur during the next 5 to 10 years will be the result of existing infections. Therefore, the epidemic **cannot** be materially reduced in this time frame by any reduction in new HIV cases. Worldwide, millions of HIV infections will progress into AIDS during the 1990s.

Is it your impression that some of your friends and associates *still* regard HIV/AIDS as someone else's problem? HIV/AIDS has invaded *all* segments of society worldwide! It is EVERYONE'S problem!

The 1990s are the second decade of HIV disease/AIDS. The prevalence of HIV infection and new AIDS cases will continue to increase dramatically. The number of AIDS cases in the United States is, according to the CDC, underreported by 15% to 20%. More people have died in the United States of AIDS in any 2 years from 1988 through 1994 than died during the 8 years of the Vietnam War. In the United States, between 100 and 200 people a day are

BOX 10.2

THE HIV/AIDS PANDEMIC HAS LIMITS

Epidemics or pandemics typically reach a point of saturation whereby incidence levels off under 100% of the population. This happens because some people either are naturally immune or avoid exposure to the disease. Thus AIDS will not wipe out entire populations, but the point of saturation for HIV (number of susceptible persons infected) probably varies substantially from population to population and cannot be predicted with any precision.

becoming HIV-infected and about 160 a day are diagnosed with AIDS. One person dies of AIDS in the United States about every 13 minutes; worldwide, at least one every minute.

OLD FORMULA FOR ESTIMATING HIV INFECTIONS

The estimated prevalence of HIV infection in the United States is an important measure of the extent of the nation's HIV disease/AIDS problem. Initial estimates on the number of HIV-infected people were based on the CDC formula: for every diagnosed case of AIDS, there are 50 to 100 people who are HIV-infected. The estimate was crude, but data essential for greater specificity were lacking. This was a new plague and no one was prepared for it. A workable definition for what constituted an AIDS patient had to be agreed upon. Surveillance networks also had to be set up to gather information on areas of highest incidence, who was being infected, and routes of transmission.

NEWER FORMULA FOR ESTIMATING HIV INFECTIONS

A newer formula proposed by the CDC for use in determining the number of HIV-infected persons is as follows:

National Number of Persons Living With AIDS (1994)	Number of PLWA in Your City (1994)

$$\frac{170{,}000}{1{,}200{,}000} \times \frac{\text{(e.g.,) } 1{,}000}{X} = 170{,}000$$

(Estimated national number of HIV-infected persons.)

$$X = 1{,}200{,}000{,}000$$

$$X = \frac{1{,}200{,}000{,}000}{170{,}000}$$

$$= 7{,}509$$

(About 7,509 persons in this sample city are HIV-infected.)

Single or Multiple Exposure Categories

In Table 10-2, the number of AIDS cases is presented with respect to *single* or *multiple* exposure categories. For example, under *Single Mode of Exposure*, heterosexual contact accounts for 6% of all AIDS cases. Under *Multiple Modes of Exposure*, 3% of AIDS cases occurred among injection drug users who also had heterosexual contact. In other words, Table 10-2 lists the numbers and percentages of all reported AIDS cases broken down into six categories of people who contracted AIDS from a single risk mode of exposure and 24 categories of people who contracted AIDS from multiple risk modes of exposure. Note that of the total number of adult/adolescent AIDS cases, 81% occurred from **single risk** modes of exposure. Of this 81%, 52% occurred among men who had sex with men and 20% among injection drug users.

A composite representation of all AIDS cases by exposure category reported for 1994 is seen in Figure 8-1.

BEHAVIORAL RISK GROUPS AND STATISTICAL EVALUATION

Behavioral Risk Groups and AIDS Cases

As the pool of AIDS patients grew in number during 1981–1983, individual case histories were separated into **behavioral risk groups**. The early case histories of AIDS patients clearly separated people according to their social behavior and medical needs. AIDS patients were placed into the following six risk behavior categories: (1) homosexual and bisexual men; (2) injection drug users; (3) hemophiliacs; (4) blood transfusion recipients; (5) heterosexuals; and (6) children whose parents are at risk. Each of these groups is considered to be at risk of HIV infection based on some common behavioral denominator. That is, those within these groups represented a higher rate of AIDS cases than people whose needs or behaviors excluded them from these groups. However, because there is some mixing between individuals in behavorial risk groups, HIV infection has gradually spread to lower-risk behavioral groups. Over time the behavioral risk groups

TABLE 10-2 Adult/Adolescent AIDS Cases by Single and Multiple Exposure Categories, Reported through December 1994, United States

Exposure Category	AIDS Cases No.	(%)
Single Mode of Exposure		
1. Men who have sex with men	229,830	(52)
2. Injection (IJ) drug use	88,396	(20)
3. Hemophilia/coagulation disorder	4,420	(1)
4. Heterosexual contact	26,519	(6)
5. Receipt of transfusion of blood, blood component or tissue	8,840	(2)
6. Receipt of transplant of tissues/organs	8	(0)
7. Other/undetermined	30	(0)
Single Mode of Exposure Subtotal	358,043	(81%)
Multiple Modes of Exposure		
1. Men who have sex with men; IJ drug use	26,519	(6)
2. Men who have sex with men; hemophilia	93	(0)
3. Men who have sex with men; heterosexual contact	4381	(1)
4. Men who have sex with men; receipt of transfusion/transplant	2,850	(1)
5. IJ drug use; hemophilia	125	(0)
6. IJ drug use; heterosexual contact	16,932	(4)
7. IJ drug use; receipt of transfusion	1,199	(0)
8. Hemophilia; heterosexual contact	40	(0)
9. Hemophilia; receipt of transfusion/transplant	735	(0)
10. Heterosexual contact; receipt of transfusion/transplant	783	(0)
11. Men who have sex with men; IJ drug use; hemophilia	29	(0)
12. Men who have sex with men; IJ drug use; heterosexual contact	2,410	(1)
13. Men who have sex with men; IJ drug use; receipt of transfusion/transplant	440	(0)
14. Men who have sex with men; hemophilia; heterosexual contact	8	(0)
15. Men who have sex with men; hemophilia; receipt of transfusion/transplant	30	(0)
16. Men who have sex with men; heterosexual contact; receipt of transfusion/transplant	179	(0)
17. IJ drug use; hemophilia; heterosexual contact	23	(0)
18. IJ drug use; hemophilia; receipt of transfusion/transplant	33	(0)
19. IJ drug use; heterosexual contact; receipt of transfusion/transplant	485	(0)
20. Hemophilia; heterosexual contact; receipt of transfusion/transplant	25	(0)
21. Men who have sex with men; IJ drug use; hemophilia; heterosexual contact	6	(0)
22. Men who have sex with men; IJ drug use; hemophilia; receipt of transfusion/transplant	12	(0)
23. Men who have sex with men; IJ drug use; heterosexual contact; receipt of transfusion/transplant	83	(0)
24. IJ drug use; hemophilia; heterosexual contact; receipt of transfusion/transplant	4	(0)
25. Men who have sex with men; inject drug use; hemophilia; heterosexual contact; receipt of transfusion/transplant	2	(0)
Multiple Modes of Exposure for AIDS Cases	57,420	(13)
Risk Not Reported or Identified	26,519	(6)
Total AIDS Cases	441,982	(100)

(Source: For exposure categories. CDC HIV/AIDS Surveillance Report, June 1994:1–25. Figures are based on latest total AIDS cases reported to CDC)

have been aligned and defined according to age, exposure category, and sex. (See Table 10-2)

A review of AIDS cases by sex, age at diagnosis, and race/ethnicity reported through December, 1994 in the United States, shows that white, black, and Hispanic males between the ages of 20 and 44 make up 80% of all male AIDS cases. Between ages 20 and 59, they make up 96% of all male AIDS cases. Of the total number of male AIDS cases, 56% are white, 26% are black, and 15% are Hispanic.

Collectively, 88% of female AIDS cases occur between ages 20 and 59. Of the total number, 52% are black, 25% are white, and 20% are Hispanic. A greater race/ethnicity disproportionality occurs among females than among males. For example, there are twice the number of black female than white female AIDS cases, yet there are about seven times more white females than black females in the United States. There were 73 AIDS cases among every 100,000 black women in the United States while the rate for white women was 5 per 100,000. This means that black women are nearly 15 times more likely than white women to contact AIDS (73 ÷ 5 = 14.6) Black and Hispanic females make up 75% of all female AIDS cases in the 20 to 59 age group. In the under-5 to over-65 age group, black and Hispanic females make up 73% of the AIDS cases but account for less than 10% of the female population.

Of the 105,990 AIDS cases in the United States reported to the CDC, for 1993, 58,295 or 55% occurred among racial and ethnic minorities. Of these, 38,544 occurred in the black population, 18,888 in the Hispanic population, 767 in the Asian-Pacific Islanders, and 339 in American Indians and Alaska natives. The CDC reports that of the 1993 AIDS cases, racial and ethnic minorities accounted for three-fourths of AIDS cases among adult and teenage women, and 84% of the cases involving children aged 12 and under (MMWR, 1994).

Statistical Evaluation of Risk Behavioral Group AIDS Cases

Pediatric AIDS Cases— Through early 1995, only two states had not reported a pediatric AIDS case, North Dakota and Wyoming. By early 1995, over 6,000 pediatric AIDS cases were reported and over 3,000 have died from AIDS. Pediatric AIDS cases represent about 1.3% of the total number of AIDS cases to date. Of the pediatric AIDS cases, about 5% were/are hemophilic children who received HIV-contaminated blood transfusions or blood products (pooled and concentrated blood factor VIII injections). About 5% of pediatric AIDS cases occurred in nonhemophilic children who were transfused with HIV-contaminated blood. Ninety percent of pediatric AIDS cases received the virus from HIV-infected mothers who transmitted it to them either during the fetal stage, as the newborn passed through the birthing canal, or from breast milk soon after birth. Eventually, 95% of HIV-infected newborns will result from parental transmission (transfusion-related cases will drop). In 2% of pediatric AIDS cases, the route of HIV infection can not be determined.

Children of color make up 15.4% of all children in the United States but account for over 50% of pediatric AIDS cases. Whites make up 70% of children and account for 24% of pediatric AIDS cases. Hispanics make up 11% of children and account for 20% of pediatric AIDS cases. By the year 2000, it is estimated that there will be between 80,000 and 100,000 pediatric orphans in the United States.

Adult/Adolescent AIDS Cases— By the end of 1994, some 442,000 AIDS cases and over 260,000 AIDS-related deaths were reported to the CDC. Cumulative through 1994, 7% of AIDS cases have occurred among the heterosexual population, Table 10-3 (for 1993, due to the new AIDS definition 9% of cases were heterosexual), 31% occurred among injection drug users and their homosexual and heterosexual partners, and 53% occurred in the male homosexual/bisexual population.

Figure 10-1 shows that the percentage of AIDS cases for ethnic related adult/adolescent groups are in striking contrast to the population percentages of each group. For example, whites make up 80% of the population and represent 54% of adult/adolescent AIDS cases. Blacks make up less than 13% of the population but represent 28% of the adult/adolescent AIDS cases. Hispanics make up 6% of the population but represent 17% of the adult/adolescent AIDS cases.

Collectively, blacks and Hispanics make up about 19% of the population but make up 44% of adult/adolescent and 77% of pediatric AIDS cases **reported**. Thus, blacks and Hispanics contribute disproportionately high percentages to the total number of reported AIDS cases.

TABLE 10-3 Adult/Adolescent Behavioral Risk Groups, Race and Sex: Percent of Total AIDS Cases—United States, 1994

HIV/AIDS	No. of Cases[a]	% of Cases
Exposure Group		
Homosexual/bisexual male	42,651	53
Injection drug user (IDU) (women/heterosexual men)	20,118	25
Homosexual/bisexual IDU	4,828	6
Hemophiliac	805	1
Heterosexual contact	5,633	7
Transfusion Related	1610	2
None of the above	4828	6
Total	80,473	100.0
Race/Ethnicity (all cases)		
White (non-Hispanic)	37661	46.8
Black (non-Hispanic)	28,166	35
Hispanic	13,680	17
Other	966	1.2
Sex (adults only)		
Male	70,011	87
Female	10,461	13
Age Group (yrs)		
13–19	402	0.5
20–24	2,414	3.0
25–29	12,474	15.5
30–39	36,213	45.0
40–49	20,118	25.0
50–59	6,438	8.0
60 and above	2,414	3.0

[a]Total in each category = 80,473 = 100% of cases for 1994.
(Adapted from AIDS Surveillance Report, June,1994)

Figure 10-2 is a United States map of all AIDS cases reported to the CDC through the year 1994. Note, the highest incidence of AIDS cases occurs along the coastal regions.

Behavioral Risk Groups and Percentages of HIV-Infected People

Through mid-1995, investigators at the CDC found that HIV infection remained largely confined to the populations at recognized behavorial risks: homosexual men, injection drug users, heterosexual partners of injection drug users, hemophiliacs, and children of infected mothers. In the general population, rates for HIV infection include 0.04% for first-time blood donors, 0.14% for military applicants, 0.33% for Job Corps entrants, 0.19% to 0.87% for child-bearing women, and 0.30% for hospital patients. Data reported by the CDC in 1990 indicated that while the number of new AIDS cases increased by 5% in cities, it had increased by 37% in rural areas. This trend continues.

Comments on a Variety of Individual Behavioral Risk Groups

It must be kept in mind that because a group of people is at risk for HIV does not mean that these people are predestined to become infected. People are placed within these groups because of their social behavior, a behavior that has been associated with a high-, medium- or low-risk of becoming HIV-infected. Essentially there is no zero-risk group because a scenario can always be formulated to show that under certain circumstances one or more members of that group could become HIV-infected.

The point of placing people in behavorial risk groups is not to offend them but to provide a warning that certain behavior might make them more vulnerable to HIV infection. It is not the race or ethnic group that people belong to that places them at high or low risk for infection, it is their behavior.

The fact that AIDS was first identified in 1981 in seemingly well defined behavioral groups (homosexual men, injection drug users, hemophiliacs, Haitian immigrants) probably contributed to a false sense of security among people who did not belong to any of these groups. However, as information about HIV and AIDS accumulated, it became clear that HIV was transmitted in body fluids. This had grave implications for all social groups. On reflection, the people in the original high-risk groups simply had the bad luck of being in the way of a newly emerging infectious agent as it first began to spread. It is highly probable that in the different behavioral risk groups there were lifestyle or medical history factors that increased the efficiency with which the virus was transmitted.

Homosexual Males— In 1981, 100% of all AIDS cases reported to the CDC occurred in homosexual males. By the first half of 1991,

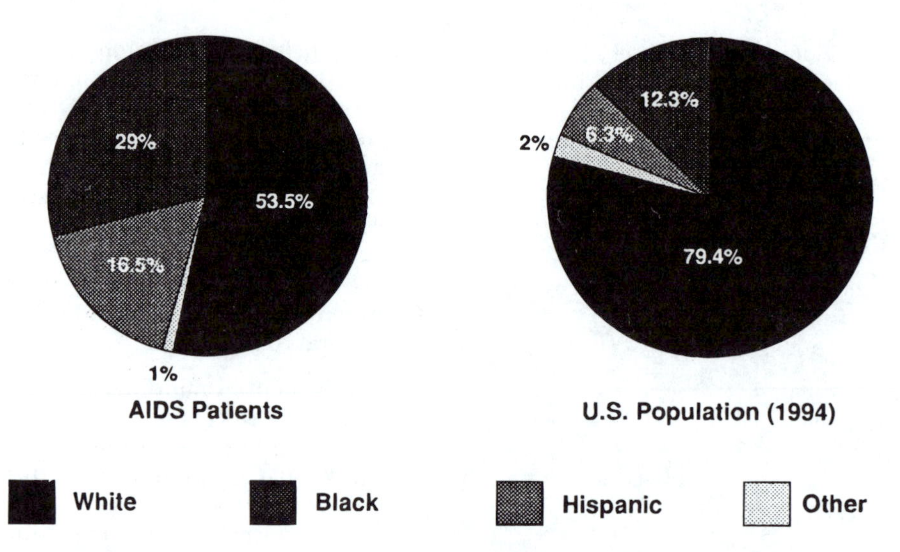

FIGURE 10-1 Racial and Ethnic AIDS Patient Classification. Adult AIDS cases show a disproportionate percentage among blacks and Hispanics. Over 46% of reported AIDS cases occur among racial and ethnic minorities. The figures reflect higher rates of AIDS in blacks and Hispanic injection drug users and their sex partners. Percentages of the population are based on the numbers of AIDS cases in the United States reported to the CDC through December 1994. U.S. population data (about 261,000,000).

about 56% of all AIDS cases occurred in homosexual males. For 1993, 46% of the 105,990 new AIDS cases occurred in gay males. It appears that in the first years of the 1990s, the number of gay male AIDS cases, as a percentage of all AIDS cases is decreasing as the number of cases associated with injection drug use increases. However, there are indicators of a *second wave* in the HIV/AIDS epidemic among gay males. Young gay men who have come of age since the emergence of AIDS appear to perceive the disease as a problem of older gay men and have not adopted safer sex behaviors to the same extent as older men. In a survey by Robert Hays and colleagues (1990; 1992), of gay men aged 18 to 25, 42% reported having engaged in unprotected anal intercourse in the previous 6 months. In a study of 258 gay men aged 17 to 25 conducted at gay dance clubs in San Francisco, 12% were found to be infected with HIV (Lemp, 1991). Finally, studies show that a significant percentage of gay men who had originally adopted safer sex behaviors are "relapsing" to unsafe sex (Stall et al., 1990; Lemp et al., 1994).

As most people who have attempted to change behavior know, it is difficult to maintain new behavior patterns over a long period of time. Increasing attention and concern has been focused on the issue of relapse. High seroprevalence levels among homosexual men (estimated to be 50% in high incidence cities such as San Francisco) make relapse to risky behaviors a significant source of new infections and justifies continued interventions to reinforce behavior change.

Size of the Homosexual Community. Estimating the size of the homosexual population continues to be a problem for the CDC. Because of the lack of available information on sexual practices, the CDC has relied on the 1948 Kinsey report, *Sexual Behavior in the Human Male,* for its estimate that 2.5 million (10%) American males are *exclusively* homosexual, while another 2.5 to 7.5 million have *occasional* homosexual contacts. These numbers are refuted by some recent surveys like the 1992 National Opinion Research Center that reports that among males, 2.8% are exclusively gay, and among women, 2.5% are exclusively lesbian. Judith Reisman argues in her 1990 book, *Kinsey, Sex and Fraud,* that male homosexuals make up about 1% of

Geographic distribution of AIDS cases reported in 1994, United States
Each point represents 10 cases. All points are displaced slightly to preclude identification of counties with small numbers of reported cases.

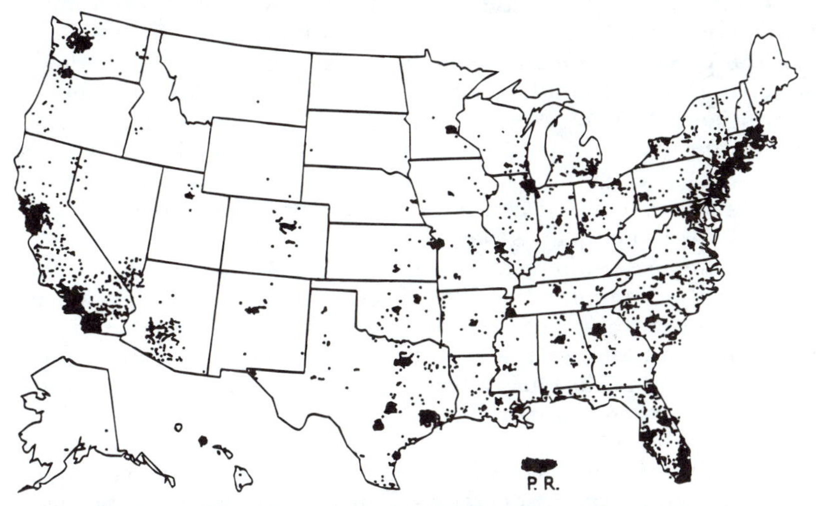

HIV/AIDS Surveillance Report, Centers for Disease Control and Prevention

FIGURE 10-2 Surveillance Report showing the Approximate Location of AIDS Cases that Occurred in the year 1994

the population. The group, Coloradans for Family Values and the Washington-based Family Research Institute believe about 3% of the male population is exclusively gay. In the late 1980s, Congress approved two national surveys of sexual behavior but this action was stopped in the Senate.

Using data collected from HIV testing conducted in 1986 and 1987, the CDC estimates that 20% of exclusively homosexual men are HIV-infected. This means (depending on whose numbers are used) that between 500,000 and 625,000 gay males are HIV-infected. For bisexuals and men with infrequent homosexual encounters, the CDC tabulates a prevalence rate of 5%, meaning that between 125,000 and 375,000 of this population are HIV-infected (Booth, 1988). Approximately 6% of all IDU-associated AIDS cases occur in the homosexual/bisexual male population. These cases may reflect HIV transmission either by contaminated syringes or sexual activity.

Injection Drug Users— According to the CDC, as many as 33% of the nation's 1.2 million injection drug users may be HIV-infected. This behavioral risk group contains the nation's second largest group of HIV-infected and AIDS patients. An association between injection drug use and AIDS was recognized in 1981, about 2 years before the virus was identified. AIDS in IDUs and hemophiliacs offered the first evidence that whatever caused AIDS was being carried in and transmitted by human blood. From the first reported IDU AIDS cases in 1981 through mid-1995, 29% of all adult/adolescent AIDS cases occurred in IDUs. Of IDUs, 74% listed IDU as their *only* risk factor for HIV infection; 26% were also homosexual/bisexual. According to a study by Hahn and colleagues (1989), 52% of women and 25% of men with AIDS were/are IDUs.

IDUs have been reported in all 50 states and the District of Columbia. Fifty-two percent now based on 29% of 442,000 end of 1994 of the accumulated 128,180 IDU AIDS cases occurred in New York and New Jersey. Among the adult/adolescent heterosexual AIDS cases over half had sexual partners who are/were IDUs.

Rates for IDU-associated AIDS varied widely by area: rates in Puerto Rico, New Jersey, New

York, and the District of Columbia were greater than 10 per 100,000; in 22 states, rates were lower than 1 per 100,000 population.

About 55% of all IDU-associated cases were reported in the Northeast, which represents about 20% of the population of the United States and its territories. The South reported 20% of IDU-associated AIDS cases, 5% from the Midwest, and the West reported the remaining 20%.

The rate of IDU-associated AIDS continues to be higher for blacks and Hispanics than for whites. Except for the West, where rates for whites and Hispanics were similar, this difference by race/ethnicity was observed in all regions of the country and was greatest in the Northeast. J. Peterson and colleagues (1989) reported that among *heterosexual* men, injection drug use accounts for 83% of black, 87% of Hispanic, and 45% of white AIDS cases. Overall, IDU-associated AIDS cases represented 16.3% of all AIDS cases in whites, 52.7% in blacks, 55.5% in Hispanics, 6.3% in Asians/Pacific Islanders, and 29.0% in American Indians/Alaskan Natives.

Sex Partners and Children of IDUS. AIDS cases associated with injection drug use involve not only IDUs themselves but also their sex partners and children. IDU accounts for most AIDS cases in heterosexual men, women, and children. In New York, 70% of IDUs are men and 50% of their sex partners are women who do not use drugs. These women typically have two children before being diagnosed with HIV infection. Female sex partners of male IDUs form a bridge across which the AIDS virus is transmitted into the heterosexual population (Thomas, 1989). As the HIV-infected mothers die of AIDS, their children become orphans. HIV-infected children languish in hospital nurseries because foster parents fear becoming HIV-infected themselves. David Michaels and colleagues (1992) report that by the end of 1995, maternal deaths caused by the HIV/AIDS epidemic will have orphaned an estimated 24,600 children and 21,000 adolescents in the United States. Unless the course of the AIDS epidemic changes dramatically, by the year 2000, the overall number of motherless children and adolescents in the United States will exceed 140,000. About 50,000 orphans will live in 6 cities, New York, Newark, NJ, Miami, San Juan, P.R., Los Angeles, and Washington, DC. Worldwide there will be 10 million orphans. In 1991, an estimated 13% of children's and 9% of adolescents' mothers died of HIV/AIDS-related diseases. These numbers are expected to reach 17% and 12%, respectively, by 1995. The vast majority of these motherless youth will come from poor communities of color.

Heterosexuals— The spread of HIV in the general population is relatively slow, yet potentially it is the source of the greatest numbers of HIV/AIDS cases.

Data from the CDC through mid-1995 indicated that between 6% and 7% of all the AIDS cases in the United States occurred within the heterosexual population. But this must be placed in perspective. Although 6% of anything may be a significant number, by mid 1995 it stood for over 28,000 adult/adolescent/pediatric AIDS cases. Most of these heterosexual AIDS cases occurred in persons or the sexual partners of individuals with an identified behavioral risk. Relative to the general adult population, the number of heterosexual AIDS cases is only a fraction of 1%.

According to the CDC, of the heterosexual population (143 million) *without* an identified behavior risk, 0.021% or about 30,000 are HIV-infected.

In the United States, CDC data for 1993 and1994 indicate that 3% of men and 35% of women contracted HIV from people of the opposite sex. Worldwide, mid 1995, heterosexuals make up 75% of the 20 million HIV-infected people. Over half of these people live in Sub-Saharan Africa (about 12.8 million). North America (2.2 million), Latin America (1.8 million), East Asia (3.2 million), and Africa account for 96% of global HIV infections. The World Health Organization (WHO) projects that by the year 2000, up to 90% of all HIV infections globally will be transmitted heterosexually. Most HIV infections in North America have been transmitted homosexually to men who practiced receptive anorectal intercourse, whereas most of those occurring in Africa and parts of

POINT OF INFORMATION 10.1

HETEROSEXUALLY ACQUIRED AIDS—UNITED STATES, 1993

From 1991 through 1992, persons with AIDS who were infected with HIV through heterosexual transmission accounted for the largest proportionate increase in reported AIDS cases in the United States. During 1993, a total of 105,990 persons aged 13 years and older with AIDS were reported to CDC (pediatric AIDS, 968).

From 1985 through 1993, the proportion of persons with AIDS who reported heterosexual contact with a partner at risk for or with documented HIV infection increased from 1.9% to 9.0%, respectively. During the same period, the proportion of cases attributed to male-to-male sexual contact decreased from 66.5% to 46.6%, while the proportion attributed to injection drug use among women and heterosexual men increased from 17% to 28%. In 1993, AIDS cases attributed to heterosexual contact ($n = 9,288$) increased 130% over 1992 ($n = 4,045$). Cases in all other exposure categories combined increased 109% in 1993.

In 1993, most heterosexually acquired AIDS cases were attributed to heterosexual contact with an injection drug user (IDU) (42.3%) or with a partner with HIV infection or AIDS whose risk was unreported or unknown (49.7%). Men were more likely than women to report contact with a partner with HIV infection or AIDS whose risk was unreported or unknown (60% versus 44%); this group may include persons whose sex partners were IDUs or bisexual men for whom risk was not known or reported and persons whose sex partners were themselves infected heterosexually.

Compared with 1992, during 1993 the number of cases associated with heterosexual contact with an IDU ($n = 3,916$) increased 79%, and the number of cases associated with heterosexual contact with a partner with HIV infection or AIDS whose risk was unknown or unreported ($n = 4,617$) increased 195%. Increases also occurred in the number of cases associated with heterosexual contact with a bisexual man (171%), a person with hemophilia or other coagulation disorder (200%), or a transfusion or transplant recipient (132%). However, the number of cases in these latter three categories is small, and they represent a decreasing proportion of all heterosexual contact cases.

In 1993, heterosexual HIV transmission accounted for 6,056 AIDS cases reported among women (median age: 33 years) and 3,232 cases among men (median age: 38 years). In addition, 55% of men and 50% of women were non-Hispanic black, and 23% of men and 24% of women were hispanic. Rates were higher for non-Hispanic blacks (20 per 100,000 population) and Hispanics (10 per 100,000) than for non-Hispanic whites (1 per 100,000). During 1992 and 1993, persons aged 13 to 29 years accounted for 25% and 27%, respectively, of heterosexual contact cases, while representing 18% of total adolescent and adult AIDS cases each year. In 1993, over 50% of the new cases of AIDS among men, over 75% among women, and 84% among children occurred in minority populations,particularly within African-American and Hispanic communities.

The highest proportions of cases associated with heterosexual contact during 1993 were in the South (42%) and Northeast (31%); these areas also accounted for 24% and 53%, respectively, of cases reported among heterosexual IDUs ($n = 28,687$). States reporting the largest number of heterosexually acquired AIDS cases in 1993 were Florida (1,772 cases), New York (1,336), and New Jersey (885).

(Adapted from *MMWR*, 1994)

the Caribbean have been transmitted heterosexually to both women and men during vaginal intercourse. Heterosexual transmission accounts for a growing proportion of HIV/AIDS cases in Europe and Latin America, and is proliferating at explosive rates in parts of Thailand and India (Aral et al., 1991). Homosexual transmission still predominates in North America, but heterosexual transmission is increasing.

Hemophiliacs— There are about 20,000 hemophiliacs in the United States. At least half are HIV positive. Over 98% received HIV in blood products that were essential to their survival. By mid-1985, an HIV blood screening test was put into effect nationally. From that point, the risk of HIV infection from the blood supply has been significantly lowered but a small risk still exists. Scandals in a small risk still exists. Scandals in knowingly selling HIV-positive blood for transfu-

POINT OF INFORMATION 10.2

ACQUIRED IMMUNODEFICIENCY SYNDROME—UNITED STATES, 1994

During 1994, health departments reported to CDC 80,473 cases of acquired immunodeficiency syndrome (AIDS) among persons in the United States. This was 24% fewer AIDS cases than for 1993 (105,990). The number of cases reported in 1993 and 1994 was greater than that reported in 1992 (49,106). The increase in numbers of AIDS cases followed the expansion of the AIDS surveillance case definition for adolescents and adults implemented on January 1, 1993.

Of the total 80,473 reported cases, 79,456 (99%) occurred among adolescents and adults (i.e., persons aged ≥13 years) and 1,017 among children aged <13 years. Women, blacks and Hispanics, and persons in the South and Northeast accounted for higher percentages of reported cases during 1994 than during 1993. Among cases for which risks were reported, the largest decline in the proportion of reported cases occurred among homosexual/bisexual men.

The decline in the number of AIDS cases reported in 1994 compared to 1993 was predictable. Following the expansion of the surveillance definition on January 1, 1993, a substantial increase occurred in the number of AIDS cases reported, predominantly reflecting the reporting of persons with conditions diagnosed before that date and who were not eligible for reporting until these conditions were added to the surveillance definition. However, after these cases had been reported, the number of reported cases began to decrease, and during 1994, the numbers of AIDS cases reported by quarter became relatively stable.

The findings for 1994 indicate a continuation of trends for certain population groups, including an increase in the proportion of cases accounted for by women and racial/ethnic minorities, a decrease in the proportion accounted for by homosexual/bisexual men, and an increase in the number of cases in children. These patterns may reflect the evolution of the HIV epidemic but also may have been influenced by the differential effects of the expansion of the surveillance definition among different populations and in different geographic areas (*MMWR*,1995a).

sions and in production of the blood factor essential for hemophiliacs have surfaced in France, Germany, the United States, Canada, and Japan in the 1990s. (For discussion, see chapter 8, "Epidemiology and Transmission of the Human Immunodeficiency Virus."

From 1982 through 1994, 3,132 adult/adolescent, 143 sexual partners of hemophiliacs, and 249 hemophilic pediatric AIDS cases have been reported. Almost all of these cases are the result of HIV infections that occurred prior to 1985.

Prostitutes— The term prostitute is used in preference to the more recently coined "sex worker." No single term can adequately encompass the range of sex for money/drugs/friendship/accommodation transactions that undoubtedly occur worldwide. However, the term prostitute is at least relatively clear in referring to those who are directly involved in trading sex, Whereas the term sex worker may encompass a wide range of individuals directly and indirectly involved in such sexual transactions. In the United States, prostitutes represent a diverse group of people with various lifestyles. About 31% of female IDUs admit to engaging in prostitution. They need money to support their drug habit, pay rent, and eat. Cities with large numbers of IDUs subsequently have large numbers of prostitutes. Evidence is overwhelming—IDU, prostitution, and HIV infection are strongly associated.

In a multicity study, HIV antibody was detected in 13% of 1,378 female prostitutes; **80% of the infected prostitutes reported using injection drugs** (Darrow et al., 1988). For prostitutes *without* histories of injection drug use, HIV seroprevalence was 5%; HIV infection in this group was greater among blacks and Hispanics and among those who had had more than 200 nonpaying sex partners. The point is that **non-drug using prostitutes in the United States play a small role in HIV transmission**. This is believed to be because of the low incidence of HIV infection among their male clients and on the insistence by many prostitutes that their clients use condoms (Felman, 1990). In Africa and Asia, however, prostitution plays a major role in HIV transmission.

Military— The incidence of HIV infection can be measured best in groups that undergo routine serial testing. Because active duty military personnel and civilian applicants for the service are routinely tested for HIV antibody, there is a unique opportunity to measure the incidence of HIV infection in a large, demographically varied subset of the general population.

Since October, 1985, all military personnel on active duty, as well as all civilian applicants for military service, have undergone mandatory testing for HIV antibody. Over the next 2 years, the armed forces screened 3.96 million people for exposure to HIV. Of the 3.96 million tested, 5,890 (0.15%) were HIV-positive. This total included active duty personnel, members of the National Guard, members of reserve units, and would-be recruits. The recruits who tested positive have been barred from entering the service. Those carrying HIV who are already in uniform are allowed to stay in the service as long as they remain asymptomatic. They are, however, ineligible for overseas duty and must undergo close health monitoring.

The Navy has the highest incidence of HIV, with 2.5 per 1,000 people. The rate in the Army is 1.4 per 1,000; in the Marines, 1 per 1,000; and in the Air Force, 0.99 per 1,000. The higher rate in the Navy may reflect that Navy personnel are based primarily on the East and West Coasts, which have the highest number of AIDS cases.

Women— In rural America, HIV/AIDS due to heterosexual sexual transmission is increasing faster than in any other part of the country. Women most at risk are ethnic minorities and the disadvantaged. Among sexually active teenagers, college students, and health care workers nationwide, nearly 60% of the heterosexual sexual spread of HIV is among women (Pfeiffer, 1991).

In 1982, it was thought that all female AIDS cases were associated with injection drug usage. It soon became apparent that some of these women had become infected through heterosexual sexual contact with HIV infected males. Additional AIDS cases from heterosexual transmission appeared in 1983 and the percentage of female cases in the heterosexual category has continued to increase. The trend in heterosexual sexual transmission may serve as a marker for future trends in HIV transmission.

HIV/AIDS women are of special interest because they are the major source of infection in infants. In 1993, about 96% of HIV-infected children, aged 0 to 4 years, got the virus from their mothers (*MMWR*, 1993b).

At the end of 1988, women made up 6,964 or 9% of the total adult AIDS cases in the United States. By the end of 1993, women accounted for 11.3% or 44,431 cases (Table 10-4). An additional 15,200 cases occurred in 1994. Fifteen thousand plus womens AIDS cases are expected in 1995. At least 50% of these cases have been reported since 1989. And they have been reported from all 50 states and territories. About 75% of these women are between the ages of 13

TABLE 10-4 Reported AIDS Cases for Women, United States

Year	Number		
1981 (From June)	6		
1982	47		
1983	144		
1984	285		
1985	538		
1986	980		
1987	1,701		
1988	3,263		
1989	3,639		
1990	4,890		
1991	5,732		
1992	6,571	% Increase	
1993	16,514[a]	1992–1994	Total
1994	15,200	151[b]	Through 1994
1995	(Projected)		(59,631)
			Through 1995
			(74,000)
Men	390,000 (1981–1994)		
Total	474,000 (mid-1995)		

[a]The large increase in women's AIDS cases for 1993 over previous years was due to the January 1, 1993 implementation of the new definition of AIDS. Fifty-two percent of cases are associated with IDU. Most of the remaining cases occurred in women who are sexual partners of IDUs.

[b]Reported male AIDS cases for 1993 were up 105% (*MMWR*, 1994).

and 39 and some 25% are over age 40 (Guinan, 1993). In 1990, female AIDS cases were and continue to be twice as frequent among black women than among white and over three times that of Hispanic women (Figure 10-3). The number of reported male and female AIDS cases across the United States for 1994 is seen in Figure 10.4A1 and A2. The number of all AIDS cases for 1993 is seen in Figure 10.4B.

Among the most alarming statistics to emerge is that transmission of HIV through heterosexual intercourse accounts for 35% of female cases of AIDS compared with only 3% of male cases. Of the total reported cases acquired through heterosexual contact in the United States, 66% are women.

Figure 10-5 presents the source of women's AIDS cases in 1993 and in 1994. In 1994, 60% of all new female HIV infections in the United States occurred in women by the age 20 (Cotton, 1994).

To identify women at risk accurately, physicians need to be aware of the known demographic, epidemiological, and transmission risk factors related to HIV in women. Another consideration is the person's state of residence. Puerto Rico has the highest incidence of AIDS in women, followed by New Jersey, New York, the District of Columbia, Florida, Connecticut, Maryland, Delaware, Massachusetts, Rhode Island, Georgia, and South Carolina (Guinan, 1993).

Figure 10-6 shows the risk factors of the sexual partners of 8,534 women who contracted their infection through heterosexual intercourse. Many women may not be aware that their partners are in these behavioral risk categories, but those who are should be given the opportunity to discuss the risks and should be counseled to undergo testing. These data illustrate the importance of obtaining as much information as possible concerning the patient's sexual partners.

As the frequency of HIV/AIDS increases in women, the question of whether AIDS will explode in the heterosexual community of the United States becomes more a question of when the number of female AIDS cases will equal male cases. Worldwide, women accounted for 25% of all HIV-infected adults in 1990. By 1992, that percentage had risen to 40%. The World Health Organization predicts that by the year 2000, women will constitute the majority of HIV-infected adults (Figure 10-7) (Driscoll, 1992). For 1993, the WHO reported that *two* women are becoming HIV-infected *every minute*, that's over 1 million per year (Butler, 1993). The WHO estimates that over 9 million women will be HIV-infected by the end of 1995 and over 2 million will have AIDS.

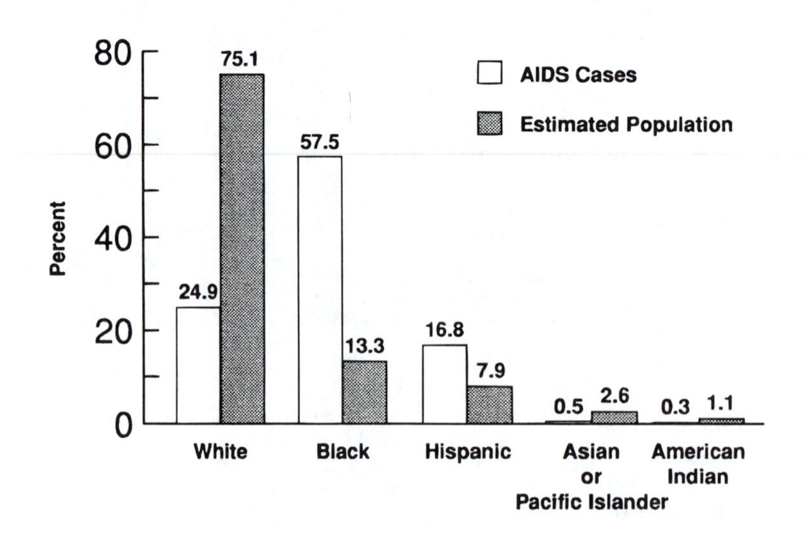

FIGURE 10-3 Incidence of AIDS Cases Among Women of Different Ethnic Groups. Worldwide, every minute, two women become HIV-infected, and every two minutes, a woman dies of AIDS. (Source: Courtesy of CDC, Atlanta, 1993)

Adolescent/Adult Women AIDS Annual Rates per 100,000 Population
United States—Cases Reported in 1994

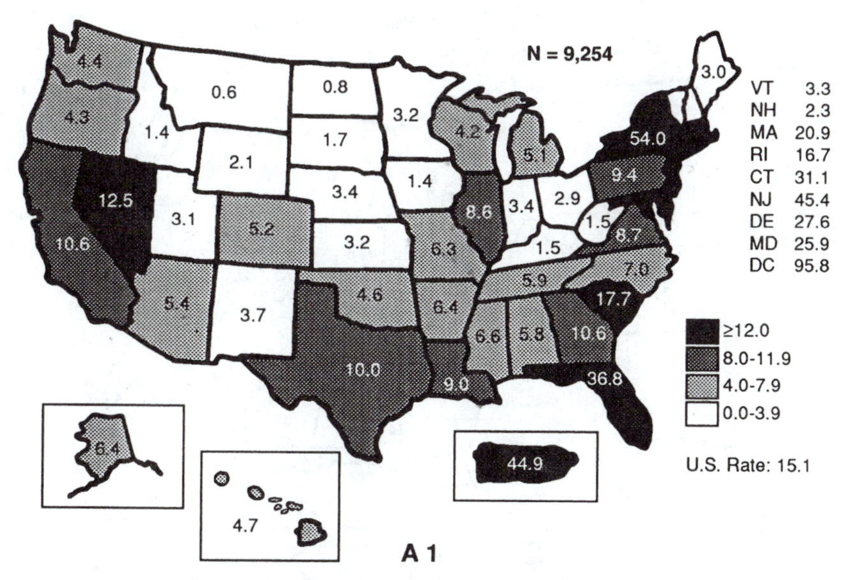

Adolescent/Adult Men AIDS Annual Rates per 100,000 Population
United States—Cases Reported in 1994

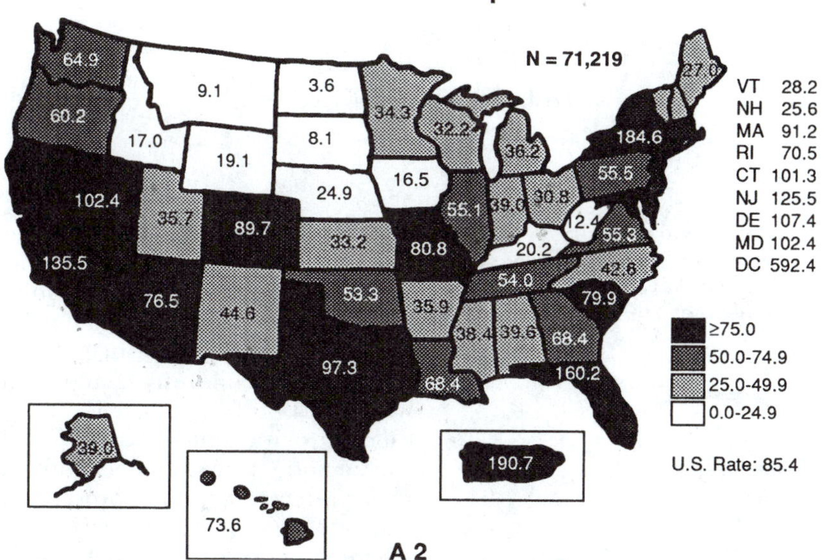

FIGURE 10-4 **A1,** Rates of Reported AIDS Cases per 100,000 Population Among Adolescent and Adult Women by State of Residence—United States, 1994. **A2,** Rates of Reported AIDS Cases Per 100,000 Population Among Adolescent and Adult Men by State of Residence—United States, 1994. **B,** One Year of New AIDS Cases, Adults/Adolescents Across the United States, Reported for 1993. (Total AIDS cases for 1993, 105,990) *(Source: Courtesy of CDC, Atlanta)*

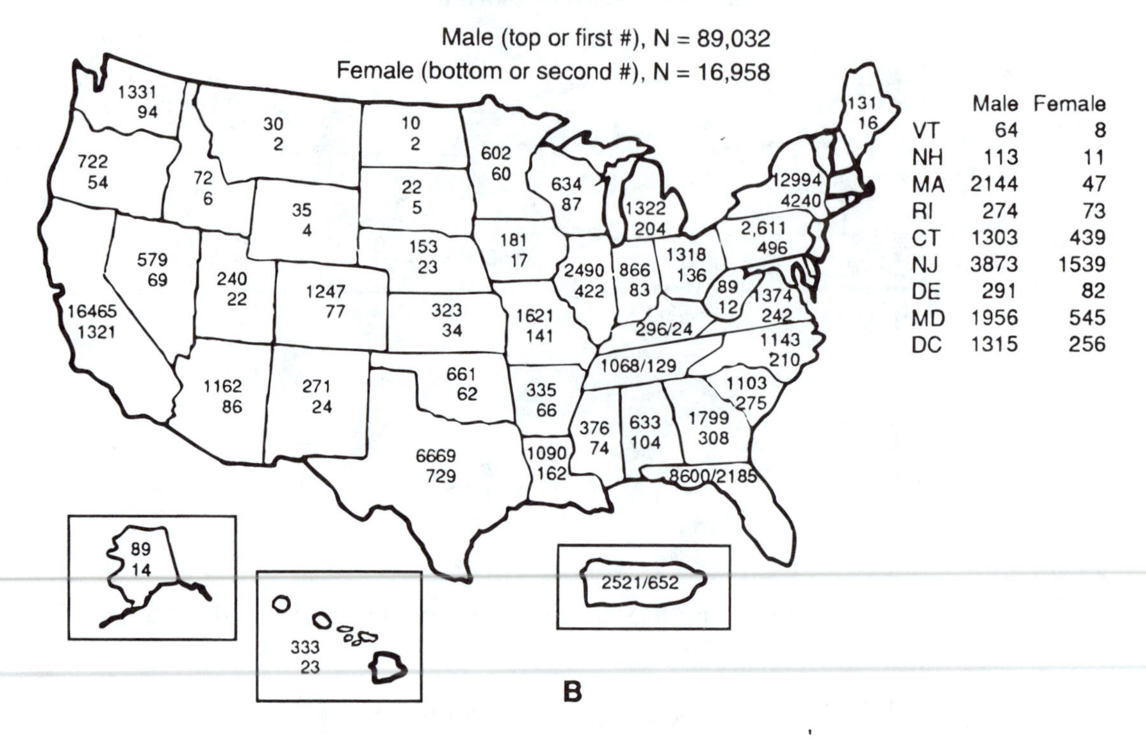

FIGURE 10-4 *(continued)*

FIGURE 10-5 Major Sources of HIV Infections in Women. (*Source: U. S. Centers for Disease Control and Prevention, AIDS in the World, top number for 1993, bottom number for 1994.*

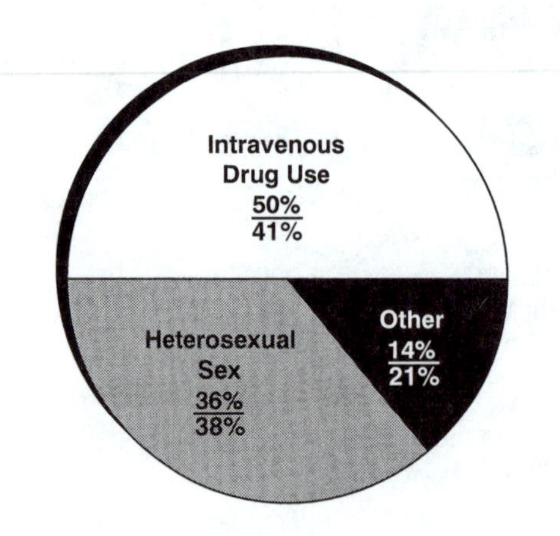

Transmission Categories. Injection drug use (IDU) has, since the beginning, been the major route of HIV transmission for women. Fifty-two percent of all female AIDS cases are among IDUs. It is a principal link to other adults and to children. Heterosexual contact with an HIV-infected male is the second highest route of transmission at 35%. This category can include sexual contact with male IDUs, males infected by blood products, and males who are bisexual. Female IDUs and sexual partners of male IDUs make up the largest number of HIV-infected women of child-bearing age. Blood transfusions and use of clotting factor make up 6% of female AIDS cases, and, in 7% of cases the cause was undetermined.

HIV infection has occurred in a substantial number of women exposed only occasionally to semen from a single HIV-infected male. To

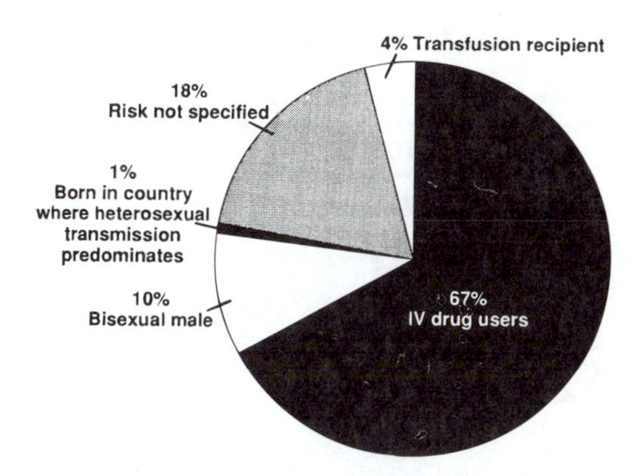

FIGURE 10-6 Risk Category of Sexual Partners of Women with Heterosexually Acquired AIDS, through 1994, United States. While the majority of women who contracted AIDS through heterosexual intercourse had partners who were injection drug users, 33% acquired HIV from partners with other risk factors. Many women may not be aware that their partners are in these risk categories. (Adapted from Guinan, 1993)

date there is only one case of transmission through artificial insemination reported in the United States, but several other cases are known to have occurred (Joseph, 1993). Four of eight Australian women who received semen from a single infected donor became infected. Infected semen had been injected into the uterus through a catheter. In another case of HIV exposure, 10 out of 17 women became infected through vaginal intercourse with one HIV-infected man (Allen et al., 1988).

Special Problems. Heterosexual women are at far greater risk of contracting AIDS during heterosexual intercourse than heterosexual men for several reasons.

1. During vaginal contact, women are exposed to semen carrying significant quantities of lymphocytes. Conversely, men are exposed to small amounts of potentially infected vaginal fluids and cervical secretions (fewer lymphocytes).

POINT OF INFORMATION 10.3

WOMEN WITH AIDS—UNITED STATES, 1994

In 1994, of the 79,456 persons aged ≥13 years reported with AIDS, 14,302 (18%) occurred among women—nearly threefold greater than the proportion (534 [7%] of 8,153) reported in 1985; in addition, the proportion of cases among women has increased steadily since 1985. The median age of women reported with AIDS in 1994 was 35 years, and women aged 15 to 44 years accounted for 84% of cases. More than three fourths (77%) of cases among women occurred among blacks and Hispanics, and rates for black and Hispanic women were 16 and seven times higher, respectively, than those for white women.

In 1994, the Northeast region accounted for the largest percentage of AIDS cases reported among women (44%), followed by the South (36%), West (9%), Midwest (7%), and Puerto Rico and U.S. territories (4%). In the Northeast, most cases among women occurred in urban areas; 1.4% of women with AIDS in the Northeast resided outside metropolitan areas compared with 10.2% of women who resided outside metropolitan areas in the South. Of all AIDS cases among women, 61% were reported from five states: New York (26%), Florida (13%), New Jersey (10%), California (7%), and Texas (5%).

In 1994, 59% of AIDS cases among women were reported based on criteria added in the 1993 expanded AIDS surveillance case definition. This total included 7181 women with severe HIV-related immunosuppression (CD4+ T-lymphocytes <200 cells/μL or percentage of total lymphocytes <14), 557 with pulmonary tuberculosis, 376 with recurrent pneumonia, and 164 with invasive cervical cancer.

In 1994, 41% of women with AIDS reported injecting-drug use; 38%, heterosexual contact with a partner at risk for or known to have HIV infection or AIDS; and 2%, receipt of contaminated blood or blood products; 19% had no specific HIV exposure reported. Of all women with AIDS who were initially reported without risk but who were later reclassified, most had heterosexual contact with an at-risk partner (66%) or a history of injecting-drug use (27%). In 1994, of the 5,353 women reported with AIDS attributed to heterosexual contact, 38% reported contact with a male partner who was an injecting-drug user; 7%, a bisexual male; 2%, a partner who had hemophilia or had received HIV-contaminated blood or blood products; and 53%, a partner who had documented HIV infection or AIDS but whose risk was unspecified (*MMWR*, 1995b).

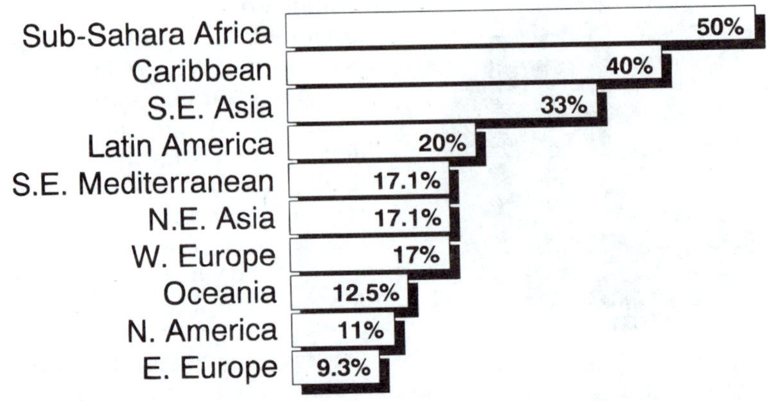

FIGURE 10-7 Incidence of HIV-Infected Women Worldwide. *(Source: U. S. Centers for Disease Control and Prevention, AIDS in the World, 1993. No appreciable change in 1994.)*

2. The mucosal surface area available for HIV penetration is significantly smaller in men than in women. The entire vagina and cervix are of a mucosal nature. In men, the urethra is the only mucosal surface area exposed to female secretions.
3. During the act of sexual intercourse, the vaginal mucosa often suffers microscopic abrasions, drawing lymphocytes to the area. This makes vaginal tissue more susceptible to HIV-positive semen. Abrasions do not normally occur within the male urethra.
4. There are more HIV-infected men than women. In Western Europe, Australia, and North America the ratio of HIV-infected men to HIV-infected women is about 6:1. (Aggleton et al., 1994) Because of the greater number of infected men, the sexually active woman is at increased risk. This is particularly true if the woman has multiple partners and lives in an area with a large population of HIV-infected men.

Special concerns of HIV/AIDS Women. *First,* HIV/AIDS has a profound impact on women, both as an illness and as a social and economic challenge. Women play a crucial role in preventing infection by insisting on safer sexual practices and caring for people with HIV disease and people with AIDS. The stigma attached to HIV/AIDS can subject women to discrimination, social rejection, and other violations of their rights.

Women need to know that they can protect themselves against HIV infection. Women have a traditionally passive role in sexual decision making in many countries. They need knowledge about HIV and AIDS, self-confidence, and the skills necessary to insist partners use safer sex methods.

Efforts to influence women to practice safer sex must also be joined by efforts to address men and their responsibility in practicing safer sex.

POINT OF VIEW 10.1

A LEGACY FOR HER DAUGHTER

In 1990, Patrica Kloser,the director of the only AIDS clinic in the United States devoted entirely to the needs of women (personal communication, 1990), related that one of her most moving experiences involved a women with AIDS who was knitting a scarf for her 2-year-old daughter.The woman said that she wanted to leave *"some legacy"* for her daughter. Kloser said, "I couldn't tell her that her daughter, also infected, wouldn't live long enough to appreciate the legacy." (Patricia Kloser is Clinical Director of AIDS Services and Attending Physician in the Department of Infectious Disease and Internal Medicine, University of Medicine and Dentistry of New Jersey, Newark.)

Second, women get pregnant. Women who are ill and discover they are pregnant need information about both the potential impact of pregnancy on their own health and maternal—fetal HIV transmission.

Third, women have the role of mothering. From this role come two important consequences. First, when a woman becomes ill with HIV disease or AIDS, her role as caretaker of the child or children or other adults in the household is immediately affected. The family is severely disrupted and each family member has to make adjustments. Second, the mother must cope with her own life-threatening illness while she also deals with the impact of the disease on her family. Demographic studies show that many HIV-infected or AIDS women have young children; and these women are often the sole support of these children.

Fourth, a woman's illness may be complicated further by incarceration and the threat of foster care proceedings. If the mother is healthy enough to care for her child, she must still cope with the complex issues of medical and home care, school access, friends, and family stress.

Fifth, worldwide, an estimated 3 million women will die of AIDS during the 1990s, and over 15 million will have become HIV-infected (Douglas, 1994). Yet little is known about the course and consequences of HIV infection among women and about the appropriate standards for their clinical care. What is known about HIV disease has been derived from studies on men, who for the most part differ from women in race, income, and risk behavior. What female-derived information there is on HIV disease in women comes mostly from studies on pregnant women which have focused primarily on perinatal issues. Because relatively few studies have been done on HIV-infected women, little is known about the pharmacokinetics of HIV/AIDS drugs in women, nor is it clear whether gender influences specific illnesses. For example, does HIV infection increase cervical and vaginal disease and pelvic inflammatory disease (PID)? Why are certain opportunistic diseases more aggressive and damaging to females? And how are the drugs used to treat opportunistic infections metabolized in women?

On July 23, 1992, the International Community of Women Living with HIV/AIDS was formed. The Community intends to disseminate women-specific information to seropositive women worldwide and to establish an international "calling list" so that HIV-positive women need never be alone when traveling. Information can be obtained from: Kate Thomson, c/o Positively Women, 5 Sebastian Street, London EC1V 0HE, United Kingdom; tel.: 44-71-490-5515; fax: 44-71-490-1690.

Female HIV/AIDS Deaths— These deaths rose from 18 cases in 1981 to 1,668 in 1988, to 25,213 by the end of 1992 (Buehler et al., 1992), and to 31,363 by the end of 1994, and over 35,800 will have died by the end of 1995. In New York City, AIDS has been the leading cause of death of women between ages 25 to 34 for several years. It is now the leading cause of death in women between the ages of 25 and 34 and the second leading cause of death in women between the ages of 20 and 44 nationally. AIDS is the leading cause of death for black women between the ages of 15 and 44 in New Jersey and New York.

Preventing HIV Infection

Women have been told to reduce their number of partners, to be monogamous, and to protect themselves by using condoms. But these goals, generally speaking, do not fit the realities of women's lives or they may not be under their control.

Women who have more than one partner in their lifetime often practice serial monogamy, remaining with one partner at a time. People living as couples reduce the number of their sexual partners. Still, in many phases of life, sex is practiced with new partners in new relationships. American women, on average, are single for many years before their first marriage; they might be single again after a divorce; they might marry again; and, in later phases especially, they might be widowed. For some women, multiple partners throughout life are an economic necessity; and urging them to reduce the number of partners is meaningless unless the economic situation for these women is improved (Ehrhardt, 1992).

Childbearing Women— The prevalence of HIV infection in childbearing women was determined for 38 states and the District of Columbia (Gwinn et al., 1991). New York, New Jersey, Florida, and the District of Columbia have the highest rates of HIV/AIDS in women and their babies. An estimated 5,810 women with HIV infection gave birth in these states between mid-1988 and mid-1990. As of December 31, 1989, the same 39 areas had reported 95% of the perinatally acquired AIDS cases in children. Assuming that these areas accounted for the same proportion of all births to HIV-infected women, it was estimated that 6,079 such births occurred in the United States in 1989. Based on an expected 4 million total births that year, the prevalence of HIV infection was estimated to be 1.5 per 1,000 childbearing women. If the rate of perinatal transmission of infection was approximately 30%, approximately 1 in every 2,200 infants born in the United States in 1989 was infected with HIV as a result of perinatal exposure (Gwinn et al., 1991).

The perinatal incidence rate of 30% for HIV infection is second only to that for gay men. As of mid 1995, there will be an estimated 90,000 to 100,000 infected women of childbearing age in the United States, perhaps 10% know that they are infected. Women, in general, have two children before they find out they are infected (Thomas, 1989). The birth of an infected child may serve as a *miner's canary*—the first indication of HIV infection in the mother. In New York, in 1993, 25% of HIV infected babies were born to mothers who did not know they were HIV-infected.

BOX 10.3

HIV-INFECTED WOMEN: DIFFICULT CHOICES DURING PREGNANCY

She was 19 years old, a nursing student, pregnant, and HIV-positive, She spent 4 1/2 months of pregnancy in constant fear for herself and for her baby. She waited, her health began to falter, then she decided to have an abortion.

Several studies have reported that HIV-positive women who preceived their risk of infecting their fetus to be greater than 50% were more likely to abort than those who perceived a lower risk. HIV-positive women who chose to continue their pregnancy cited the desire to have a child, strong religious beliefs, and family pressure (Selwyn et al., 1989).

For women who are HIV-positive, pregnancy poses difficult choices. Besides the possibility that the pregnancy may influence the progression of HIV disease or mask the presence of symptoms,having a child poses other questions such as: Can the mother cope with a normal or infected child? and, Who will care for the child if the mother becomes too ill or dies?

The World Health Organization estimates that worldwide, by the year 2000, 10 million children will be orphaned because of HIV/AIDS.

Reproductive Rights. These are central to a woman's right to control her body. The choice of becoming pregnant or terminating the pregnancy are continually disputed.

However, as more women become HIV-infected and give birth to infected children, childbearing may come under the surveillance of the state. Women of childbearing age may be among the first groups to undergo mandatory testing as part of an attempt to control the birth of infected newborns.

Reproductive rights take on new meaning with HIV-infected pregnancies. The state has traditionally expressed an interest in protecting the rights of the fetus. This interest was transcended in the 1973 *Roe v. Wade* decision when the Supreme Court recognized a woman's right to choose an abortion. The court ruled that a woman's right to privacy must prevail against the state's interest in protecting the future life of the fetus. The state's interest in fetal survival tends to diminish, however, when the mother is infected with HIV (Franke, 1988). (See Chapter 7, page 146 for recent information on preventing HIV infection of the fetus.)

Pediatric Cases— Pediatric AIDS cases make up about 1.3% of the total number of reported AIDS cases in the United States. This proportion bears a striking similarity to the incidence of cancer in children. But, unlike cancer or the other major causes of death in children whose contributions to childhood mortality have remained stable over the years, the impact of HIV infection is increasing. For infants and young children, AIDS is already among the 10 leading causes of death, surpassing all other infections, and is likely to be among the five leading causes of death within the next several years.

There is evidence that HIV was present in female IDUs as early as 1977 because their babies developed AIDS (Thomas, 1988). As the number of HIV-infected women of child bearing age rises, so does the number of HIV-infected babies. Currently 6 to 7 thousand HIV-infected women give birth in the United States.

Pediatric AIDS, in the United States is most widespread among blacks, Hispanics, and the poor of the inner cities (Figure 10–8). Ten metropolitan areas account for more than 50% of all cases: New York, Miami, Newark, Los Angeles, San Juan, Washington DC, West Palm Beach, Philadel-phia, Nassau/Suffolk, and Jersey City. New York City, Newark, and Miami report the largest numbers. The epidemic is also spreading into smaller communities; pediatric AIDS cases have been reported in all 50 states and two territories.

Factors that influence intrauterine or perinatal HIV transmission are not known; but, influencing factors do exist because one mother gave birth to an HIV-infected child followed by an uninfected child who was followed by an infected child (Dickinson, 1988)!

Because newborns who test HIV-positive may not be HIV-infected, infected mothers are advised not to breast-feed these children. The reason a newborn can test positive and not be infected is because the mother's HIV antibodies can enter the fetus during gestation. Because of the presence of maternal HIV antibody, the newborn may appear to be infected but is not. The HIV antibody will be lost with time and the child will revert to **seronegativity** (no HIV antibody in the serum).

Rate of Transmission. The rate of HIV transmission from mother to child is 30% to 50%. The Public Health Service and 16 other national health organizations have recommended that HIV testing be offered to all women at risk prior to or at the time of pregnancy. (Pre- and post-counseling of at risk females who want to become pregnant or have become pregnant is covered in Chapter 13.)

College Students— Between April, 1988, and February, 1989, the blood of 16,863 students, enrolled at 16 large universities and three private colleges was tested for HIV antibodies.

Figure 10-8 Pediatric AIDS cases—United States, 1994. The number of pediatric AIDS cases in proportion to the ethnic population is presented in percent. (*Source*: CDC, Atlanta, GA, 1994)

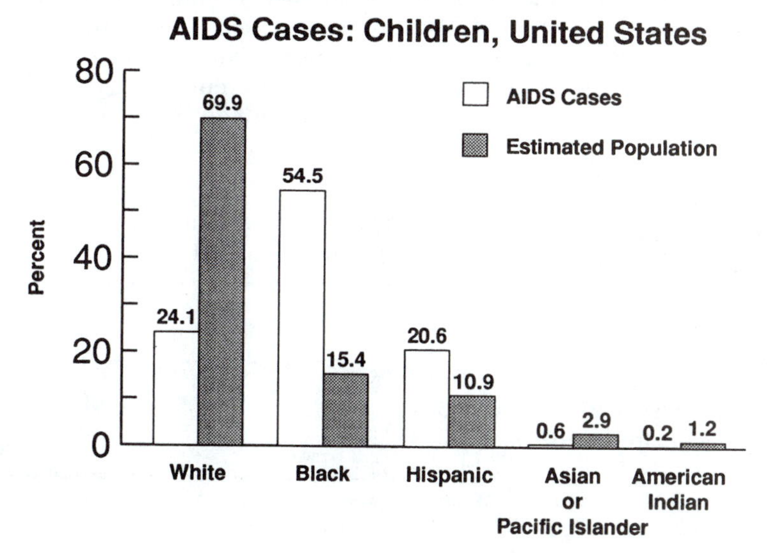

Thirty students, 28 males and 2 females, tested HIV-positive for an overall rate of 2 per 1,000 or 0.2%. With 12.5 million students enrolled in American colleges and universities, the rate of 2 in 1,000 means there are about 25,000 HIV-infected college students.

The study was conducted by the CDC with The American College Health Association (Gayle et al., 1990). Because the samples were not identified, students who tested positive could not be informed. All blood samples from 10 of the 19 campuses were HIV-negative. At five campuses the rate of HIV-positive blood ranged from four to nine samples per 1,000. In contrast, the rate of HIV in the general heterosexual population is about 0.02% and the rate for military personnel in about the same age group tested over a similar time period was 0.14%.

The important question is **why** college students have a rate of HIV infection 10 times higher than the general heterosexual population. Are college students less well informed than the general heterosexual population?

Surveys indicate that college students are well educated about HIV/AIDS. Why, then, the higher rate of infection? Perhaps it's the age-old dilemma of information versus behavior. They know what to do—but they don't do it. There is a difference between knowledge and action based on that knowledge. College students have always had information on drug use, alcoholism, pregnancies out of wedlock, and sexually transmitted diseases; but, this knowledge has not appreciably reduced at-risk behaviors. STDs are at an all time high in teenage and college students.

College Students and National Issues. In April of 1994, The Roper College Track poll asked undergraduate students at 4-year colleges and universities, "What are the national issues you are most concerned about?" Their overwhelming response was AIDS. Of the top 10 issues listed most frequently, 50% of students listed AIDS as their main concern, followed by crime at 34%, drugs 21%, quality of education 20%, cost of health care 19%, moral values and race relations at 17% each, the budget deficit 16%, and environmental damage and poverty each at 15%.

Teenagers— There was a time when safer sex meant not getting caught by your parents. With time, sexually transmitted diseases and in particular HIV/AIDS have changed the meaning of safer sex. Today, over half of teenagers (aged 13 to 19) in the United States have had sex by the time they reach 16, and 7 in 10 are sexually active by 19. Many enter the sexual arena unprepared for the responsibility of their actions (Table 10-5). About 1 million teenage women become pregnant, outside of marriage, each year. In a 1990 nationwide survey, 19% of high school students have had four or more sex partners by their junior year and 29% had four or more by their senior year (*MMWR*, 1992c). Every 30 seconds a teenager somewhere in the United States is infected with an STD. Nine percent of American girls become mothers before turning 18, and one in four teens will contract an STD before finishing high school. In April of 1992, the *MacNeil/Lehrer Report* estimated that 40,000 to 80,000 teenagers will become HIV-infected during the 1990s. Yet, AIDS cases are relatively rare among 13- to 19-year-olds. This is because of the 10-year time average from HIV infection to AIDS diagnosis. In 1984, there were 39 reported teenage AIDS cases, by 1991 there were 789 reported cases. Through 1994, there were 3,290 (0.7% of the total AIDS cases). Between 1990 and 1992 the number of AIDS cases in 13- to 24-year-olds increased by 77% (House Select Committee, 1992). It is projected that after 1994 the number of teenage AIDS cases will double annually (Black et al., 1990; Burkhart, 1991). This means that regardless of available information on prevention, there has been a continuing increase in HIV infections within the

TABLE 10-5 Sexually Active Teenagers by High School Year and Age (%)

High School Year	Age Group	Female	Male	Combined
9th Grade	14–15	31.9	48.7	39.6
10th Grade	15–16	42.9	52.5	47.6
11th Grade	16–17	52.7	62.6	57.3
12th Grade	17–19	66.6	76.3	71.9

(Source: CDC HIV/AIDS Surveillance Report, November 1991:1–18)

preteen and early teen population! There are about 28 million teenagers between the ages of 13 and 19. There are another 18 million people ages 20 to 24, and about 22 million between the ages of 25 and 29. That's 68 million people between the ages of 13 and 29. Eighty-six percent of all STDs occur in the age group of 15 to 29. It has been estimated that 34% of all adults with AIDS were infected with HIV as teenagers.

The total number of HIV-infected teenagers is unknown. But it is known that 56% of teenagers who were tested for HIV infection did *not* return for their results!

Federal health agencies estimate that teenagers make up about 20% of the HIV-infected population. They are a silent pool for eventual cases of AIDS. About 20% of the total number of AIDS cases in the United States occur in people ages 20 to 29 (over 88,000 through 1994). Most of these people, given the 9- to 15-year period before being diagnosed with AIDS, were infected as teen-agers! About 50% of HIV-infected teenagers come from six locations: New York, New Jersey, Texas, California, Florida, and Puerto Rico. The overall male-to-female ratio of AIDS cases in the United States is now about 7:1; but, among 13- to 19-year-olds, the ratio is 3:1.

In New York City, teenagers account for 29% of all New York AIDS cases. Nationally persons aged 20 to 29 account for 20% or 1 in 5 of all U.S. AIDS cases. AIDS is the sixth leading cause of death among persons aged 15 to 24 and fourth among women aged 25 to 44 years (*MMWR*, 1995). Sixty percent of new HIV infection in women now occurs during their adolescent years. Over 40% of AIDS cases among women have occurred between the ages of 13 and 24. Over 500,000 people in the United States under the age of 25 are HIV-positive.

Teenagers of color account for 59% of reported teen AIDS cases. Among males, white teenagers account for 47% of reported AIDS cases, followed by blacks (30%) and Hispanics (21%). Among females, black teenagers account for 56%, white for 27%, and Hispanic for17% Teenage females, unlike their adult counterparts, are more likely to become infected with HIV through sexual exposure than through injection drug use. A program that followed a large cohort of HIV-infected adolescents found that although 85% of females contracted HIV infection through heterosexual intercourse, very few were aware that their male partners had HIV infection at the time of their exposure (Futterman et al., 1992). Worldwide, Faustin Yao (1992) reports that 20% to 25% of all new HIV infections are occurring among teen-agers. Of the 20 million HIV-positive people worldwide at mid-1995, 10 million became HIV-infected between the ages of 15 and 24.

Teenage women are leading the next wave of the HIV epidemic worldwide. In Asia, Africa, and North America HIV infections are increasing at an alarming rate among young women, with the highest rates now being found in the 15- to 19-year age group. Many more young women than young men are being HIV-infected worldwide.

Helene Gayle (1988) states that the proportion of teen females with AIDS is greater than for adult females; and the proportion of teen females infected via heterosexual contact is greater than for adult females. A 1993 study at Montefiore Medical Centre, New York, found that of HIV-positive teenage girls, 85% had contracted the virus through sex with males; 26% reported having anal sex either for contraceptive purposes or to retain vaginal virginity. One new face of the epidemic in the United States may be reflected in the behavior of teenage women.

For 1993, and 1994, the breakdown for HIV infection among teenagers was as follows: males who have sex with males account for 29%, patients with hemophilia and other coagulation disorders account for 31%, heterosexual contact represents 14%, intravenous drug use 17%, and nonhemophilia-related transfusions and organ donations 9%.

David Rogers, vice chairman of the National Commission on AIDS (which dissolved in 1993) said, "We have let issues of taste and morality interfere with the delivery of potentially life-saving information to young people."

Do you think he is correct? What is the down side of his statement? (class discussion)

RUNAWAY TEENAGERS: THE HOMELESS. An estimated 1 to 2 million runaway teenagers are homeless each year.These youth may engage in behaviors such as having multiple sexual partners, exchange of sex for money or drugs, and unprotected sexual intercourse that place them at risk for HIV infection. HIV seroprevalence studies among homeless youth have shown rates that are higher than adolescents in other settings (Rotheram et al., 1992).

David Allen and co-workers (1994) report that in general HIV infection rates among the homeless youth populations were comparable with persons attending STD clinics. In nine of 16 sites, HIV seroprevalence rates among homeless youth were higher than the median rates of youth attending STD clinics within the same city. These studies can only hint at how far HIV has infiltrated specific groups of teenagers.

If you are a teenager or know of one who needs help or has HIV/AIDS questions, call: **NATIONAL TEENAGERS AIDS HOTLINE** 1-800-234-8336.

Prisoners— In 1992, the nation's population under correctional supervision was at an all time high of 4,435,000 adults—2.4% of the total U.S. adult population (*MMWR*, 1992a). Of this population, just over 1 million are in state and federal prisons.

Prison inmates make up a small number of AIDS cases, but a significant percentage are HIV-positive. Blood testing of inmates at 10 selected prisons indicated that 1 in every 24 prisoners is infected with the AIDS virus. This study also found that incarcerated women under age 25 were found to have higher HIV seroprevalence (5.2%) than incarcerated young men (2.3%). The rate was comparable among older women (5.3%) and older men (5.6%). Non-whites were almost twice as likely to be infected as whites. Rates varied widely among the 10 institutions from 2.1% to 7.6% for men, and 2.7% to 14.7% for women (Vlahov et al., 1991).

In general, prisoners diagnosed with AIDS were infected prior to their incarceration—most are IDUs (Francis, 1987). Infected inmates most often transmit the virus to others through homosexual and drug related activities. For that reason 21 states segregated HIV-infected and AIDS patient prisoners from the other prisoners. In September of 1989, a court order in the state of Connecticut ended their prison segregation policy. Similar antisegregation lawsuits have been filed in Alabama and Oregon.

A number of state prisons have instituted either mass screening programs or large scale blind serological surveys for HIV infection. The Federal Bureau of Prisons tests a 10% sample of federal prisoners. Other jurisdictions conduct screening or testing programs for selected groups of prisoners, such as known injection drug users and homosexuals.

The incidence of AIDS is about 14 times higher in State and Federal correctional systems (202/100,000 prisoners) than in the United States population (15/100,000 population) (Gostin et al., 1994). In 1993, the WHO reported that AIDS is responsible for 30% of all deaths in United States Prisons. It is the leading cause of death in the New York and Florida prison systems. In 1991, according to the *People With AIDS Coalition Newsline*, 66% of inmate deaths in New York and New Jersey and 50% in Florida resulted from AIDS. The *AIDS Quarterly Report* in May, 1990, stated that in 1992, 15,000 HIV-infected prisoners left the New York prison system to join the general population, and because of confidentiality laws, no one will know who they are. At Riker's Island facility in New York, of 21,000 plus prisoners, one in four are reported to be HIV-infected (National Press Release, 1989).

The Elderly— AIDS cases remain relatively low among people between the ages 65 and 90. Howard Fillit and colleagues (1989) reported that nationally 10% of the total AIDS cases occur in people over age 50. By the end of 1994 this represented 47,000 people. Three percent of AIDS occurs in people over age 60 or 13,300 people. One AIDS patient was 90 years old when diagnosed. He became HIV-infected from a blood transfusion during surgery at age 85. He became symptomatic about 4 years later and died 1 year later of *Pneumocystis carinii* pneumonia.

In *Florida*, a state with a large retired population, the number of recorded AIDS cases among the elderly has risen from 6 in 1984 to 1,341 through 1993, or nearly 4% of the state's cases.

POINT OF INFORMATION 10.4

WHERE OLDER PATIENTS WITH HIV DISEASE CAN GET HELP

The problem of AIDS in persons 50 and older has received little recognition. But a few organizations now provide literature or services aimed specifically at older patients and their physicans:

American Association of Retired Persons
601 E St. NW
Washington, DC 20049
(202) 434-2277

Publishes free fact sheet, "AIDS: A Multigenerational Crisis" (Stock No. D14942), that includes listings of referral services.

Senior Action in a Gay Environment (SAGE)
208 W. 13th St.
New York, NY 10011
(212) 741-2247

Provides a variety of services to gays in their 50s or older. Also offers training, education, counseling, and therapy and is a source of information for physicians and hospitals. Operates chiefly in the area surrounding New York City (N.Y., N.J., Conn.).

Healthcare Education Associates
70 Campton Pl.
Laguna Niguel, CA 92677
(714) 240-2179

Publishes a training manual for use in discussion groups: "AIDS and Aging: What People Over 50 Need to Know." "Leaders Guide" and "Participant's Workbook" are $13.95; workbook alone, $5.

HIV/AIDS in Aging Task Force
425 E. 25th St.
New York, NY 10010
(212) 481-7670

Arranges conferences and educational seminars; participants include physicians. Provides support for establishing task forces and seminars throughout the country.

National Institute on Aging
Public Information Office
Federal Bldg. 31 (Room 5C27)
Bethesda, MD 20892
(301) 496-1752

Publishes fact sheet, "Age Page: AIDS and Older Adults," available as a FAX transmission by calling (800) 222-2225.

Source: Feldman et al., 1994.

In general Americans over 50 are potentially at risk, sometimes without realizing it, when they begin dating following a divorce or the death of a spouse. Others are at risk because they are IDUs or continue to have multiple sex partners or have a sex partner who practices unsafe sex. Individuals who acquire HIV infection at older ages progress to AIDS, more rapidly on average, than individuals infected at younger ages (excluding pediatric cases).

The majority of AIDS cases in the elderly have occurred due to HIV-contaminated blood transfusions. It is believed that with the growing number of elderly people in the United States and better therapy for those who are HIV-infected in their early and late 50s, there will be an increasing number of elderly HIV-infected and AIDS patients who must be cared for. The male/female ratio in the age 50 and over is about 9:1 (Ship et al., (1991).

Health Care Workers— Health care workers are defined by the CDC as people, including students and trainees, whose activities involve contact with patients or with blood or other body fluids from patients in a health care setting.

The risk of HIV transmission from health care worker to patient during an exposure prone invasive procedure is remote. There is a greater and well documented risk of transmission from an infected patient to a health care worker.

As the pandemic of HIV infections continues to increase, workers in every health care field will be involved in the detection, counseling, therapy, maintenance, quantity, and

TABLE 10-6 Health Care Workers with Documented and Possible Occupationally Acquired AIDS/HIV Infection, by Occupation, Reported Through December 1994, United States[a]

	Documented Occupational Transmission[b]	Possible Occupational Transmission[c]
Occupation	No.	No.
Dental worker, including dentist	-	7
Embalmer/morgue technician	-	3
Emergency medical technician/paramedic	-	9
Health aide/attendant	1	9
Housekeeper/maintenance worker	1	6
Laboratory technician, clinical	15	14
Laboratory technician, nonclinical	2	1
Nurse	13	20
Physician, nonsurgical	6	9
Physician, surgical	-	2
Respiratory therapist	1	2
Technician, dialysis	1	1
Technician, surgical	2	1
Technician/therapist, other than those listed above	-	4
Other health-care occupations	-	2
Total	42	90

[a]Health care workers are defined as those persons, including students and trainees, who have worked in a health care, clinical, or HIV laboratory setting at any time since 1978. See *MMWR,* 1992;41:823–825.

[b]Health care workers who had documented HIV seroconversion after occupational exposure or had other laboratory evidence of occupaitonal infection: 37 had percutaneous exposure, 4 had mucocutaneous exposure, 1 had both percutaneous and mucocutaneous exposures, and 1 had an unknown route of exposure. Thirty-eight exposures were to blood from an HIV-infected person, 1 to visibly bloody fluid, 1 to an unspecified fluid, and 2 to concentrated virus in a laboratory. Fifteen of these health care workers have developed AIDS.

[c]These health care workers have been investigated and are without identifiable behavioral or transfusion risks; each reported percutaneous or mucocutaneous occupational exposures to blood or body fluids, or laboratory solutions containing HIV, but HIV seroconversion specifically resulting from an occupational exposure was not documented.

(Source: HIV/AIDS Surveillance June Report, 1994)

quality of life for the symptomatic HIV-infected and for those expressing AIDS. Although the largest number of HIV-infected people are asymptomatic, each day many of them begin to experience signs and symptoms of HIV disease; and each day new cases of AIDS are diagnosed. As the number of patients increases, additional health care workers are required to meet their needs. As this work force enlarges to meet the demands of the estimated numbers of AIDS cases in the coming years, precautions must be practiced to prevent health care workers themselves from becoming HIV-infected.

Ruthanne Marcus and colleagues (1988) reported that, across the board, health care workers exposed to HIV-contaminated blood have about a 1 in 300 chance of becoming infected. Other more recent reports place the risk of HIV infection at 1 in 250.

Health Care Workers with HIV/AIDS

By the end of 1994, the CDC had received reports of 40 health care workers in the United States (worldwide 59 cases were reported) with documented occupationally acquired HIV infection and 84 with possible occupationally acquired HIV infection (Table 10-6). Twelve of these workers have developed AIDS. Three had died by the end of 1994. The U.S. Occupational Safety and Health Administration (OSHA) has published case reports of 65 health care workers who appear to have been HIV-infected through exposure at work (*AIDS Alert,* 1993). These are small numbers when compared to some 7,000 hepatitis B transmissions to health care workers every year in the United States (Osborne, 1993).

For 69 of the 84 CDC reported health care workers classified with possible occupationally acquired HIV infection, four (6%) had occupational exposures to blood of patients known to be HIV-infected or to research laboratory specimens known to contain infectious HIV. Of the remaining 65, none reported exposure to blood or body fluids known to be HIV-infected. Of the 69 possible occupationally acquired HIV-infected workers, 54 (78%) have developed AIDS (*MMWR*, 1992b). The number of persons with occupationally acquired HIV infection is probably greater than the totals presented here because not all health care workers are evaluated for HIV infection following exposures and not all persons with occupationally acquired infection are reported.

Of the estimated 476,000 plus adult/adolescent/pediatric AIDS cases by mid 1995, about 16,600 (3.5%) are health care workers including an estimated 1,900 (0.4%) physicians, 3,618 (0.76%) nurses and 2,618 (0.55%) dentists (Toufexis, 1991). Overall, by 1995, 72% of the health care workers with AIDS, including 821 physicians, 66 surgeons, 240 dental workers, 1,877 nurses, and 161 paramedics have died. The CDC estimated in 1990 that there were at least 5,000 HIV-infected physicians (Breo, 1990). The Medical Expertise Retention Program (MERP) in San Francisco in November 1991 estimated that 7,000 to 10,000 physicians and 50,000 to 70,000 other HCWs in the United States are HIV-positive (Williams, 1991).

Like other adult AIDS patients, health care workers have a median age of 35 years. Males account for 91.6% of cases and 62% are white.

Ninety-five percent of the health care workers with AIDS were classified into known transmission categories. Health care workers with AIDS were significantly *less likely* to be injection drug users and *more likely* to be homosexual or bisexual men. Thirty-two healthcare workers have contracted HIV in work-related accidents in France and the French Association of Health Workers said that the real number of people who became HIV-infected on the job is closer to 300 (Butler, 1994).

Needlestick Injuries— Health care workers are in a quandary about the possibility of becoming HIV-infected via needlesticks. Articles such as "Needlestick Risks Higher Than Reports Indicate" or "The Risk of HIV Transmission via Needlesticks Is Low" convey conflicting impressions.

The kinds of needlesticks most likely to occur in hospital or health care settings come from disposable syringes, IV line/needle assemblies, prefilled cartridge injection syringes, winged steel needle IV sets, vacuum tube phlebotomy assemblies, and IV catheters, in that order. Needlesticks and penetration of sharp objects account for about 80% of all health care workers' exposures to blood and blood products. An estimated 1,000,000 needlesticks occur in the United States each year (Lumsdon, 1992).

A recent report indicates that 1,989 HCWs experienced 2,119 needlesticks with some amount of HIV-contaminated blood. Six of these workers became HIV-infected (*Skin and Allergy News*, 1991). This is a transmission rate of 0.30%. These data would place the risk of seroconversion resulting from such needlesticks to be about 1 in 330. In contrast, 545 HCWs received 928 mucous membrane exposures to secretions of HIV-infected patients; only one resulted in seroconversion. Although it can be concluded that the risk of HIV infection via needlestick injury is relatively low, *the risk is not zero.* Another point of view with respect to risk is that *if the probability of HIV infection is low but the severity of the disease after infection is high, then the risk is high no matter how low the probability of infection.*

Surgery and HIV Risk to Surgeons— About 27 million operations are performed annually in American hospitals. During these procedures, surgeons and operating room personnel are at risk for becoming infected with any of a variety of microorganisms and viruses that may be in the patient's blood. Patient blood contact may occur on exposed skin, by eye and mouth splashing, cuts, and needlesticks. In one study, 149 HCWs experienced 5,000 exposures (skin, mucous membrane, or body fluid) in cases where the patient was documented HIV-positive— *no* seroconversions occurred.

Needlesticks appear to be the most dangerous with respect to the transmission of blood-borne pathogens, especially HIV. Wilson and colleagues (1990) reported that the annual probability of a surgeon receiving at least one needle puncture per year is 86%. Twenty-five percent of surgeons receive nine or more punctures yearly.

Calculations based on worst-case figures estimate that if the prevalence of HIV infection in patients entering a trauma center is 5% and the risk of HIV seroconversion after puncture injury is 0.4%, the average cumulative estimated probability of HIV infection for a surgeon over a 30-year career, assuming four needlesticks a year, would be about 2% (120 needlesticks × 0.05 prevalence × 0.004 risk). In theory, risk of seroconversion increases proportionately with the number of puncture injuries sustained. Some authorities have suggested that surgeons who work with a high-risk population (e.g., trauma patients) should do so only for a limited time. The recommended time limits are yet to be determined, but may be based on number of injuries or years of service.

Pregnancy— Pregnant health care workers are not known to be at greater risk of contracting HIV infections than health care workers who are not pregnant.

Dentistry— Special precautions are recommended for dentistry. Occupationally acquired infection with hepatitis B virus in dental workers has been documented, and two possible cases of occupationally acquired HIV infection involving dentists have been reported. During dental procedures, contamination of saliva with blood is predictable, trauma to health care workers' hands is common, and blood splashing may occur.

Infection control precautions for dentistry, as outlined by the CDC, minimize the potential for nonintact skin and mucous membrane contact of dental health care workers with blood-contaminated saliva of patients. In addition, the use of gloves for oral examinations and treatment in the dental setting may also protect the patient's oral mucous membranes from exposure to blood from cuts on the dental workers' hands.

It appears that HIV transmission to health care workers does occur, but not often and virtually always where the blood or body fluid contains HIV and has been accidentally inoculated into or splashed onto the skin or membrane of the worker.

ESTIMATES OF HIV INFECTION AND FUTURE AIDS CASES

In 1987, Otis Bowen, then Secretary of Health and Human Services, said "AIDS would make black death pale by comparison."

As long as the number of newly infectious people each year exceeds the number who die, the pandemic will continue to build.

Reportability

AIDS— AIDS is reportable in all 50 states, the District of Columbia, and United States territories. AIDS surveillance has been crucial in identifying people at risk for the disease and the modes of transmission. AIDS surveillance data, together with HIV surveys, are important components of public health programs directed toward controlling HIV infection, and assist in providing the most accurate picture of the HIV epidemic in the United States.

By the end of 1993, all 50 states, the District of Columbia, and four territories (Guam, Pacific Islands, Puerto Rico, and the Virgin Islands) reported adult/adolescent cases. The CDC also reported the numbers of adult/adolescent/pediatric AIDS cases in metropolitan areas with a population of 500,000 or more. Of the 94 such cities, 14 had no reported pediatric AIDS cases in 1989. By December, 1993, all have reported pediatric AIDS cases. The 10 leading metropolitan areas for AIDS through 1994 (1 through 10) were: New York City; Los Angeles; San Francisco; Miami; Washington, DC; Chicago; Houston; Newark, NJ; Philadelphia; and San Juan. In 1993 and 1994, the nine states reporting the highest incidence of AIDS cases for adult/adolescents was, from highest to lowest: New York, California, Florida, Texas, New Jersey, Illinois, Pennsylvania, Georgia, and Massachusetts. For pediatric AIDS cases it was: New York, Florida, New Jersey, California, Texas, and tied for sixth place, Illinois,

Pennsylvania, and Massachusetts; Georgia is ninth. There were no changes in these categories in 1994.

HIV— Through 1994, only two states, Maryland and Washington, required that HIV infection reports carry the name of persons who are symptomatic (Table 10-7).

TABLE 10-7 Status of HIV Infection Reporting—United States, December, 1994

HIV Reporting Required		
Name[a]	Anonymous[b]	HIV Reporting Not Required[c]
Alabama	Georgia	Alaska
Arizona	Iowa	California
Arkansas	Kansas	Connecticut
Colorado	Kentucky	Delaware
Idaho	Maine	District of Columbia
Illinois	Montana	Florida
Indiana	New Hamphsire	Hawaii
Michigan[d]	Oregon	Louisiana
Minnesota	Rhode Island	Maryland[f]
Mississippi	Texas	Massachusetts
Missouri		Nebraska
Nevada		New Mexico
New Jersey[e]		New York
North Carolina		Pennsylvania
North Dakota		Vermont
Ohio		Washington[f]
Oklahoma		
South Carolina		
South Dakota		
Tennessee[e]		
Utah		
Virginia		
West Virginia		
Wisconsin		

All states require reporting of AIDS cases by **name** at the local/state level.

[a]Names of HIV-infected people are provided to local or state health departments.

[b]Individual reports of people with HIV infection are provided to local or state health departments. Reports may contain demographic and transmission category information but do not record identifiers.

[c]Some states receive HIV reports on a voluntary basis.

[d]Names[a] are reported to the local health department only.

[e]In 1992 New Jersey implemented legislation requiring HIV reporting by name.

[f]Requires HIV reports with names for symptomatic HIV-infected persons only.

(Source: El-Sadr et al., 1994 updated)

BOX 10.4

HIV/AIDS DATA DEFICIENCIES

Neither the United States nor any other country has an accurate count of the number of people infected by HIV. Much of the testing to date comprises small samples of high-risk groups, such as prostitutes and drug addicts, and is therefore unrepresentative of entire populations. Within countries, infection rates vary widely from region to region, further complicating the problem of generalizing from a small sample. Counting the number of AIDS cases and AIDS-related deaths is also difficult, particularly since health care systems in many countries lack the required diagnostic ability. Moreover, some governments suppress what information they have. Further improvements in data collection may reveal a crisis of even greater magnitude than is portrayed in this text.

How Many People in the United States Are HIV-Infected?

How many people in the United States are HIV-infected? And, just how many cases of AIDS are expected to occur and when? Although projections have been made, the numbers are in question. Why? They come from surveys and incidence data that lack rigorous scientific documentation. For example, publications give information such as "researchers believe that the current number of HIV-infected people ranges from 1% to as high as 10% of everyone in the nation" (Slack, 1991). But, even if this range is to be believed, the difference between 1 in every 100 versus 10 in every 100 is very significant. This range implies that the data are questionable, and this is what raises the spectrum of concern. How many people in the United States and worldwide have HIV disease and how many have AIDS? **How large a problem is the HIV pandemic?** The answers to such questions are crucial to the allocation of funds for research and medical programs and for medical preparedness of institutions that will be hit hard as the number of cases increases.

All health care institutions and personnel will be affected by the increase in AIDS cases as will allied health service and support occu-

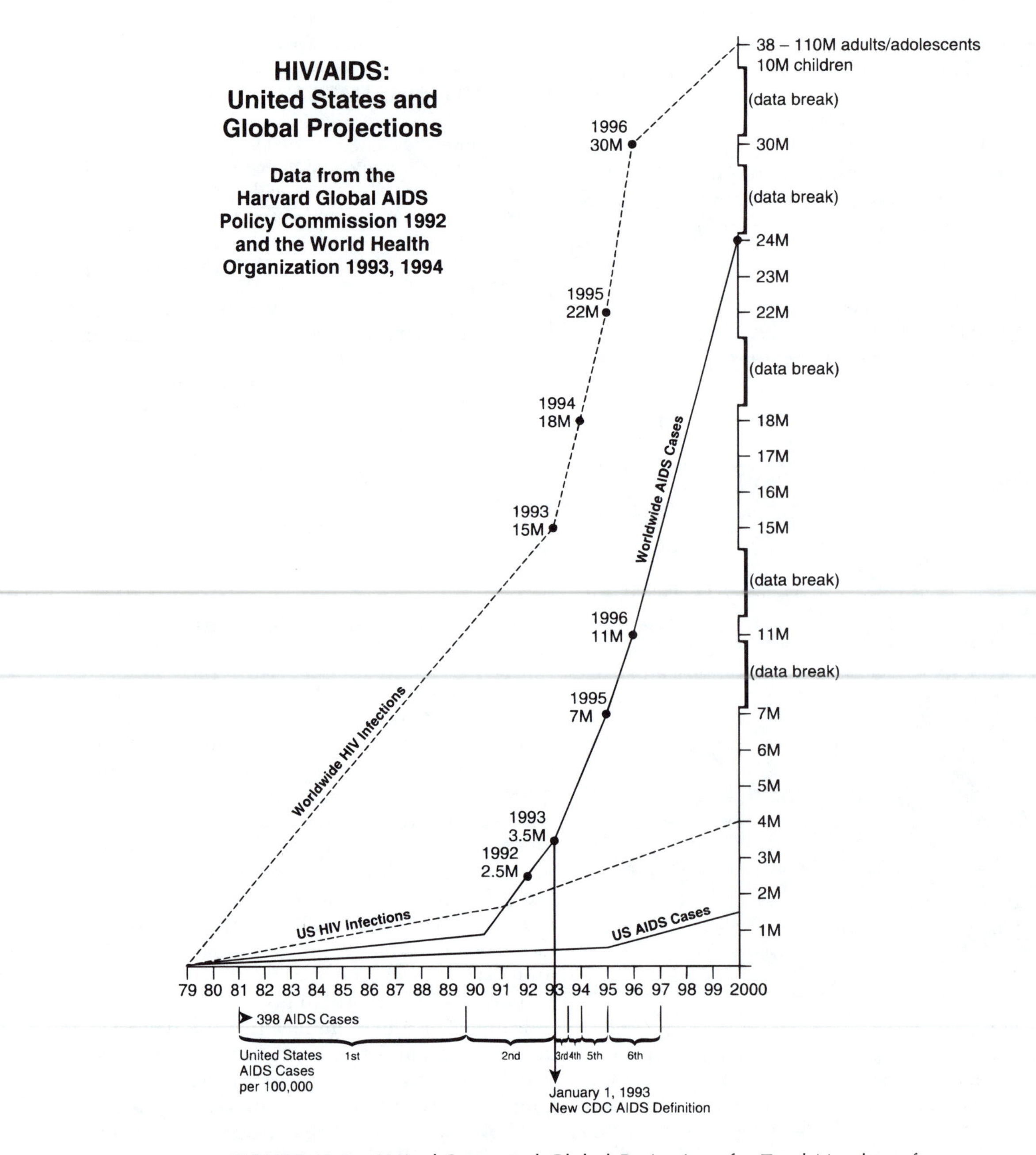

FIGURE 10-9 United States and Global Projections for Total Number of HIV and AIDS Cases. Through 1994, about 442,000 United States AIDS cases were reported to the CDC. Most of these cases were diagnosed according to the 1987 CDC AIDS definition guidelines. On January 1, 1993, the CDC changed the definition of AIDS to include all persons with a T4 cell count of **less than 200.** The new definition raised the number of AIDS cases in the

(continued on next page)

pations, insurance companies, the funeral industry, and the work force in general.

United States Estimates Lead to Confusion

AIDS is a global pandemic. By the end of 1994, over 4.5 million AIDS cases had been reported in 178 countries. Some 18 million were HIV infected by the end of 1994. Over 22 million are expected to be HIV infected by the end of 1995 along with 7 million AIDS cases.

The World Health Organization estimates that, by the year 2000, most of the 1 to 1.5 million HIV-infected people in the United States will have AIDS. Worldwide, there will be 16 times that number of AIDS cases (Figure 10-9) and 40 million cases of HIV infection. However, J. Chin and colleagues (1990), averaging the data of 14 experts, suggest that, by the year 2000, there will be about 18.3 million HIV-infected and 6.1 million AIDS cases. In 1992, a Harvard research group of 40 HIV/AIDS experts estimated that by the year 2000 there would be between 38 and 110 million HIV-infected adult/adolescents and 10 million children. By then, there will also be 24 million adult and several million pediatric AIDS cases. The estimates of HIV infections by the Harvard group is over twice that of the World Health Organization. Regardless of whose figures are more accurate, it is clear that the HIV/AIDS pandemic of the 1990s will be much worse than for the 1980s.

WHOSE FIGURES ARE CORRECT?

The Public Health Service (PHS) in 1986, estimated that 1.5 million Americans were HIV-infected (Table 10-8). The PHS and the CDC (1987) estimated that, by 1991, there would be 270,000 cases of AIDS and that 179,000 people with AIDS would have died since 1981; by 1992, 365,000 Americans would demonstrate AIDS and 263,000 would have died of AIDS. These are ominous figures about the future of AIDS in the United States, *but are they responsible figures*? In fact, by 1992 there were 206,559 reported AIDS cases and 140,282 deaths—the estimates were off by 44% and 47%, respectively.

In mid-1988, New York City's Health Commissioner, who had relied on the CDC's methodology for calculating the number of future HIV-infected AIDS cases, cut the estimated number of HIV-infected gay and bisexual men from 250,000 to 50,000—an 80% reduction. The Commissioner also reduced the total estimated number of HIV-infected New Yorkers from 400,000 to 200,000—a 50% reduction. The reason for these reductions was that the numbers of AIDS cases expected from a pool of 400,000 infected people were not happening.

A major source of conflict in attempting to track the disease via number of AIDS cases is that the CDC continues to change the definition of what constitutes an AIDS diagnosis. Also, there are major problems in reporting all

---

(continued)

United States from 1992 to 1993 by about 111%. The expected number of adult/adolescent cases for 1993, 49,100, became 105,990. This raises the number of persons living with diagnosed and reported AIDS in the United States in 1994 to over 200,000. By the year 2000, the United States is projected to have about 1.5 million AIDS cases. Worldwide, the number of AIDS cases is expected to be about 24 million. By the year 2000, 10% of all HIV infections and 12.5% of total AIDS cases will be in the United States. William Hazeltine, AIDS researcher formerly at the Dana Farber Institute, and now with Human Genome Sciences Inc. said that if prevention does not work or a cure is not found, some **1 billion** people could be HIV-positive by the year 2025. Global population on January 1, 1995 was about 5.7 billion. For the year 2000, it is projected to be about 7.5 billion people. (*Source: Harvard Global AIDS Policy Commission 1992 and World Health Organization 1993*)

TABLE 10-8 Estimated[a] Prevalence of HIV-Infected People in the United States

	Estimated Number in U.S.	Proportion Infected with AIDS Virus	Estimated Number Infected
Homosexual men	2.5 million	20–25%	500,000–625,000
Bisexual men and men with highly infrequent homosexual contacts	2.5-7.5 million	5%	125,000–375,000
Regular injection drug users (at least weekly)	900,000	25%	225,000
Occasional injection drug users	200,000	5%	10,000
Hemophilia A patients	12,400	70%	8,700
Hemophilia B patients	3,100	35%	1,100
Heterosexuals without specific identified risks	142 million	0.021%	30,000
Others, including heterosexual partners of people at high-risk, heterosexuals born in Haiti and Central Africa, transfusion recipients	N.A.	N.A.	45,000–127,000
Total			945,000–1.4 million

[a]Public Health Service in 1986 and the CDC in 1987 made the above *rough estimates.* (Source: CDC; Figures projected in 1986 remained unchanged through mid 1995. March, 1995, CDC announced 50% to 59% reduction of HIV people in the United States—from 1,200,000 to between 600,000 and 700,000)

AIDS cases to the CDC because there are those who die of AIDS who never see a physician and those who see physicians but are misdiagnosed or simply not reported to have AIDS.

A number of insurance companies, pharmaceutical manufacturers, and other industrial companies wanted more reliable prevalence figures. The demand for reliable data resulted in hiring research firms that specialize in population surveys. One such company, the Hudson Institute, reported that, in 1989, 1.9 million to 3 million Americans were HIV-infected. The 3 million estimate is double the 1986 PHS and the 1987 CDC estimates. These figures, if correct, would at least double projected total health care costs. AIDS patient care estimates then run from $50,000 for home care to $150,000 for hospital care per AIDS patient from diagnosis to death (see Chapter 15, "The Economics of AIDS).

Allan M. Salzberg, Chief of Medicine at the Veterans Center in Miles City, Montana, devised a computer model of the AIDS epidemic. It forecasts a future with 3 million American AIDS cases and 10 million infected by the year 2000 (Thomas, 1988). In mid-1989, the General Accounting Office (GAO) of the U.S. Congress reported that it analyzed 13 forecasts of the number of AIDS cases expected by the end of 1991 and found that the range of predictions was so large—from 84,000 to 750,000—that they could not be used as a meaningful guide to health services planning. The GAO concluded that a range of 300,000 to 485,000 AIDS cases by the end of 1991 was more realistic than the PHS and CDC's estimates of 270,000. (Recall only 206,000 were reported.)

James Curran of the CDC reported that blind HIV testing of Job Corps applicants revealed a rate of HIV infection 2.5 times higher than that found in military personnel. Job Corps data extrapolated to the general population would mean that there are 900,000 cases of HIV infection in the United States. Curran said that if there were 2 to 3 million HIV-infected individuals, as estimated by the Hudson Institute, the number of AIDS cases being reported would be much higher than it is.

According to the CDC projections in Figure 10-10, about 35,500 AIDS cases should have oc-

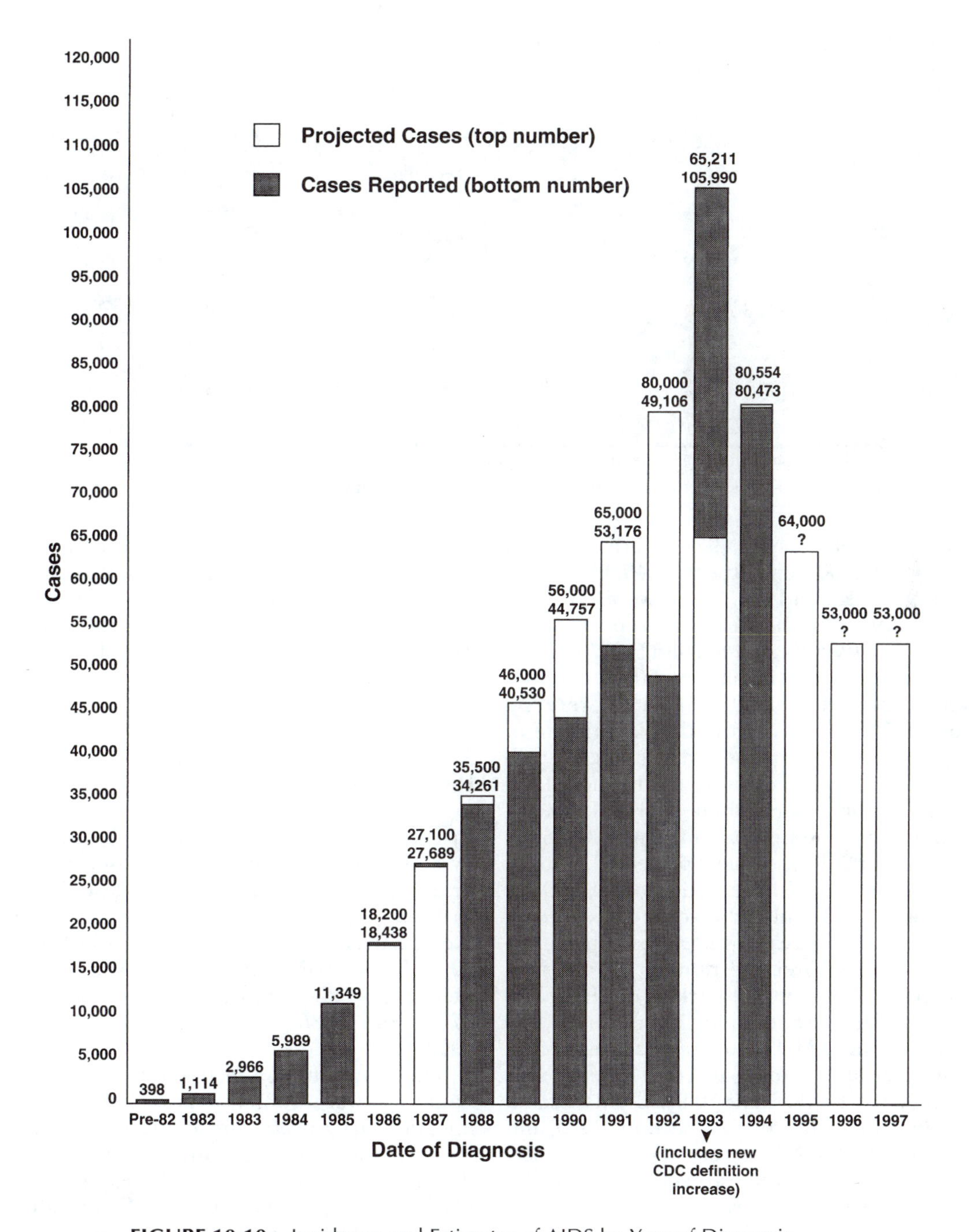

FIGURE 10-10 Incidence and Estimates of AIDS by Year of Diagnosis—United States, pre-1982 through 1997. The estimate for 1995 reflects a 25% reduction in AIDS cases from 1994 due to a drop in the backlog of persons to be identified as AIDS cases according to the 1993 definition of AIDS. Estimates for 1996 and 1997 reflect a 17% reduction from 1995 due to leveling off of AIDS cases.

TABLE 10-9 AIDS Cases Comparison—50,000 vs. 100,000

Dates in Years	Time in Months[a]	AIDS Cases by 50,000	AIDS Cases by 100,000
1987	84	First	—
Jun. 89	17	Second	First (8 years)
Nov. 90	17	Third	—
Nov. 91	12	Fourth	Second (29 months)
Nov. 92	12	Fifth	—
Mar. 93	5	Sixth	Third (17 months)[b]
Jul. 93	5	Seventh	—
Dec. 93	5	Eighth	Fourth (10 months)[b]
Oct. 94	10	Ninth	—
Aug. 95	10	Tenth	Fifth (20 months)[b]
Aug. 96	12	Eleventh	—
Aug. 97	12	Twelveth	Sixth (24 months)
		600,000	600,000

[a]Reported AIDS cases beginning 1981 through 1994. Estimated for 1995, 1996, 1997.

[b]Rapid increase in AIDS cases due to new January 1, 1993 CDC AIDS definition.

curred in 1988—34,261 (98%) were reported. In 1989, 46,000 were expected, 40,530 (88%) were reported. In 1990, 56,000 were expected and 44,757 (80%) cases were reported. In 1991, 65,000 were expected and 53,176 (82%) were reported; and in 1992, 80,000 AIDS cases were expected and 49,106 (61%) were reported. If one adds in the CDC's estimate of 15% to 20% of unreported AIDS cases, the projected and reported numbers through 1992 become more closely aligned. For 1993, before the implementation of the new AIDS definition, 65,211 cases were projected. Due to the 1993 change in the definition of AIDS, a total of 105,990 adult/adolescent cases were reported, a 37% increase over the expected and a 111% increase over the number of cases reported in 1992. After the backlog of AIDS cases based on the new definition are reported, the increase in new AIDS cases per year is expected to stabilize at a 3% to 5% increase for each year through the 1990s. Table 10-9 presents data on the time it took for the first, second, third, and fourth 100,000 AIDS cases to occur in the United States and the estimated time for the fifth 100,000 AIDS cases.

HIV/AIDS Cases in Urban Versus Rural America

In 1989, the number of new AIDS cases rose over four times as fast in the nation's *smaller* (with less than 100,000 population) cities as in its *larger* cities (with a population between 500,000 and 1,000,000), and about eight times faster than in the largest cities (populations over 1 million). Yet, in February, 1991, there were *only* four rural AIDS clinics in the United States and only one HIV/AIDS clinic solely devoted to women.

Rise in HIV/AIDS Cases Among Heterosexuals

In 1989, while the number of new cases rose by 11% among gay males, it increased by 36% or more among heterosexuals and newborns. In 1993, due to the new AIDS definition, heterosexual AIDS cases increased 130% over 1992, from 4,045 to 9,288. AIDS cases attributed to gay males or bisexual males increased 87%, from 25,864 cases in 1992 to 48,266 in 1993.

The groups most affected by the expanded definition were women, blacks, heterosexual injection drug users, and hemophiliacs. The increase was greater among women (151%) than among men (105%), and greater among blacks and Hispanics than whites. Young adults ages 13 to 29 accounted for 27% of the heterosexual cases. Overall, women accounted for about 65% of the 1993 heterosexual cases.

James Chin (1990), an epidemiologist in charge of AIDS surveillance at the WHO, predicts that by the year 2000, heterosexual transmission will predominate in most industrialized countries. The growth of the epidemic may have been slower among heterosexuals than it has been among gays or injection drug users, but it will continue to increase because HIV infection is a sexually transmitted disease and most people in society are heterosexual.

Conclusion

There is one thing on which all prognosticators agree: there is no reliable baseline from which to organize and analyze the data. There is no standard curve available to indicate the number of people from each behavioral risk group who will either become HIV-infected or develop AIDS.

There are no reliable means of obtaining data on human sexual behavior. Over the years, a constant theme has emerged from groups working on HIV/AIDS data. That is (1) extracting sensitive behavior risk information from HIV-infected or AIDS patients is difficult for even the most experienced interviewer; and (2) as HIV infection spreads beyond initially identified behavioral risk groups, assessing risk by sexual history becomes even less reliable. People do not always tell the truth when answering questions about their sexual preferences and sexual habits.

Measurement error is true for all self-report assessment devices, but it is particularly relevant to the measurement of intimate sexual behavior. The disclosure of homosexual behavior, for example, could evoke legal action and social stigma. Also, questions on the practice of anal intercourse among heterosexuals have been avoided on surveys and questionnaires. Even if questions on anal intercourse were asked, would most persons answer truthfully?

Sexual data generated from the well known Kinsey Report of 40 years ago are still being used as the best approximation of sexual practices in the United States. It does not contain 1980s and 1990s data about how many men have sex with men, yet homosexual men have the nation's highest incidence of HIV infection and AIDS. In addition, little is known about the prevalence of extramarital affairs or the practice of anal sex among heterosexuals. The National Institutes of Health was planning just such a survey (Booth, 1989; Fay et al., 1989). But political pressures have caused all such studies receiving federal funds to be placed on hold even though such information is crucial to understanding HIV transmission and prevalence.

ESTIMATES OF DEATHS AND YEARS OF POTENTIAL LIFE LOST DUE TO AIDS IN THE UNITED STATES

Deaths Due to AIDS

Former Surgeon General C. Everett Koop has said on a number of occasions that "AIDS is virtually 100% fatal." Looking back over the number of AIDS cases diagnosed and comparing them to the number of AIDS patients who have died would indicate that a diagnosis of AIDS is a death sentence. Virtually all the retrospective AIDS patients, as far back as 1952 and through 1982 have died. Figure 10-11 presents a sobering look at the numbers of AIDS patients who have died since those first CDC reported cases in 1981. They are now dying at the rate of over 3,000 a month. About 95% of those diagnosed with AIDS in 1981 have now died. And about 65% of AIDS cases diagnosed up through 1992 have died. In New York City, 17 people a day die from AIDS.

The majority of AIDS deaths have occurred among homosexual/bisexual men (59%) and among women and heterosexual men who were injection drug users (21%). In 1992, less than 2% of AIDS deaths occurred in persons under age 25. Most (75%) AIDS deaths have occurred among people 25 to 44 years of age, and about 24% occurred in those over age 45. In 1992, HIV disease/AIDS became the number one cause of death among black and Hispanic men ages 25 to 44 and second among black women ages 25 to 44. (*MMWR*, 1994c). AIDS is now the leading cause of death in all Americans aged 25 to 44 (*MMWR*, 1995).

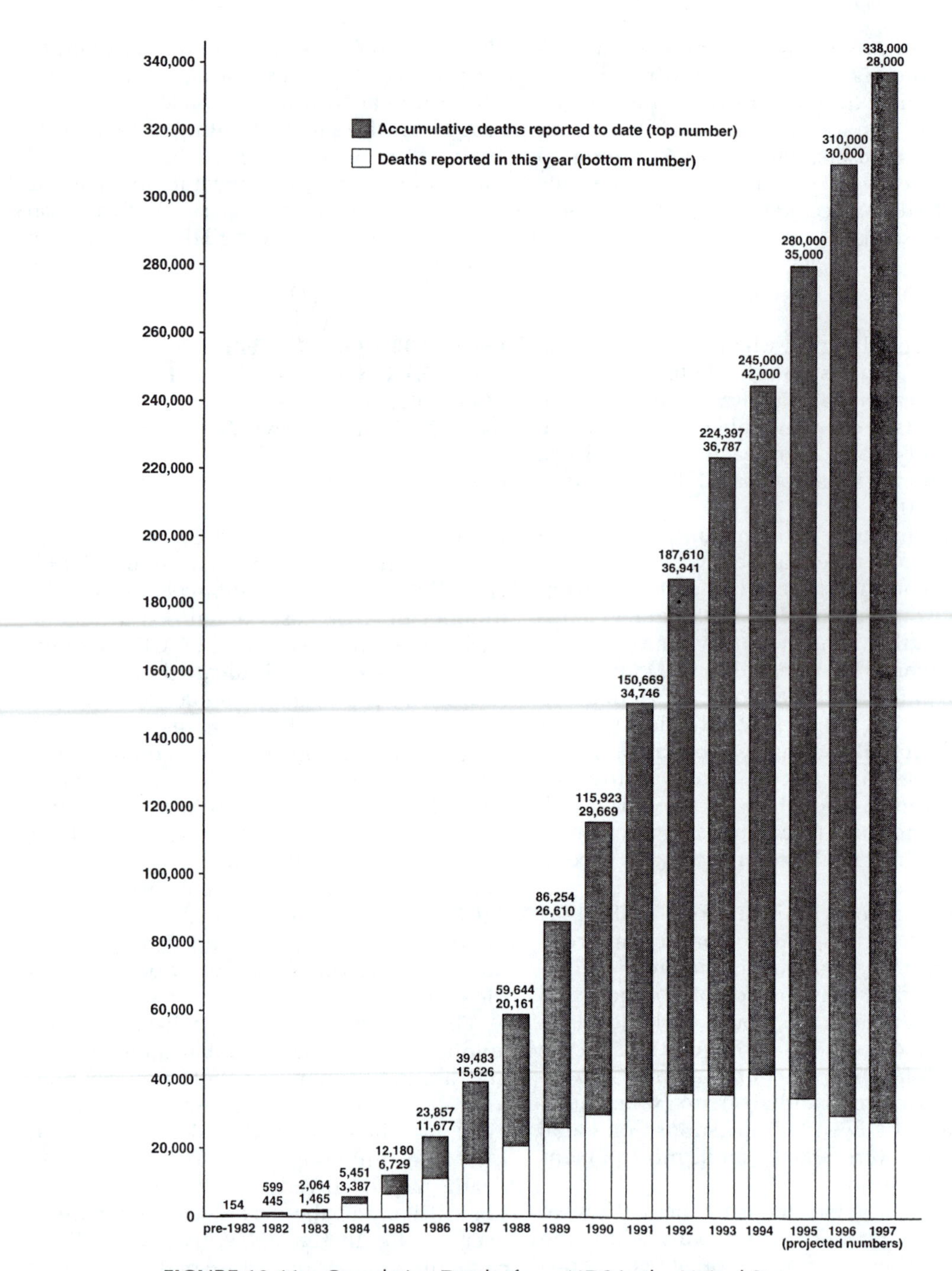

FIGURE 10-11 Cumulative Deaths from AIDS in the United States pre-1982–1994 (1995, 1996, and 1997 projected). By the end of 1988, there were about 60,000 deaths due to AIDS. By the end of 1994, there were 245,000 AIDS deaths, a 4 fold increase. About 340,000 will have died by the beginning of 1998.

TABLE 10-10 AIDS Cases and Deaths Prior to 1981 through 1995—Adult/Adolescent and Pediatric

	Adult		Pediatric[a]	
	Cases	Deaths	Cases	Deaths
Before 1981	92	30	6	1
1981	306	124	15	8
1982	1,114	445	29	14
1983	2,966	1,465	75	29
1984	5,989	3,387	111	48
1985	11,349	6,729	227	114
1986	18,438	11,677	322	156
1987	27,689	15,626	483	285
1988	34,261	20,161	586	308
1989	40,530	26,610	665	355
1990	44,757	29,669	692	381
1991	53,176	34,746	574	362
1992	49,106	36,941	585	365
1993	105,990	36,787	930	380
1994[b]	80,473	42,000	800	300
1995	64,415	35,000	700	300
1996	53,000	30,000	700	300
1997	53,000	28,000	700	300
Totals[c]	646,651	359,397	8,200	4,006

[a]Fatality rate: Adults and pediatrics about 53% each. Rate of death has dropped for adults from 65% to 53% due to the large increase in the 1993 number of AIDS cases.

[b]The numbers for 1995 are estimates which reflects a 25% reduction of AIDS cases for 1994 as the backlog of the 1993 AIDS definition cases became reported. Numbers for 1996 and 1997 are estimated.

[c]Total number of AIDS cases and deaths due to AIDS reported to the CDC; about 30% of cases and deaths are not reported.

According to the CDC (1993), deaths from HIV disease/AIDS is underreported by 25% to 33%. Although most deaths occurred among whites, proportional rates have been highest for blacks and Hispanics. During 1992, the number of deaths per 100,000 population, aged 25–44 years, was 136 for black men and 42 for white men. It was 12 times as high for black women as for white women. In proportion, since 1985, the rate of death was higher for women than for men (*MMWR*, 1993). By the year 1990, 86,254 AIDS patients died (Table 10-10 and Figure 10-11). By mid 1995, over 260,000 AIDS patients had died. White death rates from most other leading causes of death declined or remained relatively stable for men and women aged 25–44 years, the death rate due to AIDS has steadily increased. In 1993, AIDS was the leading cause of death among men aged 25 to 44 years in nine states (highest to lowest incidence): New York, Florida, New Jersey, California, Georgia, Maryland, Massachusetts, Connectiut, and Rhode Island. In 1993, AIDS became the fourth leading cause of death for women.

Prevalence and Impact of HIV/AIDS

However the impact of the disease is measured—by deaths, AIDS cases, or monetary losses—it is just beginning. The worldwide impact during the 1990s will be 5 to 10 times that of the 1980s. As this process unfolds, the United States will find itself progressively more involved with prevention programs and with the political changes that HIV/AIDS will bring about in countries with a high incidence of HIV/AIDS.

SUMMARY

In 1981, the CDC reported the first case of AIDS in the United States, and, from that time onward, has constantly tracked the prevalence of AIDS cases in different geographical areas and within different behavioral "risk" groups. In all behavioral risk groups, the common denominator is the exchange of body fluids, in particular blood or semen. The heterosexual population at large is considered to be at low risk for HIV infection in the United States. As of 1993, all states and the District of Columbia, Puerto Rico, and the Virgin Islands have reported AIDS cases in people who have had heterosexual contact with an "at-risk" partner. The geographic distributions of women with AIDS who were the sex partners of bisexual men or men who used injection drugs were similar to those of men with AIDS from these two groups. In contrast, the geographic distribution of men who reported heterosexual contact with a woman who used injection drugs was different from that of women with AIDS who were IDUs.

A major problem exists in attempting to determine the number of HIV-infected people. Several different approaches have been used by the CDC to estimate the total number of

HIV infections. These estimates can be evaluated by examining their compatibility with available prevalence data.

With respect to race and ethnicity, the cumulative incidence of AIDS cases is disproportionately higher in blacks and Hispanics than in whites. The ratio of black to white case incidence is 3.2:1 and the Hispanic to white ratio 2.8:1. This racial/ethnic disproportion is also observed in HIV-positive blood donors and in applicants for military service. Even among homosexual and bisexual men and IDUs, where race/ethnicity-specific data are available, blacks appear to have higher seroprevalence rates than whites.

With regard to prostitution, in a large multicenter study of female prostitutes, black and Hispanic prostitutes had a higher rate of HIV infection than white and other prostitutes. This disproportion existed for both prostitutes who used injection drugs and for those who did not acknowledge injection drug use.

The risk of new HIV infections in hemophiliacs and in people who receive blood transfusions has declined dramatically from 1985 because of the screening of donated blood and heat treatment of clotting factor concentrates. Evidence also indicates an appreciable decline in the incidence of new infections in homosexual men. However, the risk of new infections appears to remain high in IDUs and in their heterosexual partners. In several metropolitan cities, the prevalence of HIV infection in IDUs has been increasing.

AIDS surveillance and HIV seroprevalence studies indicate that a significant proportion of HIV infection among women in the United States is acquired through heterosexual contact. Because more men than women are HIV carriers, a woman is more likely than a man to have an infected heterosexual partner. The predominance of heterosexually acquired HIV infection in women of reproductive age has important implications for vertical HIV transmission to their offspring: nearly 30% of children with AIDS were infected by mothers who acquired infection through heterosexual contact.

Studies conducted by the CDC along with the American College Health Association revealed that in 1989, two college students per 1,000 were HIV-infected.

There are some 5.3 million health care workers in the United States. Even though they are supposed to adhere to Universal Protection Guidelines set down by the CDC for their protection, a significant number are exposed to the AIDS virus annually. A relatively small number of those infected have progressed to AIDS.

Estimating the number of HIV-infected people in the United States continues to be a numbers game. Various agencies and private industries have, for different reasons, attempted to determine the number of HIV-infected people. The numbers from the different groups vary widely. However, the 1986 CDC estimated numbers of 1 to 1.5 million HIV-infected people may be too high. However, the number of new AIDS cases occurring each year is within 10% to 20% of the CDC estimated figures.

REVIEW QUESTIONS

(Answers to the Review Questions are on page 481.)

1. How did the CDC estimate the numbers of HIV-infected people in the United States? In what year was this done? In retrospect, how accurate were their estimates?
2. Collectively, what percentage of male and female AIDS cases occur between the ages of 20 and 59?
3. Black and Hispanic females make up what percentage of the total female AIDS cases? What is their percentage of the United States female population?
4. What percentage of all female AIDS cases occur between ages 20 and 44?
5. Why are people placed in potential HIV risk groups?
6. True or False: The time it takes for HIV-infected people to become AIDS patients is different for each ethnic group, risk group, and exposure route. Explain.
7. What percentage of all U.S. HIV-infected IDUs are in the New York–New Jersey region?
8. What percentage of newborns from HIV-infected mothers are HIV-infected?
9. Eventually, what percentage of HIV-infected children will result solely from HIV-infected mothers?

10. What is the rate of college students currently HIV-infected? Is this more or less than the rate for military personnel? Explain.
11. Compare the college student rate of HIV infection with the rate of HIV infection for the general U.S. population.
12. What is the risk of a health care worker converting to seropositivity after exposure to HIV-contaminated blood?
13. What single job-related event causes the greatest risk of HIV infection among health care workers?
14. What percentage of the total number of AIDS cases in the United States represents health care workers?
15. Are health care workers more apt to become infected with the hepatitis B virus or the AIDS virus?
16. In May of 1989, four states had no reported pediatric cases. Name these four states. What might this imply about HIV infection in these states?
17. In mid-1989, the government's General Accounting Office said ________ cases of AIDS will have occurred in the United States by the end of 1991. How many did the CDC predict?
18. Do you think people of the United States openly and truthfully discuss their sexual habits with survey personnel? What does the text say?
19. How many AIDS patients were estimated to die by the end of 1992?
20. By mid-1989, data on AIDS deaths indicated that of AIDS patients diagnosed between 1981 and mid-1985, ____% had died.
21. True or False: White children account for 75% of all pediatric AIDS cases.
22. True or False: Over half of the female AIDS cases are in black women.
23. True or False: The majority of HIV-positive Native American women have been infected through behaviors associated with injection drug use.

REFERENCES

AGGLETON, PETER, et al. (1994). Risking everything? Risk behavior, behavior change, and AIDS. *Science,* 265:341–345.

AIDS Alert. (1993). Which accidents infect health care workers with HIV? 8:49–64.

ALLEN DAVID et al. (1994). HIV infection among homeless adults and runaway youth, United States, 1989–1992. *AIDS,* 8:1593–1598.

ALLEN, J.R., et al. (1988). Prevention of AIDS and HIV infection: Needs and priorities for epidemiologic research. *Am. J. Public Health,* 78:381–386.

ARAL, SEVGI O., et al. (1991). Sexually transmitted diseases in the AIDS era. *Sci. Am.,* 264:62–69.

BLACK, STANTON B., et al. (1990). HIV risk behaviors in young black people: Can we benefit from 30 years of research experience? *AIDS and Public Policy J.,* 5:17–23.

BOOTH, WILLIAM. (1988). CDC paints a picture of HIV infection in U.S. *Science,* 242:53.

BOOTH, WILLIAM. (1989). Asking America about its sex life. *Science,* 243:304.

BREO, DENNIS L. (1990). The slippery slope—Handling HIV-infected health workers. *JAMA,* 264:1464–1466.

BUEHLER, JAMES W., et al. (1992). The reporting of HIV/AIDS deaths in women. *Am. J. Public Health,* 82:1500–1505.

BURKHART, DYMPNA. (1991). Who said the sexual revolution is over? *Med. Asp. Human Sexuality,* 25:9.

BUTLER, DECLAN. (1993). Who side is focus of AIDS research? *Nature,* 366:293.

BUTLER, DECLAN. (1994). HIV health workers need better protection. *Nature,* 369:173.

CHIN, J. et al. (1990). Projections of HIV infections and AIDS cases to the year 2000. *Bulle. WHO,* 68:1–11.

COTTON, PAUL. (1994). U.S. sticks head in sand on AIDS prevention. *JAMA,* 272:756–757.

DARROW, W.W., et al. (1989). HIV antibody in 640 U.S. prostitutes with no evidence of intravenous (IV) drug abuse. *Fourth International Conference on AIDS.* Bio-Data Publishers: Washington, DC.

DICKINSON, GORDON M. (1988). Epidemiology of AIDS. *Int. Ped.,* 3:30–32.

DRISCOLL, CHARLES E. (1992). Women with HIV: Update 1992. *Female Patient,* 17:11–12.

EHRHARDT, ANKE A. (1992). Trends in sexual behavior and the HIV pandemic. *Am. J. Public Health,* 82:1459–1464.

EL-SADR, et al. (1994). *Managing Early HIV Infection: Quick Reference Guide for Clinicians.* Agency for Health Care Policy and Research. Publication #94-0573, Rockville, MD.

FAY, ROBERT E., et al. (1989). Prevalence and patterns of same-gender sexual contact among men. *Science,* 243:338–348.

FELDMAN, MITCHELL, et al. (1994). The growing risk of AIDS in older patients. *Patient Care,* 28:61–72

FELMAN, YEHUDI M. (1990). Recent developments in sexually transmitted diseases: Is heterosexual transmission of HIV a major epidemiologic in the spread of AIDS? III: AIDS in Sub-Saharan Africa. *Cutis*, 46:204–206.

FILLIT, HOWARD et al. (1989). AIDS in the elderly: A case and its implications. *Geriatrics*, 44:65–70.

FRANCIS, DONALD P. (1987). The prevention of acquired immunodeficiency syndrome in the United States. *JAMA*, 257:1357–1366.

FRANKE, K. (1988). Turning issues upside down. *In AIDS: The Women* (Eds., I. Rieder and P. Ruppelt), San Francisco: Cleis Press.

FUTTERMAN, DONNA, et al. (1992). Medical care of HIV-infected adolescents. *AIDS Clin. Care*, 4:95–98.

GAYLE, HELENE. (1988). Demographic and sexual transmission differences between adolescent and adult AIDS patients, U.S.A. *Fourth International Conference on AIDS.*

GAYLE, HELENE et al. (1990). Prevalence of HIV among university students. *N. Engl. J. Med.*, 323:1538–1541.

GOSTIN, LAWRENCE, et al. (1994). HIV testing, counseling and prophylaxis after sexual assault. *JAMA*, 271:1436–1444.

GUINAN, MARY S. (1993). AIDS: Your patients are at risk. *Menopause Manage.*, 11:10–18.

GWINN, MARTA, et al. (1991). Prevalence of HIV infection in childbearing women in the U.S.: Surveillance using newborn blood samples. *JAMA*, 265:1704–1708.

HAHN, ROBERT A., et al. (1989). Prevalence of HIV infection among intravenous drug users in the United States. *JAMA*, 261:2677–2684.

HAYS, ROBERT B., et al. (1990). High HIV risk-taking among young gay men. *AIDS*, 4:901.

HAYS, ROBERT B. (1992). AIDS and gays: Look for a second wave. *Med. Asp. Human Sexuality*, 26:61.

HIV Guideline Panel. (1994). Managing early HIV infection. *Am. Fam. Phys.*, 49:801-814.

HIV/AIDS Surveillance Report. (June 1994). 6:1-25.

House Select Committee on Children, Youth and Families. (1992). A decade of denial: Teens and AIDS in America. Washington, D.C., May.

JOSEPH, STEPHEN C. (1993). The once and future AIDS epidemic. *Med. Doctor*, 37:92–104.

LEMP, GEORGE. (1991). The young men's survey: Principal findings and results. A Presentation to the San Francisco Health Commission, June 4.

LEMP, GEORGE. et al. (1994). Scroprevalence of HIV and risk behaviors among young homosexual and bisexual men. *JAMA*, 272:449–454.

LUMSDON, KEVIN. (1992). HIV-positive health care workers pose legal, safety challenges for hospitals. *Hospitals*, 66:24–32.

MARCUS, R., et al. (1988). AIDS: Health care workers exposed to it seldom contract it. *N. Engl. J. Med.*, 319:1118–1123.

MICHAELS, DAVID, et al. (1992). Estimates of the number of motherless youth orphaned by AIDS in the United States. *JAMA*, 268:3456–3461.

Morbidity and Mortality Weekly Report. (1990). HIV prevalence, projected AIDS case estimates. *Workshop*, Oct. 31–Nov. 1, 1989. 39:110–119.

Morbidity and Mortality Weekly Report. (1991). The HIV/AIDS epidemic: The First 10 Years. 40:357–368.

Morbidity and Mortality Weekly Report. (1992a). HIV prevention in the U.S. correctional system, 1991. 41:389–391, 397.

Morbidity and Mortality Weekly Report. (1992b). Surveillance for occupationally acquired HIV infection—United States, 1981–1992. 41:823–824.

Morbidity and Mortality Weekly Report. (1992c). Selected behaviors that increase risk for HIV infection among high school students—United States, 1990. 41:236–240.

Morbidity and Mortality Weekly Report. (1993a). Update: Mortality attributable to HIV infection among persons aged 25–44 years—United States, 1991 and 1992. 42:869–873.

Morbidity and Mortality Weekly Report. (1993b). Update: Acquired immunodeficiency syndrome—United States, 1992. 42:547–557.

Morbidity and Mortality Weekly Report. (1994a). Update: Impact of the expanded AIDS surveillance case definition for adolescents/adults on case reporting—United States, 1993. 43:160– 170.

Morbidity and Mortality Weekly Report. (1994b). Heterosexually acquired AIDS—United States, 1993. 43:155–160.

Morbidity and Mortality Weekly Report. (1994c). AIDS among racial/ethnic minorities—United States, 1993. 43:644–655.

Morbidity and Mortality Weekly Report. (1995a). Update: AIDS—United States, 1994. 44:64–67.

Morbidity and Mortality Weekly Report. (1995b). Update: AIDS among women—United States, 1994. 44:81–84.

OSBORNE, JUNE E. (1993). AIDS policy advisor foresees a new age of activism. *Fam. Prac. News*, 23:1,45.

PETERSON, J.L., et al. (1989). AIDS and IV drug use among ethnic minorities. *J. Drug Issues*, 19:27–37.

PFEIFFER, NAOMI. (1991). AIDS risk high for women; care is poor. *Infect. Dis. News*, 4:1,18.

REISMAN, JUDITH. (1990). *Kinsey, Sex and Fraud: The Indoctrination of a People.* Huntington House Press: Lafayette, LA.

ROTHERAM-BORUS, M. et al. (1991). Sexual risk behaviors, AIDS knowledge, and beliefs about AID Samong runaways. *Am. J. Public Health*, 81:208–210.

RYDER, ROBERT, et al. (1994). AIDS orphans in Kinshasa, Zaire: incidence and Socioeconomic consequences. *AIDS*, 8:673–679.

SELWYN, PETER A., et al. (1989). Knowledge of HIV antibody status and decisions to continue or terminate pregnancy among intravenous drug users. *JAMA,* 261:3567–3571.

SHIP, J. A., et al. (1991). Epidemology of AIDS in persons aged 50 years or older. *J. Acquired Immune Deficiency Syndrome,* 4(1):84–88.

Skin and Allergy News. (1991). HIV risk in health settings remains "Extremely" remote. Nov.:8.

SLACK, JAMES D. (1991). *AIDS and the Public Workforce: Local Government Preparedness in Managing the Epidemic.* Tuscaloosa: The University of Alabama Press.

STALL, R., et al. (1990). Relapse from safer sex: The next challenge for AIDS prevention efforts. *J. Acquired Immune Deficiency Syndromes,* 3:1181.

THOMAS, PATRICIA. (1988). Official estimates of epidemic's scope are grist for political mill. *Med. World News,* 29:12–13.

THOMAS, PATRICIA. (1989). The epidemic. *Med. World News,* 30:41–49.

TOUFEXIS, ANASTASIA. (1991). When the doctor gets infected. *Time,* 137:57.

VLAHOV, D., et al. (1991). Prevalence of antibody to HIV-1 among entrants to U.S. correctional facilities. *JAMA,* 265:1129.

WEISFUSE, ISAAC C., et al. (1991). HIV-1 infection among New York City inmates. *AIDS,* 5:1133–1138.

WILLIAMS, PATRICIA. (1991). Job fears may impede care for seropositives. *Med. World News,* 32:39.

WILSON, J., et al. (1990). Keeping your cool in a time of fear. *Emergency Medical Services,* 19:30–32.

YAO, FAUSTIN K. (1992). Youth and AIDS: A priority for prevention education. *AIDS Health Promotion Exchange No. 2,* Royal Tropical Institute, The Netherlands:1–3.

CHAPTER

11

Prevalence of HIV Infection and AIDS Outside the United States

Chapter Concepts

- Worldwide, about 26 persons a minute become HIV-infected.
- In Africa, HIV is mainly transmitted heterosexually.
- Prostitution is a major route of HIV transmission in Africa.
- It is estimated that there will be a 20% decline in population in East Africa by the year 2001 due to AIDS.
- In Europe, France and Italy have the two highest rates of AIDS cases, respectively.
- Mexico ranks eighth in the number of AIDS cases in the world.
- Cuba mandates national screening for HIV-infected people.
- Former Soviet Union reported its first AIDS case in 1988.
- China reported its first AIDS case in 1989.

There are enormous disparities in the quality of life for people born in different parts of the world. The Third World contains three fourths of the Earth's population. There 87% of all births and 98% of all infant and childhood deaths occur. One in 10 people suffers from a tropical disease; 190 million children are undernourished; and 10 million people die of acute respiratory and diarrheal infections each year.

With regard to HIV disease/AIDS, data from the World Health Organization (WHO) suggests that Americans are in a relatively enviable position. Although the people in the United States have lived through 14 years of HIV transmission, the current rate of new infections in the United States appears to be stabilized (World Health Organization, 1992). This is not true for persons living in many countries in the developing world where the HIV epidemic progresses unchecked.

Seventy-five percent of the world's estimated 22 million (through 1995) HIV-infected persons live, or have lived, in developing countries; this will soon increase to an estimated 90%. The global epidemic has intensified despite a massive prevention effort. In many countries with high infection rates, education campaigns have spread the news about HIV, but this has not led as yet to a decrease in the frequency of high-risk sexual behavior adequate to halt the epidemic (Berkley, 1992).

GLOBAL PATTERNS OF HIV TRANSMISSION

The most important news to come from the Seventh, Eighth, and Ninth International Conferences on AIDS (1991 through 1993) was bad news. While Western nations believe the number of new HIV infections has leveled off, data from the WHO clearly show that the heterosexual spread of HIV in Asia and Africa constitutes an epidemic that threatens the very fabric of those continents.

The WHO describes four distinct patterns of HIV transmission:

Pattern I: Predominantly homosexual men and injection drug users (IDUs); gradual increase in heterosexual and perinatal transmission; North America, Western Europe, Australia and New Zealand

Pattern II: Predominantly non-IDU heterosexuals; female to male ratio approaches or surpasses 1:1; perinatal transmission a major problem; sub-Saharan Africa, parts of the Caribbean, and parts of Asia

Pattern I/II: Currently evolving from predominantly homosexual and bisexual to heterosexual transmission; Brazil, Honduras, and Chile

Pattern III: HIV infection still relatively uncommon; infected homosexual men, prostitutes, and IDUs are a rapidly growing problem in some areas; Eastern Europe, North Africa, the Middle East, parts of Asia and the Pacific Islands

These four patterns, although useful conceptually, provide only a broad brush-stroke outline of the current status of the epidemic in a particular area and do not necessarily represent the future of the epidemic in that area. Because HIV infection occurs disproportionately in certain behavioral high-risk groups, seroprevalence may differ markedly between neighboring countries, urban and rural areas within a country, or social strata within an urban population (Holmes, 1991).

GLOBAL PREVALENCE OF HIV INFECTION AND AIDS

Various sources, including the WHO's global program on AIDS, estimated that, by the end of 1994, there were about 5 million AIDS cases worldwide. In late 1992, the Harvard Global AIDS Policy Coalition estimated that, from 1981 to 1992, the number of HIV-infected people worldwide increased from 100,000 to 12.9 million: 7.12 million men, 4.7 million women, and 1.1 million children. By the end of 1995, there will be 22 million HIV-infected and over 7 million AIDS cases (Figure 11-1). By the end of 1996 there will be an estimated 30 million HIV-infected and about 11 million AIDS cases.

Projections to the year 2000 anticipate an increase in adult/adolescents infections at the rate of between 48 and 189 new HIV infections per minute. That means 38 million to 110 million new HIV-infected adults/adolescents. In addition, they estimate 10 million new cases of HIV-infected children. They also project 24 million adult/adolescent AIDS cases by the year 2000. (see Figure 10-10). Through mid-1995, an estimated 75% to 80% of HIV infections worldwide were due to heterosexual behavior and 15% were due to homosexual behavior. Injection drug use, and the use of con-

BOX 11.1

THE GLOBAL COURSE OF THE HIV PANDEMIC

During the 1990s, as many as 94 million people may become HIV-infected. This is in addition to an estimated 18 million infected by the end of 1994. About 85% of the new infections will occur in developing countries, about half in Africa. The epidemic will spread fastest in Asia and South America, setting the stage for a large increase in AIDS cases after the year 2000.

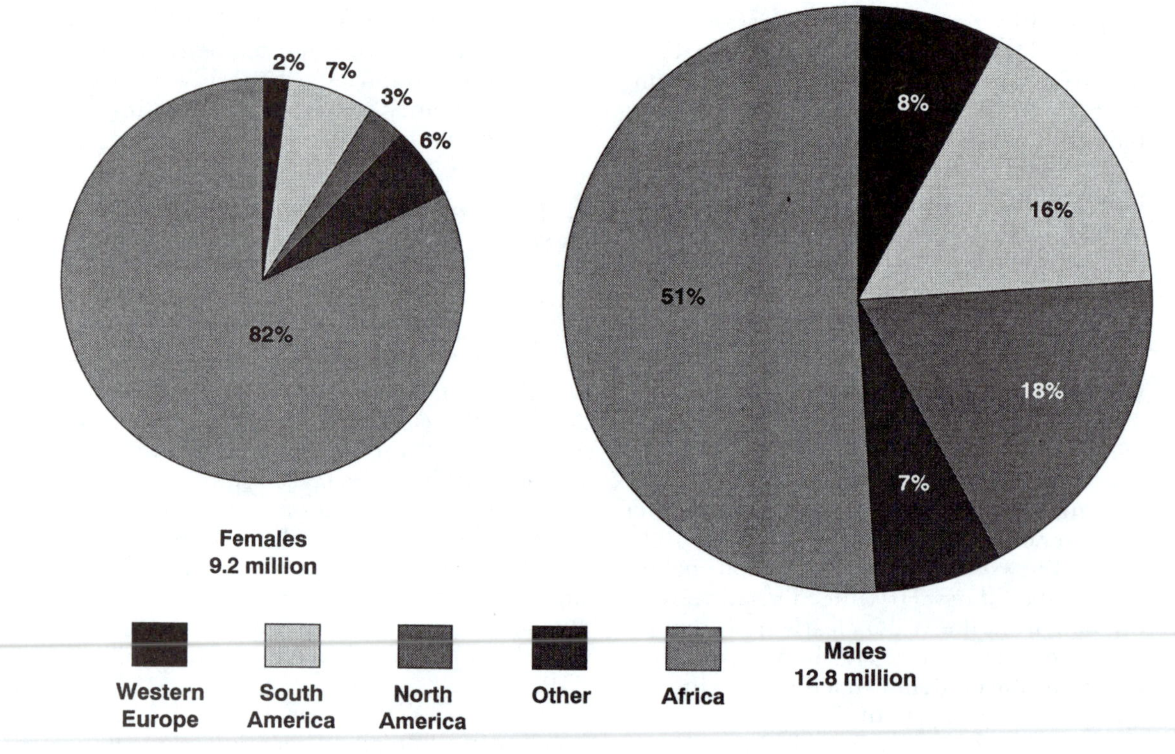

FIGURE 11-1 Global Distribution of HIV-Infected Adults. As of mid-1995, about 20 million people were HIV-infected worldwide; 36% were women (Lancet, 1993). By the end of 1995, the number is expected to rise to 22 million. The large increase over the past 2 years and in future years is and will continue to be attributed to the marked increase in HIV seroprevalence being reported in Africa and Asia.

taminated blood or breast feeding make up a small percentage of HIV infections worldwide.

The WHO projections differ from the Harvard group. The WHO projects that 30 million adults and 10 million children will be HIV-infected by the year 2000 and that there will be 5 million adult and 1 million pediatric AIDS cases (Chin, 1900; Chin et al., 1990).

The history of HIV infection suggests that about 90% to 95% of those infected will become AIDS patients within 9 to 15 years. In the beginning of 1991, there were 179 countries reporting to the WHO on AIDS. One hundred and sixty countries on the seven continents have reported AIDS cases to the WHO. Figure 11-2 presents a global overview of the number of HIV-infected people.

THE ECONOMICS OF PREVENTING HIV INFECTION IN DEVELOPING COUNTRIES

According to the World Bank's *World Development Report 1993: Investigating in Health*, the annual spending in developing countries for the prevention of HIV infection is less than $200 million. In sub-Saharan Africa, the total amount spent is about $90 million. That translates into less than 20 cents per person for the region with the greatest burden of HIV/AIDS in the world. Although only 10% of this prevention money comes from local resources in sub-Saharan Africa, internally generated revenues support 85% of all health costs. National health budgets are already strained, and any

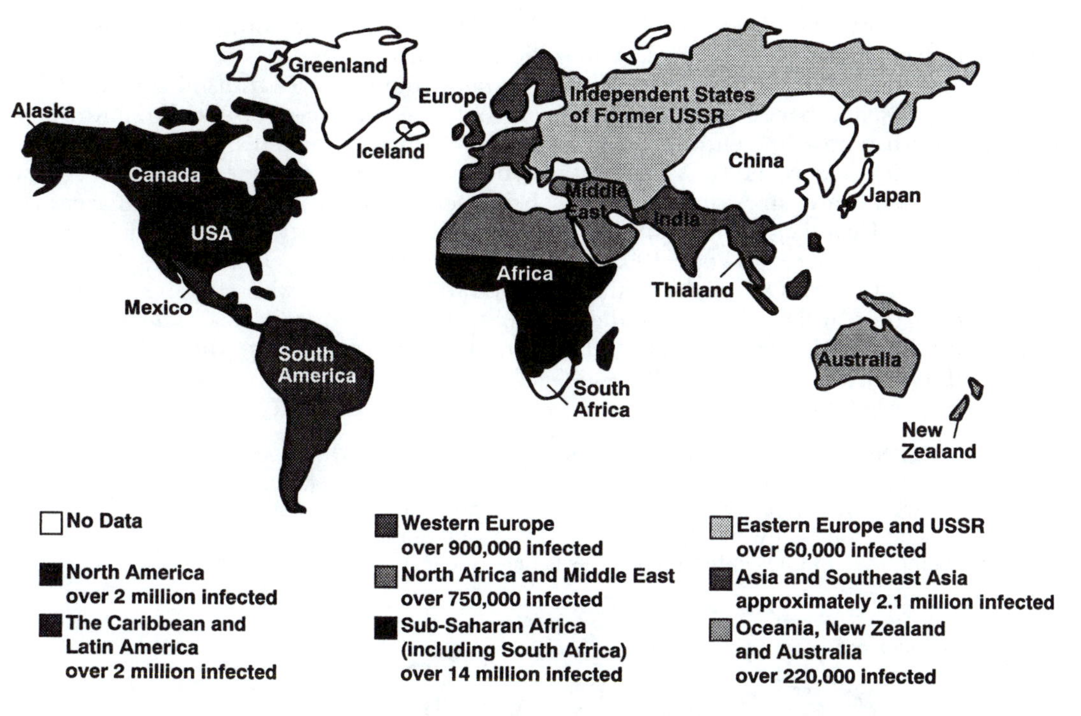

FIGURE 11-2 Estimated Global HIV Infections through 1995 (total 22 million). This map shows the global proliferation of the AIDS virus. Although sub-Saharan Africa has the greatest number of HIV-infected people, other regions are catching up. (*Adapted from Palaca, 1991*)

additional money to be allocated to medical care for AIDS patients must come from external donations.

The reality is that the resources, whether from in-country budgets or donor sources, are already far too small to undertake even the prevention effort alone. At the Ninth International AIDS Conference (June, 1993), Michael Merson, head of the World Health Organization's Global Program on AIDS, estimated that a 10-fold increase (to $2 billion) of funds spent on preventing the spread of HIV and other sexually transmitted diseases would avert 10 million new HIV infections by the year 2000 (Biggar, 1993).

THE SPREAD OF AIDS OUTSIDE THE UNITED STATES

The AIDS pandemic has demonstrated unprecedented speed in its diffusion. Whereas the great cholera pandemics took nearly 20 years to sweep across Europe, HIV/AIDS has reached most of the world within 7 years. The question now is whether research, behavior modification, and education—all of which require international cooperation—will be able to meet the AIDS challenge.

A brief summary concerning the number of AIDS cases in Africa, the Americas, Europe, and Asia is presented.

AFRICA

By the end of 1994, the United Nations Health Agency estimated that sub-Saharan Africa had over 3 million AIDS cases and that over 2 million Africans had already died from AIDS. Africa, with about 12% of the world's population, is now *reporting* about 25% of the world's AIDS cases. It is estimated to have nearly 70% of the total number of HIV-infected adults and 90% of the world's HIV-infected children (DeCock et al., 1993). Sixty percent of HIV infections occur in the 15- to 24-year-old age group. About 5,000 Africans become HIV-infected each day; that is 208 per hour or 3.5 per minute. The highest number of cases have been reported from urban areas in central, eastern, and southern Africa (Figure 11-3). About half of all reported AIDS cases in Africa originate from East Africa—Uganda, Kenya, Tanzania, Rwanda, and Burundi (Barongo et al., 1992).

Through 1995, the WHO and the United Nations estimate there will be about 14 million HIV-infected adult/adolescents and 900,000 infected children in Africa. The WHO estimates by the year 2000 there may be 40 million HIV-infected adults and as many as 10 million orphans.

Major routes of HIV transmission in Africa are heterosexual, mother-to-child, and transfusions with unscreened blood. The latter is being reduced as blood for transfusion is now being screened in most major urban areas.

Between 20% and 30% of sexually active adults between the ages of 20 and 40 are believed to be infected with HIV in some urban areas of sub-Saharan Africa. The HIV seroprevalence in rural areas, where the majority of the population lives, remains much lower but is increasing (*PAAC*, 1990).

FIGURE 11-3 Map of Africa. AIDS began to appear in Central Africa at about the same time it was being recognized in the United States. Increasing numbers of cases have been reported in urban centers in Zaire, Zambia, Rwanda, Uganda, Tanzania, and Burundi. HIV infection among prostitutes in these countries is high (see text for details).

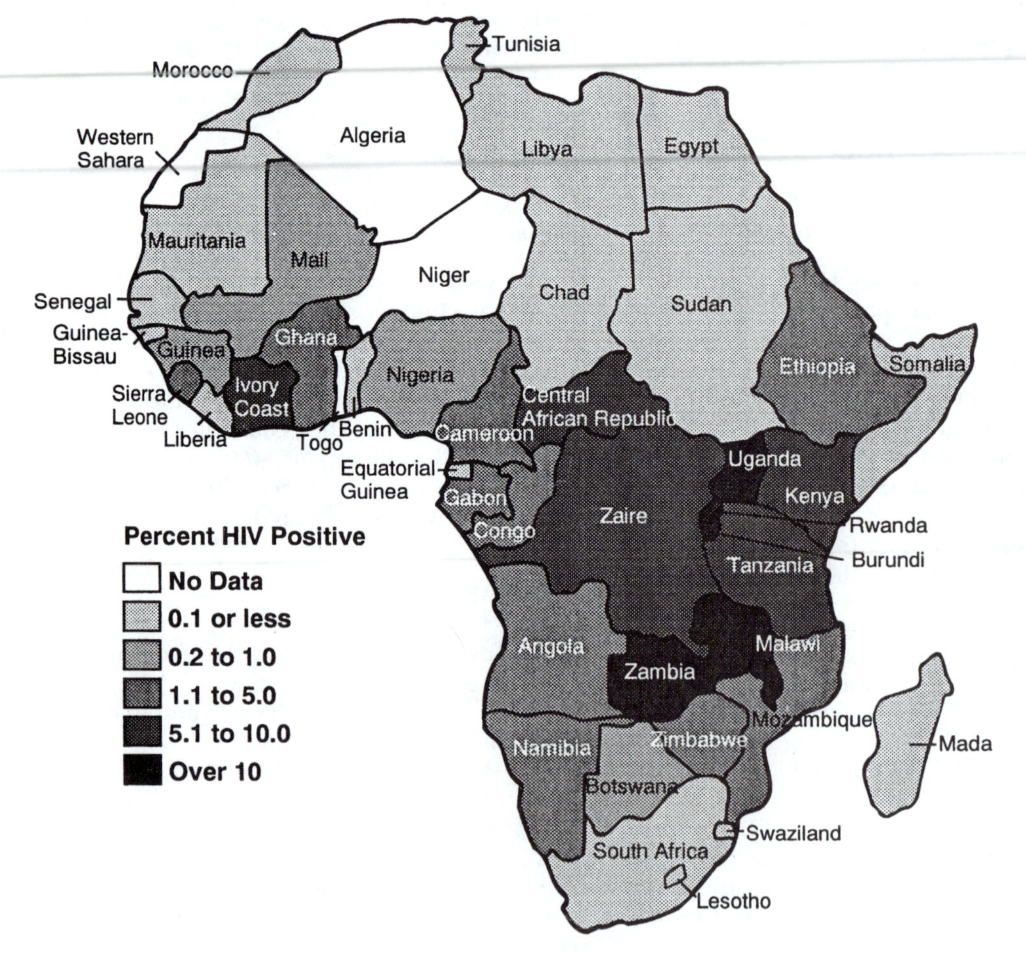

There was a report in 1960 of a young white patient who was treated in 1959 for Kaposi's sarcoma. The investigator stated that this may have been the first case of AIDS in Africa (Sonnerfeld, 1990).

AIDS in Africa was officially recognized among the indigenous African population soon after it was recognized in the United States. Some investigators contend that AIDS was present in Africa in the 1970s. It was reported that a Danish surgeon contracted AIDS in Zaire in 1976; and Vandepitte and colleagues (1983) diagnosed the disease in a Zairean visitor to Europe in 1976. Saxinger and colleagues (1985) found HIV antibodies in samples collected in the West Nile region of Uganda between 1972 and 1973. There is also a report of a husband and wife in Uganda having AIDS in 1976. These are believed to be the first reported AIDS cases in Uganda.

In 1986, for a variety of political and economic reasons such as possible international discrimination and fear of loss of tourist trade and foreign investments, only nine of Africa's 51 countries reported that they had AIDS patients. Yet, in 1987, Jonathan Mann stated, "No area in the world is more affected by HIV than Africa." The WHO estimates that one in three of the 40 million people in Southern Africa will be HIV-infected by the year 2010.

HIV Transmission in Africa

The WHO estimates by the end of 1995, 67% of the world's 22 million plus HIV-infected people will live in Africa. That is over 14 million HIV-infected people. Likewise, Africa has 67% of the total AIDS cases or about 4.7 million cases. Over 9 million HIV-infected adults live in sub-Saharan Africa. Available evidence suggests that it is unlikely that the spread of HIV will be brought undercontrol in the near future (De Cock et al., 1994). About 66% of HIV infections occur in those under age 25.

Injection drug use has traditionally been a rarity in sub-Saharan Africa. However, there are indications that the practice may be catching on, particularly in port areas and among educated and affluent city-dwellers.

Other areas hard hit by the epidemic are those of central and east Africa. These areas account for one-sixth of the region's population but between half and two-thirds of its infections. Here, in several towns and cities, about one-third of all men and women aged 15 to 49 are estimated to be HIV-positive.

Heterosexual Contacts—Data from AIDS studies in Zaire and Rwanda show about an equal number of men and women with AIDS. The major risk factor in HIV transmission appears to be related to the number of heterosexual partners one has. In Rwanda, one in four women of childbearing age is HIV-positive (Commenges et al., 1992). In some cities, 30% of pregnant women are HIV-infected (De Cock et al., 1994).

Contraception: Use of Condoms by Rwandans—It is the interaction and passage of fluids, particularly beer and milk, in the form of social exchange or gift, which constitutes, for Rwandans, the essential social bond. Blockage of the flow through the individual body or between bodies was traditionally considered to be pathological. The practice of kunyaza, a form of wet sex, in which the female is aroused to secrete copiously before penetration, is closely linked to fundamental Rwandan notions of self in relation to other. Sex follows the mode of flow, blockage, and the ideal of reciprocity. Children are built *in utero*, over time, through repeated intercourse and mixing of fluids. A condom would block this essential flow of fluids, thus contradicting a most basic cultural notion (Taylor, 1990).

In Kigali, Rwanda, 30% of adults are HIV-infected. In Uganda, there is one doctor for every 23,000 people and one hospital for every 20,000 people. Leaders in Uganda do not believe condoms will solve the AIDS problem.

In late 1993, one in every eight Ugandans was HIV-infected—that's about 2 million of 17 million Ugandans. And 300,000 have AIDS. In some districts in Uganda, over half of all deaths is due to AIDS and 9 out of 10 of those deaths occur in people under age 35. In countries like Uganda, where a mother often has to walk 20 miles to get an aspirin for her sick child, the practical problems of getting a constant supply of condoms and learning to use them properly may never be resolved. As one young Uganda said to the Health Minister, "You tell

BOX 11.2

AIDS IN AFRICA

CBS Interviewer (CBS I): They don't often say it, but a lot of scientists around the world have been watching the spread of AIDS in central Africa with a mixture of horror and fascination. Horror because of the sheer numbers of infected; fascination because the region is a kind of human laboratory for studying heterosexual transmissions. The fact is, among African heterosexuals, the disease is spreading much more rapidly than among heterosexuals in the West. At the same time, central African countries like Uganda look back at the West with embarrassment and anger. They're embarrassed by talk of African promiscuity. And they are angry when outspoken scientists like Dr. Robert Gallo of the National Cancer Institute say that while no one can prove where AIDS began, and isolated cases do appear early in the West, all scientific signposts still lead to an origin in Africa.

Response from Head of AIDS Education For Uganda (AEFU): We don't have homosexuals and drug addicts. We don't have them. So this disease must be foreign. If anyone's to blame, it's Western homosexuals and drug addicts.

CBS I: And then there was this man, who was too sick even to give us his name. This scene may well be a dark vision of the future for all of Uganda. It was just a few years ago that the disease was first noticed in this province. "Slim disease," they called it, the disease that makes you thin. And at first, everyone thought that it would stay here. But the disease didn't stop in the provinces. It traveled this road toward the capital city because this is the highway used by the truck drivers. John Nsambo is bringing coffee back from the region around the lake, the neighboring countries of Zaire and Burundi (Figure 11-3). The AIDS virus may well be part of his cargo, and his trip up the highway tells a lot about the way the disease began to spread. As he heads toward the city, he stops at four or five truck stops along the way. At every truck stop, the women are waiting. By now, as many as 76% of them are infected with the virus. Some of them are ordinary prostitutes, one-night stands. Others are what Ugandans call temporary wives, a woman supported by several regular customers who drop by before heading home to the principal wife. Here and in the rest of Africa, AIDS is a completely heterosexual disease.

CBS I: Whatever the reason, it took only 2 years for AIDS to make its way up the highway from Lake Victoria into the capital city, Kampala. It moved with lightning speed through the suburbs, the workers, the housewives, still affecting men and women equally, moving straight on to the city's educated professionals, what Ugandans call their "Mercedes Benz set." Some studies show that in parts of the city, 20% of the young people are already infected, and at the current rate, all of them will be infected in just 10 years.

What does that mean to the future of Uganda if this disease is concentrating among the professional people?

AEFU: Well, it is a disaster. It will mean that young people from the age of about 18 to 40, the bread-winners, the well-to-do, will die off.

CBS I: So you could lose an entire generation?

AEFU: We could, yes. We could lose the entire generation unless something drastically is done about it.

CBS I: While American hospitals worry about the thousands, the millions of dollars they'll spend treating AIDS, here at Mulago they worry about enough money to buy rubber gloves for the health workers or a few disposable needles. Here, when they give a man or woman a blood test for AIDS at $1.75, they've just spent the entire per capita health budget for the year. (In the United States, 500 dollars per year are spent on each citizen's health care.)

A Sister at the N'Sambya St. Francis Hospital has one of Uganda's five machines for screening blood to be used in transfusions; just a fraction of the number of machines in New York City alone. The day we were there, she tested blood samples from donors, and the results were 28% positive. But when the donors who tested positive came to get their results, if they looked healthy, they weren't told they were carrying the virus. The doctors said there was no point in giving someone a possible death sentence when you have no counselors to help them deal with the news. Even if it means they spread the disease to others, the doctors say, one cruelty doesn't justify another. One woman who tested positive saw 10 doctors; no one told her the truth.

CBS I: This male worries too. He's from Rakai, and he's been ill for months. It was an 8-hour ride to get to the doctor. But the doctor he is going to see is the witch doctor who will charge him 5 months of his wages for just one treatment. The doctor and his associate, who is called the professor, begin the treatment with a magical X-ray. They toss some coins and keys and produce an instant diagnosis. They say they can tell from the demons in the dark if the patient has AIDS, or slim disease, and that they'll adjust the prescription accordingly; though when we were there, it was always the same concoction of herbs and roots.

—— POINT OF INFORMATION 11.1 ——

AIDS CAUSES BUSINESS FAILURE

In Kasheni, a Tanzanian village bordering Lake Victoria, a village chairman turns the pages of a worn personal file in which he keeps photographs of villagers who have died. Among the snapshots of family groups is a photo of fit and smiling young men who made up the local football team. More than half have died of AIDS. He recalls a market in nearby Rukunyo, where Tanzanian and Ugandan traders did brisk business in second-hand clothing, bicycles, and other goods. Then people began to fall ill. It was discovered that the illness was AIDS, traders drifted away, the market died, and the surrounding bars and hotels closed their doors.

me that AIDS can make me ill in 10 years, but 25 people died here the past weekend. My father died young of TB . . . and my brother, out of school for three years, still has no job. Can AIDS really make life worse?"

Prostitution—The major route of HIV transmission in Africa is prostitution. Unofficial estimates by mission doctors in Kampala, Uganda, put the prevalence of HIV infection among the city's prostitutes at 70%; and at 20% in other adults (Culotta, 1991)!

A research team from the University of Nairobi, Kenya, the University of Manitoba, Canada, and the Institute of Tropical Medicine in Belgium tested 535 Nairobi prostitutes in January, 1985, and found that 348, or 65% of them, were HIV-positive. Of the remaining 185, by 2 years later 120 of them had become HIV-positive. Thus, of the original 535 prostitutes in 1985, 504 were HIV-positive by 1987 (Niftrik, 1988). According to surveys, each Nairobi prostitute averages 1,000 male sexual partners per year, most of whom are truck drivers going inland from the port of Mombasa.

One of the highest concentrations of HIV/AIDS cases in Africa is found along the route from Uganda to Zaire. Reports indicate 27% to 60% of prostitutes in Kinshasa, Zaire, are HIV-positive; and 88% of prostitutes in Rwanda are infected (Quinn, 1988). Thirty-seven percent of prostitutes in Kinshasa age 20 and older were HIV-infected; only 8% female nonprostitutes of the same age were infected. There is little reason to believe that similar situations do not exist in other equatorial African capitals. According to *Inside South Africa*, 60% of prostitutes in Entebbe and Kampala in Uganda tested in a combined study were found to be HIV-positive.

Condom use among prostitutes is infrequent. Only 23% of prostitutes say they have ever used condoms. Prostitutes say that customers refuse to use condoms or refuse to pay if made to wear a condom; "We die either way—of starvation or of AIDS." Condoms in Zaire cost less than one penny each but the demand for them is so low, health care workers can not even give them away!

Some blacks in South Africa see the human immunodeficiency virus threat as a plot by whites to preserve apartheid by persuading blacks to use condoms, thus reducing the blacks' pregnancy rate.

In Tanzania (East Africa), the men of Dar es Salaam have a unique phrase for AIDS: *"Acha Iniue Dogedego Siachi,"* a Kiswahili translation of "Let it kill me as I will never abandon the young ladies." Women as well as public health officials are understandably concerned. One young prostitute said, "Even if I take precautions, how can I be completely safe while I have no control over so many things—including my own husband"? (Earickson, 1990)

Socioeconomic Impact— The frequency of AIDS cases is highest among the upper class and the revenue-producing population. These are male and female Africans 20 to 40 years old—the bread-winners, the food-producers, the backbone of the African labor force. In Luska, Zambia, 33% of blood donors between age 30 and 35 were HIV-positive; 68% of skilled Zambian copper-belt workers were HIV-positive. In Nairobi, Kenya, 2% of all medical personnel tested positive.

Deaths due to AIDS are occurring so rapidly that African funerals which normally last up to a week are in jeopardy of being shortened. One of the reasons is that, as the labor force decreases, fewer relatives of the deceased can be spared time off for the lengthy traditional funeral. It has been estimated that there would be a 20% decline in population in East Africa by the year 2001.

BOX 11.3

TRIBAL TRADITION, LUSKA, ZAMBIA

Throughout Africa, polygamy has been culturally tolerated for centuries. The custom is still practiced in many black African states.

Sanford Mweupe looks back on the days when he had only two wives to worry about. So do the two wives. Domestic life has been strained since events led to what was delicately referred to as "the confusion."

In 1988, after his brother died, Mweupe was chosen by the family's elders to perform a ceremony called "ritual cleansing." According to tribal tradition, the brother's two widows had to be purged of their husband's spirit by having sex with a member of his family.

Mweupe's brother had died of AIDS, and the widows may also have been infected. Mweupe's wives pleaded with him not to keep the tradition, but the elders insisted he cleanse the widows and then take them as his wives. He was warned by modern doctors, but a traditional healer assured him it would be safe.

Mary Mweupe was pregnant with her third child—her husband's 18th—when Mweupe's brother died.

Mweupe took some precautions. He took his brother's widows to a traditional healer who gave them injections and said they were free of AIDS. He also brought some condoms over to his brother's house on the day the families gathered for the ceremony.

He said "I wanted to use them, but the grandmother of one of the widows saw them and she said this would not be according to the tradition. She said the widows would not be cleansed. I was afraid she would tell other people and make me a laughingstock, so I did not use them."

After the families drank beer in his brother's yard, Mweupe and the two widows retired inside. He stayed with them for a week. He agreed to go beyond his cleansing duties and take them as his wives, assuming responsibility for their five children, as well as a sixth who was born 9 months after the ceremony.

When Mweupe went home at week's end to the first and second Mrs. Mweupe, the reunion was less than warm. Mweupe told his wives that he should not sleep with them because of the possibility of infection. But after a time they insisted. They said he was their only husband—who else could they sleep with?

The consequences are still unclear, because Mweupe and the brother's widows have not been tested for the HIV virus.

(Adapted from John Tierney, The New York Times, Sept. 17, 1990)

Obstacles to fighting AIDS in Africa were set out forcefully by N'Galy Bosenge, director of the National AIDS Program in Zaire, as he addressed the Fifth International Conference on AIDS (1989).

First among the obstacles is poverty. "We lack resources not only for AIDS, but for health in general . . . The situation in Europe and North America—where homosexuals and [injection] drug users are well-defined risk groups—make it easy to target prevention and control programs. But apart from prostitutes, there really are no risk groups in Africa; 90% of cases are from the general population."

Will Africa's Experience Be Repeated Elsewhere?

Conditions in Africa that contributed to the AIDS disaster included sexual behavior patterns conducive to the spread of HIV infection, high incidence of STDs, nonuse of condoms, government inattention to the problem in its early years, and contaminated blood supplies in some places. Whenever such conditions prevail, the African experience is likely to be repeated. In certain Latin American and Asian countries, conditions resemble those of Africa.

BOX 11.4

HIV/AIDS IN UGANDA

One in four young adults is HIV-infected in Uganda's cities. In Roki, a district in Southern Uganda, where the first AIDS cases were diagnosed, over 50% of adults are HIV-positive. Every family in Roki has lost someone—a mother, father, or child. There are over 400,000 orphaned children in Roki due to AIDS (Figure 11-4).

BOX 11.5

BOGUS HIV CERTIFICATES IN KENYA

Nairobi—Kenyatta Hospital is selling HIV-negative certificates, according to the Dutch gay publication *De Gay Krant*. The certificates, supplied within 15 minutes, are going for the rough equivalent of $40, and no medical tests are done. The report states that the certificates are valuable to people who wish to become foreign laborers or visit the United States, where HIV-seropositive immigrants and visitors are not generally permitted to enter the country.

There, the future course of AIDS threatens to follow Africa's (*United States Department of State*, 1992).

FIGURE 11-4 Grieving for Lost Children. A sole Ugandan parent grieves at the graveside. He mourns the loss of seven children and grandchildren who have died of AIDS. (Photograph by E. Hooper, World Health Organization, Geneva)

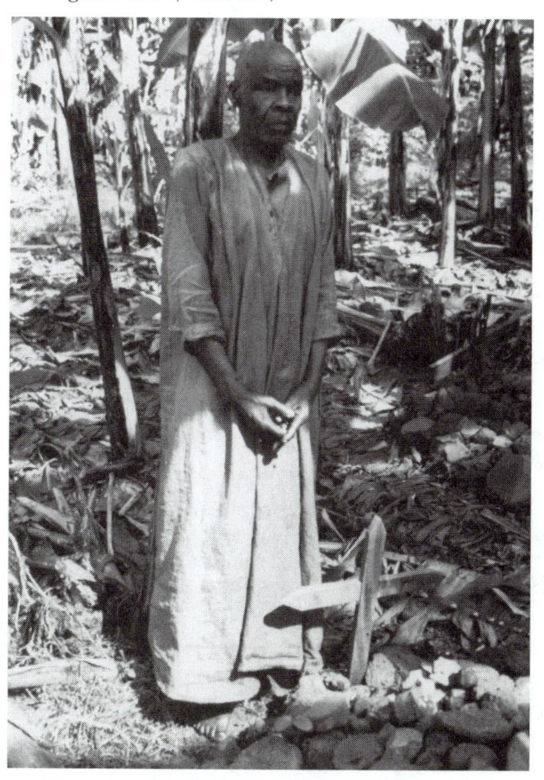

THE AMERICAS (NORTH, SOUTH, AND CENTRAL)

By the end of 1994, over 600,000 AIDS cases and 300,000 deaths were reported by 35 countries and 14 nonindependent units in the Americas, representing less than 20% of the world total AIDS cases. Approximately 78% of the AIDS cases in the Americas have been reported by the United States. Puerto Rico has the second highest overall rate of AIDS cases in the Americas.

In North America and many urban areas of Latin America, most AIDS cases occur among homosexual or bisexual men between the ages of 20 and 49 and among injection drug users. Over 50% of homosexual men in some urban areas have been infected. The proportion of cases involving heterosexual contact in these areas is estimated at about 5%. In some areas of Latin America, especially in the Caribbean, there is an increasing trend towards heterosexual transmission which now accounts for the majority of new HIV infections in some places (*PAACNOTES*, 1990).

Canada

The first reported case of HIV/AIDS in Canada was diagnosed in 1979. In July of 1993, Canada changed their definition of AIDS to follow the CDC's January 1, 1993 definition with the exception that Canada does not include T4 cell counts to **diagnose** AIDS cases (*Canadian Quarterly Surveillance Update*, July, 1994). Through September 1994, the Federal Centre for AIDS received reports on 10,391 AIDS cases, 9,779 males and 612 females. These included 10,279 adults/adolescents and 112 children (Figure 11-5.) A total of 6,930 have died. Adult cases in Canada are defined as ages 15 to 65; pediatric, less than age 15. About 19% of total cases occurred in the 15- to 29-year age group with a 10- to 15-year delay in the onset of AIDS, one in five people with AIDS were infected as teenagers. As in the United States, the largest number of AIDS cases occur in the 30- to 39-year age group (4,572 or 44% of AIDS cases).

Michael Chretien, the chairman of a 1988 report entitled "AIDS: A Perspective for

Canadians," said that Canada lags behind the United States in incidence of AIDS cases by 2 or 3 years. About 70% of AIDS cases occur in three cities: Montreal, Toronto, and Vancouver. Twenty-five percent of Canadians live in Montreal and Toronto.

About 80% of AIDS cases are among homosexual and bisexual males. Less than 1% of AIDS cases involve heterosexuals or injection drug users. About 6% of AIDS cases are women. The report on AIDS issued by the Royal Society of Canada opposes mandatory testing for HIV infection, and supports antidiscrimination legislation, education on condom use, and dispensing clean needles to drug addicts.

Mexico

In 1988, Mexico ranked eighth in total number of AIDS cases reported to the WHO. By June of 1994, Mexico had reported a total of 8,353 AIDS cases. Thirty-four percent of AIDS cases are in Mexico City, 64% are in provincial towns and cities, and 2% are in the outlying areas. Most affected are middle and upper class Mexicans. Mexico now ranks second to Brazil for AIDS cases in Latin America (*United States Department of State*, 1992; Pan American Health Organization, 1994).

As elsewhere in the world, most AIDS cases occur in the 25 to 45-year age group. About 66% of the female AIDS patients became HIV-infected via blood transfusions and 33% from heterosexual contact. Of men with AIDS, 93% became infected through sexual activities. Of these, 56% are homosexuals, 27% are bisexuals, and 10% are heterosexuals. IDUs account for less than 1%, apparently because of the high cost of injection drugs (Sternberg, 1989).

Latin America and the Caribbean

By the end of 1988, over 10,000 AIDS cases from Latin America and the Caribbean had been reported to the WHO. In 1994, over

FIGURE 11-5 Total Reported AIDS cases in Canada by Age Group and Sex Canada (N = 10,689: reported deaths 7,471). Data reported to December 31, 1994. (Source: Division of HIV/AIDS Epidemiology, BCDE, Laboratory Centre for Disease Control, Health Canada)

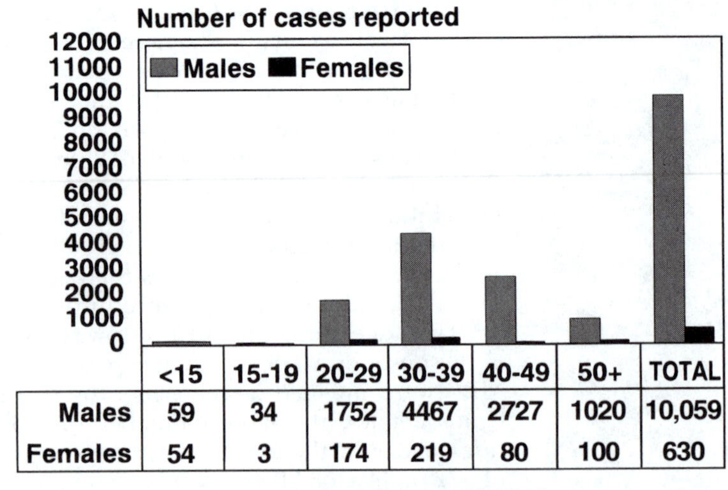

	<15	15-19	20-29	30-39	40-49	50+	TOTAL
Males	59	34	1752	4467	2727	1020	10,059
Females	54	3	174	219	80	100	630

Women (n = 630) %

Heterosexual Contact	58.2
Injection Drug Use	11.9
Blood Recipient	11.6
Perinatal	7.8
Clotting Factor	2.1
Occupational Exposure	0.2
No Identified Risk	8.2

Pediatric (n = 113) #

Perinatal Transmission	55
Blood Recipient	34
Clotting Factor	8
No Identified Risk	3

115,000 cases were reported. It is estimated that 30% to 50% of cases are not reported. Mann believes they are underreported by about 60% (Mann, 1988). The concentration of AIDS cases here, as elsewhere, is largely in urban areas. Through 1986, virtually all AIDS cases occurred among homosexual males and IDUs. Nearly all Caribbean islands have reported at least one case of AIDS. Rates range from a low of 0.33 per 100,000 people in Cuba to a high of 159 per 100,000 in Bermuda. Six islands—Bahamas, Barbados, Bermuda, Jamaica, Trinidad and Tobago—account for 90% of all AIDS cases in the Caribbean. Taking the region as a whole, the cumulative rate per 100,000 people is 11 compared with 33 in the United States and three in Britain. Early cases of AIDS in the Caribbean were reported in Haiti in 1979 and in Trinidad in 1983. In Haiti, one recent study found one in 10 pregnant nonprostitutes to be HIV-infected (Palaca, 1991).

Transmission— Modes of HIV transmission in the Caribbean are similar to those in the United States and *also* to those in Africa. Initial cases tended to be among homosexual and bisexual men. But, as the pandemic has progressed, the mode of HIV transmission has become increasingly heterosexual; it is now the dominant mode. The male to female ratio in 1992 was about 2:1 and decreasing. About 9% of AIDS cases reported to the Caribbean Epidemiology Centre from 19 member islands (excluding Cuba, Haiti, the Dominican Republic, and the French-speaking islands) are among children under 5.

The majority of AIDS cases in Bermuda are associated with IDUs, which are not a problem in most of the other Caribbean islands. On several islands, female prostitutes are HIV-infected; and in Jamaica they constitute 11% of all AIDS cases. Some migrant farm workers, who work in the United States for 3 to 6 months each year, have become HIV-infected through heterosexual contact while abroad and have developed AIDS. They represent 14% of all cases in Jamaica.

Virtually all Caribbean islands now have HIV control programs which include screening of blood donors, public education, and counseling. Cuba has been unique in undertaking national screening and in isolating HIV-infected people in a sanatorium.

Cuba

As of early 1994, Cuba stopped its quarantine of people who test HIV-positive. Reasons for Cuba's reversal of policy on testing everyone for HIV is not known. Prior to this change in policy, everyone old enough to have sex was tested—*no exceptions.* By December of 1993, over 90% of 11 million people had been tested. Of these, 710 men and 297 women tested positive and were being confined in 13 sanatoriums. The government paid every sanatorium resident the salary he or she received prior to confinement. Almost all send money home to their families.

Except for cigarettes, everything was free—pots and pans, coffee makers, phone calls, detergent, rice, beans, zidovudine, antibiotics, and condoms.

Within the sanatorium, no one taught abstinence; no one expected people to give up sex.

Beginning 1995, at least 245 of the 1,007 had AIDS; 148 have died.

Cuba's experience has shown that there are effective, albeit draconian, public health measures for controlling the spread of HIV/AIDS.

Brazil

> Equating AIDS with death can blunt a campaign's effectiveness. If you say "AIDS kills," street kids say, "It's just another thing that kills us. The police kill us too." Killing is not serious to them.
>
> *Ana Filquerias*

With the exception of Haiti, Brazil ranks highest in Latin America for HIV infections. At the Fourth International Conference on AIDS (1988), Brazilian Health Minister Borges da Silveira said that Brazil had 4,946 cases of AIDS. By 1995, Brazil had over 50,000 AIDS cases. It is now estimated that 1 million out of a population of 157 million Brazilians are HIV-infected. Two-thirds of all families live below the poverty level of $900 a year. Private insur-

POINT OF INFORMATION 11.2

CHOOSING TO DIE FROM AIDS

On May 16, 1994, *Newsweek* carried the following story.

By the time he was 20, Luis Enrique Delgado was fed up. The police had been harassing him for five years over his long hair, his crucifix earring and his contempt for the rules and rituals of Cuban society: military service, work brigades, May Day parades. He just wanted to listen to the heavy-metal band Metallica, hang out with his girlfriend and be left alone. Only one place in Cuba seemed to offer what he was looking for. He left his farm town in 1990 to visit a friend at an AIDS sanitarium near Havana and had the friend extract some blood with a syringe. Another patient then injected the HIV-laced blood into his vein. Now starting to waste away, Delgado explains: "We gave ourselves AIDS to liberate ourselves from society and those laws about obligatory work, and live in our own world."

Delgado is one of a dozen young heavy-metal fans—known as *frikis* ("freaks") or "rockers"—who claim to have shot up infected blood. He and three others spoke to *Newsweek* last month in Pinar del Rio, 125 miles west of Havana. Six other patients at a sanitarium there appear with Delgado on a video recently smuggled out of Cuba, saying that they, too, voluntarily received the AIDS virus. Vladimir Ceballos, one of two young film students now in Miami who shot the video for a documentary, says he has the names of 25 young people from Pinar del Rio who injected HIV and knows of some 55 more from there, all now dead.

ers throughout Brazil *do not* pay for AIDS treatment. In 1985, 3% of AIDS cases were women; for 1993 it was over 20%.

In Brazil, surveys show that men are aware of the AIDS threat, but are reluctant to use condoms, currently the most effective barrier to virus transmission during sex. In Rocinha, Rio's largest slum, 77% of sexually active male respondents to a survey said they never used condoms.

In addition to objections on grounds of pleasure, Brazilian men fault condoms for their high price and their poor quality. Priced out of reach of Brazil's poor majority, a pack of three condoms cost the equivalent of 1 kilogram (2.2 pounds) of rice or 2 kilograms of black beans.

Brazil, with a population of 157 million, has seven free clinics for HIV testing.

About 70% of AIDS patients live in Sao Paulo or Rio de Janeiro, but AIDS is spreading into the rural areas. Blood banks are contaminated and 74% of the hemophiliacs in Rio de Janeiro are HIV-infected. Government figures show that in Rio de Janeiro, 34% of professional blood donors are HIV-infected.

EUROPE

In 1993, most European countries expanded their AIDS case definition to that used in the United States. In Spain, the new definition was introduced on January 1, 1994. By the end of 1994, over 120,000 cases of AIDS, representing about 3% of the world's total, were reported from 38 countries in Europe (Table 11-1). This number represents an increase of about 71% over the 1990 number of AIDS cases. Over 50% of AIDS persons have died. The number of cases reported in central and eastern Europe remains low. The two countries with the largest number of AIDS cases are France and Italy (Figure 11-6).

About 85% of AIDS cases in Europe occur in homosexual males and IDUs. Women account for about 14% of total AIDS cases. And, over half of the women who have AIDS are IUDs (Smith et al., 1994). Regional differences in Europe are similar to those in the United States. The prevalence of AIDS cases in Europe is strikingly different from north to south and east to west. In Denmark, Sweden, and the United Kingdom, 70% to 90% of the total number of AIDS cases occur in the homosexual male population. At the beginning of 1992 in Southern Europe, in Italy 66% and in Spain over 50% of AIDS cases occurred in IDUs.

AIDS cases were first reported in France in 1978 (Coles, 1988). In 1994, the greater Paris area still had the largest number of AIDS patients. Of these, 70% were homosexual males and 7% were IDUs. However, as in the United States, homosexual AIDS cases have declined. In France, they went from 78% in the early 1980s to 53% in 1987. IDUs, on the other hand,

TABLE 11-1 The Incidence of AIDS in Europe

Country	Cumulative through March 31, 1990	Cumulative through 1994
Albania	0	1
Austria	415	1,156
Belarus	0	10
Belgium	651	1,664
Bulgaria	7	26
Croatia	1	70
Czechoslovakia	23	50
Denmark	573	1,450
Estonia	0	4
Finland	58	162
France	9,718	33,040
Germany	4,672	12,550
Greece	295	920
Hungary	34	159
Iceland	13	34
Ireland	142	401
Italy	6,068	23,860
Latvia	0	10
Lithuania	0	6
Luxembourg	26	84
Malta	14	31
Moldova	0	4
Monaco	2	26
Netherlands	1,189	3,155
Norway	153	401
Poland	35	225
Portugal	410	1,851
Romania	478	3,353
Russian Federation	26	141
San Marino	1	1
Slovak Republic	0	8
Slovenia	0	33
Spain	5,295	25,301
Sweden	406	1,061
Switzerland	1,255	3,702
Ukraine	0	29
United Kingdom	3,157	9,525
Yugoslavia	120	361
Total	35,236	123,465

Cumulative AIDS cases reported by 38 countries and estimated cumulative incidence rates per million population—World Health Organization (WHO) European Region, through March 31, 1990 and mid-1994. (SOURCE: WHO Surveillance Program, Geneva)

increased from 6% in the early 1980s to 17% in 1987.

Jean-Baptiste Brunet, of Claude Bernard Hospital in Paris, said the number of AIDS cases in Europe by mid-1988 was 12,221 and was doubling about every 11 months. By the end of 1993, 81,000 AIDS cases were reported. Brunet reported that the incidence of AIDS cases among IDUs in Spain, France, and Italy is increasing at an annual rate of 16%. In 1985, 7% of Europe's AIDS cases were IDUs. In 1988, 30% of AIDS cases were IDUs. It is estimated that 1 million people in 30 European countries are HIV-infected. AIDS has killed about 17,000 people in France and about 9,300 in Italy through 1994. In Paris, 40% of AIDS deaths occur in males between ages 25 and 44.

ASIA AND SOUTHEAST ASIA

The Asian and Pacific regions include over 50 countries and are home to over half the world's population (Moodie et al., 1993).

Through mid-1995, 44 countries in Asia had reported 250,000 AIDS cases. The WHO estimated that by the end of 1995 over 4 million Asians will be HIV-infected. By the year 2000, an estimated 10 million Asians will be HIV-infected. By the year 2000 it is estimated that between 4 million and 8 million Asian children will have been orphaned by the disease. Many of the initial cases were linked to people who had been to areas where HIV disease and AIDS were more prevalent. The AIDS virus is believed to have entered Asia in the mid-1980s. Thus far, relatively few AIDS cases have been reported to the WHO from Asian nations. However, the WHO's Global Program on AIDS (GPA) states that the rate of new HIV infection is rising dramatically—so fast, in fact, that, even though the disease was virtually unknown only a few years ago, by the end of this decade more Asians than Africans are expected to become infected each year (Palaca, 1991).

The Former Soviet Union

The former Soviet Union has only recently been alarmed by an increasing number of AIDS patients. The first case of AIDS was reported in 1987. Until 1990, Soviet officials still regarded AIDS as a Western problem. Foreign Ministry spokesman Gennady I. Gerasimov called AIDS "a scourge of God for the downfallen morals in our world." In November 1988, the Soviet Union reported its first AIDS associated death, a 29-year-old woman. But by the end of 1992, 600 AIDS cases had been re-

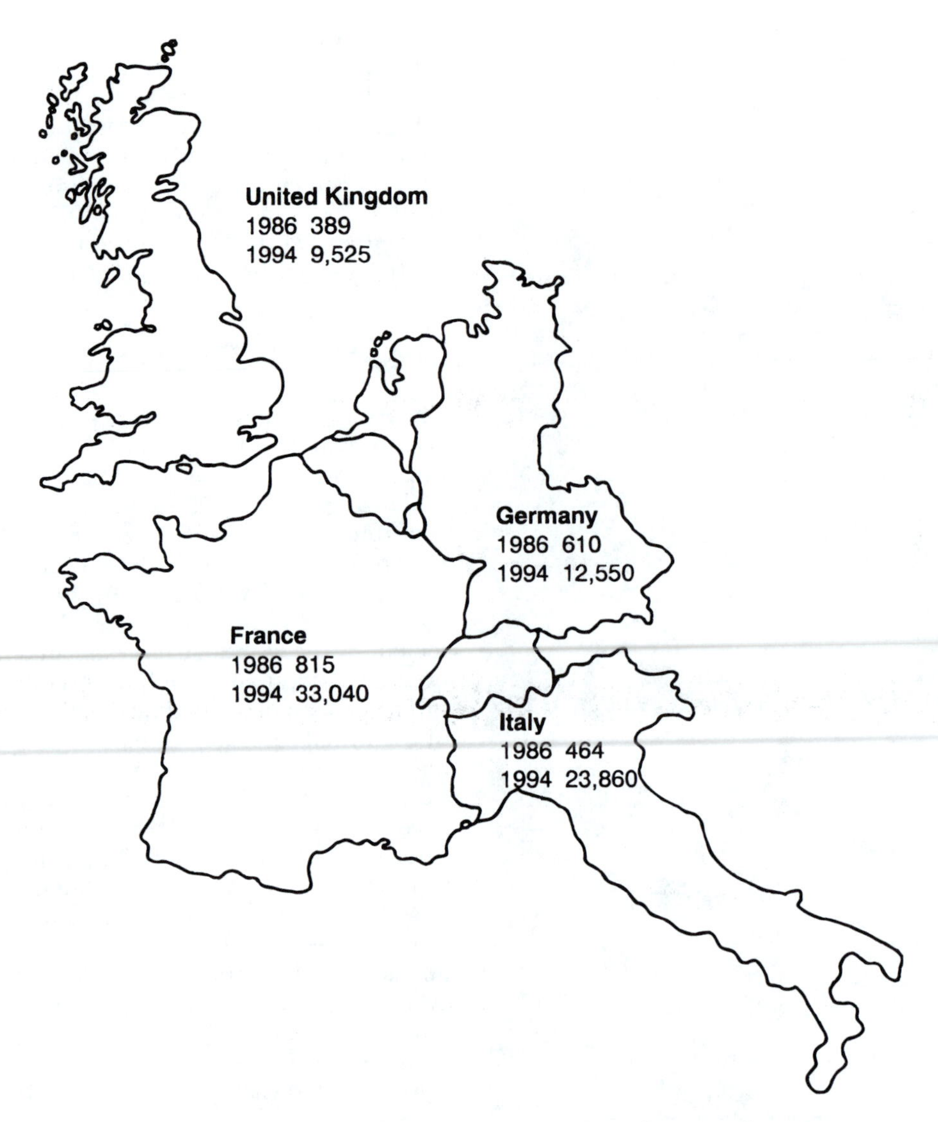

FIGURE 11-6 AIDS Cases in Western Europe through 1994. The number of new AIDS cases in Western European countries increased 19- to 30-fold over the number diagnosed in 1986. The numbers under each Western European country represent diagnosed AIDS cases in 1986 and in 1994. AIDS cases in these countries are mostly in metropolitan areas.

ported. Health officials also estimated there were over 20,000 HIV-infected.

In March of 1989, the Soviet Health Minister said that AIDS was a threat similar to that posed by nuclear weapons. In February, 1989, Gerasimov cautioned the world that the Soviet Union would now require foreigners who planned to stay there for more than 3 months to show certificates proving they were HIV-free. In late 1994 the Russian Parliament approved documents compulsory HIV screening of foreigners (Butler, 1994).

Soviets receive prison sentences of up to 8 years for transmitting the virus and 5 years for exposing someone else to the virus in cases where transmission does not occur. Soviet law

BOX 11.6

POLAND'S HIV/AIDS EPIDEMIC

The rapid spread of HIV disease/AIDS in Poland is directly linked to a form of homemade heroin called *campuk*. It is easily and cheaply made in the kitchens of Polish homes. Campuk consists of poppy straw, acetone, ammonia, and water. After boiling to reduce the broth, the left-over residue consists of 25% heroin, 50% morphine, and 25% codeine—*it is highly addictive.* The problem is compounded because injection needles are scarce and so those addicted share needles. There are between 300,000 and 600,000 injection drug users in Poland. Few treatment facilities are available with even fewer medical supplies and too few medical staff to make a difference. Over 10,000 physicians left Poland in 1990. A single day clinic in Warsaw treats 25,000 addicts a year; 75% are HIV-positive. Because drugs are in limited supply, only the fatally ill receive zidovudine. It is not unusual to have people die of AIDS within 2 years of diagnosis. The only hospital in Warsaw has a ward with 20 beds for AIDS patients but only eight can be accommodated because of staff shortages.

EDUCATION

The population is not well educated on the various aspects of HIV/AIDS. As a result, many believe the disease is casually transmitted. Those who are known to be HIV-infected or have AIDS are shunned like lepers. Townspeople chase the sick from their towns.

PROSTITUTION (COMMERCIAL SEX WORKERS)

From January to October 1990, 500,000 Polish women lost their jobs and turned to the streets. Officially, 10,000 are registered prostitutes; however, the figure is probably much higher. Some of the women do not tell their clients they are HIV-infected or have AIDS.

One of these women said that in 2 or 3 hours she could make 3 months' salary. This woman bragged of having clients from New York, Sweden, and Finland. Warsaw is becoming the prostitution capital of Eastern Europe.

(Source: *AIDS Quarterly*: *The Crisis in Poland,* WGBH Educational Foundation)

BOX 11.7

ONE MAN STARTS THE RUSSIAN AIDS EPIDEMIC

In 1981, the engineer returned to Elista carrying HIV. He married. The virus spread to his wife. She had a child. The child was infected, became sick, and in 1988 was sent to the hospital. Doctors did not know the child carried the virus.

In the hospital, the child received drug injections. The same drug was given to other children by doctors and nurses who used the **same syringe** because they thought children are sterile.

Some of these HIV-infected children were transferred to larger hospitals.

At each of those hospitals, the pattern was repeated. New cases appeared 300 miles away in hospitals in Volgograd, Rostov-on-Don, and Stavropol. A total of 260 children and several of their mothers became HIV-infected before this chain of events was stopped.

Russian medical authorities realized there had not been a single case of AIDS infection in the area before this outbreak of HIV infections. When authorities recognized the disease, they began exhaustive medical detective work to track the epidemic to its source.

In 1989, more than 140,000 people were tested for evidence of infection. The investigation led to the Russian engineer.

empowers authorities to test anyone suspected of carrying the AIDS virus.

Pakistan

In mid-1989, Health Minister Amir Haider Kazmi announced that HIV-antibody tests would be given to all foreigners living in Pakistan and to citizens who had lived abroad. By December of 1993, 26 cases of AIDS had been reported to the WHO. Pakistan borrowed about $17 million to purchase the necessary testing equipment.

China

China reported its first case of AIDS in November 1988, a male who had had a homosexual relationship with an HIV-infected foreigner. None of the previous 31 cases of

AIDS in China had originated there; they had involved HIV-infected foreigners visiting China. By August, 1990, the national newspaper reported that China, with a population of over 1 billion people, had a total of 305 cases of AIDS. Ninety-one of the newest AIDS cases involved heroin addicts in southwest Yunnan Province (Zheng et al., 1994).

In early 1990, Yunnan Province had 95% of all known HIV-infected people in China. Beijing had the next largest number. In order to halt further cases of HIV infection, the Beijing government asked the people to determine if their words and deeds conformed to the standards of the People's Republic and whether they knew what to do and what not to do when making contact with foreigners to avoid HIV infection.

Chinese officials dismiss the idea that the use of condoms might be able to control HIV infection.

With help from the World Health Organization, China is working out a 3-year program (1990–1993) for HIV/AIDS prevention and control. The program is designed to prevent HIV infection by conforming to global policies and strategies, and keeping in line with Chinese policies and local exigencies. There are now over 50 laboratories in 29 provinces conducting HIV-antibody testing on prostitutes, injection drug users, and other high-risk groups. In addition to beginning a national education campaign, China is also concerned about sterilizing techniques in some hospitals. Hospitals in major cities have just started to use disposable needles, but many still do not. Health care workers are now urged to follow strict guidelines in sterilizing syringes and needles.

India

It is now estimated that there are over 1.6 million HIV-infected people in India. Through 1993, 500 AIDS cases had been reported. Estimates on HIV-infection rates in India are difficult to make, but there are signs that an epidemic is at hand. In larger cities such as Bombay and Madras, about 20% of prostitutes or commercial sex workers are infected. In Bombay, the WHO estimates there are 250,000 HIV-infected people. There are an estimated 200,000 women working as prostitutes; 30% to 50% are believed to be HIV-infected. It is estimated that each prostitute has about five clients in a 24-hour period!

The new data show that HIV has spread to over 1 million people in India, far beyond the port cities of Bombay and Madras where it first entered, and is beginning to threaten rural populations, which are virtually defenseless because of a lack of information and condoms. Vulimiri Ramalingaswami of the All India Institute of Medical Sciences in New Delhi said that India is "sitting on top of a volcano" (Dickman, 1991). Snood (1990) reported that some Indian hospitals have banned AIDS patients and some doctors hesitate to treat them. In Delhi, nearly all physicians refuse to treat AIDS patients. V. Sharma, of the Malaria Research Center, Delhi, India (1994) reports that by the year 2000 India could have 1 million AIDS patients.

Thailand

According to the WHO, Thailand, with its 56 million people, is the most AIDS-prone country in Southeast Asia, mainly because of widespread prostitution and injection drug use. By the end of 1994, Thailand health officials believe that about 1 million people were HIV-infected. In some areas of Thailand, 23% of pregnant women and 10% to 15% of military draftees have tested HIV-positive (Dickman, 1991). Projected estimates indicate that 4 million people may be HIV-infected by the year 2000.

Japan

By January of 1995 there were about 750 AIDS cases in Japan. Most cases thus far have been in men with hemophilia reported to have received contaminated factor VIII. Around 1990 the rate of heterosexual infections in Japan began to rise dramatically, marking the beginning of a new trend in the pattern of HIV transmission in that country. In 1990 under half of all reported HIV infections and AIDS cases in Japan were in women; by 1992, women outnumbered men by about three to two.

Oceania

By January of 1995, over 5,500 AIDS cases were reported from Oceania. Oceania along with Eastern Europe, the Middle East, and North Africa thus far account for only about 1% of all reported AIDS cases. While the prevalence of HIV infection is still low in most of these countries, indigenous transmission is occurring and HIV infections are being recognized among people with multiple sexual partners and those who use injection drugs, A.

SUMMARY

The United States now accounts for about 40% of reported AIDS cases worldwide. But many countries, for political and economic reasons, underreport their AIDS cases. Thus the total number worldwide is an estimate and the real number remains unknown. The WHO estimated that there were between 5 and 10 million HIV-infected people worldwide in 1992. But, the Harvard Global AIDS Policy Coalition estimated the number of HIV-infected persons worldwide to be 12.9 million. It is estimated that by the end of 1996, there will be 30 million HIV-infected persons.

AIDS cases have been reported from all seven continents and from 160 countries. Africa has been reporting increasing numbers of AIDS cases from about 1985. HIV transmission in Africa is primarily between heterosexuals and from infected mothers to offspring. Injection drug use and homosexual activities are considered rare in Africa. There are some reports of blood transfusion cases of HIV infection in Africa, but they are relatively few.

The point is that HIV infections continue to increase in all nations reporting to the CDC or the WHO. The largest number of AIDS cases have yet to appear. Will the separate nations be prepared to handle the many medical, economic, social, and political problems that will accompany the tremendous drain on national resources?

REVIEW QUESTIONS

(*Answers to the Review Questions are on page 482.*)

1. Worldwide, what is the estimated rate of HIV infection?
2. What is the primary route of HIV transmission in Africa?
3. Name the two countries in Europe with the highest number of AIDS cases.
4. What is the incidence of new AIDS cases in Europe?
5. What route of HIV exposure is becoming the most prevalent throughout the United States and Europe?
6. Of the countries presented, which appears to have the largest rate of HIV transmission by bisexual males? Which country is isolating HIV-infected people in sanatoriums? Which countries mandate that foreigners must have certificates proving they are **not** infected with HIV?
7. Name the two European countries in which over 50% of AIDS cases occur in IDUs.

REFERENCES

BARONGO, LONGIN R., et al. (1992). The epidemiology of HIV infection in urban areas, roadside settlements and rural villages in Mwanza region, Tanzania. *AIDS*, 6:1521–1528.

BERKLEY, SETH F. (1992). AIDS in the global village. *JAMA*, 268:3368–3369.

BIGGAR, ROBERT. (1993). Editorial: When ideals meet reality—the global challenge of HIV/AIDS. *Am. J. Public Health*, 83:1383–1384.

BUTLER, DEALAN. (1994). Hopes and doubts mired Paris AIDS summit. *Nature*, 372:308.

CHIN, J. (1990). Current and future dimensions of the HIV/AIDS pandemic in women and children. *Lancet*, 336:221–224.

CHIN, J., et al. (1990). Projections of HIV infections and AIDS cases to the year 2000. *Bull. HO*, 68:1–11.

COLES, PETER. (1988). French government recognizes need for AIDS health campaign. *Nature*, 335:2.

COMMENGES, DANIEL, et al. (1992). Estimating the incubation period of pediatric AIDS in Rwanda. *AIDS*, 6:1515–1520.

CULOTTA, ELIZABETH. (1991). Forecasting the global AIDS Epidemic. *Science*, 253:852–853.

DeCock, Kevin, et al. (1993). Clinical research, prophylaxis, therapy and care for HIV disease in Africa. *Am. J. Public Health,* 83:1385–1388.

DeCock, Kevin, et al. (1994). The public health implications of AIDS Research in Africa. *JAMA,* 272:481–486.

Dickman, Steven. (1991). AIDS threatens Asia. *Nature,* 351:682.

Earickson, Robert J. (1990). International behavioral responses to a health hazard: AIDS. *Social Sci. Med.,* 31:951–952.

Holmes, King K. (1991). The changing epidemiology of HIV transmission. *Hosp. Pract.,* 26:153–178.

Lancet. (1993). Heterosexual AIDS: pessimism, pandemics and plain hard facts. 341:863–864.

Mann, Jonathan, et al. (1988). The international epidemiology of AIDS. *Sci. Am.,* 259:82–89.

Moodie, Rob, et al. (1993). Confronting the HIV epidemic in Asia and the Pacific: successful strategies to minimize the spread of HIV. *AIDS,* 7:1543–1551.

Niftrik, Jack van. (1988). AIDS in Africa. *Med. Interface,* 1:12–17.

Palaca, Joseph. (1991), WHO AIDS program: moving on a new track. *Science,* 254:511–512.

Physicians Association for AIDS Care. (1990). WHO Projects 6,500,000 HIV Cases Worldwide. July/Aug.: 177, 211.

Pan American Health Organization. (1994). *AIDS Surveillance in the Americas.* June 10: 94,015.

Quarterly Surveillance Update. AIDS in Canada. Jan. 1994:1–30.

Quinn, Thomas C. (1988). Epidemiology of HIV-1 and HIV-2 in Africa. *Excerpta Medica,* Sept.: 42–48.

Saxinger, W. C., et al. (1985). Evidence for exposure to HTLV III in Uganda before 1973. *Science,* 227:1036–1038.

Sharma, V. P. (1994). Malaria and AIDS. *Nature,* 369:700.

Smith, Eloe, et al. (1994). The AIDS epidemic among Scandinavian women, 1980–1990. *AIDS,* 8:689–692.

Snood, S. (1990). AIDS patients are safe to treat. *Nat. Med. J. India,* 3:149.

Sonnerfeld, E. D. (1990). First AIDS case in South Africa? *South African Med. J.,* 78:4.

Sternberg, Rachel. (1989). Fighting taboos, fighting AIDS. *Am. Med. News,* Feb.: 3, 25–28.

Taylor, C. C. (1990). Condoms and cosmology: the fractal person and sexual risk in Rwanda. *Social Sci. Med.,* 31:1023–1028.

United States Department of State. (1992). *Global AIDS Disaster: Implications for the 1990s.* Publication No. 9955.

Vandepitte, J., et al. (1983). AIDS and cryptococcosis. *Lancet,* 1:925–926.

World Development Report 1993: Investing in Health. Washington, D. C.: World Bank, April 1993. World Bank Report 11778.

World Health Organization Global Programme on AIDS. (1992). *Current and Future Dimensions of the HIV/AIDS Pandemic: A Capsule Summary, January 1992.* Geneva, Switzerland: World Health Organization. Publication WHO/GPA/RES/SFI/92.1.

Zheng, Xiwen, et al. (1994). Injecting drug use and HIV Infection In Southwest China. *AIDS,* 8:1141–1147.

CHAPTER 12

Testing for Human Immunodeficiency Virus

CHAPTER CONCEPTS

- ELISA means enzyme linked immunosorbent assay; it is a screening test for HIV infection.
- Western blot is a confirmatory HIV test.
- The ELISA test has been used to screen all blood supplies in the United States since March 1985.
- HIV screening tests can produce both false positives and false negatives.
- A positive ELISA test only predicts that a confirmatory test will also be positive.
- False positive readings result from a test's lack of specificity.
- There is a relationship between the incidence of HIV in the population being tested and the number of false positives reported. The higher the incidence, the fewer the false positives.
- Several new screening and confirmatory HIV tests are now available.
- The polymerase chain reaction test is the most sensitive HIV test currently available.
- AIDS cases have been reported in all 50 states.
- HIV testing for the most part is on a voluntary basis.
- Compulsory HIV testing is used in the military, prisons and in certain federal agencies.

Public HIV/AIDS clinics in the United States are becoming overwhelmed with requests for HIV testing. Most of the requests are repeats. But at least half of the CDC-estimated 1.5 million HIV-infected persons in the United States have never been tested. They have not been tested because of fear, lack of access, or lack of education.

REASONS FOR HIV TESTING IN THE UNITED STATES

HIV testing in the United States is done to prompt behavior change, to provide entry into clinical care, if necessary, to provide a starting

BOX 12.1

AN ASSUMPTION OF AIDS WITHOUT THE HIV TEST: IT SHATTERS A LIFE

San Francisco— For six years, a 53-year-old gay male lived in the nether world of AIDS. He stopped working, suffered the painful side effects of experimental drugs and waited to die.

Now his doctors say he never had the disease.

His health shattered by AIDS treatment, his livelihood lost, he filed a $2 million claim against Kaiser Permanente health maintenance organization. He claims he underwent sustained treatment for full-fledged AIDS without receiving an HIV test.

His attorney said, "For six years he thought that the most he had was six months to live. So everyday he'd wake up and think 'Is this the last day of my life?'"

To begin, this male says he checked into a San Jose hospital affiliated with Kaiser in 1986 with respiratory problems and doctors told him he had pneumocystis pneumonia, considered a sure sign of AIDS at the time.

He underwent tests but **was not** given one to determine the presence of HIV, the virus associated with AIDS.

In 1986, he began taking the drug zidovudine in high doses, which gave him a chronic headache, high blood pressure and peripheral neuropathy—permanent pins and needles pains from his calves to his feet. He is battling an addiction to Darvon and other prescription drugs.

Under doctors' orders, he quit his job as a skin care technician and lives on government welfare and disability benefits of $600 a month.

(Associated Press, 1992)

point for partner notification and education, and to protect the nation's blood supply. There is an immediate need to change our perception about being HIV-positive so that people feel good about taking the test to protect themselves and others, rather than the discrimination that now exists against those who have taken the test.

AIDS is diagnosed by evaluating the results of clinical findings during a physical examination, and by laboratory analysis of blood samples for the presence of antibodies to HIV. Until early 1983, the causative agent of AIDS was unknown. Up to that time, infection could only be determined after the person began to express the signs and symptoms associated with AIDS. Once the virus was identified, a means of detecting viral exposure was developed. There is still no single diagnostic test for AIDS. All **screening** tests to date measure the absence or presence of antibodies against HIV. HIV counseling and testing are important components of HIV prevention programs.

IMMUNODIAGNOSTIC TECHNIQUES FOR DETECTING ANTIBODIES TO HIV

Refinements in the field of immunological testing, serology, and the study of antigen–antibody reactions have produced test names that reflect the component parts of the test being used. In most cases, tests are based on the detection of antibodies present in the serum, in this case antibodies to HIV. One immunological test uses enzyme-labeled antibodies. An enzyme is connected to an antibody; after the enzyme–antibody unit complexes with its specific antigen, the presence of the antigen can be determined by adding a reagent that will form a colored solution if antibody to HIV is present. This is called the **enzyme immunoassay** (EIA) test. An EIA test was adopted in 1983 for the detection of HIV antibodies. It is the now called **enzyme linked immunosorbent assay** (ELISA, el-i-sa).

Recently, a technique has been developed that uses fluorescently labeled antibodies against HIV-specific antigens. This technique, called the fluorescent antibody technique, and others are described.

ELISA-HIV ANTIBODY TEST

The initial application of the ELISA test outside the research laboratory, was used primarily in large-scale screening of the nation's blood supply. ELISA testing of the existing blood supply and all newly donated blood began in the United States in March 1985. The ELISA test is used as a screening test because of its low cost,

BOX 12.2

PRETEST PATIENT INFORMATION

It is important that you read and understand the following information before having the HIV antibody test.

The HIV antibody test is a blood test. It was first used in 1985 to screen donated blood. **This test is not a test for AIDS. But a positive result does mean that there is a high probability an HIV-infected person will eventually develop AIDS.**

Only anonymous test results remain absolutely confidential.

What Does the Test Reveal?

The test reveals whether a person has been exposed to HIV. The test detects the presence of HIV antibodies, an indication that infection has occurred. It does not detect the virus itself nor does it indicate the level of viral infection, only that one has been infected.

It is important to find out whether you are HIV-positive or negative so that you can prevent spreading the virus to others and seek early medical intervention.

What Tests Will Be Done?

Wherever the test is done, the procedures are similar. A blood sample is taken from the arm and analyzed in a laboratory using a test called *ELISA* (*enzyme linked immunosorbent assay*). If the first ELISA test is positive, the laboratory will run a second ELISA test on the same blood sample. If positive, another test, called Western blot, is run on the same blood sample to confirm the ELISA result.

What Do the Test Results Mean?

See Table 12-1.

Positive Result: A positive result suggests that a person has HIV antibodies and may have been infected with the virus at some time. People with

TABLE 12-1 The Meaning of Antibody Test Results

A Positive Results	B Negative Results
If you test positive, it does mean: 1. Your blood sample has been tested more than once and the tests indicate that it contained antibodies to HIV. 2. You have been infected with HIV and your body has produced antibodies. If you test positive, it does *not* mean: 1. That you have AIDS. 2. That you necessarily will get AIDS, but the probability is high. You can reduce your chance of progressing to AIDS by avoiding further contact with the virus and living a healthy lifestyle. 3. That you are immune to the virus. Therefore, if you test positive, you should do the following: 1. Protect yourself from any further infection. 2. Protect others from the virus by following AIDS precautions in sex, drug use, and general hygiene. 3. Consider seeing a physician for a complete evaluation and advice on health maintenance. 4. Avoid drugs and heavy alcohol use, maintain good nutrition, and avoid fatigue and stress. Such action may improve your chances of staying healthy.	If you test negative, it does mean: 1. No antibodies to HIV have been found in your serum at the time of the test. Two possible explanations for a negative test result exist: 1. You have not been infected with HIV. 2. You have been infected with HIV but have not yet produced antibodies. Research indicates the most people will produce antibodies within 6 to 18 weeks after infection. Some people will not produce antibodies for at least 3 years. A very small number of people may never produce antibodies. If you test negative, it does *not* mean: 1. That you have nothing to worry about. You may become infected, be careful. 2. That you are immune to HIV. It has not yet been shown that anyone is immune to HIV infection. 3. That you have not been infected with the virus. You may have been infected and not yet produced antibodies.

(Adapted from the San Francisco AIDS Foundation)

a positive result should assume that they have the virus and could therefore transmit it:

- by sex (anal, vaginal, or oral) where body fluids, especially semen or blood, get inside the partner's body;
- by sharing injection drug "works" (needles, syringes, etc.);
- by donating blood, sperm, or body organs; or
- to an unborn baby during pregnancy or to a newborn by breast feeding.

Negative Result: If it has been 4 to 6 months since the last possible exposure to HIV, then a negative result suggests that a person is probably not infected with the virus. However, **false negatives** can occur. For example, if the test was too soon after HIV exposure, the body may not have had time to produce HIV antibodies. **Collec-tively, studies show that 50% of HIV-infected persons seroconvert (demonstrate measurable HIV antibodies) by 3 months after HIV infection and 90% seroconvert by 6 months. A small percentage seroconverted at 1 year or later. Most important, a negative result does not mean that you are protected from getting the virus in the future—your future depends on your behavior.**

Inconclusive Result: A small percentage of results are inconclusive. This means that the result is neither positive nor negative. This may be due to a number of factors that have nothing to do with HIV infection, or it can occur early in an infection when there are not enough HIV antibodies present to give a positive result. If this happens, another blood sample will be taken at a later time for a retest.

How Accurate Is the Test Result?

The result is accurate. However, as with any laboratory test, there can be false positives and false negatives.

False Positive: A small percentage of all people tested may be told they have the HIV antibody when, in fact, they do not. This can be due to laboratory error or certain medical conditions which have nothing to do with HIV infection.

False Negative: Some people are told that they are not HIV-infected when, in fact, they are. This can happen when the test is taken too soon after being infected—the body has not had time to produce HIV antibodies. This is called the **window period**.

Should the Test Be Performed?

Whether to have the test done is a personal decision. However, knowing your antibody status can help you address some very difficult questions. For example, if the test is negative, what lifestyle changes should be made to minimize risk of HIV infection? If the test is positive, how can others be protected from infection? What can be done to improve your chances of staying healthy?

(Source: Roche Biomedical Laboratories, Inc.)

standardized procedures, high reproducibility, and rapid results.

The ELISA test is now semi-automated. It uses an antigen derived from HIV cultivated in human cell lines. One such line is the human leukemia cell line **H9**. Whole viruses isolated from H9 **are disrupted** into subunit antigens for use. The subunits of HIV are then bound to a solid support system.

Two solid support systems are used in the seven ELISA screening test kits licensed in the United States. Some attach the antigens onto small glass beads (Figure 12-1A), while others fix the antigens onto the sides and bottoms of small wells (micro wells) in a glass or plastic microtiter plate (Figure 12-1B). The serum to be tested is separated from the blood and is diluted and applied to the HIV-coated solid support systems (Figure 12-2). The ELISA test takes from 3.5 to 4 hours to perform (Carlson et al., 1989) and costs between about $7 in state sponsored virology laboratories and about $60 to $75 in private laboratories.

In accordance with FDA recommendations, effective June 1992, blood collection centers in the United States began HIV-2 testing on all donated blood and blood components. The CDC does not recommend routine testing for HIV-2 other than at blood collection centers (*MMWR*, 1992).

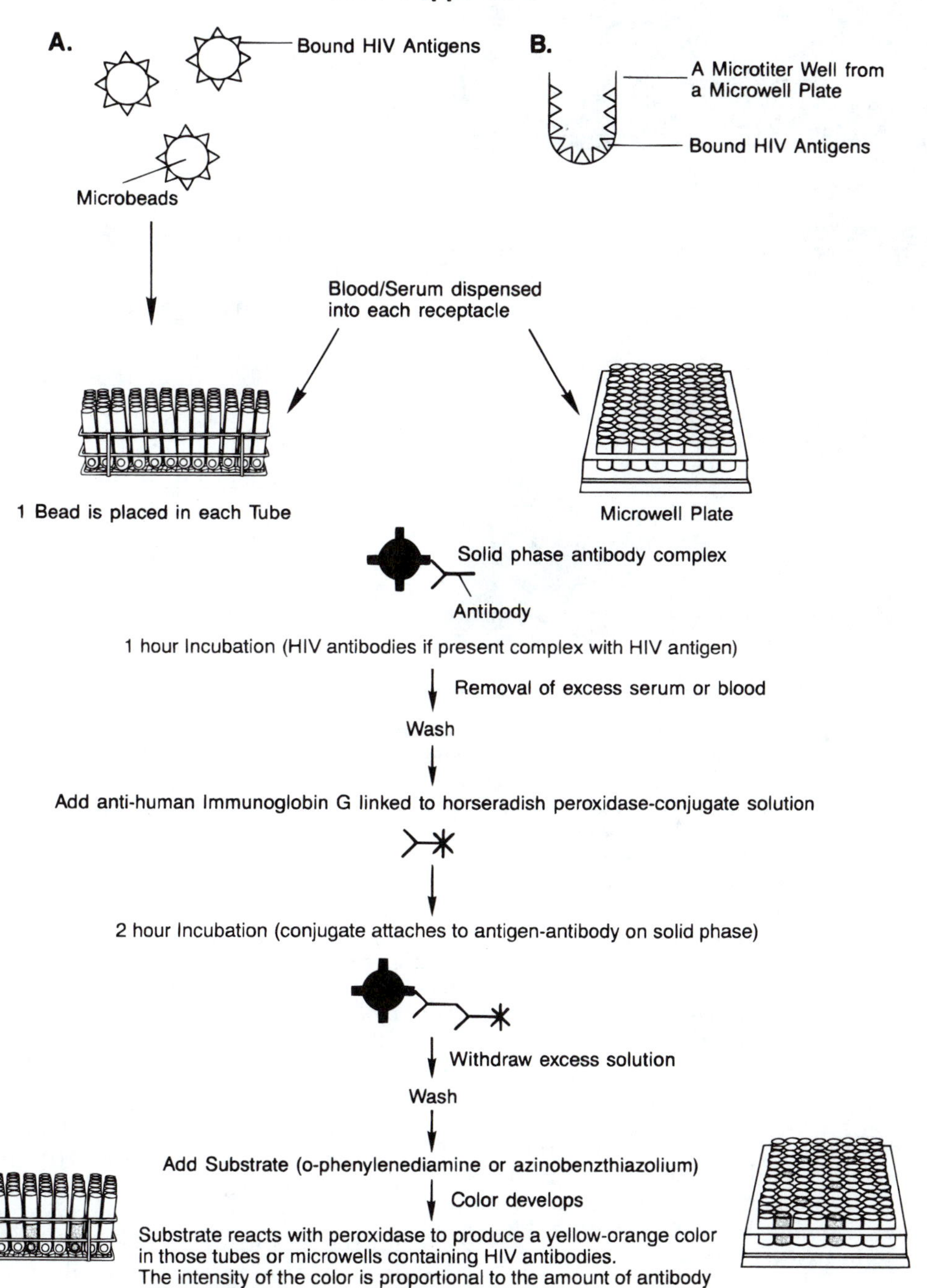

FIGURE 12-1 The ELISA Test. **A**, Microbeads with attached antigen in test tubes. **B**, Antigens bound to walls and bottom of microtiter wells.

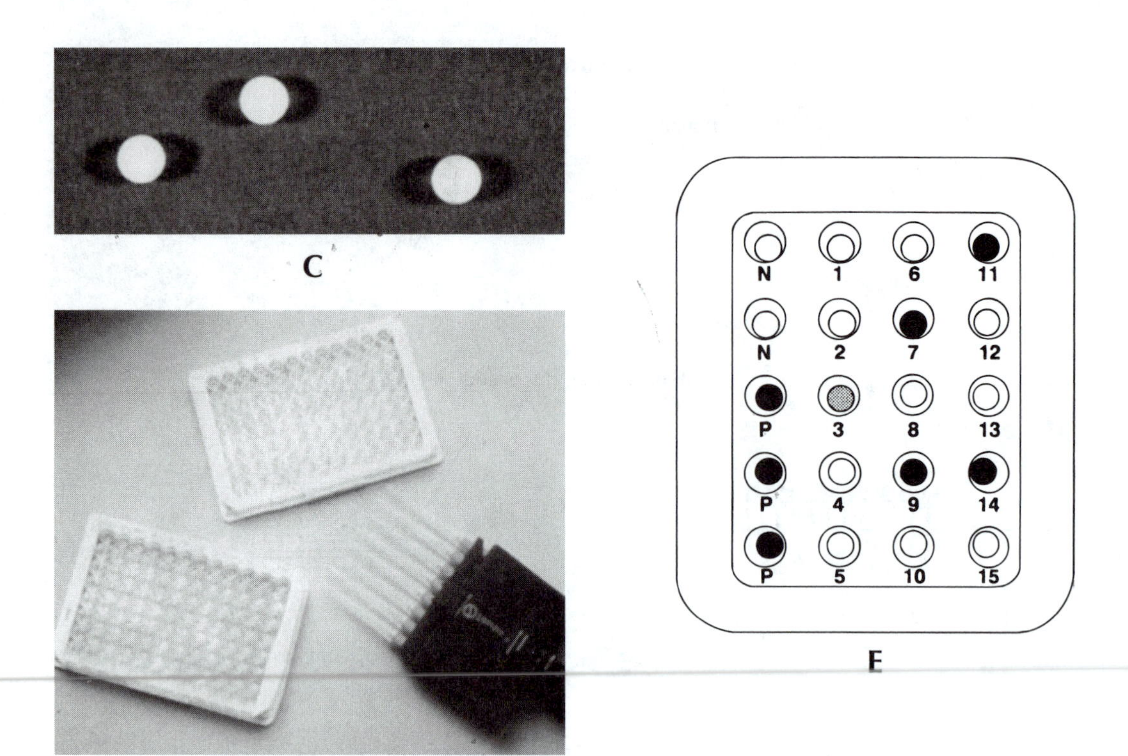

FIGURE 12-1 *(continued)* **C**, Microbeads are 7 mm in diameter. The test takes between 2.5 and 4 hours to perform. **D**, Microwell plates showing positive (yellow) and negative (clear) test results. The microtiter dispenser handles eight microwells at a time. **E**, Specimens positive for HIV antibody have a deeper color in this microwell tray. Serum specimens from 15 patients were tested for antibodies to HIV. Two negative and three positive control specimens are provided in the first column. In wells 7, 9, 11, and 14, the dark yellow color change, matching the color in the three positive control wells, indicates that the specimens are positive. Well 3 shows a weakly reactive result. The remaining specimens showed no color change and were interpreted as negative for HIV antibodies. (Adapted from Fang et al., 1989) (**C** and **D** *Courtesy of Roche Biomedical Laboratories, AIDS Testing Brochure*)

Understanding the ELISA Test

The ELISA test determines if a person's serum contains antibodies to one or more HIV antigens. Although there are some minor differences among the FDA licensed kits, test procedures are basically similar.

Problems with ELISA Test

Any HIV screening test must be able to distinguish those individuals who are infected from those who are not. The underlying assumption of an ELISA test is that all HIV-infected people will produce detectable HIV antibodies. However, the HIV-infected population in general does not produce detectable antibodies for 6 weeks to 1 or more years after HIV infection. Most often, HIV antibody is present within 6 to 18 weeks. Thus, HIV-infected people can test HIV-negative. **This is a false negative result**. In some HIV-infected persons, as their disease progresses, the virus ties up the available antibody. Testing at this time would also produce false negative results.

False-positive reactions may also occur. This means that the person's serum does not contain antibodies to HIV but the test results indicate that it does.

Purpose for ELISA Test

Because the original purpose of the ELISA test was to screen blood, the sensitivity (ability to detect low-level color formation; see Figure 12-1) of the test was purposely set high. It was reasoned that it was better to have some false positives and throw away good blood rather than to take in any HIV contaminated blood. Thus the ELISA test is a **positive predictive value** test. It only predicts that the serum tested will continue to test positive when a test with greater specificity, called a **confirmatory test**, is done.

In 1985, during the first month of donor screening, 1% of all blood tested HIV-antibody positive. On ELISA retesting of these samples, only 0.17% (17/10,000) were HIV-antibody-positive. On subjecting these samples to a confirmatory test, only 0.038% (4/10,000) were actually HIV-positive. These early tests produced about 24 false positives for every true positive result. The main reason for such a high false positive rate or **lack of specificity** was that something other than HIV produced an antibody or other substance that reacted with HIV antigen causing the HIV test to appear positive.

People may test false positive who have an underlying liver disease, have received a blood transfusion or gamma globulin within 6 weeks of the test, have had several children, have had rheumatological diseases, are injection drug users, or have received vaccines for influenza and hepatitis B (Fang et al., 1989; MacKenzie et al., 1992). In each case, the person may have antibodies that will cross-react with the HIV antigens giving a false-positive reaction. Other reasons for false positives are laboratory errors and mistakes made in reagent preparations for use in the test kits.

Although high sensitivity tests eliminate HIV-contaminated blood from the blood supply, there is a downside to high sensitivity testing when proper procedure is *not* used. People told that they have tested positive have become emotionally distraught. Former Senator Lawton Chiles of Florida, at an AIDS conference in 1987, told of a tragic example from the early days of blood screening in Florida. Of 22 blood donors who were told they were HIV-positive by the ELISA test, seven committed suicide.

There continue to be false positive reactions among blood donors and low-level risk populations because of a *low prevalence* of HIV infection in such populations. The American Red Cross Blood Services laboratories report that using current ELISA methodology, a specificity of 99.8% can be achieved (*MMWR*, 1988a).

Positive Predictive Value— The positive predictive value of the ELISA test indicates the percentage of true positives among total positives in a given population. To safeguard against false-positive tests, the CDC recommends that serum that tests positive be retested twice (in duplicate). If both tests are negative, the serum is considered HIV-antibody-negative and further tests will only be done should signs or symptoms of HIV infection occur (Figures 12-3A and 12-3B). If one or both of the tests is positive, the serum is subjected to a confirmatory test, usually a Western blot (WB) (Figure 12-4). At blood banks, if the initial ELISA test is positive, the blood is discarded. If an individual's serum subjected to a confirmatory test is positive, the person is considered to be HIV-infected.

Although confirmatory tests can be used to determine true- positive results, they are too labor intensive and expensive to be used in screening a large population. Thus the positive predictive value of an ELISA test is an important first step in large-scale screening. Recall, however, that the predictive value depends on the prevalence of HIV infection in the population tested. The higher the prevalence of HIV infection in a given population, the more likely a positive ELISA test is to be a true positive; and conversely, the lower the prevalence of infection, the less likely a positive ELISA test is to be a true positive.

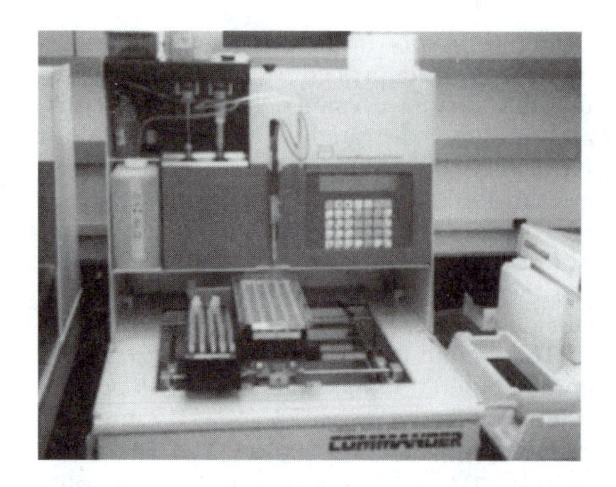

A

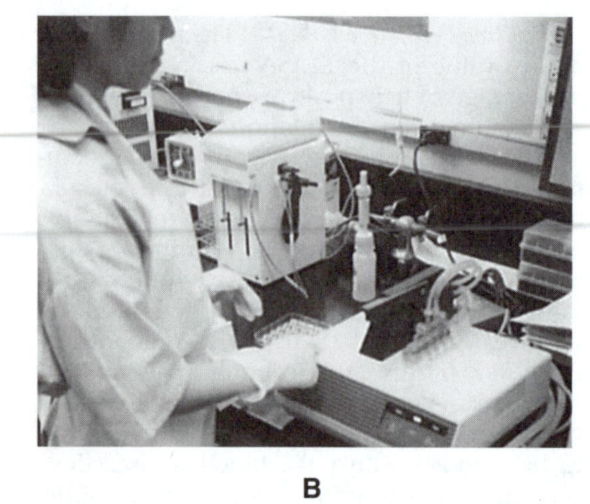

B

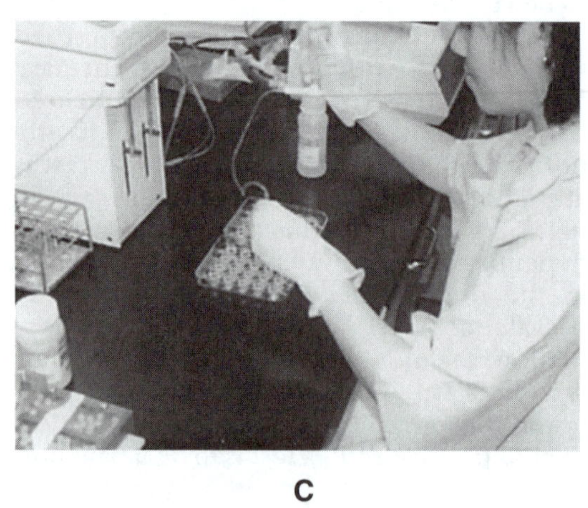

C

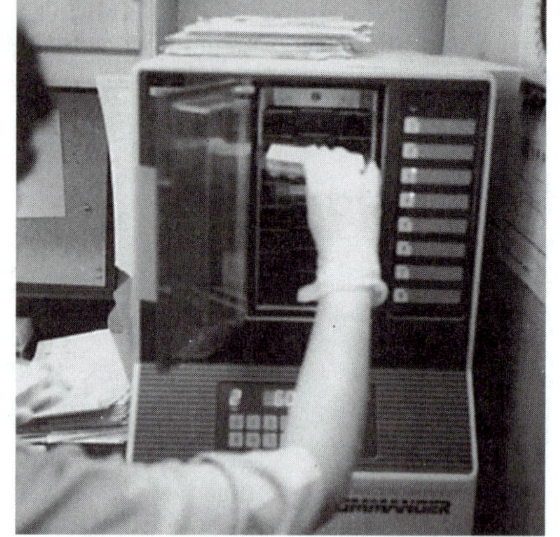

D

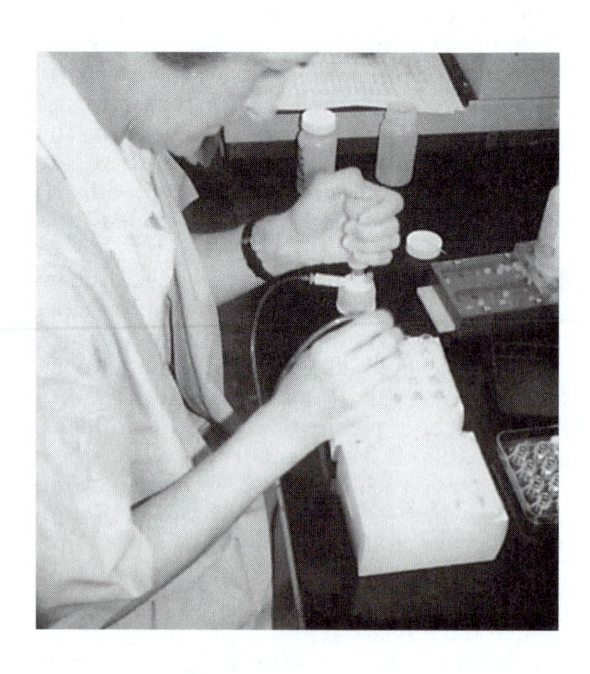

E

WESTERN BLOT ASSAY

The gold standard for determining a true-positive HIV-antibody test is still the **Western blot** (WB). This test is a method in which individual HIV proteins are used to react with HIV antibody in a person's serum. It should be understood that the WB test is not a **true** gold standard because it is not 100% certain, but it can come close to 100% if properly used.

Human cells in which HIV is being cultured are lysed or broken open, and the mixture of cell components and HIV components (proteins) are separated from each other. The viral proteins are placed on a polyacrylamide gel which then gets an electrical charge. The electrical current separates the viral proteins within the gel. This is called **gel electrophoresis**. The smallest HIV proteins will move quickly through the gel, separating from the next larger size, and so on.

Each different protein will arrive at a separate position on the gel. After proteins of similar molecular weight collect at a given site, they form a band; and these bands are identified based on the distance they have run in the gel. Because each band is a protein produced as a product of a different HIV gene, the gel band patterns give a picture of the HIV genes that were functioning and the location of each gene's products on the gel (Figure 12-4 and Table 12-2). The protein or antigen bands within the gel are "blotted," that is, transferred directly, band for band and position for position, onto strips of nitrocellulose paper (Figure 12-4).

Once the antigen bands have been formed, serum that is believed to carry HIV antibodies is placed directly on them. That is, a test serum is added directly to antigen bands located on the nitrocellulose strip. If antibodies are present in the serum, they will form an antigen–antibody complex directly on the antigen band areas. After the strip is washed, the HIV antibody– antigen bands are visualized by adding enzyme-conjugated antihuman immunoglobulin G to the strip. Then the substrate or color agent is added. If antibody has complexed with any of the banded HIV proteins on the nitrocellulose strip, a color reaction will occur at the band site(s) (Figure 12-4). Positive test strips are then compared to two control test strips, one that has been reacted with known positive serum and one that has been reacted with known negative serum.

In contrast to the ELISA test, which indicates only the presence or absence of HIV antibodies, the WB strip qualitatively identifies which of the HIV antigens the antibodies are directed against. The greatest disadvantage of the WB test is that reagents, testing methods, and test-interpretation criteria are not standardized. The National Institutes of Health (NIH), the American Red Cross, DuPont company, the Association of State and Territorial Health Officers (ASTHO), and the Department of Defense (DoD) define a positive WB differently.

It can be concluded from the criteria set up by different organizations to define a positive result that although the WB may be the gold standard of confirmatory testing, there is **no** agreement on what constitutes a positive WB test (Miike, 1987).

The WB procedure is labor-intensive, takes longer to run (12 to 24 hours), and is therefore more costly than the ELISA test. The WB is **less sensitive** than the ELISA **but more specific**.

FIGURE 12-2 (*facing page*) Semi-Automated ELISA Test. **A**, Serum samples are individually machine diluted 1 to 400. This includes the dilution of positive serum negative samples supplied with the test kit. Beads containing the HIV antigens are placed into the individual sample holders. Antibodies, if present in the individual sera, attach to the HIV antigens. **B,** Excess serum is withdrawn from each sample and the beads are washed. **C,** The antihuman immunoglobulin-horseradish enzyme conjugate is added to each prepared sample. **D,** The samples are incubated. **E**, Each sample receives the chromogen or substrate (o-phenylenediamine or azinobenzthiazolium). A yellow-orange color appears in samples that contain antibodies to HIV. (*Courtesy of Florida Health and Rehabilitative Services, Office of Laboratory AIDS Unit, Jacksonville*)

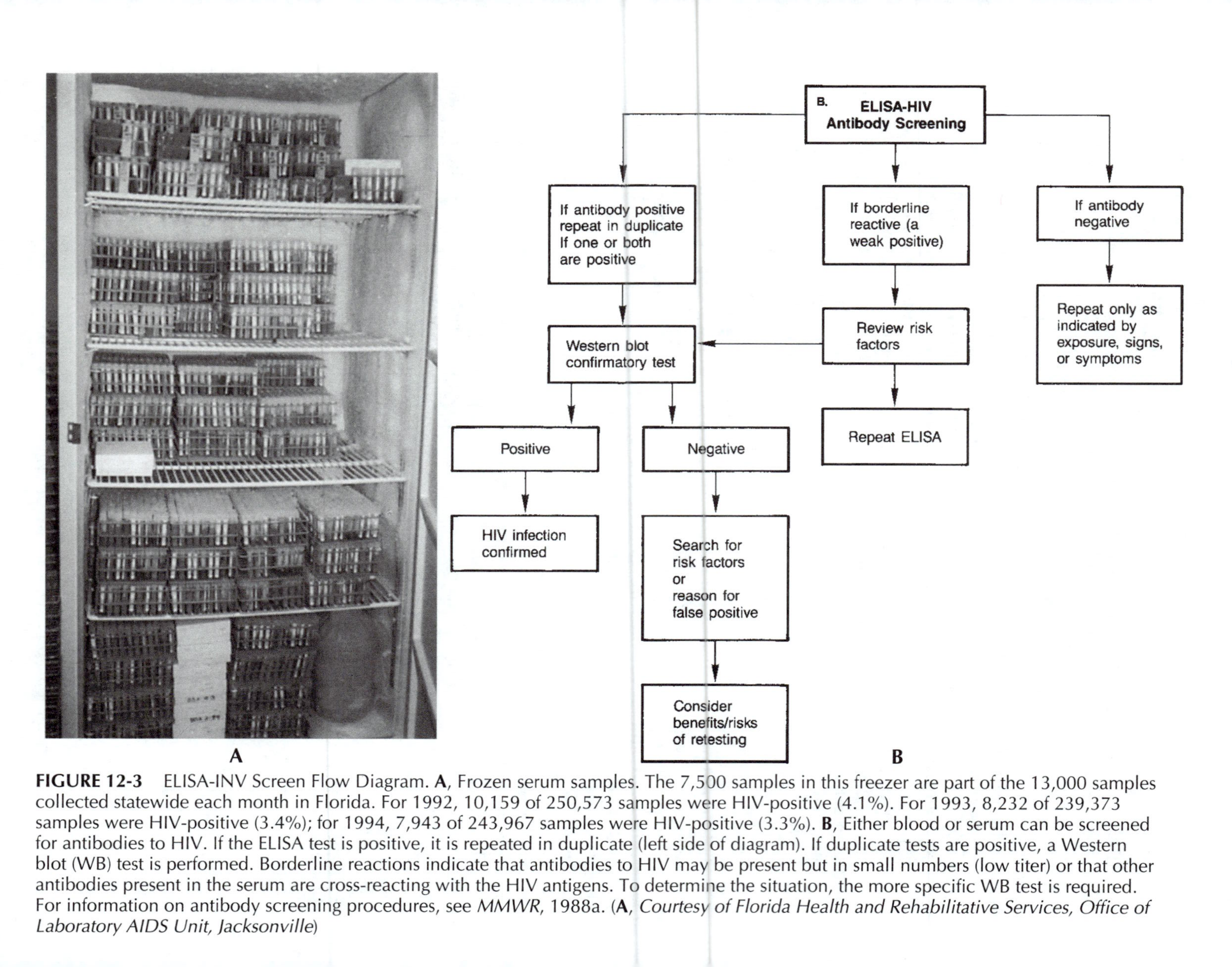

FIGURE 12-3 ELISA-INV Screen Flow Diagram. **A**, Frozen serum samples. The 7,500 samples in this freezer are part of the 13,000 samples collected statewide each month in Florida. For 1992, 10,159 of 250,573 samples were HIV-positive (4.1%). For 1993, 8,232 of 239,373 samples were HIV-positive (3.4%); for 1994, 7,943 of 243,967 samples were HIV-positive (3.3%). **B**, Either blood or serum can be screened for antibodies to HIV. If the ELISA test is positive, it is repeated in duplicate (left side of diagram). If duplicate tests are positive, a Western blot (WB) test is performed. Borderline reactions indicate that antibodies to HIV may be present but in small numbers (low titer) or that other antibodies present in the serum are cross-reacting with the HIV antigens. To determine the situation, the more specific WB test is required. For information on antibody screening procedures, see *MMWR*, 1988a. (**A**, *Courtesy of Florida Health and Rehabilitative Services, Office of Laboratory AIDS Unit, Jacksonville*)

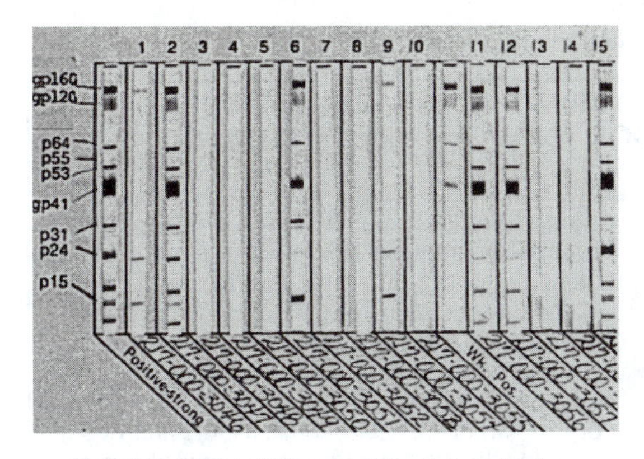

FIGURE 12-4 Western Blot Strips. Each WB strip contains nine separate antigenic proteins of HIV. Human serum or blood can be applied directly to the strips. See text for details on reactions. Because false positives can sometimes occur with the ELISA test, additional testing is needed to evaluate specimens which are repeatedly reactive by ELISA. The Western blot is more specific but less sensitive than the ELISA and is recommended for blood banks and organ donor centers. Its clinical usefulness in trials to aid in evaluating specimens which are questionably positive by other methods has been proven. It is not a screening test because it lacks a high level of sensitivity. (*Courtesy of Roche Biomedical Laboratories, AIDS Testing Brochure*)

A test's **sensitivity** is its capacity to identify **all** specimens that **have** HIV antibodies in them. A test's **specificity** is its capacity to identify **all** specimens that **do not have** HIV antibodies in them. Because the WB lacks the sensitivity of the ELISA test, it is not used as a screening test. Despite the high specificity of the WB, false positives do occur, but they occur less frequently than with ELISA tests because the WB is only run on serum or blood already suspected of containing HIV antibodies.

Relative Costs of ELISA and Western Blot Tests

The cost incurred to identify each true-positive HIV individual in a population with a 10% prevalence for HIV infection is presented in Table 12-3. Cost estimates are for tests performed on a contractual basis, that is, for screening large numbers of people versus testing of individuals. Note that the difference is quite significant.

TABLE 12-2 Description of Major Gene Products of Human Immunodeficiency Virus

Gene Product[a]	Description
p17/18[b]	GAG[c] protein
p24/25	GAG protein
p31/32	Endonuclease component of POL[d] translate
gp41	Transmembrane ENV[e] glycoprotein
p51/52/53	Reverse transcriptase component of POL translate
p55	Precursor of GAG proteins
p64/65 p66	Reverse transcriptase component of POL translate
gp110/120 gp120	Outer ENV glycoprotein
gp160	Precursor of ENV glycoprotein

[a]Number refers to molecular weight of the protein in kilodaltons; measurement of molecular weight may vary slightly in different laboratories.

[b]Where two bands on acrylamide gel are to close for easy identification, they are presented as such, p51/53, etc.

[c]GAG = core.

[d]POL = polymerase.

[4]ENV = envelope.

(Adapted from *MMWR*, 1988a)

OTHER SCREENING AND CONFIRMATORY TESTS

There are a variety of HIV antibody and HIV antigen detection tests now on the market and others are on their way. A few of these tests have been singled out because they are currently in use or because of their potential to make a contribution in the field of HIV antibody–antigen testing methodology. A new test undergoing development measures plasma HIV-DNA.

Immunofluorescent Antibody Assay

The **immunofluorescent antibody assay** uses a known preparation of antibodies labeled with a fluorescent dye such as fluorescein isothiocyanate (FITC) to detect antigen or antibody. In the direct fluorescent antibody test, fluorescent antibodies detect specific antigens in cultures or smears. In the indirect fluorescent

BOX 12.3

THE PERFORMANCE RATE FOR THE COMBINED ELISA AND WESTERN BLOT HIV TEST—IS 99% ACCURACY GOOD ENOUGH? THE ANSWER: NO!

The Centers for Disease Control and Prevention (CDC) states that the two tests used to identify HIV— the ELISA and the Western blot (WB)—used in combination, have a better than 99% overall accuracy rate, but only if they are performed repeatedly. (The exact rate is unknown and the CDC states that it has no data on just how many false positives versus false negatives occur!) This **rate** is the percentage of correct test results in all specimens tested. With a 99% rate, if a population of 10,000 were tested, 9,900 would receive correct results, but 100 would receive erroneous results—either false positives or false negatives—including indeterminates.

If 99% accuracy is used as an example, then false positives would have to be less than 6/10ths (0.6%) of the erroneous results, because the CDC estimates that 0.6% of Americans are HIV-positive. That is, if false positives accounted for fully 0.6% of the errors, then the 0.6% of people who are HIV-positive would all be false positives, and that is not the case. However, if one assumes that only 0.2% are false positives, this leaves 0.8% as false negatives. So, of those same 100 people with erroneous results, 20% would be false positives and 80% would be false-negatives. False negative people are an unwitting threat to sex partners. But there is still another ramification: using the CDC estimate that 0.6% of Americans are HIV-positive, in a population of 10,000, thats 60 Americans that would test positive! This 60 must include all the false positives, 30, leaving only 30 people actually infected. This leads to the following conclusion: using a 99% accuracy, one finds as many false positives as true positives.

Even if the results of both AIDS tests, the ELISA and WB, are positive, the chances are only 50-50 that the individual is infected. This is why people with HIV-positive results must be tested repeatedly over the following 6 months to 1 year. The error rate at 99% accuracy is high with only two tests. (The CDC's *Morbidity and Mortality Weekly Report* shows an overall performance rate of only 98.4% on the Western blot alone—a lower accuracy than that used in this example. Even with repeated HIV-positive tests, the rare person may just be a false-positive tester.

The implications resulting from a false-positive test are broad for people tested at random. For example, a person was recently HIV-tested for a routine insurance examination. Because he or she had no behavioral risk factors and was in excellent health there was no concern about testing HIV-positive. The major concern was testing falsely positive— that risk, with a 99% accuracy testing procedure, is 30 out of 10,000 (0.3%). This may appear to be a low risk, but it isn't if you are one of the 30—after all, some 30 people out of 10,000 will be false positive. The results can destroy one's personal and professional life; other people believe your test results even if they are later found to be in error. It's like the newspaper scenario: retractions are found in small print on the back page— somewhere.

There is also the danger that false-positive people will not feel the need to avoid sex with truly infected people— a good route to infection.

But there is also room for optimism in these statistics. An individual who is a random false positive can find hope in them. This does not mean that he or she can take chances with other people's lives, of course, so each person must behave as though he or she is actually infected. But, inwardly, the random false HIV-positive individual can be cautiously optimistic.

The occurrence of even a small number of false positive HIV tests can have profound implications. This is especially true when testing blood donors, since false-positive results waste resources in discarded blood units and require verification of positive results using more expensive tests. A false negative result, indicating that an individual is not infected, can have serious consequences for the blood recipient. Therefore, attempts to improve tests are a continuous challenge.

antibody test, specific antibody from serum is bound to antigen on a glass slide.

The indirect procedure is modified for use in detecting antibodies to HIV. Cells that are HIV-infected will have HIV antigens on their cell membranes and will later fluoresce when the antihuman fluorescent conjugate is added.

A diluted sample of a person's serum is placed on a slide prepared with HIV antigens and incubated to allow antibody-antigen re-

TABLE 12-3 Incurred Costs to Identify True Positive HIV-Antibody-Containing Sera in a Population with a 10% Prevalence of HIV-Antibody-Infected People

Price of testing under negotiated contracts:
Low estimate: $4.41 per specimen tested
High estimate: $7 for each ELISA, $60 for each Western blot
Price for individual testing: $47.50 for each ELISA, $121 for each Western blot
Best case:
Number of true positives: 9,920
Number of ELISAs performed: 100,000
Number of Western blots performed: 9,960 + 900 = 10,860
Low estimate: $4.41 × 100,000 divided by 9,920 = $44
High estimate: $7 × 100,000 plus $60 × 10,860 divided by 9,920 = $136.25
Individual testing: $47.50 × 100,000 plus $121 × 10,860 divided by 9,920 = $611.30

(Adapted from Miike, 1987; adjustment reflects charges through 1994)

action if there are HIV antibodies in the serum. The slides are then rinsed to get rid of excess serum and other materials. Fluorescent antihuman antibody is then placed on the slide and incubation allows antihuman HIV antibody complexing to occur. The slide is again rinsed and dried. Fluorescence, if any, is observed using a special fluorescence microscope. The indirect fluorescent antibody (IFA) test is now used in many laboratories as a screening procedure. Inasmuch as the sensitivity and specificity of the IFA test are similar to the Western blot, this method has been proposed as an alternative confirmatory test for positive ELISA results. The IFA method is relatively simple and is one of the quickest tests available.

In late 1992, the FDA approved Fluorognost for marketing, the first assay for HIV-IFA confirmation and screening.

The assay allows doctors to do in-office tests for antibodies to HIV in human serum or plasma. As opposed to the Western blot test, the current standard confirmation test, Fluorognost posts almost no indeterminate test results. In addition, the test takes only 90 minutes to complete, while the Western blot takes from 12 to 24 hours to process. This FDA-approved test allows smaller health care facilities, emergency rooms, and doctors' offices to conduct in-office HIV screening and confirmation with accuracy, ease, and low overhead.

Recombigen HIV-1 Latex Agglutination Test

Recombigen, a 5-minute HIV antibody test that requires no special equipment, was FDA approved in December, 1988. The test is designed for use with serum, plasma, or whole blood. Patient samples are placed on a card along with positive and negative controls that come with the kit. Each serum sample is combined with a suspension of latex microspheres (beads) coated with CBre3, a recombinant protein containing the most immunogenic segments of the HIV envelope glycoprotein gp120 and the transmembrane protein gp41. The ingredients are then mixed for 3 minutes either by tilting the card manually or by carefully mixing the solution on the card. If antibodies to HIV are present in a sample, they will form complexes with the protein-coated beads causing a visible agglutination reaction.

Positive readings should be confirmed with a Western blot assay. The accuracy of the test is thought to be comparable to that of other conventional screening assays.

Polymerase Chain Reaction

Interactions between HIV and its host cell extend across a wide spectrum, from latent to productive infection. The virus can persist in cells as unintegrated DNA, as integrated DNA with alternative states of viral gene expression, or as a defective DNA molecule. Deter-mining the fraction of cells in the blood that are latently or productively infected is important for the understanding of viral pathogenesis and in the design and testing of effective therapies. Determining the number of infected cells in a heterogeneous cell population and the proportion of those cells that are carrying the virus but not producing new viruses requires the identification of the proviral DNA and viral mRNA in single cells.

The **polymerase chain reaction (PCR)** is a technique by which any DNA fragment from a single cell can be exponentially multiplied to an amount large enough to be measured. The PCR is now being used to diagnose a number of infectious diseases. For HIV testing, the technique used is to copy a segment of proviral DNA found in cells such as T4 lymphocytes and macrophages that carry the latent virus. The PCR is so sensitive that it can detect and amplify as few as six molecules of proviral DNA in 150,000 cells or one molecule of viral DNA in 10 μl of blood. This level of sensitivity is unparalleled by any other technology.

Finding these few molecules of DNA to copy and amplify is, as the saying goes, like finding a needle in a haystack. The needle in this case is the proviral DNA molecule. It is only a miniscule fraction of the total DNA content of a given cell and far less when mixed in with the DNA of over one million cells as used in some HIV PCRs.

One of the first uses of the PCR in HIV/AIDS research was to show that HIV was present in its latent form in people who were suspected of being infected but did not produce HIV antibodies. The HIV provirus was detectable in their cells. The PCR's most recent use has been in the detection of HIV provirus in newborns of HIV-infected mothers (Rogers et al., 1989).

In 1993, researchers reported that, in HIV-infected persons, 4% to 15% of peripheral blood lymphocytes were infected with HIV. The percentage of these cells that contained HIV mRNA, an indicator of viral replication, ranged from less than 1% to 8%. The data indicate that, in HIV-positive individuals, a significant proportion of peripheral blood lymphocytes are infected with HIV, but that the virus is in a latent state in the majority of these cells.

Now that there are some good therapies available to treat opportunistic disease which help slow the onset of AIDS, the diagnosis of individuals who carry the provirus is critical because they may benefit from early treatment. The PCR test will become even more important with the advent of an HIV vaccine. Vaccinated people will become HIV-antibody-positive. The PCR test will be used to identify those who are truly HIV-infected.

How PCR Works— The PCR (Figure 12-5) was developed by Kary Mullis and colleagues at Cetus Corporation (Mullis et al., 1987; Keller et al., 1988). The procedure requires the synthesis of **oligomer primers** (short 16 to 25 nucleotide sequences of DNA) that will hybridize or bind to the segment of DNA to be copied. The primer is required because the polymerase enzyme used to copy the desired DNA sequence needs an initial DNA sequence of nucleotides to add on to.

In the case of the HIV provirus, the primers need to hybridize to a DNA sequence adjacent to the gene area to be copied—for example, the GAG gene DNA sequence that produces the p24 protein. Because DNA is double-stranded, a primer molecule is attached to each strand (Figure 12-5). After primer attachment, a polymerase enzyme (usually Taq 1) is added. The polymerase enzymes, using the primers as starting points, add one nucleotide at a time as they copy their single DNA strands.

After each strand of the DNA segment has been copied at a temperature of 70°C, the reaction is heated to 93°C to separate the newly synthesized strands from the original DNA strands. This is called denaturation. The temperature is then cooled to 37°C to permit the additional primer molecules to attach (anneal) to the newly synthesized DNA sequences and the original DNA sequences (Figure 12-5). After primer attachment, the temperature is raised to 70°C and the polymerase enzyme molecules, starting at the primer sites, copy each strand of DNA. At the end of this second cycle there are four copies of each of the original DNA single strand sequences. By repeating the cycles of denaturation, annealing, and synthesis, the original DNA sequence can be amplified exponentially according to the formula 2^n where n is the number of cycles.

Single-Use Diagnostic Test

In late 1992, the FDA also approved a rapid (10-minute) screening test for detecting HIV antibodies. This test is a single-use diagnostic system (**SUDS**). According to the manufacturer, in clinical trials the test had a sensitivity of 99.9% and a specificity of 99.6%, which is comparable to other approved HIV tests used by clinical laboratories. This test can be used in a physician's office, and requires no special equipment and only minimal staff training. The process involves taking a small quantity of serum or plasma and mixing it with an antibody capture reagent. It is then poured into a test cartridge with HIV antigens, followed by a wash step and the addition of enzyme–antibody and a chromogen. Results are available in approximately 10 minutes. Positive results, indicated by a blue-colored window, should be confirmed with other assays.

Saliva and Urine Tests

By the end of 1994, there were at least nine **serum** HIV antibody **screening** tests and four confirmatory tests available in the marketplace. Because HIV antibodies are present in body fluids other than blood (e.g., urine and saliva), HIV antibody assays have been developed for their use. Collecting samples of urine and saliva is noninvasive, easier, less dangerous, and less expensive. Such tests are particularly useful in developing nations where there is a shortage of refrigeration and sterile equipment (Constantine, 1993); Frerichs et al., 1994).

Saliva and urine tests have not yet received FDA approval for use in the United States. However, home saliva tests for HIV are available. When FDA approved, they will sell for about $30.00.

HIV Gene Probes

Gene probes or genetic probes are an idea borrowed from methodologies used in recombinant DNA research. The idea is to isolate a DNA segment, make many copies of it, and label these copies with a radioisotope or other tag compound. If the DNA sequence copied is contained in any of the HIV genes, then the labeled copies of this DNA sequence can be used to hybridize or attach to DNA of cells that contain HIV DNA. This method of DNA probe analysis eliminates the need of searching for HIV gene products or antibodies to these products to prove that a person is HIV-infected.

At least two HIV-specific probes are on the market. One uses a radioactive sulfur label on the DNA for detection (^{35}S). This probe hybridizes to about 50% of the entire HIV genome and most specifically hybridizes to the HIV polymerase region. A second probe, also using ^{35}S, is an **RNA probe**. It is being used to detect HIV RNA in peripheral blood or tissue samples. RNA probes for in situ hybridization allow detection of one HIV-infected cell out of 400,000 uninfected cells. Specifically, the assay detects the presence of HIV in whole white blood cells as soon as the virus begins to replicate. The ^{35}S-labeled probes enter the white blood cells and combine with HIV; the procedure does not require DNA extraction and results are obtained in just over 1 day (Kramer et al., 1989).

Passive Hemagglutination Assay

There continues to be an urgent need for an inexpensive, accurate assay for anti-HIV screening in the developing world. Scheffel's results (1990) indicate that the **passive hemagglutination assay (PHA)** is a good candidate. The assay is simple to perform and requires no expensive equipment or precision pipettes. The reagents appear very stable even in adverse conditions. However, the assay requires a minimum of 3 hours before a reading can be made.

The accuracy of the assay is reportedly excellent, with 100% sensitivity on some 890 anti-HIV-positive serum samples and sensitivity equal to or better than the second-generation ELISA.

The PHA uses stabilized human group O red blood cells that have been coated with HIV core protein, p24 and envelope glycoprotein, gp41. For long-term stability, the antigen-coated cells are placed in phosphate buffer and vacuumed to dryness (lyophilized). For use, the dried cells are reconstituted in phosphate buffer.

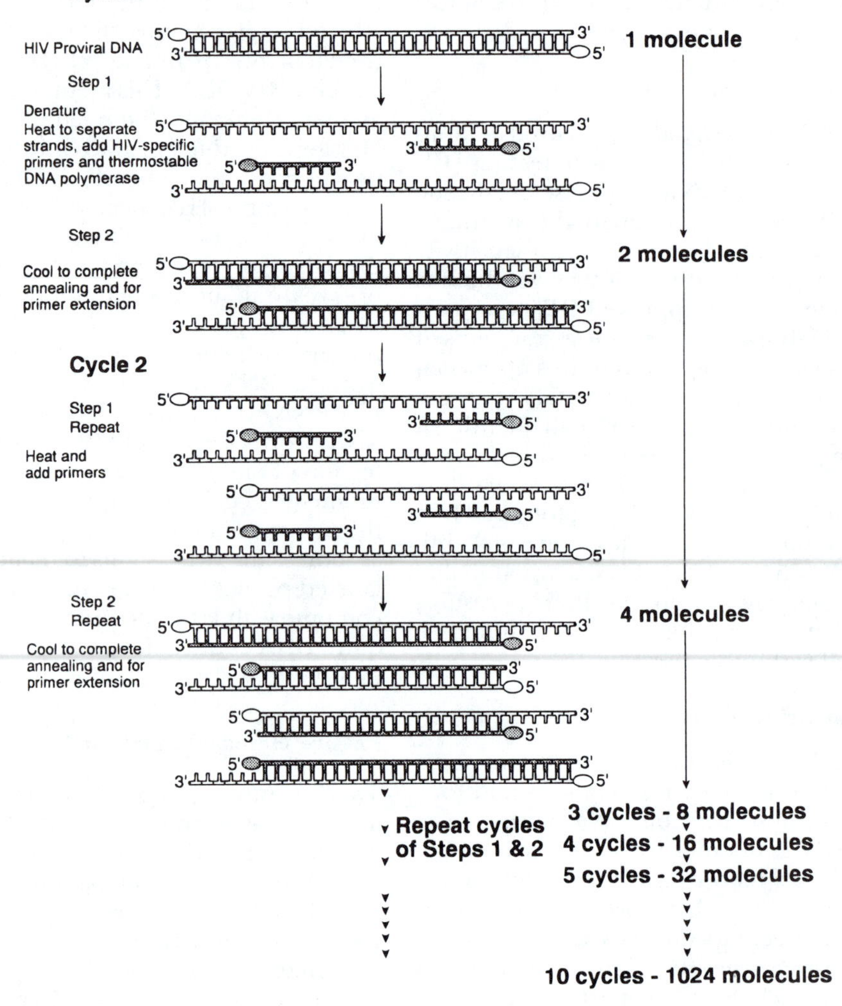

FIGURE 12-5 Polymerase Chain Reaction. A source of DNA containing the sequence to be amplified is mixed with two primers, nucleotide triphosphates and the DNA polymerase Taq 1 (Taq 1 is a DNA polymerase derived from the bacterium *Thermus aquaticus*). The primers are synthetic oligonucleotides of *known sequence*. Therefore, the boundaries of the DNA sequence to be copied are already known. *Cycle 1:* Primers are added in excess (1 million-fold). Using DNA polymerase, the primers are extended by DNA synthesis. The first cycle takes about 5 minutes. *Cycle 2:* The product from cycle 1 is denatured, reannealed, and primer extension occurs once again. This cycle takes place as many as 50 times so that the primer-extended sequence increases thousands of times. The original DNA sequence can be amplified exponentially according to the

(continued on facing page)

Two drops of phosphate buffer are placed in the microwell of a test plate. To this is added a small amount of a person's serum. After gentle mixing, one drop of HIV coated red blood cells (RBCs) is added, mixed, and incubated at room temperature for at least 3 hours. Hemagglutination patterns, stable for 72 hours, are read by eye and compared to a chart or scale that reads from negative to 3+ for HIV infection.

Measuring HIV RNA

The polymerase chain reaction, as described above and shown in Figure 12-5, can be used to detect HIV RNA in the early stages of HIV infection. This test measures the RNA of HIV, which indicates the number of free viral particles and reflects how much viral replication is going on in an infected individual. When used for blood samples, the test findings are expressed as the number of copies of HIV RNA in each milliliter of blood plasma. Further studies are necessary to ensure reliability and accuracy of the test, define its range of day-to-day variation, standardize the test, and clarify the correlation of test results, level of tissue viral load, and disease stage.

The most significant implication of this finding is that since reducing viral load appears to correlate with clinical benefit, RNA test results may be able to serve as surrogate markers for the progress of HIV disease.

DETECTION OF HIV INFECTION IN NEWBORNS

Early detection of HIV infection in newborns and children is important because it may prevent unwarranted toxicity from the use of antiretroviral agents in children who are not infected, and it can allay the fears of parents with potentially afflicted but uninfected newborns. However, early diagnosis of HIV infection in children born to HIV-positive women is difficult owing to the presence of maternal IgG antibody in the newborn which may persist until the child is about 2 years old (Table 12.4). Thus serological detection of HIV infection in neonates is complicated by the presence of immune complexes, consisting of passively transferred maternal antibodies and HIV antigens. Steven Miles and colleagues (1993) have used a rapid assay designed to disrupt these immune complexes in order to permit the detection of a specific HIV antigen. Their preliminary work correctly identified p24 antigen in the blood of 29 of 29 children. These children tested HIV-positive, but when the maternal antibodies were treated to separate the p24 antigen present (the antigen would be present because the virus was present), they found p24 antigen. Children who were HIV-positive but lacked the presence of the p24 antigen were falsely positive—they contained only the mother's HIV antibodies. Although this technique is simple to perform and accurate when compared to other methods of HIV detection in newborns, additional testing of this technique is required before adoption. If a mother is known to be HIV-infected, cells from the newborn can be subjected to HIV blood culture or polymerase chain reaction tests. These two techniques, although very accurate, are not yet ready for the screening of

---

(continued)

formula 2^n, where n is the number of cycles. In theory, 25 PCR cycles would result in a 34 million-fold amplification. However, since the efficiency of each cycle is less than 100%, the actual amplification after 25 cycles is about 1 to 3 million-fold. The size of the amplified region is generally 100 to 400 base pairs, although stretches of up to 2,000 bases can be efficiently amplified. In HIV-infected cells, the DNA template is a specified region within the provirus (Keller et al., 1988).

Viral DNA can also be specifically amplified with some additional steps. The RNA template in infected cells is either viral mRNA or packaged virion RNA. And a different enzyme is used to amplify the RNA (Q beta replicase).

TABLE 12-4 Diagnosis of Infection in HIV-Exposed Infants

Age	Test	If Test Is Positive	If Test Is Negative
1 month	HIV culture or PCR[a]	Repeat test to confirm diagnosis of infection	Repeat test at age 3–6 months
3–6 months	HIV culture or PCR[a]	Repeat test to confirm diagnosis of infection	Test with ELISA at age 15 months
15 months	ELISA	Repeat test at age 18 months	Repeat test at age 18 months
18 months or older	ELISA	Child is infected[b]	Child is not infected[c]

[a]If HIV culture and PCR are unavailable, p24 antigen testing may be used after 1 month of age.

[b]Serological diagnosis of HIV infection requires two sets of confirmed HIV serological assays (ELISA/Western blot) performed at least 1 month apart after 15 months of age.

[c]Confirmation of seronegativity requires two sets of negative ELISAs after 15 months of age in a child with normal clinical and immunoglobulin evaluation.

(*Source:* El-Sahr et al., 1994).

all newborns. They can detect the presence of HIV in the first few days of life.

FDA BAN ON HOME HIV ANTIBODY TEST KITS

As of early 1995, the FDA has still refused to permit the marketing of home use kits to detect HIV antibodies. The kits basically work using a fingerstick blood sample or a saliva assay. Some companies wanted to develop a mail-in blood test sample with a telephone counseling service. One argument in favor of home kits is that 30% of people who want to be HIV tested would do so only in the privacy of their own homes.

The FDA counters with its concerns about the lack of face-to-face counseling following test results, the need to collect enough blood to allow confirmatory testing, the need to ensure the safe disposal of lancets used to prick the finger, and the need to ensure proper physician follow-up. For mail-in tests, which would involve collecting blood at home and sending it in for testing, there are additional concerns. Foremost among them is the need to design mailers to prevent blood samples from contaminating postal workers (Weiss, 1988).

REPORTING HIV INFECTIONS

In April of 1992, the CDC suggested that all states consider implementing programs requiring physicians to report names of HIV-positive patients.

Reporting HIV infection is useful in directing HIV-related prevention activities such as patient counseling, partner notification, and referral for appropriate medical management. HIV infection reports are also useful for guiding pediatric medical and social support programs. Prevention activities and medical management of patients can be carried out without requiring HIV reporting, but an HIV reporting system provides a means of maintaining HIV-related prevention activities (*MMWR*, 1988b).

All 50 states and the District of Columbia require health care providers to report new cases of AIDS to their state health departments. As of March 1 1993, 35 states required reporting of HIV-infected people (Table 10-7). The 35 states that require HIV reporting have over 50% of the population and accounted for 50% of reported AIDS cases through mid-1995. Twenty-five of the 35 states require the patient's name (Table 10-7). These 25 states account for about 16% of all reported AIDS cases and require information to include sex, age, and race/ethnicity; 19 states ask for the mode of transmission; six ask for clinical status and three require CD4 T cell count. As of mid-1995, only 11 states classified HIV/AIDS as a sexually transmitted disease and only 12 states authorized physicians to inform partners of HIV/AIDS patients (*Medical Tribune*, 1991).

BOX 12.4

THE PHYSICIAN'S DILEMMA

While on vacation, a physician came upon a motorcycle accident. He administered cardiopulmonary resuscitation for 45 minutes to one of the riders, who was bleeding from the mouth. After the man died, the physician asked the emergency department doctor in charge, who was a personal friend, to test the deceased for HIV.

The doctor said he needed consent. The physician said, "The guy died. I have a wife and kids."

The incident prompted this physician to raise the issue of testing without informed consent. This brings up the pro and con issues on informed consent. After reading the *Pro* and *Con,* decide where you stand on the issue.

Pro: *Physician*: "Consent for every test we do is a nice luxury, but we don't do it for syphilis or hepatitis B. Only with this disease have we departed from public health policy. The majority with HIV are not aware they're infected. Not in the history of medicine have we chosen a policy to protect the infected."

Con: *Physician*: "It's extremely paternalistic. We should be trying to get patients involved in their care and give them informed choices on what is possible. I favor consent on any test. I am afraid that liberal HIV testing laws and policies are being fostered out of physician self-interest rather than patient need.

Doctors don't like HIV particularly, and they don't like people who have HIV infection. They want a way to be in control. They want to know the patient's status, and their reasons are less medical or for the patient's best interest than for the physician's."

Your Position: (class discussion)

WHO SHOULD BE TESTED FOR HIV INFECTION?

Testing for antibodies to HIV is an important first step in establishing a diagnosis of HIV infection. Since testing every person is counterproductive, the decision to test must be based on people's risk behaviors and/or symptoms. As to who **needs** to be HIV tested; a complete history and physical examination will give the best answer to this question. Decisions based on individual indications are often more appropriate than decisions based on one's classification (i.e., all pregnant women or all single men between 20 and 49 years of age). Initial assessment for current or past behaviors (within the past 10 years) should include:

1. Persons with **risk behaviors** such as:
   a. Anal sexual activity, male or female
   b. Injection drug use
   c. Frequent casual heterosexual activity
   d. Encounters with prostitutes
   e. Previous treatment for sexually transmitted diseases (*Condyloma acuminata* (genital warts), herpes simplex virus, gonorrhea, syphilis, *Chlamydia*)
   f. Blood transfusions, especially before 1985
   g. Sexual activity with partners having any of the above
   h. Infants born to women involved in any of the above
2. Persons with **symptoms** such as:
   a. Fever, weight loss (unexplained)
   b. Night sweats
   c. Severe fatigue
   d. Recent infections, especially thrush and shingles (varicella-zoster)
3. Persons with **signs** (based on physical exam) such as:
   a. Weight loss
   b. Enlarged lymph nodes and/or tonsilar enlargement
   c. Oral exam (candidiasis, oral hairy leukoplakia)
   d. Skin lesions (e.g., Kaposi's sarcoma, varicella-zoster, psoriasis)
   e. Hepatosplenomegaly (enlarged liver)
   f. Mental status examination showing changes.

Knowledge of HIV infection status allows infected persons and their infected partners to seek treatment with retroviral agents, prophylaxis against *Pneumocystis carinii* pneumonia, tuberculosis skin testing and tuberculosis prophylaxis (if appropriate), and other types of therapy and vaccines that may delay or prevent the opportunistic infections associated with HIV infection. Such measures have been shown to delay the onset of AIDS in infected persons and to prolong the lives of persons with AIDS. Counseling and testing may help some persons change high-risk sexual and drug-use behaviors thereby preventing HIV transmission to others.

Entry into Foreign Countries

An increasing number of foreign countries require that foreigners be tested for HIV prior to entry. This is particularly true for students or long-term visitors. Information available through 1994, reveals that 30 of 45 foreign countries require an HIV test prior to entry, on arrival, or on application for residency. Before traveling abroad, check with the embassy of the country to be visited to learn entry requirements and specifically whether or not HIV testing is a requirement. If the foreign country indicates that U.S. test results are acceptable "under certain conditions," prospective travelers should inquire at the embassy of that country for details (i.e., which laboratories in the United States may perform tests and where to have results certified and authenticated) before departing the United States. For a copy of HIV Testing Requirements for Entry into Foreign Countries, send a self-addressed, stamped, business-size envelope to: Bureau of Consular Affairs, Room 5807, Department of State, Washington, DC 20520.

Testing for HIV Infection

With AIDS cases being reported from almost all the countries of the world, and with about 1.5 million HIV-infected and over 500,000 AIDS cases in the United States by the end of 1995, the question of HIV testing on either a voluntary or a mandatory basis cannot be ignored. Perhaps the decision on *who* is to be tested should be decided by society since everyone is at risk.

The case in which a Florida dentist, David Acer, is believed to have infected six of his patients has led members of Congress, the Senate, and others to demand changes in HIV testing and confidentiality procedures. Under current policy, people are tested only with their *informed* consent. Although the *number* of people who test positive is reported to the CDC, their names are not. No attempts are made to track down contacts of infected individuals.

Marcia Angell, executive editor of the *New England Journal of Medicine*, wrote in 1991 that it was time to adopt a traditional public health approach to HIV/AIDS. She said, "Tracing and notification of the sexual partners of HIV-infected persons, and screening of pregnant women, newborns and hospitalized patients and health care professionals are warranted. This should be adopted only if steps are taken to protect HIV-infected people from discrimination and hysteria. Jobs, housing and insurance benefits, for example, should be protected by statute."

Regardless of protection, it has been estimated that 10% to 28% of persons in the United States and between 18% to 30% in Australia choose not to be HIV-tested. These percentages most likely are in keeping with personal attitudes toward HIV testing in the other developed countries (Clezy et al., 1992).

Benefits of HIV Testing— Testing for the presence of HIV antibodies or antigens as early as possible when HIV is suspected can provide substantial health benefits. The infected person can be better treated for other infections if his or her HIV status is known. For example, 2% of HIV/AIDS patients in the United States contract tuberculosis. Unless otherwise indicated, HIV-infected patients with a past or present positive TB test should receive isoniazid as early as possible because active TB may be the first sign of AIDS. If other diseases occur prior to isoniazid treatment, treatment for those diseases may interfere with the therapy for TB and vice versa.

The presence of HIV in people with syphilis may also alter the recommended therapy and follow-up. Influenza and pneumococcal polysaccharide vaccines are recommended for *all* people infected with HIV. The recommendation for pneumococcal immunization explicitly states that the vaccine be given as early in the course of HIV infection as possible to maximize antibody response (Rhame et al., 1989). In addition, the early detection of asymptomatic HIV infection provides an even more important health benefit: a chance for a lifestyle change to reduce stress. This would lessen the chance of acquiring other microbial infections

BOX 12.5

BOXER STRIPPED OF FEATHERWEIGHT TITLE AFTER POSITIVE HIV TEST

It took Ruben Palacio 12 years to win a world title. On the eve of his first defense, he became the first champion to test positive for HIV. The British Boxing Board of Control said, "We can't risk the life of another boxer by letting him fight. It's a kind of disease that can be spread via blood contact, and boxing is a sport where that is likely to happen."

Palacio is the first active world title holder known to have tested positive for the AIDS-causing virus. Esteban DeJesus, who held the WBC lightweight boxing title in the 1970s, contracted AIDS after his retirement and died in 1989.

HIV testing has been a routine part of the pre-fight medical examination in Britain for several years. In February 1990, African heavyweight champion Proud Kilimanjaro of Zimbabwe was barred from a fight with Britain's Lennox Lewis because he refused to give details of an HIV test to the British Boxing Board of Control.

His manager said, "This brings the HIV thing into perspective. Instead of going home with the largest paycheck of his life, he is going home with an HIV test result that means he will die."

that may stimulate the immune system, activate HIV to reproduce and destroy T4 cells, and begin AIDS progression. However, too few of the HIV-infected are aware of their infections, and so, do not take these precautions.

Competency and Informed Consent— Competency is often used interchangeably with capacity; it refers to a person's ability to make an informed decision. For example, to consent to medical treatment, a person must be mentally capable of comprehending the risks and benefits of a proposed procedure and its alternatives. While a health care provider can assess competence, a legal finding of competency is often required based on the testimony of a mental health professional. Mental illness by itself does not indicate that a person is incompetent to make medical decisions. Various degrees of mental incapacity may occur with HIV infection, requiring an assessment of competency. AIDS dementia complex (ADC) occurs in approximately 70% of HIV-infected patients at some point in HIV disease/AIDS and may interfere with the patient's capacity to provide an informed consent.

Informed Consent

Informed consent is not just signing a form but is a process of education and the opportunity to have questios answered. The concept of informed consent includes the following components: full disclosure of information, patient competency, patient understanding, voluntariness, and decision making. The process of obtaining informed consent involves appropriate facts being provided to a competent patient who understands the information and voluntarily makes a choice to accept or refuse the recommended procedure or treatment.

When the concept of informed consent is applied clinically, complexities arise regarding both the content and the process. The concept contains ambiguous requisites such as "appropriate" facts, "full" disclosure, and "substantial" understanding. The process is affected by many variables including the communication skill and range of practice style of the physician; the maturity, intelligence, and coping strategies of the patient; and the interaction between the physician and the patient (Hartlaub et al., 1993).

Testing Without Consent

In 1994, 22 states had laws that allowed HIV testing without informed consent under certain conditions. The required conditions vary and include:

1. Patient or other authorized person is unable to give or withhold consent.
2. Test result will help determine treatment.
3. Patient is unable to give consent, and physician can document that a medical emergency exists and that the test is needed for diagnosis and treatment.
4. Test is needed to protect the health of other patients or health workers.
5. Several states require post-test counseling.
6. In 34 states, teenagers must have signed parental consent to be HIV tested.

Generally, HIV antibody testing without consent is legally considered battery. Legal liability for "unlawful touching" may result from performing an HIV antibody test without consent. Such a procedure may also constitute an illegal search.

Question: Are federal and state governments overly stressing personal privacy at the expense of prevention? (Defend your answer with examples/situations.)

Mandatory HIV Testing

Many people advocate mandatory HIV screening for everyone. They believe that this is the best way to stop the transmission of HIV. Perhaps this attitude is a reflection of fear. Mandatory premarital syphilis screening has often been cited as a precedent for premarital HIV screening. The logic appears to be: we screen for syphilis, but HIV infection and AIDS are a lot worse; therefore we should screen for HIV infection to prevent the spread of AIDS.

It can be answered that *syphilis is curable*; yet history reveals that syphilis screening has turned out to be ineffective and unnecessary. For example, in 1978, premarital syphilis screening found only 1% of the total number of new syphilis cases in the United States at a cost of 80 million dollars. Over the past dozen years, many of the 50 states have dropped this screening program and others have indicated that they will follow. Still, in 1988, legislation was pending in 35 states that would require premarital HIV testing. Louisiana, Illinois, and Maryland passed mandatory testing legislation; by 1989, all three states repealed that legislation.

Why Mandatory Testing?

Mandatory testing is for the protection of a certain group or the public at large. Although it is not anonymous, results are kept confidential on a need-to-know basis. Mandatory testing for HIV continues to be angrily debated primarily because of the possibility of error when running large numbers of test samples,

BOX 12.6

IMPACT OF MANDATORY HIV TESTING ON PHYSICIANS AND NURSES

Physicians and nurses in 13 northern and central New Jersey hospitals responded to an anonymous four-page survey containing 16 questions relating to the following scenario:

> "Assume a law has been passed requiring yearly HIV testing of all health care workers. Those that test positive will be prohibited from performing certain procedures and activities and, if employed by a hospital, clinic or medical school, will not be dismissed but may be reassigned. Attempts may be made to trace patients who might have contracted HIV from the health care worker."

Results: Approximately three-fourths of all surveyed health professionals stated that a mandatory testing policy would persuade individuals in their profession not to work in high-prevalence areas. Among those who currently work in high-prevalence HIV/AIDS areas, only 51% said that they would definitely or probably remain in the area should such a policy be instituted. Among those practicing surgery or performing invasive procedures, 7% currently avoid HIV-positive patients, and an additional 34% said that they would do so under the proposed testing policy. Finally, 4% of these professionals currently advise others to stop working in high-prevalence areas, and an additional 22% state that they would definitely do so if the proposed policy were instituted.

Conclusion: An HIV testing policy would create a shortage of physicians and nurses in high-prevalence HIV/AIDS areas. (Source: Passannante et al., 1993)

Update: In late 1994 new CDC guidelines called for health-care workers performing "exposure-prone" procedures to be tested for HIV and HBV, and recommended that **patients** of infected health care workers be notified of the workers' status.

Thirty-eight states have passed regulations simular to the CDC's recommendations (AIDS Alert, 1994).

POINT OF VIEW 12.1

CAN MANDATORY HIV SCREENING BE JUSTIFIED?

Paul Goldschmidt (1993) states that an argument often invoked to justify mandatory HIV screening refers to the social responsibility. The argument goes that, even if testing is of little help to those already infected, it is necessary to avoid further contamination. Every effort should be made to protect others from infection; however, screening will not achieve this.

Alleviating human suffering is the common goal of medicine, and emotional support is offered in an atmosphere of confidentiality and trust. Systematic screening dramatically contradicts this principle; it may reveal information about an individual who has expressed no wish to obtain it. Furthermore, a breach of confidentiality could ultimately lead to an individual being branded as dangerous and ostracized. Instead of using knowledge to avoid suffering, it is created by confronting unwilling individuals with the possibility of developing a fatal and incurable disease.

People infected with HIV face an irreversible destruction of their immune system. **None of the attempted treatments have been shown to inhibit virus replication effectively, or to limit the destruction of the immune system.** Can mandatory screening be justified as helping those infected, when, under these circumstances, to be made aware of one's HIV infection can be detrimental. HIV-infected people face the prospect of a complete disruption of their personal and professional lives and the anguish of probable physical suffering leading to death. If the individual has given informed consent, or freely chosen to consult a physician, the medical team can be emotionally supportive. However, there is no justification for screening those who have never asked, or consented to, HIV testing.

Goldschmidt argues that mandatory screening can not be scientifically or ethically defended, so why is the pressure for mandatory screening so strong in the United States? (class discussion)

Update 1995: "The findings of the Protocol 076 (zidovudine pregnancy study) offer the hope of preventing a devastating disease in children," wrote Harold Jaffe, MD, director of AIDS research at the CDC (Jaffe, 1994). "The challenge now is to implement effective ethical, and practical public health strategies to turn the success of this clinical trial into a public health success."

The study, which involved 477 pregnant women infected with HIV, showed that just 8.3% of the infants born to the women who took zidovudine (AZT) were infected with the virus, while 25.5% of the infants born to the women who did not take zidovudine were infected with the virus.

The efficacy of zidovudine in preventing HIV transmission has changed the issue of pregnancy testing from a philosophical disagreement over patients' rights to privacy to a referendum on the responsibility of public health officials to use means at their disposal to prevent the spread of HIV. The point of contention is whether testing of pregnant women should be mandatory or voluntary.

The prevailing view among health officials is that the testing should be voluntary. But a number of vocal public health officials and medical ethicists favor mandatory, "routine" testing of pregnant women.

Arthur Caplan, MD, director of the Center for Bioethics at the University of Pennsylvania, said, "It's one thing to have voluntary testing when there are no cures, it's another matter when there's a way of preventing transmission. I don't believe that voluntary testing is going to be effective in picking up women that might be HIV-positive and don't think they're at risk. They're not going to be tested and you're not going to find them."

Opponents of mandatory testing argue that mandatory testing of pregnant women—like mandatory screening of health care workers for HIV—is inefficient and unconstitutional (AIDS Alert, 1994).

Would Paul Goldschmidt argue for or against mandatory HIV testing of pregnant women? What is your position with regard to HIV testing of all pregnant women?

inadvertent loss of confidentiality, and lack of overall benefit to those who are found to be HIV-positive.

Mandatory HIV testing is routine for blood donors, military and Job Corps personnel, federal prisoners, and people seeking immigration. In Florida, Georgia, Illinois, Nevada, Rhode Island, and West Virginia, HIV testing is mandatory for people convicted of prostitution. However, many prostitutes are back on the streets before their test results are in. In many cases, the prostitutes could not be found for follow-up counseling. In Duval County Florida, county judges agreed to impose a 30-day jail term for convicted prostitutes, a time period long enough to get their test results and provide counseling. Prostitutes have to sign the test results sheet. They are released as soon as they do.

Under Florida law, a prostitute who knows he or she is carrying the AIDS virus but continues to offer sexual favors can be jailed for 1 year.

At least nine states (California, Colorado, Illinois, Indiana, North Dakota, Ohio, Oregon, South Carolina, and West Virginia) have mandatory HIV testing for sex offenders (*Intergovernmental AIDS Report*, 1989).

Fear of Mandatory Testing— If a massive mandatory screening test program was implemented, would it be possible to keep results confidential? What would be done with the information? For example, would the state prevent an uninfected person from marrying an infected one? Officials fear that mandatory testing will drive many people who might have volunteered for anonymous testing underground and away from the health care system. These people will be lost to the counseling and education that would benefit them and others. The reason for going underground would be fear of discrimination and social ostracism if found to be HIV-infected.

TABLE 12-5 Groups that Favor Voluntary Testing of People at Elevated Risk for HIV Infection

1. Presidential Commission on the HIV Epidemic
2. Oversight of AIDS Activities Committee, Institute of Medicine
3. Centers for Disease Control and Prevention
4. U.S. Public Health Service
5. Canadian National Advisory Committee on AIDS
6. National Institute of Allergy and Infectious Diseases
7. San Francisco AIDS Foundation

These are only a few of many groups that favor voluntary testing and counseling of high-risk groups as defined by the CDC.

BOX 12.7

WILL MOST PEOPLE AGREE TO BE HIV TESTED IF THEIR PHYSICIANS RECOMMEND IT?

Brady Allen (1991) of Baylor University Medical Center suggested that most patients would agree to be tested if their physicians recommended it and if they believed that the results would remain confidential. If a high-risk patient refuses to be tested, however, the physician can suggest continuing the discussion at a follow-up appointment or can refer the patient to a counselor. Brady believes that the availability and benefits of early intervention therapy provide a strong incentive for testing. "Knowing one's status also offers many nonmedical benefits, such as the ability to make more informed decisions regarding sexual practices, marriage, childbearing and employment." Physicians must emphasize that although the test result becomes part of the patient's file, the result cannot be disclosed to anyone unless the patient agrees to it or the law requires it.

A case can be made that a compulsory program could maintain strict confidentiality even with large numbers of people being tested. But it would appear that the political powers and public in general are not ready for broad-scale compulsory screen testing in the United States.

Confidential, Anonymous, and Blinded Testing

Both confidential and anonymous testing involve the use of informed consent forms which are, to date, with exception of the U.S. military, Job Corps workers, and certain criminals, done on a voluntary basis. Blinded testing **does not,** because of procedure, require informed consent.

Confidential HIV Testing— A consent to HIV testing must be given freely and without coercion. The volunteer does not have to provide any information unless he or she wants to. Individuals to be tested in a state laboratory complete a HIV Antibody Form. The consent form explains in simple terms what the pres-

POINT OF INFORMATION 12.1

CIVIL LIBERTIES VERSUS SAVING LIVES

Nowhere was the trade-off between civil liberties and saving lives more vivid than in the 1994 session of the New York State Legislature. Two bills were proposed: One would have required doctors to notify parents of the results of the HIV tests now performed anonymously on all newborns. The other bill would have set up a counseling program urging mothers to find out the status of their infants. Neither was passed.

Objections to the first bill came from AIDS activists and civil libertarians who argued that, since an HIV-positive newborn always has an HIV-positive mother, telling a mother the results of her child's HIV test would violate her right to privacy. It was also opposed by a subcommittee of the state's AIDS Advisory Council, which said care cannot be mandated "through coercion."

A Different Perspective

Some pediatricians see the problem differently. They say that the tempo of HIV infection in babies does not offer the luxury of persuasion. At six weeks, an HIV-p[ositive infant may look normal but be desperately in need of drug treatment. Some children infected at birth are now living until age 13 or 14. If it is known that the mother is HIV-positive and the infant is also, it will not be lost in the first months. If it is not known the baby dies.

While the debate centers on testing at birth, a far better time to test mothers and inform them of the results would be during pregnancy. If HIV-positive women were identified while pregnant, found and treated, it might be possible to prevent some of their infants from becoming infected. In February of 1994, a joint French-American clinical trial showed a 67.5% reduction in transmission risk among infants whose mothers began taking zidovudine during pregnancy. The numbers are not insignificant: each year, nearly 7,000 HIV-positive mothers deliver babies in the United States, and about 25% to 30% of their infants become infected with the virus.

ence of HIV antibody does and does not signify. It explains the uncertain medical outcome and potential social and legal implications of a positive test result. The consent form assures confidentiality but warns that the result is part of the patient's medical record, to which others may have access under certain conditions. Some centers provide completely anonymous testing; this option is available to the patient and his or her physician.

The following example demonstrates one of the problems with confidential testing. A young homosexual male with signs of oral thrush agreed to an HIV test. Later that day, he called and asked that his blood *not* be sent to the lab. He was a teacher in a parochial school and feared the results would be revealed. His sample was set aside, but the laboratory courier mistakenly took it for testing. The result was positive, yet no one could tell the patient. A malpractice attorney said to make certain all records of the test were deleted and to send the patient a letter urging him to return for a blood test. He never appeared (Wake, 1989).

Many national agencies and committees favor a confidential screening and counseling program that includes all individuals whose behavior places them at high risk of HIV exposure (Table 12-5). These agencies recommend that the following eight groups seriously consider volunteering for periodic HIV antibody testing:

1. Homosexual and bisexual men
2. Present or past injection drug users
3. People with signs or symptoms of HIV infection
4. Male and female prostitutes
5. Sexual partners of people either known to be HIV-infected or at increased risk of HIV infection
6. Hemophiliacs who received blood clotting products prior to 1985
7. Newborn children of HIV-infected mothers
8. Emigrants from Haiti and Central Africa since 1977

Anonymous HIV Testing— This is also a form of voluntary testing. It differs from confidential testing only in that those who request anonymity receive a bar coded identification number. They provide no personal information and they come back at a predetermined time to find out if their test number is positive or negative. No follow-up occurs.

Blinded HIV Testing— This occurs when blood or serum is available for HIV testing as a result of another medical procedure wherein the patient's blood has been drawn for analysis. In this case, the demographic data have been recorded and can be used for epidemiological studies even if the name of the individual is withheld and a bar code is used. In 1988, the CDC asked for a blinded study of all 1989 newborn blood samples taken in certain cities in 30 states for metabolic studies. The name and other demographics of each newborn were recorded on the label of each tube. After the metabolic tests were completed, the name was changed into a bar code and leftover blood was sent to a state HIV testing center.

New York began a study of this type in 1987. Since then, New York has blind-tested about 250,000 newborns. The statewide incidence rate for HIV-infected newborns is 0.7%, or seven per 1,000. The incidence is 1.3% in New York City, between 0.1% to 0.2% for upstate New York, and close to 2% in the Bronx.

In voluntary testing, the reason for the test, how it is administered, and the persons right to privacy and confidentiality must be explained. This allows the person the choice of taking or refusing the test and giving or not giving demographic data.

SUMMARY

HIV infection can be detected in two ways: first, by HIV antibody testing prior to the signs and symptoms of AIDS; and second, by physical examination after symptoms occur.

The test most often used to screen donor blood at blood banks and individuals referred to testing centers is the ELISA test. ELISA (enzyme-linked immunosorbent assay) is a highly sensitive and specific test that determines the presence of HIV antibodies in a person's blood or serum. The ELISA test was first used in 1985 to reduce the number of HIV-infected blood units for blood transfusions.

Because the ELISA test is only a predictive test which gives the percentage chance that a person is truly positive or truly negative, serum from those who test positive is retested in duplicate. If still positive, the serum is then subjected to a Western blot (WB) test. The WB is a confirmatory test. If it is also positive, the person is said to be HIV-infected.

Other screening and confirmatory tests are available. The indirect immunofluorescent antibody assay (IFA) is relatively quick and easy to perform. Although it can be used as a screening test, it is generally used as a confirmatory test. The test is similar to the ELISA test except that the analysis is made by looking for a fluorescent color, indicating the presence of HIV antibodies, with a dark field light microscope.

The Recombigen HIV-1 Latex Agglutina-tion test requires no special equipment and can be performed in 5 minutes. This test can be a major contribution in Third World countries that do not have the equipment or trained personnel to run ELISA and WB tests.

The polymerase chain reaction (PCR) is a process wherein a few molecules of HIV proviral DNA can be amplified into a sufficient mass of DNA to be detected by current testing methods. It can determine if newborns of HIV-infected mothers are truly HIV-positive.

Gene probes are also being used to detect small HIV proviral DNA sequences in cells of people who are HIV-infected but not yet making antibodies.

The CDC recommends that people in high-risk groups volunteer for HIV testing if there is any reason to suspect they may have been exposed. Broad-scale testing in low-risk populations is not advocated because the rate of false positives rises with decreasing rates of HIV infections.

Many people have voiced opinions that HIV testing should be mandatory for all people in high-risk groups. They believe that identifying HIV carriers is the way to stop HIV transmission. However, mandatory premarital testing has failed to stop the spread of syphilis. But, nearly everyone agrees that voluntary HIV testing and counseling should be available to anyone who wants it. For those who want to be tested, there are at least two routes to consider: voluntary confidential and voluntary anonymous. In the first, people give their names and addresses and the test results become a confidential part of their medical records. In the latter, no personal identification information is asked for; a bar code (number) is used to label the blood sample.

REVIEW QUESTIONS

(*Answers to the Review Questions are on page 482.*)

1. What is the acronym for the most commonly used HIV antibody test and what does each letter stand for?
2. What basic immunological assumption is this test based on?
3. Does a single positive HIV antibody result mean the person is HIV-infected? Explain.
4. Is there a specific test for AIDS? Explain.
5. What is currently the most frequently used HIV confirmatory test in the United States?
6. What is the name of one additional confirmatory test in use in the United States?
7. How is HIV antibody detected in the ELISA test?
8. True or False: All newborns who are antibody positive are HIV-infected and all go on to develop AIDS. Explain.
9. What is the greatest shortcoming of the ELISA and WB tests?
10. What are the two major problems in interpreting ELISA test results?
11. What two factors may account for false-positive and false-negative results?
12. What is the relationship between false-positive results and prevalence of HIV in the population?
13. In an HIV screening test, what is a positive predictive value? Why is it called a predictive value?
14. What is the current gold standard of confirmatory tests in the United States?
15. What is the major problem in using this test?
16. Why is the polymerase chain reaction (PCR) considered so useful in HIV testing? Name two situations when PCR can be significant in HIV testing.
17. True or False: A variety of home use HIV antibody test kits are available in the United States. Explain.
18. Using the ELISA test, when are HIV antibodies first detectable?
19. How early are HIV antigens detectable in human serum?
20. What are three benefits of early identification of HIV-infected people?
21. Name the four kinds of testing privacy available to people who want to take an HIV test.
22. What is the major difference between an anonymous and a blind HIV test?
23. Why would someone want an anonymous test?
24. True or False: The ELISA serological test is adequate to confirm HIV infection.
25. True or False: Pre- and post-HIV-antibody test counseling is recommended any time an HIV antibody test is performed.

REFERENCES

AIDS Alert. (1994). AZT study reinvigorates debate over mandatory testing. 9:133–135.

Allen, Brady. (1991). The role of the primary care physician in HIV testing and early stage disease management. *Fam. Pract. Recert.*, 13:30– 49.

Angell, Marcia. (1991). A dual approach to the AIDS epidemic. *N Engl J Med*, 324:1498–1500.

Belongia, Edward A., et al. (1989). Premarital HIV screening *JAMA,* 261:2198.

Carlson, Desiree A., et al. (1989). Testing for HIV risk from therapeutic blood products. In: *Pathology and Pathophysiology of AIDS and HIV Related Diseases* (Eds. Jami J. Harawi and Carl J. O'Hara), St. Louis: C.V. Mosby Co.

Clezy, K., et al. (1992). AIDS-related secondary infections in patients with unknown HIV status. *AIDS*, 6:879–893.

Constantine, Niel T. (1993). Serologic tests for the retroviruses: Approaching a decade of evolution. *AIDS*, 7:1–13.

El-Sahr, W., et al. (1994). *Managing Early HIV Infection: Quick Reference Guide for Clinicians.* AHCPR Publication No. 94-0573. Rockville, MD.

Fang, Chyang T., et al. (1989). HIV testing and patient counseling. *Patient Care*, 23:19–44.

Frerichs, Ralph R., et al (1994). Saliva-based HIV-antibody testing in Thailand. *AIDS*, 8:885–894.

Goldschmidt, Paul. (1993). Systematic screening for HIV infection. *AIDS*, 7:740–741.

Hartlaub, Paul, et al. (1993). Obtaining informed consent: It is not simply asking "do you understand?", *J. Fam. Pract.*, 36:383–384.

Hegarty, J.D., et al. (1988). The medical care costs of human immunodeficiency virsu infected children in Harlem. *JAMA,* 260:1901–1905.

Intergovernmental AIDS Report. (1989). Illinois court overrules mandatory HIV testing for prostitutes and sex offenders, 2:1–18.

JAFFE, HAROLD, et al. (1994). Reducing the risk of maternal-infant transmission of HIV: a door is opened. *N Eng J Med,* 331:1222.

KELLER, G.H., et al. (1988). Identification of HIV sequences using nucleic acid probes. *Am. Clin. Lab.,* 7:10–15.

KRAMER, F.R., et al. (1989). Replicatable RNA reporters. *Nature,* 339:401–402.

MACKENZIE, WILLIAM R., et al. (1992). Multiple false positive serologic tests for HIV, HTLV-1 and hepatitis C following influenza vaccination, 1991. *JAMA,* 268:1015–1017.

Medical Tribune. (1991). Beware of blanket AIDS solutions. June:14.

MERCOLA, JOSEPH M. (1989). Premarital HIV screening. *JAMA,* 261:2198.

MIIKE, LAWRENCE. (1987). *AIDS Antibody Testing.* Office of Technological Assessment Testimony To The U.S. Congress. Oct.:1–21.

MILES, STEVEN A., et al. (1993). Rapid serologic testing with immune-complex-dissociated HIV p24 antigen for early detection of HIV infection in neonates. *N Engl J Med,* 328:297–302.

Morbidity and Mortality Weekly Report. (1988a). Update: Serologic testing for antibody to human immunodeficiency virus. 36:833–840.

Morbidity and Mortality Weekly Report. (1988b). HIV infection reporting—United States. 38:496– 499.

Morbidity and Mortality Weekly Report. (1992). Testing for antibodies to HIV-2 in the United States. 41:1–9.

MULLIS, KARY B., et al. (1987). Process for amplifying, detecting, and/or cloning nucleic acid sequences. (U.S. Patent No. 4,683,195). *Official Gazette of the U.S. Patient and Trademark Office,* Volume 1080, Issue 4, July.

PASSANNANTE, MARIAN R., et al. (1993). Responses of health care professionals to proposed mandatory HIV testing. *Arch. Fam. Med.,* 2:38– 44.

RHAME, FRANK S., et al. (1989). The case for wider use of testing for HIV infection. *N Engl J Med,* 320:1242–1254.

ROGERS, MARTHA F., et al. (1989). Use of the polymerase chain reaction for early detection of the proviral sequences of human immunodeficiency virus in infants born to seropositive mothers. *N Engl J Med,* 320:1649–1654.

SCHEFFEL, J.W. (1990). Retrocell HIV-1 passive haemagglutination assay for HIV-1 antibody screening. *J. Acquired Immune Deficiency Syndromes,* 3:540–545.

WAKE, WILLIAM T. (1989). How many patients will die because we fear AIDS? *Med. Econ.,* 66:24– 30.

WEISS, RICK. (1988). Improving the AIDS test. *Sci. News,* 133:218–221.

WOFOY, C. B. (1987). HIV infection in women. *JAMA,* 257:2074–2076.

CHAPTER

13

Counseling for HIV Testing, HIV Disease, and AIDS

Chapter Concepts

- Some states now have mandated pre- and post-HIV test counseling for everyone who wants to take the test.
- Drug abusers present special problems for HIV counselors.
- Counselors must prepare the counselee for both a positive and negative test result.
- Lack of confidentiality remains the most serious objection to HIV testing.
- The major problem of confidentiality is: To whom does the physician or counselor have the greater moral obligation—the HIV-positive patient or others the patient may place in danger?
- Does the public have a right to know who is HIV-infected?

A disease is a condition of the body but it affects the human spirit as well. If you live with aches, pains, stiffness, and fatigue, if you are physically limited in what you can do, if your appearance has changed, and if, in addition, you fear for your life, your thoughts and feelings about yourself and others are inevitably affected. Distressful thoughts and feelings about yourself and others can undermine your life as much as, or even more than, your illness. Emotional stress can be reduced through proper counseling.

COUNSELING FOR HIV TESTING

Perhaps more than any other disease, AIDS is about human interactions. HIV is transmitted during the most intimate moments. Diagnosis results in immediate and powerful emotional responses, often long before physical symptoms occur. At the moment, medical care and emotional and practical support are the only weapons available in the fight against HIV/AIDS.

The greatest need at the present time is effective counseling of those at both high and low risk of HIV infection. Several million Americans have already been tested for the presence of HIV antibodies. According to medical health counselors, even considering whether to be tested often constitutes a crisis in a person's life, a crisis that becomes monumental if the test results are positive. Given the complexity of the testing process and its social implications, a number of state health departments require that pre- and post-test counseling accompany all HIV antibody testing.

State regulations on the issue of counseling HIV test clients vary widely and the definition of adequate counseling remains imprecise. HIV/AIDS counseling should cover the **purpose, limitations, risks**, and **benefits** of testing.

PURPOSE

Primary HIV Counseling Objective

Regardless of the patient's HIV antibody status, the primary objective of counseling is to provide an education that will help people avoid behaviors which may place them or others at risk of infection. Ideally, counseling should reduce anxiety, alleviate depression, lessen self-destructive impulses, and help people cope with the mental and physical stress associated with the need to be tested. A recent CDC report (1993) states that, although it is unlikely that a single episode of HIV counseling will result in the immediate and permanent adoption of safer behaviors, *client-centered* HIV counseling and attendant prevention services (i.e., referral and partner notification) do contribute to the initiation and maintenance of safe behaviors.

CDC-Supported Counseling and Testing Centers

The Centers for Disease Control and Prevention (CDC) provides support to 65 HIV prevention programs through health departments in 50 states, eight territories, and the District of Columbia. The critical component of the CDC's prevention program is support for HIV counseling and testing services (CTS). Each calendar quarter, the 65 programs report to the CDC aggregate data on: (1) the number of pretest counseling sessions, HIV antibody tests, positive tests, and post-test counseling sessions; (2) type of testing site (public or private); (3) risk category; (4) age group; and (5) sex and race/ethnicity (*MMWR*, 1991). By 1993, there were over 5,000 CTS listed in the 65 programs.

From 1985 through September 1989, the programs performed approximately 2.5 million HIV antibody tests; 6.0% were positive. In 1990, the 65 programs accounted for 1.4 millions tests; 3.7% were positive (*MMWR*, 1991). In 1991, the federal government allocated $100 million to state and local health agencies to provide testing and counseling programs in public clinics. Additional financial support was provided in 1992, 1993, and 1994.

Client-Centered Counseling

To fulfill its public health functions, HIV counseling must be client-centered, that is, tailored to the behaviors, circumstances, and special needs of the person being served. Risk-reduction messages must be personalized and realistic. Counseling should be:

1. Culturally competent (i.e., program services provided in a style and format sensitive to cultural norms, values, and traditions that are endorsed by cultural leaders and accepted by the target population);
2. Sensitive to issues of sexual identity;
3. Developmentally appropriate (i.e., information and services provided at a level of comprehension that is consistent with the age and the learning skills of the person being served); and
4. Linguistically specific (i.e., information is presented in dialect and terminology consistent with the client's language and style of communication).

Counseling should be provided not only in *terms* and *language* that people understand, but also, it should progress at a speed that is comfortable for the individual.

HIV counseling *is not a lecture.* An important aspect of HIV counseling is the counselor's *ability to listen* to the client in order to provide assistance and to determine specific prevention needs.

Although HIV counseling should adhere to minimal standards in terms of providing basic information, it should not become so routine that it is inflexible or unresponsive to particular client needs. **Counselors should avoid providing information that is irrelevant to their clients and should avoid structuring counseling sessions on the basis of a data collection instrument or form.**

Counseling HIV-infected persons and persons with AIDS can induce all kinds of feelings, including ones we do not always enjoy having—fear, repugnance, revulsion, anger, despair, resentment, hopelessness. The feelings themselves are not the problem, but a lack of awareness and understanding of these feelings means they can become obstacles to effectively counseling those most in need.

Counseling Anecdotes on Language and Terms

1. A heterosexual client at an HIV/AIDS clinic and the counselor became involved in a discussion of the client's sexual behavior. The counselor was concerned and somewhat confused when the client insisted that anal intercourse was not a risky sexual behavior. The counselor responded with a set of facts that led to the inescapable conclusion that anal intercourse was a *very* risky sexual behavior. The client said, "Gee, you wouldn't think that having sex *once a year* would place you at high-risk for HIV infection!" It was immediately obvious to the counselor that the client's lack of understanding resulted from confusing the words *annual* and *anal.*
2. A counselor said to a young woman during a conversation on HIV infection, "You know how one comes in contact with the virus during sex—you get it from coming into contact with *semen.*" The woman responded, "Oh, I'm safe then. I don't have sex with sailors." (She obviously thought the counselor said seamen.)
3. A young woman was told by her Ob/Gyn that she was in danger of contracting HIV infection because she was *sexually active.* She responded, "**No sir, I'm not sexually active. I lie very still when I'm having sex.**" (Clearly this young woman misunderstood the meaning of the term 'sexually active' in the clinical setting.)

Counselors should aid people who want to be tested by reinforcing positive feelings and by encouraging them to recall successful responses to previous stressful events in their lives. These responses can then be used as signals for handling situations that may arise.

BOX 13.1

COUNSELING MY FIRST HIV-POSITIVE PATIENT

Betty needed post-test counseling; she was HIV-positive. Sitting behind my desk, I dryly reviewed the implications of the test results and didn't let her get a word in edgewise.

She never came back for a follow-up appointment. She refused to return phone calls.

I reached Betty about a year later. She told me she had been disappointed and angry about my cold presentation of the facts and my apparent lack of interest in her feelings.

She taught me the need for better communication, and she taught me the need to be flexible in dealing with HIV-positive patients. Thank you, Betty.

LIMITATIONS

Pre-test HIV Procedures

Pre-test HIV counseling provides an opportunity for the counselor to educate people who believe they have a need to be tested. Pre-test procedures can be separated into three areas: (1) education; (2) taking sexual behavior and drug history information; and (3) counseling.

Education— Counselors should use available information on the epidemiology of HIV infection pitched at a level that can be understood. They should cover the routes of HIV transmission, methods of reducing risk, and methods of testing. This information can be presented in a variety of ways: printed material, a group lecture format, or audio- and videotapes. The topics that ought to be presented according to the 1988 American Medical Association Physician's Guidelines are listed in Table 13-1. This list of topics covers the spectrum of information necessary for a good education on HIV infection, the damage it creates, how it is transmitted, and how to avoid infection.

Sexual Behavior and Drug History— If more than one person is attending the general education session, after group session information is provided participants should be told that the remaining part of the pretest procedures are confidential and will be conducted one-on-one and face-to-face.

Sometimes a client will request permission to have another person present during the counseling session. Many people find support and added comfort in a friend's presence. In some cases, however, the client may have been coerced. The counselor may, through a series of questions, determine why the other person is present and proceed from that point.

During the face-to-face session the counselor must ask specific questions about the client's sexual behavior and drug use. The questions must be straightforward, worded in a way that will be understood, and posed in a nonjudgmental tone of voice. Questions on sexual behavior and drug use will help in determining if the person is at risk for exposure or has been exposed to HIV. For some counselors, asking questions and discussing another's sexual and drug abuse behavior is uncomfortable. Yet it is crucial if there is to be any modification of that behavior. The sexual and drug abuse history are the two most important means of determining whether someone is at increased risk for HIV infection.

TABLE 13-1 Pre-test Educational Information

1. AIDS is caused by a virus called human immunodeficiency virus or HIV.
2. HIV infects the body and gradually damages the immune system.
3. The AIDS virus is spread by the exchange of blood, semen, and possibly vaginal secretions during sexual intercourse.
4. Offer the concept of high-risk vs. low-risk HIV exposure situations.
5. Groups of people are considered to be at high risk because of their sexual and drug use behaviors.
6. The AIDS virus is spread through the exchange of blood when syringes and intravenous drug needles are shared.
7. Prior to 1985, when blood screening began, the virus was spread through transfusion of infected blood.
8. Infected pregnant women can pass on the virus to their unborn children.
9. The AIDS virus is not spread by casual contact.
10. Abstinence or monogamy among partners known to be uninfected provides the surest protection against sexual transmission.
11. The more sexual partners one has, the greater the risk of exposure.
12. Unprotected sex with partners who have AIDS, who are antibody-positive, or who have engaged in high-risk behaviors is dangerous and should be avoided.
13. The proper use of a latex condom during intercourse probably provides protection since it minimizes direct contact with bodily fluids.
14. Sexual activities that could cause cuts or tears in the lining of the rectum, penis, or vagina should be avoided.
15. Having sex with male or female prostitutes should be avoided.
16. Sharing needles or syringes with anyone should be avoided.

HIV Risk Reduction— HIV counseling is more than providing routine information. Counseling should include the development of a personalized, negotiated HIV risk-reduction plan. This plan should be based on the client's skills, needs, and circumstances, and it must be consistent with the client's expressed or implied intentions to change behaviors. HIV counseling should not consist of the counsellor "telling" the client what he or she needs to do to prevent HIV infection/transmission, but instead should outline a variety of specific options available to the client for reducing his or her own risk of HIV infection/transmission. The counselor should confirm with the client that the risk-reduction plan is realistic and feasible—otherwise, it is likely to fail.

When negotiating personalized risk reduction, counselors should be especially attentive to information provided by the client, especially information about past attempts at pre-

POINT OF INFORMATION 13.1

SEXUAL ISSUES IN HIV/AIDS COUNSELING

Point I

Discussing sexual issues can be uncomfortable even for the most sophisticated counselor. However, the urgent need to ensure that people stop practicing high-risk sexual behavior requires professionals to introduce sex education into their clinical practice. The issue of sexual practices should be discussed with every individual who is already sexually active, who is contemplating becoming sexually active, who is not absolutely certain that he or she has been in a sexually exclusive relationship for the past 15 years, or who is not absolutely certain that his or her partner has not used injection drugs or had a blood transfusion within the past 15 years. Thus adolescents, individuals in sexually nonexclusive relationships, newly separated or divorced adults, and anyone contemplating having sex with a gay or bisexual man, injection drug user, or transfusion recipient need to learn about safer sexual practices. It has become appropriate—in fact, essential—for therapists to ask questions such as: "How did you feel when you first heard that you might have to change your sexual behavior in order not to become HIV-infected?" or "How do you feel about the fact that HIV is sexually transmitted?" or "When you think about safer sex, what thoughts and feelings do you have?" Most important, the counselor should ask: "What are you doing to protect yourself and your sexual partners from HIV infection?" (Shernoff, 1988)

Point II

Regardless of sexual orientation, people cannot be *absolutely* certain about the drug use or sexual history of their sex partners. Because the period of HIV latency may last for 10 or more years, people may unknowingly transmit or expose themselves to HIV, erroneously believing that they are not at risk because they are currently in a stable, sexually exclusive relationship.

Interpreting data from the studies of Kinsey and colleagues in the 1940s and those of Hunt in the 1970s, Janet Shibley Hyde (1992) found that only 2% of American men are *exclusively* homosexual during their lifetime and that 25% are bisexual at some point. These data suggest that the majority of men who are or have been homosexually active in the United States may not identify themselves as gay. Many remain in heterosexual marriages, possibly hiding their homosexuality from their wives. Thus many women may falsely assume that they are safe from the risk of contracting HIV. For example, a woman client learned in one day that her husband of 15 years had AIDS, that her marriage had not been a sexually exclusive relationship, and that her husband's relationships outside the marriage had been with men. The crisis was compounded by the need to decide what to tell their 14-year-old son regarding his father's illness, and worries that she herself might have been exposed to HIV.

In attempting to assess whether a client is at risk for HIV, counselors must ascertain what the client's current sexual practices are, as well as what they were in the past. Simply asking "Are you gay?" is not sufficient. Health care professionals cannot assume that a client who is not openly gay has not engaged in sex with other men. For example, a married man with numerous symptoms who had never been transfused, who reported no history of shared needle use or other risk factors for exposure to HIV, and who stated he was not gay baffled his physician. However, when the man was questioned by a counselor as to whether he had ever had sex with other men, he stated that he had a long history of homosexual activity (Shernoff, 1988).

ventive behaviors that were unsuccessful (e.g., intentions to use condoms but failure to do so) and those which were successful. Identifying and discussing previous prevention failures helps to ensure that a risk-reduction plan is realistic, attentive to the client's prevention needs, and focused on actual barriers to safer behaviors. Identifying previous prevention successes (e.g., successful negotiation of condom use with a new sexual partner) offers the counselor the opportunity to reinforce and support positive prevention choices.

Sexual Behavior. With regard to sexual behavior, the counselor might begin the session by saying: "In order for me to give you the very best information, I need to ask you some specific questions about your sexual lifestyle. Your answers to these questions may be embarrassing to you and even painful. They may bring back memories you wish to forget. But complete and honest answers are in your best interest. Everything said here will remain between the two of us."

The counselor may determine the client's sexual orientation by inquiring: "Do you have sex with men, women, or both?" This type of question demonstrates that (1) the counselor realizes that people have different sexual preferences; and (2) the counselor is prepared for the client's response. Questions generally asked about sexual behavior by a counselor are listed in Table 13-2.

Drug Abuse. On completion of the sexual activity survey, the counselor needs to address the connection between drug use and HIV transmission and finish up by stating that drug use by the client or his or her sexual partner is an important factor in evaluating the risk of HIV infection. Questions on personal drug abuse and listed in Table 13-3. Both IDU and non-IDU drugs are listed because all drugs can impair the senses and may lead to a change in sexual behavior and ultimately to HIV exposure. It is difficult to practice safer sex when under the influence of drugs.

BOX 13.2

SEX UNDER THE INFLUENCE (SUI)

Have you ever been a victim of SUI? Sex under the influence can be as deadly as DUI, driving under the influence.

1. Judgment is the first capacity affected by alcohol.
2. What you do unprotected now may hurt you later.

The sentence you get if you get caught unprotected may be death (AIDS).

(This statement hangs in the Counseling and Testing waiting room of an HIV/AIDS clinic.)

TABLE 13-2 Sexual Practice History

Questions for Men and Women:

1. Do you have a history of sexually transmitted diseases?
2. Have you had more than one sex partner in the last 14 years?
3. Do you know the sexual history of each of your sex partners?
4. Was any sex partner an injection drug user?
5. Were any of your sex partners sexually involved with an injection drug user?
6. Was any sex partner hemophilic?
7. Have you ever practiced anal intercourse? Was a condom used?
8. Have you ever practiced oral sex? Was semen swallowed?
9. Have you ever had a blood transfusion? When?
10. Have you ever had sexual intercourse with someone who was HIV-infected or who later developed AIDS?
11. Have you ever been paid for sex?

Questions for Men:

1. Have you ever had anal intercourse with another man? Were you receptive, insertive, or both?
2. Are you bisexual?
3. Have you ever had sexual intercourse with a female injection drug user (or suspected she was)?
4. Have you ever had sexual intercourse with a male or female prostitute?
5. Do you practice oral–vaginal sex?
6. Do you practice oral–anal sex?
7. Do you practice penile–vaginal sex?

Questions for Women:

1. Do you practice anal intercourse?
2. Have you ever had sexual intercourse with a bisexual male (or suspected he was)?
3. Have you ever had sexual intercourse with an injection drug user (or suspected he was)?
4. Do you practice oral–penile sex?
5. Do you practice oral–anal sex?
6. Do you practice vaginal–penile sex?

Special Problems for Drug Counselors. In a report from the First Interdisciplinary Conference on HIV Antibody Testing Counseling in 1987, it was stated that counselors face special problems in dealing with injection drug users (IDUs). IDUs may take the test but fail to return for results or counseling. Already burdened by addiction, they are unlikely to change unhealthy behaviors without substantial intervention.

BOX 13.3

A DAY IN THE LIFE OF A DRUG USER

Janet Johnson-Wise, MSW

For most HIV providers, the lives of injection drug users are foreign at best and stigmatized at worst. This response is based both on the covert nature of drug use and on societal prejudices about drug users. A glimpse into the daily life of a "street addict" challenges these presumptions and can inform educators, counselors, and clinicians.

Street addicts, unlike more mainstream, functional drug users, often resort to theft because they have few other options for obtaining money to buy drugs and because the powerful dictatorship of addiction demands that users compromise their values in its service. Coming out of youth, poverty, and fragmented lives, street addicts often lack education and have few marketable job skills that offer alternatives to theft. Once addicted, a combination of the cost of drugs and unremitting drug craving keeps them poor and unable to compete in the job market. Even with the will to fight addiction, the social network on the street offers little support for this difficult process, and government priorities offer little hope of getting drug treatment.

The following portrait represents a "typical" day in the life of Laura, a heroin-using drug injector living in a city in the United States. Laura is a 32-year-old black single mother. After years of suffering incest, she ran away from home when she was 16. Soon she was selling her body to get money for food and shelter, and she continued to live on the streets for two years before becoming pregnant and then marrying. Now divorced and with three children, Laura is an unemployed high school dropout living in what appears to be an unbreakable cycle of crime, sex, and drug addiction. While not all drug users fit Laura's profile, many share her fear, hopelessness, and frustration.

Hustling

Laura awakens with a start to face another day in the streets and immediately checks the clock. Time is critical to the addict. If it is too early the dealers won't be out yet, and the mall will not open before Laura goes into withdrawal, becoming too sick to "get a good hustle going" (steal merchandise to sell so she can buy drugs). Today Laura is relieved. It's only noon.

Laura's work team consists of three people: two shoplifters—Laura and Mary—and the driver—John—who is available to make a quick getaway. First the team visits the mall, stealing just enough to buy drugs to "take the sick off" (prevent withdrawal). Then they sell the goods, "cop" (purchase drugs), and "get off" (use the drugs). As Laura shoots her share of the drugs, she is already worrying about getting back to the stores to complete her hustling for the day.

John waits in the car ready to pick up Laura and Mary at the first sign of trouble. Today, the women return walking "all wide-legged"; they have scored big. In the car Laura and Mary raise their skirts and begin to pull merchandise from their girdles.

At this point, everybody is happy. They place the stolen clothing under the back seat of the car, drive cautiously away, and find a "fence" to buy the stolen goods.

Taking the Sick Off

After using drugs for more than 10 years, Laura knows all the "dope men" (dealers) in town, who has the best dope, and who will not "burn" them (give them drugs that they later discover to be baking powder or some other false substitute). Mary, a newcomer, wants to go back to the safety of her home to use the drugs. John and Laura, however, know that as soon as the drugs are in their possession, each will begin to experience pseudo-withdrawal symptoms, and the urgency to use the drugs will become overwhelming.

The team ends up in the "shooting gallery" (a place to rent drug-using equipment and inject drugs), a squalid building across the street from where Laura had purchased the dope. Each team member pays the "gallery boss" $2.00 for rental of the "hype" (the syringe) and the place.

Atop a grimy table lay about 15 or 20 syringes, several greasy jars and cups, a whole slew of bottle tops, and some bleach. John and Laura scurry about trying to clear off a small space where they can "cook" (liquefy powdered heroin or cocaine) the drugs and "fire up" (inject). They consider cleaning their needles, but there is not enough bleach, so they shoot up without using it.

Nighttime

After the need to avoid withdrawal has been satisfied, the team gets back to the mall. They continue hustling until they accumulate enough

BOX 13.3 *(continued)*

to cover the rest of the day and night. This time they simply fence the goods and split the money.

Now it's everyone for themselves. Laura's kids have been home alone since they got out of school at 3:00. John has to go see his parole officer. Mary has to clean the house before her mother returns.

Laura buys more drugs. She knows to save at least $5.00 to buy hot dogs, bread, and pork `n beans for the kids. She questions the nutritional value of these foods, but knows that her habit won't allow her to do anything else. The kids are glad to see Laura when she returns and are happy about the food she has managed to buy.

There have been many times that Laura has gotten so high that she hasn't even remembered that the kids needed food. Times when Laura has had to have sex with guys so she could get some cocaine to mix with the heroin. On days like that, there was no money for food. Laura consoles herself with the thought that at least she has always come back to the children.

Throughout the evening Laura continues to get high, hour after hour until all the drugs are gone. At 2:00 AM, she sits on the side of the bed with tears in her eyes and wonders how long she can keep up this life. As she falls into a stupor, she thinks to herself, "Maybe it'll be over this time, maybe I won't ever have to wake up and face that jungle again. But, God, if I do wake up, please let it be by noonday."

Rehabilitated IDUs who test positive may revert to drugs as a means of coping with the fear of illness or death. In general, IDUs, who are impoverished and socially alienated, tend to distrust government or institution-sponsored information. Their suspicions must be offset by physicians, rehabilitation counselors, and former addicts who convey interest, consistency, and empathy.

Most important, the report pointed out the importance of realistic expectations for IDUs, setting both short-term and long-term goals, such as encouraging use of clean needles and condoms while working to control the IDU's chemical dependency. The report makes two other interesting points about IDUs. First, males and females resist safer sex practices for different reasons. Some men are concerned with maintaining their macho image and therefore refuse to use condoms, which they perceive as conflicting with virility. Women may be reluctant to ask their partners to use condoms for fear of jeopardizing the relationship that offers their only option for housing, food, and often human contact. Second, about 50% of pregnant IDUs who test positive complete their pregnancy despite the risk that the child may be born infected and develop AIDS (Selwyn et al., 1989). These HIV-positive pregnant women also appear more likely than male IDUs to be concerned about the health of their child and the response of their friends and family.

TABLE 13-3 Drug Abuse History

Types of Drugs Used:
Alcohol
Amphetamines and other stimulants
Barbiturates and other sedatives
Cocaine (crack and all other forms)
Hallucinogens
Heroin
Marijuana
Other available IV drugs

If the person admits to drug abuse, it provides an opportunity to help him or her enter a drug treatment program.

BENEFITS

Pre-test Counseling

Good counseling skills are essential to the outcome of the HIV antibody testing procedure. One of the most important aspects of counseling is establishing a rapport with the counselee. Honest, nonjudgmental concern and positive regard for the counselee will create an atmosphere conducive to the open expression of his or her feelings and attitudes. The CDC recommends that individuals listed in Table 13-4 receive pre-test counseling and HIV testing. If they have received a general background presentation on HIV infection as suggested under *Education* and have given their sexual and drug abuse histories, the counselor may begin by asking: "Why do you feel you want to be tested?" If the counselor is faced with a person who has not received HIV infection education, he or she may proceed by asking: "What do you know about the AIDS virus; how it is transmitted?" For purposes of this discussion, it is assumed that the person has received the educational information.

With preinformed clients, the counselor needs to know:

1. Why they want to take the test
2. When they think they were exposed
3. How they were exposed to the virus

This information, along with a review of the person's sexual behavior and drug history, will help the counselor to assess the level of risk for HIV infection. The level of risk assessment can be useful in helping a person decide whether to take the test.

Prior to a final decision on whether to take the HIV test, the counselor should explain the HIV antibody test that will be used. He or she should also explain that the average time after exposure before antibodies are detected in the blood is 6 to 18 weeks. In some cases that time period can be extended to over a year. A test which appears negative during this time period may be a false negative. It should be explained that the test is recommended at 3 to 6 months after presumed exposure. However, testing can be done immediately and repeated in 3 to 6 months if it will help to manage the person's fears and anxieties.

If the test is negative at 6 months, it means that the person is most likely *not* HIV-infected but it does not mean the person is immune to HIV infection. If in fact they have been exposed and are truly HIV-negative, they have won the infection gamble this time but they may not the next time.

A person should also be informed of the small chance that a test result may be a false positive. Also, that in a few cases the test is indeterminate and requires a second blood sample for repeat testing. Most important, the person must be informed that although antidiscrimination laws exist, he or she may be subjected to negative social reactions when others find out they have taken the test! Thus the person should be offered the choice of confidentiality or anonymity.

Test or No Test— The decision on whether to be tested can, depending on circumstances, be very difficult to make (Figure 13-1). Fear is a potent emotion and one that often overrules intelligence. For some people, even considering whether to be tested constitutes a crisis—one that is exacerbated if the results are positive and by no means ended if the results are negative.

Some people may cope better with a test result, of any kind, than living with the uncertainty of not knowing their status. A positive result may enable a person to make lifestyle changes that may slow the development of AIDS and improve the quality of life. In other cases, women at risk may want to use test results in deciding whether to become pregnant, complete a pregnancy, or breast feed an infant. If the test is positive, it may also help with a medical diagnosis in people with unexplained lymphadenopathy and mono-nucleosis-type symptoms.

Some people have a difficult time making a decision. Counseling an indecisive person can be either directive or nondirective. Directive counseling would *assist* the person with his or her decision one way or another. Nondirective counseling would prompt the person to find a way, perhaps through additional questioning and discussion, to make his or her own decision. A moral case can be made for both kinds of counseling and is worthy of class discussion.

If a decision has been made not to take the test and the counselor feels strongly that the person is at high risk for infection, he or she can ask the person to review the information covered; and if, for any reason, he or she needs more information or reconsiders, to come back in; or if the client has moved, to visit another state or private testing facility.

TABLE 13-4 Guidelines for Counseling and Testing for HIV Antibody: CDC Recommendations

1.	**Persons who may have sexually transmitted diseases**—All persons seeking treatment for a sexually transmitted disease, in all health care settings including the offices of private physicians, should be routinely[a] counseled and tested for HIV antibody.
2.	**Injection drug users**—All persons seeking treatment for injection drug use or having a history of injection drug use should be routinely counseled and tested for HIV antibody. Medical professionals in all health care settings, including prison clinics, should seek a history of injection drug use from patients and should be aware of its implications for HIV infection.
3.	**Persons who consider themselves at risk**—All persons who consider themselves at risk for HIV infection should be counseled and offered testing for HIV antibody.
4.	**Women of child-bearing age**—All women of child-bearing age with identifiable risks for HIV infection should be routinely counseled and tested for HIV antibody in all health care settings. Educating and testing these women *before they become pregnant* allows them to avoid pregnancy and subsequent intrauterine perinatal infection of their infants (30%–50% of the infants born to HIV-infected women will also be infected).
5.	**Pregnant women at risk**—All pregnant women at risk for HIV infection should be routinely counseled and tested for HIV antibody. Identifying pregnant women with HIV infection as early in pregnancy as possible is important in ensuring appropriate medical care; planning medical care for their infants; and providing counseling on family planning, future pregnancies and the risk of sexual transmission of HIV to others.
6.	**Women seeking family planning services**—All women who seek family planning services and who are at risk for HIV infection should be routinely counseled about AIDS and HIV infection and tested for HIV antibody. Decisions about the need for counseling and testing programs should be based on the best available estimates of the prevalence of HIV infection and the demographic variable of infection.
7.	**Persons planning marriage**—All persons considering marriage should be given information about AIDS, HIV infection and the availability of counseling and testing for HIV antibody.
8.	**Persons undergoing medical evaluation or treatment**—Testing for HIV antibody is a useful diagnostic tool for evaluating patients with selected clinical signs and symptoms such as generalized lymphadenopathy, unexplained weight loss, or diseases such as tuberculosis, as well as sexually transmitted diseases, generalized herpes, and chronic candidiasis.
9.	**Persons who received blood transfusions or blood products from 1978 to 1985**—All persons receiving blood or using blood products between 1978 and 1985 are at risk for HIV infection, especially if the blood or blood products were collected from areas with a high incidence of AIDS. They should be counseled about potential risk of HIV infection and should be offered antibody testing.
10.	**Persons admitted to hospitals**—Hospitals, in conjunction with state and local health departments, should periodically determine the prevalence of HIV infections in the age groups at highest risk for infection. Consideration should be given to counseling and routine testing in those age groups deemed to have a high prevalence of HIV infection.
11.	**Persons in correctional systems**—Federal prisons test all prisoners when they enter and leave the prison system. Correctional systems should study the best means of implementing programs for counseling inmates about HIV infection and for testing them at admission and discharge from the system.
12.	**Prostitutes**—Male and female prostitutes should be counseled and tested and made aware of the risks of HIV infection to themselves and others. Particularly prostitutes who are HIV antibody positive should be instructed to discontinue prostitution.

[a]Routine counseling and testing is a policy to provide services to clients before and after testing. Except where testing is required by law, individuals have the right to decline to be tested without being denied health care or other services. (Source: *MMWR*, 1987)

If the person decides to take the test, it may be of value to have him or her explain what a positive test is and what it is not. Ask: "If the test results do come back from the laboratory positive, what do you think your reaction will be? Will you tell anyone? Will you tell your sexual partner(s), your family, and your friends?" Explain that they may experience a certain amount of anxiety during the 2-week waiting period for the test results; that if they would like, they may come back in for further discussions.

On asking if there are any further questions, the counselor has the person sign a consent form (Figure 13-2) (individual state statutes should be consulted concerning voluntary consent forms for adults and minors), and a time is set for a postcounseling session wherein the test results will be discussed.

BOX 13.4

A COUNSELING CHALLENGE

(A letter written to Percy Ross, an internationally known philanthropist)

Dear Mr. Ross: My God—what am I going to do? I've been married for 12 years and have two children. The man I'm married to is not the man I thought I married. Imagine my horror waking up one morning to learn my spouse was a closet homosexual. That was three days ago. I didn't have a clue in the world that my husband was gay. But he's not only gay, he's also got **AIDS!** What if I have the disease too? My God, what am I going to do?

I'm confused and shocked and have never been so disillusioned with life. I kicked him out of the house and told him to seek sympathy with the man or men who gave him this decadent disease.

I have no skills, as I've been a homemaker my entire adult life. At 43, I'm faced with no hope or future for my children and myself, except the dreaded life of welfare. You've just got to help me Mr. Ross. We were living paycheck to paycheck when my husband was here and we have no savings. My household expenses are $735 a month.

I haven't been able to tell anyone about this nightmare I've been living with, I'm too ashamed. I feel like committing suicide, but my children need me. Help me. What am I going to do?

This and other scenarios continue to occur across the country. What can these people do? How can it be stopped?

Post-test Counseling

Providing the results of the test is just one of the functions of post-test counseling. The counselor must also attempt to determine if the person understands the results, the prospect of continuing at-risk behavior, and the need for immediate medical and psychiatric care. Post-test results should, if possible, be given by the pretest counselor and always in a face-to-face setting.

The results of the test should be given as soon as the person is settled and initial pleasantries are completed. The person has waited for 2 weeks and needs to know what the counselor knows *now.*

Disclosing HIV Status— When disclosing HIV status to a patient, include a face-to-face discussion of the psychosocial and medical effects of HIV infection, following a careful assessment of the person's psychosocial status. Discuss available therapies and social services and, where applicable, explain state requirements for reporting the infection. Discuss the potential advantages and disadvantages of voluntary disclosure to family, friends, and associates.

Urge patients to disclose their HIV status to significant others, particularly sex partners and needle-sharing partners. Emphasize the need to prevent further transmission of HIV infection.

Assess the need of the person infected with HIV for counseling and initial care, and make referrals for services that cannot be provided on-site (Disclosure Counseling, 1994).

The initial disclosure of HIV test results sets the foundation for the person's acceptance of his or her condition. The way in which a person accepts the information can affect the quality of life and willingness to care for themselves. Thus, the manner in which test results are communicated is very important to the formation of the infected person's future attitudes about how they will live the rest of their life. This is especially important now that the new AIDS definition has identified large numbers of **asymptomatic** people with AIDS. In the absence of overt signs and symptoms of HIV disease, it may be more difficult to believe you are HIV-infected. Thus, the asymptomatic person may be more apt to go directly into a stage of **denial** than someone who is symptomatic at the time test results are revealed. It has been shown that people in denial learn less about their illness, delay seeking help longer, and are less apt to cooperate with medical management or follow self-care or health behavior recommendations.

Denial is a coping strategy which helps the client maintain a positive quality of life. The denying client is not yet ready to deal directly or openly with the diagnosis. Denial should be challenged only when medical care or the health of others is compromised.

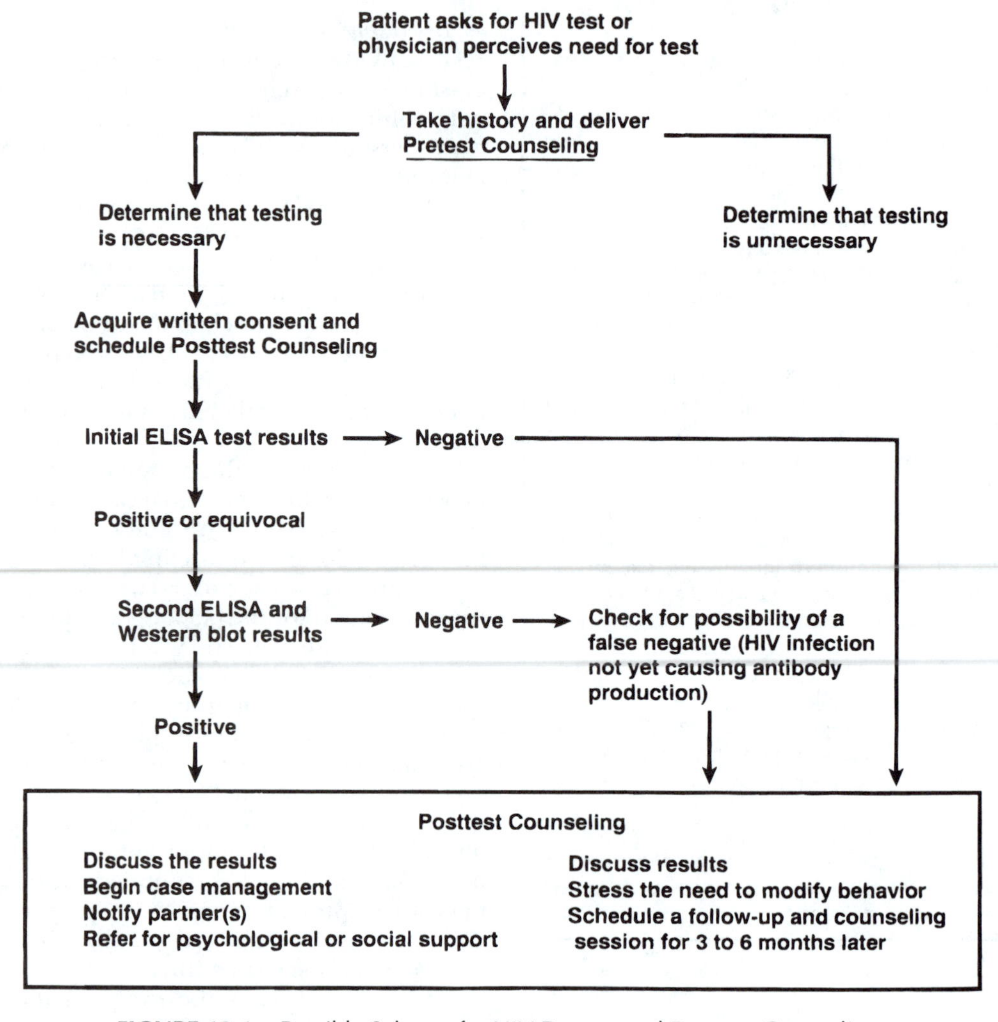

FIGURE 13-1 Possible Scheme for HIV Pre-test and Post-test Counseling. This is only a suggested scheme and the procedure will vary with individual physicians and HIV/AIDS clinics.

A Positive Test Result— A direct statement such as "Your test result came back positive" is perhaps the best approach. The statement may have to be repeated, especially if the person implied during the pretest session that he or she was most likely uninfected. After allowing time for a response, the counselor may follow up by saying "Now that you know the test is positive, can you explain what this means?" If the response is reasonably correct and he or she knows HIV antibodies are present which means HIV infection, it is reasonable to ask about feelings and thoughts. In one case, a person responded, "I lost my health—but wasn't what I really lost my freedom? How do I regain that?"

CONSENT FORM TO DO TEST FOR HUMAN IMMUNODEFICIENCY VIRUS (HIV) ANTIBODY STD, FAMILY PLANNING AND PRENATAL CLINICS — ADULTS

IMPORTANT INFORMATION REGARDING THIS TEST

This is a form that will permit the health department to test your blood for the virus that causes AIDS. The test looks for antibodies that are produced by the virus; it will not tell you if you have AIDS, or will get AIDS. The virus is called human immunodeficiency virus (HIV). For further information regarding AIDS or the HIV antibody test, please read the attached information sheet. If you still have questions about this test that the clinic staff and this form have not answered, please consult your physician or call the Florida AIDS Hotline (1-800-FLA-AIDS) between 8:00 a.m. and 5:00 p.m., before signing this form.

The antibody test is done by drawing approximately 5cc's (1 teaspoon) of blood from the arm. When the blood sample is drawn, you may have some discomfort at the site of the needlestick and a small bruise may develop. Otherwise there is no risk of physical injury.

This test is taken voluntarily. If you choose not to take the test, you will **not** lose any service to which you would otherwise be entitled. Test results will be confidential!

The test results will be available in 2 weeks, and will **only be given to you in person.** No results will be given over the telephone or by mail. A counselor may call to remind you to come to the clinic for your test result.

I understand that the test results will be part of my confidential medical record. If I am pregnant, the results of this test will also become a part of my baby's medical record. I have been informed about the AIDS (HIV) antibody test (see attached sheets). I have had a chance to ask questions which were answered to my satisfaction. I understand the benefits and risks and request this test.

Date: ______________ 19____ ________________________________

(Patient's Signature)

____

(Patient's Printed Name)

Date: ______________ 19____ ________________________________

(Witness)

FIGURE 13-2 One Type of Consent Form, State of Florida, for HIV Antibody Testing. Note that confidential implies a limited release of test result information.

If a person does not respond after hearing the results, the counselor may say, "Now that you know that you are infected, what do you think? Can we talk about it? You're very quiet. What are your thoughts at this moment?"

Reactions may vary from tears to open hostility. After the patient has settled down, it must be made clear that he or she must exercise some control over what is to happen from this point on. Reactions to a positive result will continue to ebb and rise with the flow of the conversation. Newly informed HIV-positive people may be distraught for weeks or months. Depression often occurs and thoughts of suicide are frequent. Records of a group of HIV-positive individuals revealed that 20% considered suicide during the year following their test. (Sarti, 1990).

BOX 13.5

QUESTIONS FOR THE COUNSELOR

Thousands of decisions hang on the results of a test that to most people represents a black box. Individuals who want to be tested can benefit from compassionate counseling. But counseling for this disease is not easy. There is no cure; so how does one instill hope? It brings about a protracted and tragically ugly death; so how does a counselor encourage the patient to be happy and not bitter, up and not down? With no other diagnosis does an individual face the stigma, the fear of rejection, the loss of friends, family, and autonomy. Even patients with incurable cancer are generally *not* subject to rejection by friends, family, or society. In addition, many patients with HIV infections are plagued by unresolved feelings about sexual preference and guilt about the possibility of having infected others.

The questions asked of the counselor vary. Some HIV-infected clients already know about the disease and ask relatively few questions. They bow their heads and their eyes fill with tears as they repeatedly clench and release their fists and rub their foreheads. Others have not received much AIDS education. To them, the virus is just one more sexually transmitted disease among several. When told that this infection has a high probability of progressing to AIDS, their eyes widen, their ill-at-ease smile fades, and their behavior changes. They usually begin by shifting in their chairs, trying to ask two questions at once; they become confused. They want to reject the counselor's bad news by saying things like "Are you kidding me?" or "Say what?" with a nervous grin. The initial rejection of the facts, the denial, usually grows into shock and reality at this point. The patient may well begin to ask the hard questions: How long do I have to live? Will I suffer great pain? Will I be alone? Who is going to help me? Where will the money come from to pay for hospitalization and medication? I'm too young to die; does anybody care that I'm going to die?

Survey of HIV/AIDS counselors finds that most persons being informed that they are HIV-positive want to ask questions. The questions usually fall into one or more of five categories: those relating to prognosis, life expectancy, and fear over loss of faculties, which are usually of greatest concern; those about work and finances; those about self-esteem and social issues; those about being lonely, having to move, or becoming sexually undesirable; and concerns about health issues. Sometimes these questions occur to the individual after the post-test counseling session.

Individual Reactions to a Positive HIV Test—In 1989, Robert, a 33-year-old San Francisco security guard, learned that his blood had tested positive for the AIDS virus. He resolved to fight, to take better care of himself. He entered a marathon.

When the homosexual lover of a Boston AIDS patient tested HIV-positive, he went home and committed suicide.

Reggie, a 38-year-old AIDS activist in San Francisco, resisted being tested until fatigue, weight loss, a tentative diagnosis of AIDS, and his partner of 7 years drove him to the doctor. He recalls, "I was holding out. In my denial and inability to accept what was happening, I took the test to prove my physician wrong. I wanted to wave the paper in his face. That didn't happen. I shut down emotionally." His partner, Tim, assumed that he too was HIV-infected. He quickly enrolled in a medical insurance program. California law prohibits insurers from requiring HIV antibody testing on applicants. Tim went to an anonymous testing site, had an emotional 2-week wait, and found out he was *not infected.* The emotional reactions of the two men were quite different. Tim's first reaction was one of disbelief—there had to be a mistake. Reggie said his first reaction was to feel hurt. Reggie felt the *Why Me* syndrome. He felt alone. Tim, like many others who test negative, greeted his news not with glee but with quiet relief, tinged with what might be called **survivor's guilt**. Now, having been spared the infection, he affirms, "I plan to be there when Reggie needs me most." But Reggie has reason for concern. As the disease progresses, it strains the relationship. Reggie has seen other couples in similar situations break up. The decision of Reggie and Tim to take the HIV test was traumatic; like others before them, they had to face their own vulnerability.

According to interviews with people who were told they were HIV-positive, reactions were similar to those of people who were told they had terminal cancer (Table 13-5). One person, after being told that he was HIV-positive, was asked how he felt. He responded in anger. "If someone came into your home and ripped out the electrical system, loosened the plumbing and took a sledgehammer to the inner walls, you'd be furious, wouldn't you?

TABLE 13-5 Stages of a Dying Patient

Emotion	Interpretation	Stage
Denial and Isolation	No, not me	1
Anger	Why me?	2
Bargaining	Let's make a deal (God)	3
Depression	Unfinished business	4
Acceptance	Void of feelings	5

These are the five stages presented by Elizabeth Kubler-Ross in her book, *On Death and Dying*, publisher Macmillan in 1969. People go in and out of the stages and may never reach stage 5. If they do, they have resigned themselves to death and only want simple companionship.

And if you had opened the door to that person because you trusted them, you'd feel even worse—devastated because of the destruction and betrayal by someone you trusted. How do you think I feel? I'm angry as hell—I would like to hurt someone right now!"

An AIDS patient responded in anger saying that "Loss is the critical term here. My independence is another item on a growing list of losses due to AIDS. I can't even go to a damn movie around the corner anymore! The rage and depression I feel each time an ability or choice is ripped away, or each time an example of an already lost ability rises to infuriate me, is unfathomable. It's like a hideous auctioning off of your spirit, your freedom, at ridiculous prices. You're bankrupt and there's nothing you can do about it. What's doubly depressing is knowing that it will only get worse. Of course, the final loss from AIDS is the loss of life. But along the way, if one does not succumb quickly, the losses leading to the end are insidious, infuriating, and even, sometimes, humiliating" (Rowland, 1990).

Presenting Hope. There is no easy way to tell a person that HIV infection is forever; and based on current medical knowledge, the majority of HIV-infected people will progress to AIDS. But hope can be given by explaining that many people have lived without any severe illness for as long as 10 or more years. And that in the next 10 years, there is great hope that medical breakthroughs will save their lives.

In the meantime, they must not donate blood or body organs or share personal items such as toothbrushes, razors, or anything else that might contain blood. Sexual partner(s) should be informed of HIV status and use safer sex methods. Encourage any previous sexual contact from the time of earliest HIV exposure to go in for pretest counseling.

In closing the posttest session, a counselor should attempt to have the person agree to take control of his or her life, not to transmit the virus to others, seek medical help through periodic medical evaluations, and confidentially inform his or her physician, dentist, and others on a need-to-know basis. Clearly the choices to be made rest with the HIV-positive person.

Suicide Among Persons with HIV Disease or AIDS. Throughout history, suicide has been a uniquely human response to the misery of illness and perceptions of inescapable death. Increased rates of suicide among persons with serious illness have been well documented; these risks are especially high when the illness includes a psychiatric disorder.

HIV/AIDS is a uniformly fatal condition. Persons living with AIDS (PLWAs) are frequently depressed and, in some cases, become suicidal. One individual who was told he was HIV-positive said, "I'm going to shoot myself" and he immediately left the counseling office. In November of 1992, a married couple did just that; both had AIDS. The husband, age 29, the wife, age 36, died of gunshot wounds to the head. Their suicide note said they picked a spot to die together because of its natural beauty.

In 1987 through 1989, there were 165 death certificates with both AIDS and suicide listed as causes of death. Persons with AIDS who committed suicide were 99% male, 87% white, 12% black, and 1% other races. Their median age was 35 years with a range from 20 to 69 years. There were no statistically significant differences in the age, sex, or race distribution of PLWAs who committed suicide compared with all PLWAs alive during 1987 through 1989. Suicides among PLWAs were widely distributed in the United States: California (30%), Florida (11%), Texas (5%), and New York (4%) had the most cases, but suicide among PLWAs occurred in 41 other states and the District of Columbia. In 1992, male PLWAs had a suicide rate 7.4 times higher than males in

BOX 13.6

LOSS AMONG GAY MEN

Robert Marks, Editor of *FOCUS*

HIV researchers and educators spend a good deal of time reminding a society that prefers to partition humanity into "we" and "they", that the virus does not discriminate and that people of every stripe will respond to infection in similar physical and emotional ways. This perspective is reinforced by the societal myth that the only difference between heterosexual people and gay people—the group that has been most identified with HIV disease—is the gender of sexual partners.

In fact, being gay implies much more profound psychological differences than these approaches imply, and while they may be less relevant in treatment and prevention settings, they are central in dealing with emotional response, particularly the expression of grief. In an unusual *FOCUS* article, Herman Kaal offers insights into the psychological complexity of this response among gay men in industrialized nations. His piece provides a good example of psychological detective work, laying out in all its intricacy a range of classical psychological theories that interpret HIV-related loss among gay men.

Loss upon Loss

The most important difference between gay men and others affected by HIV disease, however, is the sociological phenomenon of multiple loss. Three factors determine the conditions that have left gay men in industrialized nations vulnerable to a never-ending grief.

First, HIV disease has killed many more gay men than people in other CDC-defined categories, and the virus has infected a higher proportion of gay men in most places than members of these other groups. Second, among these identifiable groups, gay men have weathered the epidemic for the longest period of time; and third, gay men arguably comprise the group with the strongest sense of community. As Tom Grothe and Leon McKusick point out, the most important result of a multiple loss is that it interferes with the abilities of gay men to fully grieve and heal from one loss before being face with another and another and another.

In addition, while the gay identity Kaal defines is a construct of industrialized nations, according to Grothe and McKusick multiple loss is not so limited. In fact, the most dramatic example of multiple loss is among the general population in African nations, the geographic area where the epidemic is most mature.

I suggest that grief is the most enduring aspect of the epidemic. It may be the most enduring therapeutic issue as well. Kaal, Grothe and McKusick alert therapists—and, indeed, educators and medical professionals—to their great challenge. In the face of multiple loss, they must heal the community by healing the individual, and in this way, resurrect the sense of community fundamental to the mental health of the individual.

the general population. Only one woman with AIDS committed suicide (Cote et al., 1992).

Counseling Women Who Are HIV-Positive: Reproductive Concerns. Women who are HIV-infected should be counseled on their risk of progressing to AIDS and the risk of perinatal and sexual transmission. Infected women should be advised to refer their sex partners for counseling and testing. If a woman's sexual partner is not infected, the couple should be counseled on how they may modify their sexual practices to reduce the risk of HIV transmission to the uninfected partner. In addition, the couple should be told not to donate blood, organs, or sperm and should be discouraged from using IV drugs and advised against sharing needles and syringes. When seeking medical or dental care, they should inform those providers of their postive antibody status.

HIV-infected women should be advised to consider delaying pregnancy until more is

POINT OF INFORMATION 13.2

HIV DISCLOSURE WITHIN THE FAMILY UNIT

By the end of 1994, there were over 6,000 pediatric AIDS cases in the United States. The number of HIV-infected children is probably many times that, and with improving medical treatment these children are living longer. There are many more children who, although not themselves infected, have mothers and fathers who are. Unless the course of the AIDS epidemic shifts unexpectedly, the overall number of mothers, children, and adolescents infected with HIV by the year 2000 will be about 100,000. This trend intensifies the question of discussion of HIV within families.

When and how does a mother tell her child (of whatever serostatus) about her own infection? How should she tell an uninfected child about an infected sibling? These questions give rise to a range of issues within families where HIV or AIDS is present, as well as between these families and social institutions such as hospitals, schools, and churches.

Both parents and medical personnel may resist initiating discussion of HIV within the family. Often they cite the overwhelming anxiety such a revelation might bring, and children's presumed inability to understand such a devastating illness. On the other hand, children in families affected by HIV often already know the truth and give both subtle and overt signs that they want to talk.

Often it is health professionals who first urge disclosure, while family members resist. This process can begin as early as posttest counseling of infected adults. Repeated attempts may be needed to meet with people who are reluctant to hear news that the counselor **must** give. This pattern may persist, with the counselor urging greater openness, while the infected parent's initial reluctance to even know the diagnosis becomes a reluctance to tell others—especially family members.

Counselors prefer openness because of concern for the sex partners of infected patients, respect for the autonomy of infected children, and concern for the long-term well-being of uninfected children who may suddenly lose a parent or sibling to AIDS. It is often in the interests of the entire family to know about the illness of any family member. Yet, while the risk of sex partners is direct and physical, the risks of withholding such information from children are often more psychological and harder to define.

Research on pediatric cancer and bereavement in childhood has shown that relative family openness about terminal illness is beneficial. In the 1960s, cancer diagnoses within a family were frequently withheld from children, while today disclosure has become the norm. Studies of survivors of childhood cancer demonstrate that those who were told of their diagnosis early (e.g., before age 6) grow up with better psychosocial adjustment than those told later, and that children usually know even if they are told nothing. Furthermore, other studies indicate that including children in treatment decisions improves family and individual psychological adjustment.

Although little research has been done on this issue as applied to HIV disease and AIDS, clinical experience has suggested that the situation is analogous. In general, it seems that even very young children (4–6 years) want to discuss family illnesses, at their cognitive level. Younger children's concerns typically focus on separation (Will they be left alone?) and physical pain. Older children's questions range over such topics as the afterlife, etiology, social acceptance, and sexual issues.

Counselors who tend to apply the lessons of pediatric oncology and bereavement to HIV/AIDS should also consider HIV's unique social implications:

1. Most childhood HIV is acquired perinatally. A mother may feel guilty for having transmitted HIV to her child. Discussion would bring up not only guilt, but also grief, and render the illness and its prognosis more painfully real. Parents may also feel guilty for having an illness that threatens to remove them as parents, and shame for the high-risk activities that may have exposed them to infection.
2. For disadvantaged families, HIV may add to an already burdensome litany of issues, such as poverty, racial discrimination, divorce, crime, and drug dependence. Having often left these painful realities largely unspoken, from (partly adaptive) avoidance, such families may not address the emotional impact of HIV/AIDS with candor.
3. HIV/AIDS is associated with socially taboo behaviors. Parents and foster parents may remain silent for fear children's questions would lead them into uncomfortable subjects. Injection drug use, sex with multiple partners, and homosexuality are topics that many families find sensitive.

4. The social stigma of HIV/AIDS is unique. Neighbors, relatives, and schools have been known to shun families in which they suspect HIV. Parents thus keep from children what they fear the children will tell others. Despite public health education, the powerful social connotations of HIV/AIDS are unlikely to vanish soon.
5. Current HIV and AIDS treatment, while not free of side effects, do not typically cause the immediate, visible changes brought on by cancer treatments such as radiotherapy, chemotherapy, and surgery. This can make secrecy more feasible and reduce pressure for disclosure for such purposes as enlisting the child's cooperation in a "fight" against the child's own disease, or explaining to the child the effects of treatment on another.

Given these constraints, it is even more important to approach disclosure issues within families carefully.

PROCESS: Disclosure is a long-term, in fact, lifelong process requiring family members to engage in repeated discussions both on their own and with a counselor. Fostering an emotional atmosphere in which this process can begin is an essential therapeutic task. Long before HIV disease or AIDS is mentioned to children, they can be engaged in discussions that focus on their own day-to-day experience. Adults' resistance to disclosure often diminishes when good rapport is established with counselors who do not try to rush the disclosure process. Parents and children alike may go through phases of secrecy, preparation for disclosure, actual moments of more open discussion, and then back to silence, in a nonlinear progression.

OLDEST FIRST: Disclosure should generally proceed from older to younger family members. Parents and grandparents need to be comfortable with more open discussion before the topic is broached with older, then progressively younger, chidren. Discussion should be a dialogue in which all sides communicate both facts and feelings, and information at the appropriate developmental level is provided to children. This applies when family members are in relatively good mental health; in cases of cognitive or emotional disturbance, certain aspects of disclosure may never be appropriate.

PARTICULARITY: Each family and individual has unique needs with regard to disclosure. For example, older children may acquire the added emotional burden of knowing that a parent's life is threatened. Parents may resist disclosure precisely for this reason. Counselors should address these concerns, and help parents find the right moments and words for disclosure. Using clinical sensitivity, the counselor should assess the barriers to communication in each case and decide to what degree they may be adaptive.

AWARENESS: Awareness of HIV/AIDS within the family prompts widely varying reactions. One 7-year-old boy, short since birth, responded to the invitation to discuss his disease only with questions about his height. A 10-year-old girl, whose parents finally decided on telling, responded with outrage; she said she had known for years, "so why did everyone think it had to be kept secret?" A 10-year-old boy burst into tears after learning that his mother and younger brother were HIV-positive; he said he would be left all alone when everyone died.

It is best to approach disclosure as one aspect of a comprehensive, family-oriented medical and social service. For example, a mother may be more open to telling her children about HIV if she has support with estate and custody planning. Such social service interventions can go hand in hand with psychotherapeutic exploration of their meanings. To arrange for the children's future, a parent must contemplate his or her death, with all it signifies to the family.

Both parents and children can benefit from support groups that address the emotional and social stresses of HIV infection. When parents, especially, become able to address their condition and its emotional impact in group or individual psychotherapy, they can often talk about it more readily with the family. With the guidance of a clinical psychologist or a clinical trained social worker, parents can be helped to explore their own reactions to the illness, examine the questions and topics they fear most, and learn to talk about illness with their children in ways children can understand.

(Adapted from Lipson, 1993)

POINT OF INFORMATION 13.3

REPRODUCTIVE COUNSELING

During the last decade, there has been an outpouring of literature about HIV disease, but little on HIV's special impact on women. Although most HIV-infected females are of reproductive age, a void remains in our knowledge about reproductive issues and HIV disease. Most of what has been written focuses on transmission of HIV from women to their fetuses or newborns, with some information about clinical manifestations and care of HIV-infected pregnant women.

However, counselors can use this small but growing body of information, along with the broader HIV knowledge base, to counsel patients about reproductive options. While some attention has been given to the ethics of HIV-infected women having babies, there has been little discussion of the reproductive decision-making process that HIV-infected women regularly face.

Counseling in this area is based on several assumptions:

Reproductive counseling is an essential part of the primary and preventive care of HIV-infected people and should begin early in the patient–counselor relationship, preferably when the female is not pregnant. Frequently, however, this counseling takes place with a pregnant woman and so must be modified and intensified.

Even though the CDC recommends advising HIV-infected women to delay pregnancy indefinitely, many of the nonpregnant become pregnant and many HIV-infected pregnant women choose to maintain their pregnancies. People have the right to have access to all information about HIV disease and to make their own informed reproductive decisions.

Because the HIV knowledge base changes rapidly and the issues surrounding reproductive decisions making are intimate and complex, the counseling process should be continuous, not simply discussed once and checked off. As knowledge about HIV disease and its impact on pregnancy grows and as the woman develops her personal coping mechanisms, new issues will arise. The counselor must be prepared to deal with emerging issues.

Each person is unique and counseling must be individualized and shaped to each person's needs.

The framework for this counseling model is **biosocial**. With this model, the counselor can support the woman as she explores the impact pregnancy, childbirth, and childrearing would have on her, her fetus and future child, and her support network. The goal is for each female to develop her own risk-benefit analysis in order to make an informed reproductive choice.

There are five essential areas of information that should be presented: (1) the impact of HIV infection on pregnancy, (2) the impact of pregnancy on HIV disease, (3) the effect of treatment of HIV disease on the patient and her fetus during pregnancy, (4) the risk of HIV transmission from the mother to her fetus or newborn, and (5) the course of perinatally acquired pediatric HIV infection.

To summarize information on these five points, we have incomplete knowledge about the effect of HIV infection on pregnancy and about the impact of pregnancy on HIV disease. HIV infection appears to have little effect on the course or outcome of pregnancy. In pregnancies not complicated by HIV, the T4 lymphocyte count decreases throughout pregnancy and then rises after delivery. This decrease also appears to occur in HIV-infected pregnant women, but there is some evidence that the drop in T4 count may sometimes persist after delivery. Whether this accelerates the progression of HIV disease during pregnancy is not known. Little is known about the safety and efficacy of the use during pregnancy of medications for prophylaxis and treatment of HIV-related disease. However, counselors should review these issues with HIV-infected females with reproductive capacity before instituting therapy.

After providing information, answering questions, and emphasizing that much about HIV and pregnancy remains unknown, a second stage of counseling is in order, and it may or may not be appropriate during the same visit. Attempt to learn the patient's emotional and geographic relationships with her family, and expand it to include her greater support network. Ask the patient to characterize the people in her life and her relationship with each. It is important to learn who the patient lives with, who she trusts, and who knows she's HIV-infected. Does she have a partner? Is her partner HIV-infected? Does she have any children or grandchildren? Are any of them at risk for HIV infection? The goal is to help the patient identify and assess her supports and stressors. Once her network is identified, the focus can return to the patient and the biopsychosocial impact a pregnancy may have on her.

Other important questions are: What is her stage of life (e.g., adolescence, young adulthood,

POINT OF INFORMATION 13.3 *(continued)*

middle age)? In what stage is her disease? Does she have other health problems, including substance abuse? Does she have adequate housing, income, and health insurance? When was her last physical examination (try to obtain a copy before the session if one exists)?

Having done a thorough history and review of her physical, provide her with information about HIV and pregnancy, and draw a visual diagram of her concerns and available support groups. Then ask her to consider five possible scenarios:

1. She becomes ill during her pregnancy and must make decisions regarding treatments that may be life-saving to her and her fetus but potentially toxic to the fetus.
2. She does not know throughout her pregnancy and during the first 18 months of her child's life whether or not her child is HIV-infected, since it can take up to 18 months from birth to determine whether a baby is HIV-infected.
3. After her child is born, she remains asymptomatic, but her child becomes ill and possibly dies early in life.
4. She becomes symptomatic, needs hospitalization, and possibly dies, while her child remains healthy.
5. Both she and her child become ill, require hospitalization and possibly die.

With each scenario, ask versions of the following questions: How will you feel if . . .? Who will help care for your child if . . .? Who will help care for you if . . .? How will those around you (your partner, your child or children, your family and friends) feel if . . .?

This is a lengthy and intense process that lends itself to role play and discussions with other HIV-infected women who have had to make similar decisions. Emotions that typically arise during the process include a sense of loss at never having been a parent or grief at losing a child, and guilt over bearing an ill child or one she can't take care of if she becomes ill or dies. Help the patient predict her emotional response to each scenario, with the goal of helping her predict how she would cope with these feelings. How has she dealt with loss and guilt before? Would she be in danger of harming herself or someone else? If she's a substance abuser, would she increase her use of drugs or alcohol? Does she have a strong, reliable support network to help her?

Each scenario and each question can raise the patient's awareness and help her explore options. As she does this, there are several self-empowering tools the counselor can help her develop and use. The counselor should emphasize safer sex practices, not only to prevent unwanted pregnancy, but also reinfection with HIV and transmission of other STDs. If the patient is a drug user and not likely to stop, safer drug use practices should be described. The counselor can support the patient in writing her living will and appointing an appropriate health care proxy; planning for child custody in the event of inability to care for her children because of illness or death; and making medical arrangements for her children and coordinating these with her own medical care and, if necessary, that of her partner. If the patient has housing or financial difficulties or other psychosocial stresses, the practitioner should see to it that she gains access to resources and, if necessary, serve as advocate for her within the larger political system.

After all this, the woman is still left with a difficult decision. Through this intensive counseling, the counselor may hope the woman has acquired sufficient knowledge and insight to make an informed and considered decision. The counselor will also have learned a great deal, which will help in the counseling of the next patient.

(Adapted from Bermon, 1993)

known about perinatal transmission of the virus. Pregnant infected women may require additional medical and social support due to an enhanced risk of opportunistic infections and psychosocial difficulties during and after pregnancy. Also, HIV-infected women should be advised against breast feeding to avoid postnatal transmission to a child who may not be infected.

A Negative Test Result. On occasion, a person hearing that his or her test was negative becomes very quiet. Some have expressed disbelief and anger because their sexual partners tested positive. An example of the kind of reaction a person goes through when told he or she is negative is in Paul Monette's book *Borrowed Time: An AIDS Memoir.* When Paul's test came back negative, knowing that his lover

Roger's test was positive, he wrote, "When my test came back negative last month, I was overwhelmed with a sadness I hadn't expected. Coming back alive is a guilt, a terrible betrayal, a necessary starting point."

Others feel a great sense of relief and are quiet because they are grateful for the reprieve. In either case, these people must be cautioned that, although a negative test means that they are not infected, it does not mean that they are immune to infection. If their risk assessment is high, they should be told that they were fortunate this time. If they wish to remain free of HIV infection, they must change their behavior and practice risk reduction. In addition, they must also be told of the test's limits—that there is a small chance the test was a false negative if they had unsafe sex or shared IV needles within the past 6 months.

Many individuals, whether their results are positive or negative, may require long-term support to reinforce and sustain changes in their behavior that must become permanent.

PSYCHOSOCIAL ISSUES BROUGHT ON BY HIV/AIDS

HIV disease shares several characteristics with other life-threatening illnesses, most notably the progression toward death, the many physical, emotional, functional, and economic losses, and the process of psychological adjustment. Yet, certain issues associated with providing care for HIV/AIDS patients are unique. For example, there is the fear of contagion and social hostility toward primary HIV/AIDS risk groups—gay men and IDUs. The stigma and blame associated with HIV/AIDS, the infectiousness (in particular, the sexual transmissibility of HIV), the epidemic nature of infection, the youth of patients, the roller coaster course of illness, and the neuropsychological impairment, especially in late stages. These issues are irrelevant to the care of other terminally ill persons.

Lovers and friends may distance themselves out of fear of contagion or difficulty in coping with the diagnosis, or they may experience emotional exhaustion from having been exposed to too many AIDS deaths. Family members may live far away or refuse to become involved. As a result, many patients ultimately live alone. Most patients eventually deteriorate to the point of needing care on a 24-hour basis because of weakness, memory loss, confusion, diarrhea, and other impairments.

Traditional family structures are often absent, and many patients do not have the primary home caregiver required for admission to most hospice programs. For some patients, disclosing the HIV/AIDS diagnosis is tantamount to revealing to family or associates for the first time that they are gay or have used injection drugs.

Effects of Depression on HIV Disease

Accumulating evidence supports the belief held since Hippocrates that vigor, resilience, and perceived support are associated with more favorable medical outcomes. Furthermore, stress and depression have been shown to affect the immune response and, mediated by neuroendocrine mechanisms, may affect vulnerability to illnesses ranging from cancer to the common cold. So, it is reasonable to ask whether one's mental state can affect the course of HIV infection.

The clinical course of HIV disease varies widely. Some people deteriorate rapidly while others live for years, even after AIDS diagnosis. The reasons for these different rates of decline are not known, but **psychosocial** variables are on the list of possible host factors. The notion has been that one's adaptive coping or fighting spirit might somehow delay or even prevent the progression of HIV disease and, conversely, that distress and despair might measurably accelerate progression of the disease.

Jeffrey Burack and colleagues (1993) reported that overall depression and affective depression predicted a more rapid decline in T4 lymphocyte counts. This association was not attributable to baseline physiological differences. While the mechanism of the association remains unknown and cannot be addressed di-

BOX 13.7

THE THERAPIST AND THE DYING CLIENT

Jeremy S. Gaies, Psy.D. and Michael D. Knox, Ph.D.

Psychotherapy with the dying is especially challenging when clients are young adults as are many people with HIV disease. Despite its difficulties, however, such counseling frequently offers both patients and providers opportunities for growth and for learning to live more fully.

HIV-related psychotherapy does not require special expertise. However, modifications in therapeutic approach are appropriate to meet the challenges posed by the life-threatening aspects of HIV disease. This article defines therapeutic concerns for HIV-infected people facing death, adjustments therapists must make to meet these concerns, and psychological issues for therapists treating people with HIV disease.

Psychological Issues of the Patient

HIV disease shares several characteristics with other life-threatening illnesses, most notably the progression toward death, the multiple physical, emotional, functional, and economic losses, and the process of psychological adjustment. Much attention to psychological responses to terminal illness has focused on stage theories, especially that proposed by Kubler-Ross.[1] While recent theorists have questioned the conception of these responses as fixed, Kubler-Ross's five stages—denial, anger, bargaining, depression, and acceptance—are of great clinical significance when viewed as positive functions of the psyche coping with the emotional demands of the illness. Denial, for example, serves a critical protective function in allowing an individual to survive the stress of catastrophic information. Allowed to progress without impediment, denial will typically and gradually fade toward realistic assimilation of complete information.

There are also striking differences between HIV disease and other terminal diseases. Among these are the intense stigma and blame associated with AIDS, the infectiousness (in particular, the sexual transmissibility of HIV), the epidemic nature of infection, the youth of patients, the roller coaster course of illness, and the neuropsychological impairment, especially in late stages.

These characteristics of HIV disease suggest psychological issues that may be grouped into three constellations. One constellation is loss, including losses of function, health, independence, financial security, standard of living, social support, sexual freedom, mental functioning, and normal life span. A second is stress, including that associated with uncertainty of information, uncertainty of prognosis, discrimination, stigma, guilt, and anger. Much of this stress is related to rational and irrational fears of rejection, abandonment, pain, disability, loss of mental control, and transmitting HIV. A third constellation focuses on issues related to terminal disease such as fear of death and dying, and existential and spiritual aspects of life and death. A client's emotional response to these concepts will affect his or her response to the later stages of disease: a person who perceives death as a peaceful escape from mortal existence will respond differently than a patient who sees death as painful, punishing, or empty nonexistence.

Within these constellations, issues may vary in importance for different individuals and in intensity over the duration of the illness. For one person, the most significant concern will be the loss of financial resources, for another it may be the experience of physical pain or the desire to plan the funeral. Issues will change over the course of disease, as will the content of specific concerns, for example, sexual relationships or mental functioning. Appreciation of the variability and range or responses and needs among clients with HIV disease is one of the most essential aspects of the psychotherapist's preparation for providing quality care. It is particularly important for the therapists to note two aspects of HIV-related care. First, patients tend to seek therapy, even at late stages, to handle immediate needs rather than chronic concerns. Second, by the time they have reached terminal stages, many patients with HIV disease have resolved philosophical issues related to mortality and are confronting practical concerns related to dying.

Therapeutic Objectives

Although the focus of psychotherapy will vary over time, objectives always include fostering realistic hope, reducing stress, and helping the client to attain a measure of control. In the later stages of illness, for example, therapy may provide an opportunity for terminal care decision making, and funeral and memorial planning. Making decisions and taking charge of the final details may enhance client autonomy at a time when other aspects of life seem out of control.[2]

Because the emotional intensity of terminal HIV disease threatens the objectivity of practitioners, therapists are encouraged to use a structured assessment framework. The framework should be comprehensive, to ensure that issues regarding dying are not missed, and objective, to ensure that the framework is not biased toward one view of death. Among the factors assessed in a comprehensive framework are personality profile prior to illness, coping skills and styles, hope, realistic awareness of the severity of the illness, cultural and religious background, social support, self-esteem, suicide risk and other self-destructive behaviors, compliance with care, and mental functioning. To develop a comprehensive assessment, counselors should be sure they have a thorough understanding of the key issues for people with HIV disease.

Unlike most people with terminal illnesses, a high percentage of people with HIV disease experience neuropsychological impairment.[3] Clients frequently raise concerns about loss of mental functioning. Neuropsychological assessment is often warranted to identify cognitive strengths and weaknesses and to differentiate organically-based from depression-related cognitive impairment. To avoid complications related to mental incompetency, therapists should encourage clients to deal with legal, financial and health care planning and documents, such as wills, durable powers of attorney for finances and health care, and medical directives or "living wills." With more significant impairment, the therapy process itself must change, with increasing adjustment toward supportive therapy and psychosocial case management.

Adjustments in Process

Therapists must learn to be flexible when counseling people with HIV disease in the late stages of illness. Symptoms of terminal illness, which often makes regularly scheduled weekly appointments in the therapist's office difficult, may require home visits, hospital visits, and telephone sessions. Therapy may need to be interrupted at times depending on the patient's physical condition. Lack of time precludes long-term approaches, and patients frequently require greater encouragement and direction to achieve necessary tasks of closure and planning in the limited time available.

Treatment flexibility also means being open to supplementary, alternative, and modified techniques, such as art or other creative therapies, family therapy including members of a gay client's friendship network, and the use of touch. Limited physical contact is often appropriate when clients are struggling with issues of rejection, physical disfigurement, and irrational concerns regarding infectiousness. Briefly holding a client's hand or allowing a hug at the end of a session is sometimes appropriate, while strict avoidance of physical contact can confirm a client's fears that there is a reason to reject or be afraid of him or her. Adaptable therapists may also have to assume the responsibilities of mental health case managers or advocates. This decision must be based on the specific needs of patients. In general, as patients begin to lose independence, the tasks of case management increase. These tasks may include monitoring health care, ensuring social service involvement, helping to gain access to entitlement programs, and activating and supporting family and friends to care for the patient.

Because people with HIV disease tend to become financially insolvent during the course of the illness, there is often a need at later stages to lower rates of payment and to offer free treatment when health insurance is unavailable. Since therapists, especially those in private practice, are dependent on client fees, it may be advisable to set reasonable limits on the number of people with HIV disease in treatment at any one time. If appropriate, biweekly sessions might allow continued therapy while reducing the financial burden on both the client and counselor. Whatever procedure is chosen, it is imperative that therapists raise this issue with clients at regular intervals and, at all costs, avoid any situation that may be experienced by the client as abandonment.

The Therapist's Psychological Issues

Conducting psychotherapy in general can be emotionally taxing for therapists. The additional challenges of treating clients who have a stigmatized disease and are the same age or younger than the therapist can be significant. For gay therapists, many of whom have lost loved ones to HIV disease, and for seropositive practitioners, the issue of identification is even greater. Maintaining a true sense of presence with the client while maintaining separation from the client's life is critical to the psychotherapeutic relationship. Therapists can best attain the strength to be present and the objectivity to be separate by developing and enriching their own personal lives.

This balance may be threatened as the client becomes more physically ill and nears death, and the therapist experiences some degree of anticipatory grief. Anticipatory grief is a normal reaction, even for a therapist serving in a professional capacity. It is the intensity of the grief and the adaptive response to it that should be considered. The most effective response for therapists may be to acknowledge that they have feelings about the lives and deaths of their clients. It is also essential that the therapists understand that the process of dying and the psychological response to dying (both the client's and the therapist's) are natural and should be supported rather than manipulated, avoided, or suppressed.

Therapists may benefit from practicing techniques for minimizing burnout. Burnout prevention includes setting reasonable goals for therapy and for the therapist, learning to be patient, maintaining a diversity of activities outside of therapy, and finding support in one's personal and professional life. Some form of therapist support group, including a networking or educational group with a social component, may be helpful. Employing a cotherapist for group work can be an excellent way of maintaining both support and objectivity. Other burnout prevention skills include using humor, practicing relaxation, exploring one's own feelings regarding mortality and life meaning, identifying achievable goals that add a sense of purpose to work, and focusing attention every day on personal fulfillment.

Coping with the death of a patient can be a new and threatening experience, and there is little societal support for therapists working through grief about the death of a client. The most important way to cope with this loss is for therapists to be sure that they say goodbye to clients. Saying goodbye may mean actually speaking to a client before the client's death, lighting a memorial candle, setting aside a few moments for private thoughts, or attending the client's funeral.

Finding Inspiration

Providing psychotherapy to people facing the challenges of a life-threatening illness can be inspiring work, offering therapists, as well as clients, the opportunity to grow and live more fully. By sharing a client's experience of confronting the fragility of life and learning to cherish each day, for better or for worse, therapists begin to confront the vulnerability of their own lives and to acquire a deeper appreciation of living. Therapists also witness the psychological power of courage, hope, and faith. These responses awaken therapists to the great potential of human beings to adapt to life changes, an awareness that serves the therapist as an individual as well as a professional.

Jeremy S. Gaies, Psy.D. is Clinical Assistant Professor of Community Mental Health at the University of South Florida's (USF) Florida Mental Health Institute, and Staff Psychologist with American Biodyne, Inc. Michael D. Knox, Ph.D. is Professor, Chairman of the Department of Community Mental Health, and Director of the USF Center for HIV Education and Research.

References

1. Kubler-Ross, E. (1969). *On Death and Dying.* New York: Macmillan.
2. Knox, LP, and Knox, MD. (1991). *Last Wishes: A Workbook for Recording Your Funeral, Memorial, and Other Final Instructions.* Tampa, FL: Applied Science Corp.
3. Miller, EN, et al. (1990). Neuropsychological performance in HIV-1 infected homosexual men: the Multicenter AIDS Cohort Study (MACS). *Neurology,* 40:197–203.

rectly by this study, the data suggest that it can be explained neither as simply a reflection of perceived somatic symptoms nor as the result of differences in recreational drug and alcohol use. Further study is necessary to determine whether treating depression can alter the course of HIV infection.

FAMILY AND FRIENDS: STRESS FACTORS WHEN THE PERSON THEY CARE ABOUT BECOMES HIV-POSITIVE

The psychosocial impact of stress on the HIV-infected is different for each individual and is-

BOX 13.8

INFORMATION AND LEGAL GUIDELINES FOR PERSONS WITH HIV DISEASE/AIDS

Life expectancy after AIDS diagnosis is approximately 2 years. Like other patients with terminal illnesses, individuals with AIDS should be encouraged to express their wishes concerning the use or limitation of life-sustaining measures. Such decisions are crucial in early stages of AIDS because many patients experience moderate-to-severe neurological impairment that may deprive them of the power to understand, make decisions, or express their wishes long before they die.

Many professionals involved in AIDS care suggest that the question of using life-sustaining support be brought up with the patient as early as possible, even at the time that he or she first learns of the diagnosis. Some physicians may find it difficult to approach these questions with a patient who still appears healthy. Referral to a social service agency or group specifically concerned with AIDS may be helpful.

Legal Guidelines

Different types of legal documents expressing wishes about life-sustaining treatments are recognized by different states. Therefore, it may be wise to hire an attorney.

An attorney will be able to help in: (1) completing an up-to-date will for distribution of assets and settling the estate; (2) completing a living will that specifies the extent to which the patient wishes life-sustaining measures to be used in care he or she becomes mentally ill or hopelessly ill and unable to make his or her desires known; (3) preparing a durable power of attorney to designate an individual to make medical treatment decisions, such as the withholding or withdrawal of life support, in the event of mental incapacity. (Traditional power of attorney terminates when the person issuing the document becomes disabed.) The documents may be combined in a single form. Which document is most appropriate in any individual case may vary from state to state.

As of 1994, 41 states and the District of Columbia had legislation concerning a person's right to die. All states and the District of Columbia have legislation concerning a durable power of attorney. A living will can be executed in a state without specific legislation, because all states recognize the right of a competent person to refuse treatment, regardless of the consequences.

Durable power of attorney may be particularly important for the homosexual patient with AIDS who wishes to appoint a partner or mate as proxy for medical decisions. In the absence of specific legal provision, the authority to make decisions is usually transferred to the next of kin. Family members may not recognize the rights of a patient's partner as decision maker, and may resent the partner as representing a lifestyle of which they disapprove. It may be advisable to appoint more than one proxy, with the second to act if the first is unavailable when needed.

General Guidelines

1. Obtain the names, addresses, and phone numbers of the patient's physician, attorney, family, and loved ones.
2. Make funeral arrangements prior to death. Delicately determine what kind of funeral the patient wants.
3. Locate insurance policies, bankbooks, IRAs, pension funds, if any, selective service or social security numbers, safety deposit key and box, the previous year's tax return, automobile and other titles, outstanding debts, and so on.
4. Keep an account of all expenses for filing the year's tax return.
5. Specifically keep track of medical expenses—what was paid and what is still owed. The insurance company may want proof of expenses.
6. Families, friends, loved ones, or lovers are not responsible for debts left by the deceased, providing they have not signed on to accept debt responsibilities (consult an attorney about specifics).

Information about individual state laws, approprate forms, and other matters can be obtained from your local medical society or Concern for Dying, 250 West 57th St., New York, NY 10107; (202) 246-6962. Information can also be obtained from the Society for the Right to Die, 250 West 57th St., New York, NY 10107; (212) 246-6973.

An excellent booklet called, "AIDS and Your Legal Rights", is available from National Gay Rights Advocates (NGRA) which conducts litigation in the areas of AIDS, employment discrimination, freedom of speech, and domestic partnerships, primarily in the western part of the country. This booklet addresses such questions as, "I already have insurance. Can my insurer refuse to pay AIDS or ARC-related claims?", "Can an employer make me take an HIV antibody test or discriminate against me because of my results?", and "I have AIDS. What public benefits can I get?".

Because laws are constantly changing this booklet cannot give detailed information on specific laws in every state. Your local AIDS service organization or public health department will know the current laws in your jurisdiction and may be aware of litigation on your issue. Contact NGRA at (213) 650-6200 for the booklet and for help.

sues change during the course of the illness. Problems for asymptomatic HIV-infected individuals are not the same as those for terminal persons with AIDS. The most stress typically occurs at transition points such as confirmation of HIV positivity, the beginning of symptomatic symptoms, or when the need for institutional care develops.

The HIV-infected person must deal with: the stigma of HIV and associated behaviors; the real or perceived rejection by family and friends; the desire to remain anonymous because of shame or fear of rejection; not knowing how or to whom to talk about fears and concerns (Table 13-6), particularly in low-incidence areas; and few local resources in low-incidence areas or within cultures where associated behaviors are taboo.

TABLE 13-6 Common Concerns and Fears of HIV-Infected Individuals

- Leaving children behind
- Experience of real or perceived discrimination
- The possibility of having infected others in the past; continuing fears about infecting others in the future
- Loss of control over items such as who may know about one's personal choices and sexual orientation, because symptoms may reveal or raise speculation about personal matters
- A chronically uncertain future
- Fear of suffering, dying, and death
- Loneliness
- Loss of self-identity
- Loss of physical abilities
- Change in body image
- Loss of control of body functions
- Loss of independence
- Loss of mental capacity
- Bereavement—It is a mourning process for loss which typically begins at the time of an HIV-positive test result. Multiple losses are common at all stages of HIV illness.

For the family and friends, there may be a double crisis when they find out the son/daughter/friend is a drug user, homosexual, or bisexual. In this case, family/friends must cope with value conflicts as well as death and dying concerns. For parents, these revelations often force reflections on parenting practices. Parents may express guilt over permissiveness, strictness, closeness, distance, acceptance, or rejection as a way to explain or assign blame. Parents may place blame on the lover or partner for both the HIV infection and the lifestyle. Friends often become unsure of the person they thought they knew so well and may become distant.

THE WORRIED WELL

Fear of HIV infection may bring significant psychosocial stress to uninfected individuals. Regardless of behavioral risk level, such persons are referred to as the **worried well**. In such cases, individuals have fears of infection that are disproportionate to their actual risk of infection. They can experience severe anxiety reactions leading to illness, social withdrawal, or even hospitalization. In one recent event, a 35-year-old male related to the author that he had been divorced for the past 3 years and that although he is sexually aroused among women he has not had sexual foreplay or sexual intercourse since the divorce—the *reason,* "I'm just too scared of becoming infected with that damned AIDS virus." This man believed that most of the unmarried women who had sexual encounters carried the virus!

THE GRIEVING PROCESS

Grief is an emotional, psychological, and, often, physical response to the death of another. It is a period of time during which the normal state of one's own life (i.e., view of self and view of the world) is altered and out of balance. The grieving process for HIV disease and AIDS usually begins with a positive test result and varies in degree of intensity from one individual to another. The two major goals of the grieving process are: (1) restoration of the state of effective psychological functioning, and (2) redefining one's self in the face of loss: Who and what am I now?

The grieving process is not a linear process, grief does not occur according to a script, but there appear to be common items that contribute to the eventual resolution of grief: (1) the acceptance of the loss—this period is marked by a sense of unreality of the death which then gradually dissipates; and (2) feeling the pain of grief—grief pain may occur on a variety of levels: physical, psychological, emotional, and/or behavioral. The level and intensity of this pain varies from one individual to another. How and when this pain is expressed varies from culture to culture. (An excellent source of information on managing grief associated with HIV/AIDS is the May 1992 issue of *FOCUS*, Volume 7 or contact the National Clearinghouse for government publications on "Organizational Grief," Washington, D.C.)

HIV/AIDS SUPPORT GROUPS

Individuals who share a common problem such as a medical condition, life-threatening disease, or short-term crisis may benefit from support systems and mutual help. Over the last 25 years, there has been a proliferation of support groups for patients with a wide spectrum of medical and psychiatric conditions. These groups can be led by professionals, or they may be self-help groups directed by members. Professionally led support groups draw on psychotherapeutic principles but, like self-help groups, emphasize high group cohesion and low confrontation—no one blames anyone. Both types of groups stress the therapeutic value of universality, altruism, and hope (Levy et al., 1990).

COUNSELING FOR HIV-INFECTED ADOLESCENTS

To this point, counseling topics have dealt mainly with the HIV-infected adult. But there is another rapidly growing population of HIV-infected people that need caring and sensitive counseling as well—they are the adolescents. As counselors, you can expect to deal with about as many adolescent males as females; the ratio of HIV-infected males to females is 2.6 males to every female. For adults, it is about 8 males to 1 female, respectively.

Teenagers are not just older children or younger adults: adolescence is a developmental phase that occurs as one proceeds from childhood to adulthood. More changes occur between the ages of 10 and 20 than during any other period, and these may include dramatic shifts in biological and cognitive functioning. Psychosocial development shows even greater diversity as adolescents develop their own identities, experimenting with an array of sexual, moral, vocational, and political paths. This diversity frames the experience of adolescents with HIV disease, which complicates this already challenging period.

For seropositive adolescents, HIV infection can be a terrifying and mysterious intrusion into life, and teenagers react to HIV infection in a variety of ways. As with HIV-infected adults, seropositive and at-risk adolescents form a diverse group, one for which a single, formulaic approach to treatment and care is sure to result in failure. Similarly, reactions to HIV disease depend upon each youth's stage of illness, life history, social and familial support system, and levels of cognitive development, moral development, emotional maturity, and self-acceptance.

In response to these factors, counselors should pay special attention to two issues: the level of understanding and rapport. First, while many adolescents, particularly older ones, are psychologically sophisticated, counselors should assume, until proven otherwise, that they have not reached mature levels of thought. Second, as with adults, counselor rapport with adolescents is crucial to success. Achieving rapport is especially challenging since teens may see counselors as authority figures and feel that they have been forced into talking with them about something that they find terrifying or shameful.

Four specific issues that require special emphasis when counseling adolescents are: (1) disclosing HIV infection status, (2) how they respond to the news of HIV infection, (3) coping with disease progression, and (4) approaching their death.

Disclosing Infection

The issue of when and to whom to disclose the fact that they are HIV-infected is one of the first major decisions adolescents must face. Many adolescents face greater pressure to disclose because they are more likely than adults to live with family, who assume an entitlement to this knowledge, and because they are less likely than adults to have learned the resourcefulness necessary to access help. In addition, disclosure to family may be potentially more difficult among adolescents because families are legally and socially able to exert greater control over minors. Like adults, many teens fear the loss of support from family, friends, and present and future sexual partners.

For some adolescents disclosure is two-fold. Those adolescents who became infected through male-to-male or female-to-female sexual activity effectively "come out" about homosexual experimentation or orientation at the same time they disclose HIV infection status. Some support systems can tolerate the reality of HIV disease, but cannot tolerate homosexuality.

Telling a parent may be more difficult than telling a friend. The decision should be based on a thorough exploration of potential consequences. Are the parents likely to support or reject the adolescent? Will they provide emotional and financial support? Are they capable of providing such support? Does the adolescent want to tell his or her parents, or does he or she feel compelled to do so? If a youth decides to tell a parent, it may be useful to role-play the conversation to help him or her prepare for parental reactions. It may also help the adolescent for the counselor to be with him or her during the disclosure, and to have follow-up meetings to help the family adjust to the news. Referral for family therapy is another good option.

It is worth mentioning that while the involvement of a supportive adult is ideal, informing parents may not always be in the best interests of adolescents and may even be dangerous. This is particularly relevant in cases of runaway or throwaway youth.

Responding to Seroconversion

The only generality that can be made about adolescents is that each will, either overtly or covertly, have a strong reaction to the news that he or she is HIV-infected. Reactions may include anger, guilt, anxiety, depression suicidal or homicidal ideation, numbness, or terror, and, in all likelihood, all of these will be present to one degree or another.

Adolescents may have difficulty confronting HIV disease for reasons similar to adults. Unlike adults, however, many teens—particularly younger ones—have difficulty, in the absence of overt signs of infection, understanding and believing they are HIV-infected. This can be frustrating to counselors in that it adds to the difficulty of motivating changes in risk-related behaviors and ensuring compliance to medical regimens and prudent care.

Adolescents who do not fully acknowledge the implications of being HIV-infected may simply be confused or in denial. Many teens have not yet achieved the cognitive maturity level whereby full acceptance and understanding is even possible. The ability to think in abstract terms occurs slowly during the adolescent years. Until the capacity for mature thought is achieved, they frequently perceive themselves to be immortal, are pre- dominantly egocentric, and view the world in very concrete terms.

What may be common knowledge or basic information to most adults may be new to HIV-infected youth, especially if they are disenfranchised from the mainstream due to homelessness, ethnicity, or sexual orientation.

Teenagers also tend to be less deliberate in what they do or say and are less likely to follow through on actions; their impulse control and frustration tolerance may not yet be developed to the point where they can behave in a manner that ultimately serves their best interests. It is vital that counselors be ready to provide adolescents with a more mature perspective and necessary structure when the capacity to provide it for themselves is not operating. They can do this by helping adolescents to verbalize feelings and explore the consequences of planned actions. This approach will discourage acting out in potentially self-destructive ways—such as suicidal gestures, revenge towards others, or refusal to keep appointments or to take medications—behaviors that may function to camouflage feelings of fear, anger, and despair.

Finally, it is critical during this period to assist adolescents in disentangling reality from fantasy and to correct distortions stemming from internalized fears and judgments. For example, it can be difficult for teenagers to make the fine distinctions required to understand that the desire to engage in oral, anal, or vaginal intercourse did not cause infection; the act of sexual intercourse without barrier protection did.

Coping with Disease Progression

Teenagers tend to think in a concrete manner, to believe that a fixed T-helper cell number implies a specific serious illness or impending death. The idea that T-helper cell counts are a barometer of immune system function is a difficult concept for adolescents to grasp. Therefore, T-helper cell counts should not be discussed in an isolated manner; such a discussion should always be in the context of current medical status and level of functioning. To help adolescents negotiate these issues, counselors should focus on the concept of the spectrum of HIV-related illnesses, and not on fixed cutoffs for disease diagnosis and progression.

It is equally essential to provide a safe, nonjudgmental forum for teenagers to voice fears and concerns if and when T-helper cell counts fall, particularly since they may be doing everything they can to stave off such a deterioration of health. In general, adolescents are less able to permanently integrate this information without intense fear, anxiety, and defensiveness distorting their perceptions of reality, and they often requre repetition of basic facts regarding their illness. In response, counselors should repeatedly explain concepts in different ways.

As adolescents develop symptoms, they may be jolted from the denial about the severity of their symptoms. Counselors should fully explore the subjective meanings and implications of each symptom and should seek to validate these impressions while simultaneously correcting misconceptions. In particular, adolescents may need help in putting symptoms into perspective, to understand that not all infections are equally serious and not all are AIDS-defining.

Approaching Their Death

Perhaps the most agonizing area of adjustment for teens and counselors involves confronting the possibility of death. Adolescents, many of whom lack the capacity for abstract thought, have fixed ideas about death, and this lack of flexibility may raise anxiety. As with adults, teenagers may respond to this anxiety with subtle verbal and nonverbal cues. Counselors should be particularly aware of cues such as crying, anger, silence, or anxious fidgeting, which may indicate discomfort.

Discussions of death should be preceded by a thorough exploration of any preconceived notions about dying. From that base, counselors can gently and compassionately help adolescents prepare for death.

Ironically, a conversation about death is frequently a relief for adolescents. It may be a topic they have thought about, but have been afraid to verbalize for fear of upsetting family, loved ones, and friends. In keeping silent, teenagers, sensing the discomfort of others, may have actually been taking care of parents and counselors. (Adapted from Elliot, 1993)

CONFIDENTIALITY

Confidentiality and Sexual Partner Betrayal

This story took place in an HIV/AIDS clinic in the South. A husband and wife came into the clinic for an HIV test. They said the *only* reason for requesting the test was that they wanted to begin a family and hoped that nothing in their past would have led to either of them being HIV-positive. The tests were completed. The husband came in on a Monday; the wife came in that Friday.

Monday A.M.

Counselor: Mr. X, your test came back HIV-positive.

Reactions and counseling were similar to those presented in this chapter. Then Mr. X said he wanted to be the one to tell his wife; he insisted on it. The counselor agreed. Mr. X left the clinic agreeing to come back for a follow-up counseling session.

Friday A.M.

Counselor: Mrs. X, your HIV test was negative.

Mrs. X: That's wonderful news. I can't wait to tell my husband. We've been waiting for my results. I want to get pregnant immediately.

Mrs. X received HIV-negative counseling and left the clinic very happy.

Quite clearly, the husband did not tell his wife the truth about his test results. A follow-up phone call to the husband went unanswered; so did a letter from the clinic. Several months later, Mrs. X called the counselor to tell her that she was pregnant!

Question: What do you think the counselor should do now?

1. Inform the woman about her husband.
2. Take no action.
3. Call the husband and discuss the situation.
4. Threaten the husband with legal action if he does not tell his wife.
5. Your position!

Discuss the moral, ethical, and legal responsibilities of each participant.

The Public's Question

The situation surrounding confidentiality for patients infected with HIV is comparable to circumstances that dictate our reporting of sexually transmitted diseases and cancer. The reason for reporting these cases to the CDC is that valuable epidemiological data may be gathered. These data can then be used to doc-

BOX 13.9

LACK OF CONFIDENTIALITY AND PATIENT HARM

In 1985, I was the primary physician for a young man whose life was ruined by the inappropriate disclosure of a positive HIV test result. A physician ordered the test without consent and notified the local health department of the positive result. The health department notified the individual's employer and he was fired. The event became common knowledge in his rural Midwestern town and he was shunned. His landlord asked him to move. Ten days after testing, the life he had known for the past 10 years was permanently ruined and he left town. With the loss of his job came the loss of health insurance and insurability; he has been unable to obtain health or life insurance since then.

In this case, no purpose was served by taking the HIV antibody test. The patient had been diagnosed with AIDS based on the presence of opportunistic infections 6 months earlier at Cook County Hospital. He was aware of his diagnosis and its implications. He had been following safe sex guidelines for the preceding 18 months and had never donated blood or semen. (A case report by Renslow Sherer, 1988.)

A similar event happened in Jacksonville, Florida in late 1990. A young man diagnosed with AIDS moved to Jacksonville and enrolled in an area HIV/AIDS clinic. Somehow his employer found out that he was visiting the clinic and receiving zidovudine. The man was fired, asked to move out of his apartment, new friends shunned him, and he had to move out of state.

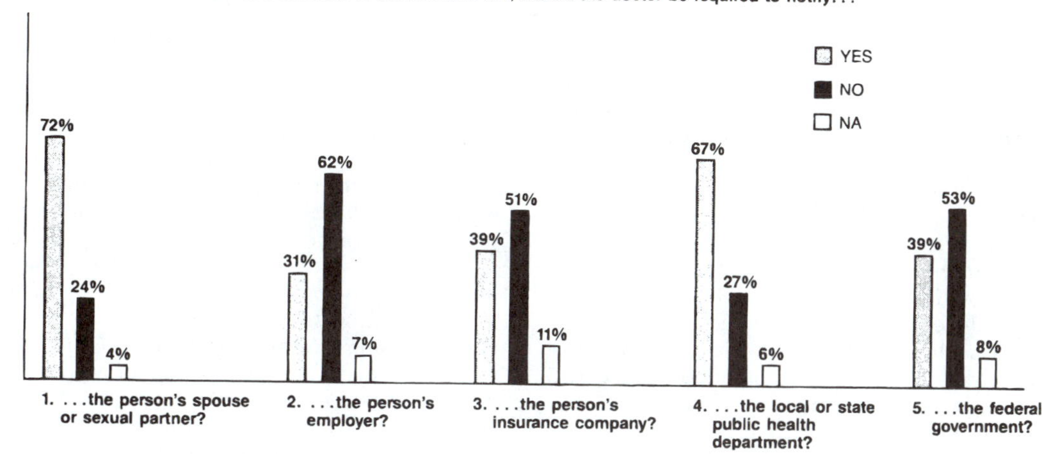

FIGURE 13-3 Confidentiality Opinion Poll in the United States. The poll was conducted by telephone for Media General-Associated Press in May 1989. The poll has a 3 point margin for error meaning that 19 times out of 20 findings should be accurate within 3 points if every adult American were asked the same questions.

ument geographical location, prevalence, routes of transmission, and those groups of people that may be at highest risk for these diseases. If these diseases are reportable for the ultimate benefit of individuals susceptible to sexually transmitted diseases and cancer, shouldn't HIV-positive people be reportable for the same reasons? It is questions such as this that are bringing about a change in public opinion concerning confidential HIV testing and use of test results.

In a mid-1989 poll taken by the Media General-Associated Press, 72% of Americans opposed strict confidentiality of HIV tests, favoring mandatory notification of spouses and health officials. In addition, 67% said the physician receiving the test results should be required to notify local or state public health officials (Figure 13-3).

The poll included 1,084 adults interviewed by telephone. Phone numbers were selected at random and the person interviewed was the adult who had the most recent birthday. About one in five of the respondents said they personally knew someone who was HIV-infected or had died of AIDS. The poll showed a growing social acceptance of individuals with AIDS compared to interviews in 1985.

About 75% said people with AIDS should be entitled to keep their jobs; and 80% said children who have AIDS should be admitted to school. Some 52% thought AIDS was likely to spread widely beyond current risk groups, while only 11% thought they were at great risk or some risk of getting AIDS; 23% thought they were at "not much risk" and 64% said "no risk at all." Two percent were unsure.

LIVING WILLS

The fact that HIV disease is not considered a terminal illness in more than half of states in the United States, makes it difficult for HIV-infected people to implement living wills. According to a review of the U.S. law surrounding this issue, the right to refuse treatment is often related to whether refusal is in response to a terminal illness. People with HIV disease face the challenge of proving that HIV disease is terminal. If they cannot, states may stop the implementation of their living wills.

BOX 13.10

MAKING TERMINAL CARE DECISIONS

Jeannee Parker Martin, R.N., M.P.H.

People with HIV disease should consider their options for terminal care early in the disease process to avoid the pressures of medical complications, such as AIDS dementia complex, and psychosocial concerns, such as diminishing financial resources. It is generally accepted that a patient is "terminally ill" when disease prognosis is 6 months or less, so the notion of terminal care should not be limited in conception to the last few weeks of life. If considered early enough, people with HIV disease may have several options about where they die and under what conditions, including in hospitals, at home, and in group residential facilities.

Factors to Consider

Where does the individual want to die? The place where someone dies may be determined by factors out of a patient's control. A good first step is to identify, through direct questioning, whether a patient has a preference about where he or she dies. Caregivers may find that patients will be relieved, instead of dismayed, by a direct approach to terminal care issues.

Does the patient want aggressive curative therapy or palliative hospice care during the final months of life? Patients in the terminal phases of illness may choose to seek curative therapy that will extend life, even when practitioners predict that these therapies will have little effect, or patients may choose only palliative care, aimed at reducing discomfort but not at fighting disease progression. Patients seeking a curative therapy may have fewer options about where to die because treatment may require special equipment and care. On the other hand, palliative therapy, which forms the basis of the hospice philosophy of care, can be provided in the patient's home, as well as in hotels, group residential settings, hospitals, skilled nursing facilities, and other sites.

What type of insurance or financial resources does the patient have now and expect to have during the final 6 months of life? The type of insurance coverage a patient has, and whether or not it changes over the course of illness, will allow access to different care options. Private insurance policies cover medically necessary care in hospitals, and, increasingly, in home care settings. Most private insurers want to provide appropriate, cost-effective care and will consider options—such as home, hospice, and residential care—even if they are not specified in their policies.

Low-income or indigent patients may become eligible for Medicaid (Medi-Cal in California), which pays for acute hospital services, skilled nursing facility care, and intermittent home health care. In some states, Medicaid may pay for group residential care, extended hour attendant or nursing care, and hospice care. Older and disabled patients may be eligible for Medicare, which covers acute hospital services, short-term skilled nursing facility care, intermittent home health care, and hospice care, but does not pay for group residential care, or extended attendant or nursing care.

Loss of job-related income, costly medications, and routine expenses such as food and shelter may diminish financial resources. Assets such as cars and homes may be sold to help pay for insurance premiums or other health-related expenses, but patients should consider how much sacrifices will affect quality of life.

What human resources are available to assist as the patient's physical or mental status deteriorates? Patients who prefer home care may be able to facilitate this care, even without insurance coverage, by organizing friends and relatives to provide round-the-clock support. This type of care requires a cohesive and reliable network of volunteers, as well as one or two individuals who are available to help organize and run this network. In addition, patients and their caregivers should consider how support services from community programs can provide additional assistance.

What cultural and religious distinctions should be considered? Patients should give credence to their own cultural and religious beliefs about death and where to die. Lack of adherence to these cultural mores may make the dying process difficult and have lasting emotional consequences for survivors.

Hospital Inpatient Care

Before they die, people with HIV disease may experience multiple episodes of acute illness requiring repeated hospitalizations. Although the focus of hospital care is generally rehabilitation to prior level of functioning, some individuals require hospital care as disease progresses and conditions deteriorate. To deal with the needs of dying HIV-infected patients, hospitals may offer designated specialty units, skilled nursing facilities for patients with long-term inpatient need, and inpatient hospice units.

Because hospitals offer care around the clock, some may feel that this is the safest environment for people whose conditions are deteriorating. They may also find a medical setting, where expert care is readily available, to be comforting and may fear that, if a patient remains at home, family members will not provide the "right" care to deal with medical emergencies, pain, or death itself.

Home Care

When offered adequate physical care and emotional support by either family, friends, or professional caregivers, most individuals choose the familiar surroundings of their homes for terminal care. Whether receiving short-term, intermittent care, extended nursing care, or hospice care, home care is most often provided by a coordinated professional health care team.

This team generally consists of the patient's attending physician, nurses, social workers, home health aides, attendants, and counselors, and addresses both physical and psychosocial needs. Specialty services, such as intravenous therapy, total parenteral nutrition, and respiratory care can be provided by most home care agencies and may be needed even during terminal phases. While family or friends may provide all or part of necessary terminal care, they usually require professional instruction and supervision.

Group Residential Care

Some communities have developed group residential hospice facilities. These homelike facilities are cost-effective because they consolidate services, such as round-the-clock attendant and nursing care, and deliver them to patients who would otherwise have to use more expensive hospital settings. Despite this, group settings often are not covered by public or private insurance programs. Skilled nursing facilities and nursing homes, while appropriate for terminal care, provide limited access to people with HIV disease.

Conclusion

Under the best circumstances, individuals will make terminal care decisions while they are mentally competent and with the help of health care professionals. They should also assign to trusted friends or relatives decision-making rights under durable powers of attorney for health care and include these people in terminal care planning. This preparation is important, because the practical aspects of terminal care are as influential in determining a patient's comfort with dying as is his or her spiritual approach to death.

Statutory definitions of what constitutes a terminal condition and a life-sustaining treatment tend to be circular. In most statutes, withdrawal or withholding of life-sustaining treatment can proceed only after several physicians certify that the person is in a terminal condition. A condition is defined as terminal only if "life-sustaining procedures"are employed to postpone the moment of death but do not improve life. Many common HIV-related treatments do not meet this definition.

Many HIV-related treatments do not meet other aspects of these definitions. In 11 states a life-sustaining procedure is defined as that which "sustains, restores, or supplants a vital function." Medication is specifically excluded from these definitions in 19 states and the District of Columbia. HIV disease is not considered terminal in 11 states because death must be "imminent," and recovery from opportunistic infections occurs too often to meet this requirement (Kortlandt, 1991).

The federal courts have frequently defined the right to die in broader terms than state statutes would imply. Case law, based on judicial decisions, has tended to be more flexible than statutory law. The federal courts have viewed the right to die in terms of the individual's right to privacy versus the state's need to prevent suicide, protect third parties, maintain the integrity of the medical profession, and preserve life. They have used the state's right to prevent suicide as a means of investigating the motives of those rejecting treatments and have ruled against withdrawal of treatment if such a decision appears to be irrational.

The federal and state courts appear to be moving toward expanding privacy rights by letting mentally incompetent as well as competent patients die. Family members and patient-designated medical decision makers are being allowed to decide to withdraw treatment. The 1990 Supreme Court decision in *Cruzan v. Harmon* established a patient's right to die if there is clear and convincing evidence that the patient would forgo treatment if mentally competent. This "substituted judgment test" and the "best interests approach"—by which the court makes decisions based on the best interests of the patient—mark an expansive trend in the law that may make it easier for people with HIV disease to have their living wills implemented (Kortlandt, 1991).

SUMMARY

In a few states, HIV testing is preceded by counseling on HIV infection, its transmission, and the types of tests available to detect HIV antibodies. Regardless of whether results are positive or negative, the person is counseled to practice safer sex and to strive to change any behavior that led to his or her visit to the testing center. Based on interviews of counselors at testing centers, the hardest client is the past or present injection drug user. Past IDUs, if positive, may revert to drug abuse with reckless abandon—a kind of suicidal behavior. The present IDU, if positive, believes he or she has *no* sane reason to give up drugs. They feel they are going to die either way.

With regard to those who take an HIV test, strict confidentiality is of the utmost importance. The literature is replete with examples of people being persecuted for taking the test—after all, if they had reason to take the test, they must be doing something wrong. In many cases, males are immediately labeled homosexuals because of the high incidence of HIV infection and AIDS in the homosexual population. Individuals who have been identified as HIV carriers and patients diagnosed with AIDS have lost their jobs, friends, families, lovers, and homes and have been denied insurance policies, bank loans, and home mortgages. Confidentiality appears to be a must in the success of any HIV testing program. It has been shown repeatedly that lack of confidentiality is driving high-risk people who might be HIV-infected away from testing centers.

REVIEW QUESTIONS

(Answers to the Review Questions are on page 483.)

1. What are the three components of HIV pretest procedure?
2. Name the two forms of counseling that can be offered when a person is indecisive about taking an HIV test.
3. What is post-HIV test counseling for?
4. People finding out that they are HIV-positive enter a stage of ______. What other stages may they go through?
5. Patients who test HIV-negative may still need counseling, because they _____.
   A. need reassurance
   B. feel guilty
   C. may become suicidal
   D. all of the above
6. Most patients will undergo testing if ____.
   A. a sexual partner is HIV-seropositive
   B. their physician recommends such and ensures confidentiality
   C. they have shared needles
   D. their physician explains their behavior has put them at risk
7. Who is primarily responsible for informing an HIV-positive patient's contacts or partners?
   A. the patient
   B. the physician
   C. a public health service agency
   D. the state health department

8. True or False: The pain associated when grief is expressed will vary from culture to culture.
9. True or False: The homosexual individual often replaces his or her family of origin with a family of choice, which may consist of lovers and close friends.
10. True or False: Support groups for HIV-infected homosexual or bisexual men should be as heterogeneous as possible with regard to disease stage.

REFERENCES

BERMON, NANCY. (1993). Family and reproductive issues. *AIDS Clinical Care,* 5:45–47.

BURACK, JEFFREY, et al. (1993). Depressive symptoms and CD4 lymphocyte decline among HIV-infected men. *JAMA,* 270:2568–2573.

COTE, TIMOTHY, et al. (1992). Risk of suicide among persons with AIDS. *JAMA,* 268:2066– 2068.

Disclosure Counseling. (1994). *JAMA,* 271:492.

ELLIOT, ALAN. (1993). Counseling for HIV-infected adolescents. *FOCUS,* 8:1–4.

HUNT, MORTON. (1974). *Sexual Behavior in the 1970s.* Chicago: Playboy Press.

HYDE, JANET SHIBLEY. (1992). *Understanding Hu-man Sexuality.* New York: McGraw Hill.

KINSEY, ALFRED C., et al. (1948). *Sexual Behavior in the Human Male.* Philadelphia: W.B. Saunders.

KORTLANDT, C.E.M. (1991). AIDS and Living Wills. *AIDS & Public Policy Journal,* 5(4): 157–66. (New York: Seward & Kessel).

LEVY, RUTH SHIPTON, et al. (1990). A group intervention model for individuals testing positive for HIV antibody. *Am. J. Orthopsychiat.,* 60:452– 459.

LIPSON, MICHAEL. (1993). Disclosure within families. *AIDS Clinical Care,* 5:43–47, 47.

MONETTE, PAUL. (1988). *Borrowed Time: An AIDS Memoir.* New York: Harcourt Brace Jovanovich.

Morbidity and Mortality Weekly Report. (1987). Public health service guidelines for counseling and antibody testing to prevent HIV infection and AIDS. 36:509–515.

Morbidity and Mortality Weekly Report. (1991). Publicly funded HIV counseling and testing—United States, 1990. 40:666–675.

Morbidity and Mortality Weekly Report. (1993). Technical guidance on HIV counseling. 42: 11–17.

PERRY, SAMUEL. (1993). Depression and HIV: How does one affect the other? *JAMA,* 270: 2609–2610.

ROWLAND, CRAIG. (1990). Losing it. *PAACNOTES,* 2:99–100.

SARTI, GERALYN M. (1990). Asymptomatic patients with HIV infection. *Postgrad. Medi.,* 87: 143–154.

SELWYN, PETER A., et al. (1989). Knowledge of HIV antibody status and decisions to continue or terminate pregnancy among intravenous drug users. *JAMA,* 261:3567–3571.

SHERER, RENSLOW. (1988). Physican use of the HIV antibody test. The need for consent, counseling, confidentiality, and caution. *JAMA,* 259:264–265.

SHERNOFF, MICHAEL. (1988). Integrating safer sex counseling into social work practice. *J. Contemp. Social Work,* 69:334–339.

CHAPTER

14

AIDS and Society: Knowledge, Attitudes, and Behavior

CHAPTER CONCEPTS

- The HIV/AIDS "devastation" is here.
- Inaccurate journalism leads to public hysteria.
- Vignettes on AIDS.
- Over 14 years later, what do we know about HIV/AIDS?
- Use of explicit sexual language on TV and in journalism.
- Goal of sex education: To interrupt HIV transmission.
- The Red Ribbon.
- Education is not stopping HIV transmission.
- Students still have misconceptions about HIV transmission.
- The general public and homophobia.
- Employees are not well informed and fear working with HIV/AIDS-infected co-workers.
- Teenagers are not changing sexual behaviors that place them at risk for HIV infection.
- First World AIDS Day observed in 1988.
- Orphaned children due to AIDS-related deaths.
- Physician–patient relationships in the AIDS era.
- Educating employees about AIDS.
- Placing the risk of HIV and infection in perspective.

Acquired Immune Deficiency Syndrome (AIDS) is an illness now characterized, according to CDC criteria, as the presence of antibody to HIV and a T4 cell count of less than 200/μL of blood, and by the presence of certain opportunistic infections and diseases that affect both the body and brain.

BLAME SOMEONE, DÉJÀ VU

With AIDS more than any other disease in history, we have found verbal mechanisms for distancing ourselves from thoughts of personal infection. AIDS statistics are published in categories, so we can identify how many gay or bisexual men, injection drug users, persons with hemophilia, and so on, have developed AIDS. Likewise, we can check which countries, states, and cities have the highest incidence of the disease, and even which racial and ethnic groups are highest among reported AIDS cases. By focusing on categories of people, have we made it possible for society to rationalize that AIDS belongs to somebody else? Have we made the thought of HIV/AIDS somewhat impersonal? Have we found a way to blame someone else?

Placing blame does not always require reason and tends to focus on people who are not considered normal by the majority. Thus minorities and foreigners are often singled out to blame for something, sometimes anything. Epidemics of plague, smallpox, syphilis, cholera, tuberculosis, and influenza have historically focused social blame onto specific groups of people for spreading the diseases by their "deviant" behavior. Blaming others leads to their stigmatization and persecution.

While the Black Death, an epidemic of bubonic plague, swept across Europe in the 14th century, blame was variously attached to Jews and witches, followed by the massacre and burning of the alleged culprits. In Massachusetts between 1692 and 1693, some 20 people were hanged or burned at the stake after being accused of having the powers of the devil. Eighty percent of those accused were women. And when Hitler blamed Jews, communists, homosexuals, and other "undesirables" for the economic stagnation of Germany in the 1930s, the result was death camps and ultimately the second World War. Now there is a new plague—HIV/AIDS. What blame comes packaged with this new disease?

Jonathan Mann, former head of the World Health Organization's Global Program on AIDS, points out that there are really three HIV/AIDS epidemics, which are in fact phases in the invasion of a community by the AIDS virus.

First is the epidemic of silent infection by HIV, often completely unnoticed. Second, after a period of incubation/clinical latency that may last for years, is the epidemic of the disease itself, with an estimated 5 million AIDS cases worldwide ending 1994, and an estimated 7 million ending 1995.

Third, and perhaps equally important as the disease itself, is the epidemic of social, cultural, economic, and political reaction to HIV/AIDS. The willingness of each generation to place blame on others when believable explanations are not readily available simply recycles history. We have been there before; we have placed blame on others and it will continue. With respect to the HIV/AIDS pandemic, blame has been disseminated among nations. And, there is no shortage of political, economic, social, or ethical issues associated with this *new* disease.

PANIC AND HYSTERIA OVER THE SPREAD OF HIV/AIDS IN THE UNITED STATES

With the 1981 announcement by the U.S. Public Health Service and the CDC that there was a new disease, AIDS quickly became a symbol for our darkest fears. Responsible public officials gave out conflicting messages; *reassurance* on one hand and *alarm* on the other. Public panic and hysteria began.

People with HIV disease and AIDS are still abused, ridiculed, and maligned. Some people believe that AIDS is divine retribution for immoral lifestyles. People who have not indulged in high-risk lifestyles (e.g., newborns and recipients of blood products) continue to be labeled as innocent victims, implying that other HIV-infected individuals are guilty of the behavior that led to their infection and therefore deserve their illness.

Families and communities continue to be divided on their beliefs and acceptance of HIV/AIDS patients. Federal and state agencies stand accused of a lack of commitment and compassion in the war against AIDS. The bottom line is that *value judgments* are associated with HIV/AIDS because the disease involves the most private areas of people's lives—sex, pregnancy, drug use, and finances.

The Fear Factor

A poster in the Swiss STOP AIDS Campaign focuses on how we think about people with AIDS:

> For the doctors, I am HIV-positive; for some neighbors, I am AIDS-contaminated; for my friends, I am Claude-Eric.

Soon after young homosexual men began dying in large numbers, a barrage of frightening rhetoric began filling the airwaves, television, the popular press, and even the most reputable scientific journals. The AIDS disaster was here. One health care administrator stated "We have not seen anything of this magnitude that we can't control except nuclear bombs."

In 1986, Myron Essex of the Department of Cancer Biology at the Harvard School of Public Health noted,

> The Centers for Disease Control and Prevention (CDC) has been trying to inform the public without overly alarming them, but we outside the government are freer to speak. The fact is that the dire predictions of those who have cried doom ever since AIDS appeared haven't been far off the mark . . . The effects of the virus are far wider than most people realize. It has shown up not just in blood and semen but in brain tissue, vaginal secretions, and even saliva and tears, although there's no evidence that it's transmitted by the last two.

In 1987, columnist Jack Anderson reported that the Central Intelligence Agency (CIA) concluded that in just a few years heterosexual AIDS cases would *outnumber* homosexual cases in the United States. Also in 1987, Otis Bowen, former Secretary of Health and Human Services, said AIDS would make the Black Death that wiped out one-third of Europe's population in the Middle Ages pale by comparison. In 1988, sex researchers William Masters, Virginia Johnson, and Robert Kolodny stated in their book, *New Directions In the AIDS Crisis: The Heterosexual Community*, that there was a possibility of HIV infection via casual transmission—from toilet seats, handling of contact lenses from an AIDS patient, eating a salad in a restaurant prepared by a person with AIDS, or from instruments in a physician's office used to examine AIDS patients.

In contrast to these reports is the 1988 article by Robert Gould in *Cosmopolitan* reassuring women that there is practically no risk of becoming HIV-infected through ordinary vaginal or oral sex even with an HIV-infected male. The vaginal secretions produced during sexual arousal keep the virus from penetrating the vaginal walls. His explanation was: "Nature has arranged this so that sex will feel good and be good for you."

ACTIONS OF COURAGE

There are far too many heroes of this pandemic to list here. And the heroes come from

BOX 14.1

AN EXAMPLE OF UNCONTROLLED FEAR

In 1986, a very ill AIDS patient on an airline flight spilled some urine from a drainage bag on the seats and carpet. Hours later, after the flight had reached its destination and the patient deplaned, several rows of seats around the area were taped off. The plane then took off for a new destination where the contaminated area would be removed. Crew members and airline union leaders expressed outrage at the exposure of passengers and crew to this threat. The clean-up crew refused to remove the carpet, even with rubber gloves. Union safety officials insisted that the materials be burned rather than just thrown away.

BUT WE HAVE LEARNED SINCE THEN, RIGHT? **WRONG!**

In April 1993, an American Airlines flight crew requested that all pillows and blankets be changed on a plane that carried a group described by an internal communication as "gay rights activists." A staff attorney for the Lambda Legal Defense and Education Fund, a gay rights organization in New York City, said the message was apparently related to fears of HIV infection and AIDS. A representative for American Airlines apologized saying that such action was completely and totally inappropriate and that American Airlines has a strict policy against discrimination of any individual or group. **But it happened.**

every walk of life and profession. So many have answered the call for help, for compassion and human kindness. But there are a few examples that might be considered either sufficiently different or unusual enough to mention. And although unusual, even these actions have been demonstrated by many.

First, in 1979, when gay pride was rising, a teenage male took a boy to the prom in Sioux Falls, South Dakota. The national media were there to record the moment; the camera lights glared as he and his date danced; gay activists were elated. It was the first time a same-sex couple had been allowed to attend an American prom. This male couple faded into obscurity—until January 1993. His death from AIDS was reported to the CDC.

The next examples of courage are about two courageous teenagers. He was a husky eighth-grader from Missouri who wore a peace symbol around his neck and was diagnosed with HIV in the summer of 1991. He recalled the day his mother called him into the house to give him the news. "I was getting ready to play baseball. I said, 'Does this mean I'm going to die?' She said, 'Not today.' I said, 'Can I go play baseball now?'".

He had only one problem with prejudice. A few parents in neighboring towns didn't want their children to play against his baseball team. **"I quit the team because I didn't think it was fair for them to not get to play because of me."**

A 13-year-old girl in Detroit who goes by the nickname of Slim has very grown-up responsibilities at home.

"It's hard, but I won't show you or let you see my pain," she said. "I was always taught to be strong."

She's had to be. Her mother, a single parent, is infected with HIV. At the same time, she learned that her sisters were also infected.

One sister died in April of 1993 at age 9. Then in November, her 6-month-old sister died. Now, another sister is battling HIV.

Through it all, she has been responsible for giving medications and intravenous feedings to everybody, around the clock.

"I want people to know what's going on. But I don't want anyone's pity."

WHOM IS THE GENERAL PUBLIC TO BELIEVE?

Because of the complexity of HIV disease, a great deal of press coverage of AIDS issues reflects what scientists say to journalists. A journalist's responsibility is to check that the facts are accurate, but not necessarily to judge their overall merit. Why should a good story be spiked just because other scientists disagree with the data interpretation? When scientists say contradictory things to the public, how can the public assess whom to believe? Science has a duty to inform and educate the public, but it must neither frighten people unnecessarily nor give them unjustified expectations. Claims of "AIDS cures" in the popular press need to be based on much more than just in vitro data. Whatever the need to attract research funding, is 5 minutes of fame ever worth a day of fear or weeks of false hopes for many? The popular press has provided HIV-infected persons with a roller coaster ride between hopelessness and fantasies of imminent cure.

As a result of journalistic promises, there was and still is a range of emotions that run from real hope of a cure to public panic and hysteria. In at least five states, children with AIDS were barred from attending local public schools. The case of 12-year-old Ryan White of Kokomo, Indiana was made into a TV movie, *The Ryan White Story*, in 1989. Many parents fail to place HIV infection in perspective. In reality, automobile accidents, voluntary and involuntary exposure to tobacco smoke, drugs, and alcohol present greater risks to their children than does casual contact with an HIV-infected person.

In some localities, police officers and health care workers put rubber gloves on before apprehending a drug user or wear full cover protective suits when called to the scene of an accident (Figure 14-1). In other communities, church members, out of fear of HIV infection, have declined communion wine from the common cup.

Since the epic announcement in 1981, HIV/AIDS has refashioned America. It is not the first epidemic to alter history; measles, smallpox, bubonic plague, polio, cholera, and

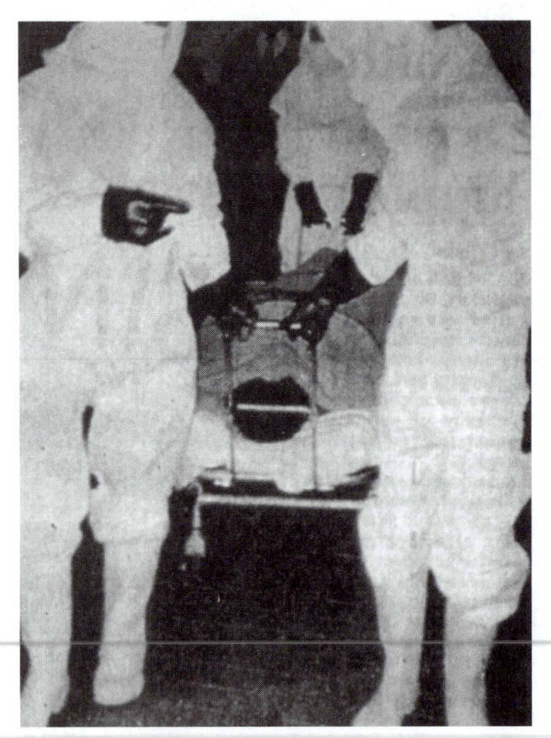

FIGURE 14-1 Ambulance Workers Protecting Themselves from the AIDS Virus at the Scene of an Accident.

other diseases have ravaged their eras. But HIV/AIDS is a disease molded to the times, one that has wedged apart the thinly concealed fault lines of American society by striking hardest at the outcasts—gay men, injection drug users, prostitutes, and impoverished whites, blacks, and Hispanics. HIV/AIDS has brought forth uncomfortable questions about sex, sex education, homosexuality, the poor, and minorities. The disease has inevitably polarized the people, accentuating both the best and worst worldwide. Many churches, schools, and communities have responded to the new disease with compassion and tolerance; others have displayed hate and reprisals of the worst kind.

As Camus wrote in *The Plague,* "The first thing (the epidemic) brought . . . was exile." Anyone who carried the disease could inspire terror. They became pariahs in society.

Hate-mongers torched the house of the Ray family and their three HIV-positive hemophilic children in Arcadia, Florida. And someone shot a bullet through the window of Ryan White's home to let the teenager know he should not attend the local high school. After he died, his 6 foot 8 inch gravestone was overturned four times and a car ran over his grave!

Early on, the federal government and its public health apparatus showed little interest in the HIV/AIDS epidemic. Former president Ronald Reagan never once met with former Surgeon General C. Everett Koop to talk about AIDS despite Koop's pleas. Koop said, "If AIDS had struck legionnaires or Boy Scouts, there's no question the response would have been very different."

Misconceptions About AIDS Linger

Despite widespread reports that casual contact does not spread the virus, families have walked out of restaurants that employed gay waiters and hospital workers have quit rather than treat HIV/AIDS patients.

In 1989, a man was barred in Anderson, Indiana from coaching his daughter's intramural basketball team because he had been diagnosed with AIDS. The 37-year-old father received the virus in a blood transfusion during open heart surgery in 1984.

Each example points out that regardless of education, the public still assumes the virus can be casually transmitted. It is fear that is being transmitted by casual contact—not the virus. How would you react if a good friend, classmate, or co-worker told you he or she was HIV-positive? What if you found out that your child's schoolmate, a hemophiliac, had AIDS? What if you were told this child had emotional problems or a biting habit? What if your work put you in direct physical contact with people who might be HIV-positive?

An AIDS diagnosis for one person resulted in his physician's refusal to treat him, his roommate left him, his friends no longer visited him, his attorney, advised him to find another attorney and his clergyman failed to be there for him. They were all afraid of "catching AIDS. In another case, a mother whose young son has AIDS sent cupcakes to his classmates on his

BOX 14.2

HOW SOME PEOPLE RESPONDED AFTER LEARNING THAT SOMEONE HAD AIDS

Vignettes on Community Behavior and AIDS

In Ohio, a man was erroneously diagnosed as being HIV-infected. Within 12 days of learning the test results, he lost his job, his home, and he almost lost his wife. The error almost cost him his life: He had planned to commit suicide on the very day he received notice that he had received the wrong test results!

In Maryland, a court of appeals upheld a lower court's ruling permitting courtroom personnel to wear gloves to prevent picking up the AIDS virus. The court did suggest that the gloves were unnecessary.

In New York, a minister said that he was in a religious "Catch-22": He wanted to show concern and compassion for AIDS patients, but there are definite biblical injunctions against homosexuality. "How," he asked, "can I support these people without supporting homosexuality?"

In Florida, Mrs. Ray, the mother of three hemophilic HIV-infected sons (Ricky, 14; Robert, 13; and Randy, 12) turned to her pastor for confidential counseling. He responded by expelling the family from the congregation and announcing that the boys were infected. As a result, the boys were not allowed to go to church, school, stores, or restaurants. Barbers refused to cut their hair. Some townspeople interviewed said they were terrified at having the boys in the community. They had to move to another town! Ricky Ray died of AIDS on December 13, 1992 at age 15. Robert, age 14, was diagnosed with AIDS in 1990; Randy, age 13, was diagnosed with AIDS in May of 1993.

In Florida, Broward County parents packed school meetings and teachers filed a class action grievance saying a student's presence endangered their health. District officials determined that the 17-year-old mentally handicapped boy with AIDS would be educated by a teacher in an isolated classroom in the school. The student received 3 1/2 years of isolated education. For the 1 1/2 years , maintenance people would not walk into the portable classroom. Instead, they would leave packages or supplies in the doorway. The teacher and an assistant got used to doing their own cleaning. The one student cost over $50,000 per year to educate.

In Duval County Florida (1990), the foster parents of a 3-year-old AIDS child who was infected by his mother, were forced to leave their church because other parents insisted that the child not be allowed to attend the church nursery. The pastor went along with the majority. When presented with CDC findings that HIV is not casually transmitted, one parent scoffed. "I called the CDC for information and they asked me what I was going to use it for." He then asked the congregation, "How can you believe anyone like that?"

In California, a young man arrived home one evening to find that the locks had been changed. A few days later he discovered that everything he had ever touched had been thrown out—clothes, books, bed sheets, toothbrush, curtains, and carpeting. Even the wallpaper had been stripped from the walls and trashed. The day before, he had told his friends he had AIDS. "Overnight, I had no friends. I slept on park benches. I stole food. I passed bad checks. No one would come near me. I was told that I had 14 weeks to live."

In a second California incident, volunteer fire fighters refused to help a 1-year-old baby with AIDS at a monastery that cares for unwanted infants. The baby was reported to be choking. Although the fire department has agreed to respond to such calls in the future, one fire fighter quit, saying he was frightened because he had not been trained to deal with victims of acquired immune deficiency syndrome.

In New Jersey, a bartender could not tell his parents or friends he had AIDS. It meant confessing that he was gay. He feared it might also mean the loss of family, friends, lovers and insurance. He was expressing signs and symptoms and paying out of pocket for medical bills rather than file an insurance claim.

In Charlotte, North Carolina, 1993, a bride wore an ankle-length chiffon dress, white above and flowered black below. She'll wear the dress again, at her husband's funeral. The groom was diagnosed with progressive multifocal leukoencephalopathy (PML), a relentless viral infection that attacks the nervous system and causes brain lesions. About 4% of people with AIDS contract the disease. No treatment exists.

A legal marriage would make the groom ineligible for Medicare and Medicaid, which he can't afford to lose. So their wedding had to be symbolic and legally nonbinding.

Both wanted a wedding as a sign of commitment. He also wanted it for psychological support: It tells him that his wife will be there as things get worse.

PML has already begun to separate the newlyweds. He has developed speech problems. Sometimes he doesn't remember what he's doing.

From the wreckage, they have clutched love.

"Love is — period," she said "We don't qualify it. We don't distinguish between heterosexual and homosexual. When love is there, the physical form it takes is just a detail."

In Texas, a father with AIDS cried while praying that his three children would not be treated as cruelly. The man, in his mid-20s, was mugged because he looked too weak to fight, hit with rocks by people who found out he had AIDS, and in one incident a man broke a bottle over his head screaming that he was out to kill AIDS. During one beating, an attacker said, "After we kill you, we will kill your wife and children in case they have AIDS."

Almost daily, similar senseless acts of violence and cruelty occur across the United States as a response to AIDS. Such episodes of panic, hysteria, and prejudice are perpetuated by the very people society uses as role models: clergy, physicians, teachers, lawyers, dentists, and so on. Philosopher Jonathan Moreno said, "Plagues and epidemics like AIDS bring out the best and worst of society. Face to face with disaster and death, people are stripped down to their basic human character, to good and evil. AIDS can be a litmus test of humanity."

The Life of Ryan White

In Kokomo, Indiana, Ryan White was socially unacceptable. He was not gay, a drug user, black, or Hispanic. He was a hemophiliac; he had AIDS. His fight to become socially acceptable, to attend school, and to have the freedom to leave his home for a walk without ridicule made Ryan a national hero (Figure 14-2).

Ryan's short life was a profile in courage and understanding. Like many other people with AIDS, Ryan tried to change the public's misconception of how HIV is transmitted. Ryan suffered most from the indignities, lies, and meanness of his classmates and his classmates' parents in Kokomo, Indiana. They accused him of being a "fag," of spitting on them to infect them with the virus, and other fabrications. Ryan said he understood that this discrimination was a response of fear and ignorance. Ryan got the virus from blood and blood products essential to his survival. Ryan's wish was to be treated like any other boy, to attend school, to study, to play, to laugh, to cry, and to live each day as fully as possible. But AIDS was an integral part of his life. AIDS may not have compromised the quality of his life, as much as the residents of his community. One day, at age 16, as Ryan talked about AIDS to students in Nebraska, another boy asked Ryan how it felt knowing he was going to die. Showing the maturity that endeared him to all, Ryan replied "It's how you live your life that counts." Ryan White died, a hero of the AIDS pandemic, at 7:11 A.M. on April 8, 1990. He was 18 years old.

Gregory Herek and colleagues (1993) determined via telephone interviews that HIV/AIDS stigma is still pervasive in the United States. They interviewed 538 white adults and 607 African-Americans. Nearly all respondents indicated some stigma. Regardless of race, men were more likely than women to support preventive policies such as quarantine and said they would ***avoid*** persons with AIDS.

FIGURE 14-2 Ryan White Died on April 8, 1990. This young male became another teenage AIDS tragedy. He gained the respect of millions across the United States before he died of an AIDS-related lung infection. (*Courtesy AP/Wide World Photos*)

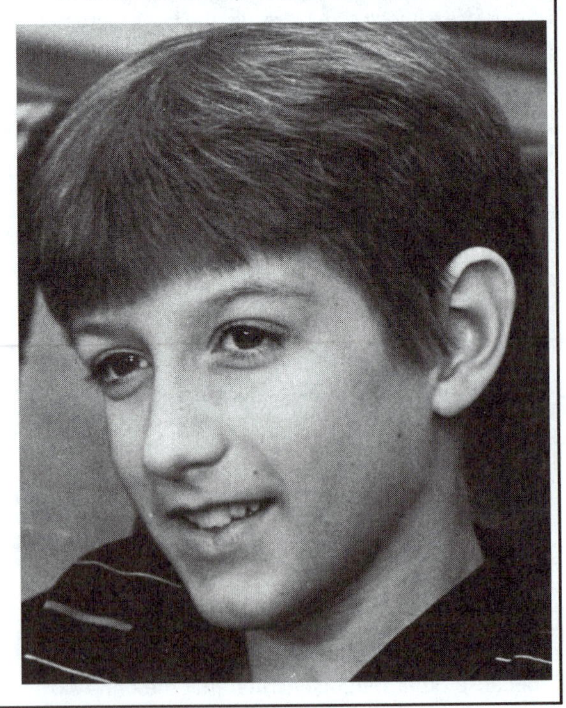

birthday. School officials would not permit the children to eat the cupcakes. The elementary school principal said the school had a policy against homemade food because it could spread diseases such as AIDS.

In Jacksonville, Florida, Leanza Cornett (Miss America 1993) using her reign as a national platform to teach about AIDS, was told by public school officials not to use the word **condom** while addressing student groups. In Bradford County, Florida she was told she could not mention the name of the disease (AIDS) in three elementary schools she planned to visit.

In Hinton, West Virginia, one woman was killed by three bullets and her body dumped along a remote road. Another was beaten to death, run over by a car, and left in the gutter. Each woman had AIDS and told people so. And each, authorities say, was killed because they had AIDS. Lawyers and advocates for AIDS patients say the similar slayings, two counties and 6 months apart, illustrate AIDS' arrival in the American countryside and the fear and ignorance it can unearth.

What Do We Know?— Mid-way through 15 years of the AIDS epidemic it is clear that the scare headlines and tactics lack substance. From what has been learned about the biology of HIV, it appears that the virus is not casually nor easily spread and will not reach the magnitude of the great plague.

The social and medical history of the AIDS epidemic parallels the syphilis epidemic. It was feared that syphilis was casually transmitted via pens, pencils, toilet seats, toothbrushes, towels, bedding, medical pro- cedures, and kissing. Immediate concern about casual transmission indicates the depth of human fears about disease and sexuality. Concerns about hygiene, contamination, contagion, pain, and death are expressions of anxieties that reveal much about contemporary society.

Fallout from AIDS— The biggest difference between HIV/AIDS and other diseases is the large amount of social discrimination. Society does not reject those with cancer, diabetes, heart disease, or any other health problems.

The AIDS pandemic has taught people about risk groups, homosexuals in particular. In some, this has promoted tolerance and understanding; in others, it has reinforced feelings of hatred. Information on HIV disease and AIDS, how it is spread and how to prevent becoming infected has, over the past 14 years, become a part of TV talk shows, movies, TV advertisements, and newspaper and magazine articles.

Phil Donohue, host of a popular TV show, said "On *Donohue,* we're discussing body cavities and membranes and anal sex and vaginal lesions. We've discussed the consequences of a woman's swallowing her partner's semen. No way would we have brought that up five years ago. It's the kind of thing that makes a lot of people gag."

The language, photography, and art work used by the media are explicit and have upset certain religious groups. They believe that open use of language about condoms, homosexuality, anal sex, oral sex, vaginal sex and so on promotes promiscuity. **Question:** How can people learn to prevent HIV infection and AIDS without talking about sexual behavior and injection drug use? Does it seem at times as if opponents of sex education would rather have people die of AIDS than have them learn about sex?

Regardless of who is correct, few could have predicted in 1980 the casualness with which these topics are presented in the media. If the AIDS pandemic has done nothing else, it surely has affected the nature of public discourse. In 1987, prior to the TV broadcast of the *National AIDS Awareness Test,* viewers were warned of objectionable material. By 1990, few if any such viewer warnings were given. It is as if to say that no one can afford to be ignorant of this information because it may save your life.

How Can Information Help?— There is great hope that information will lead the nation past its social prejudice and forward to compassion for those who are HIV-infected or have AIDS. More than any disease before, AIDS has proved that ignorance leads to fear and information can lead to compassion. The need for compassion is great.

BOX 14.3

WHEN ONE WITH AIDS COMES FORTH

Father Paul made the decision to preach on AIDS because of a phone call he had received informing him that a former parishioner was coming to Jacksonville. "George has AIDS. He will be in Church on Sunday. With your permission, he will be receiving Communion."

Father Paul granted permission and welcomed George's attendance. He sensed, however, that some might not agree to have George in church or receive Communion. In his parish a number of people refuse to believe that HIV is not transmitted by saliva from the lavitha (Communion cup).

By Sunday morning's sermon, over 60% of the congregation had learned of George.

Father Paul began his sermon, "Today's Gospel lesson, Luke 10:25-37, tells us the Parable of the Good Samaritan . . . The Parable challenges us to take stock of who our neighbors are who have needs that we can meet. . . . is it not also true that our neighbors are being harmed by AIDS? . . . Many Orthodox Christians are good about reaching out to the needy and indigent. But we are not so willing to reach out to those with AIDS."

Father Paul said that he would be dishonest if he did not admit having concerns about people receiving Communion after George. "I did not fear for myself, I feared for them, and especially for my two daughters who receive Communion regularly."

Father Paul reminded everyone about the faith of The Church. He addressed the question, "Can AIDS be contracted through casual contact and specifically from the Eucharistic Chalice?" He said, "Communion is the Body and Blood of our Lord. In the Gospel of John, chapter 6, Jesus speaks to us of His Body and Blood as being agents of life, NOT of sickness and death. Similarly, St. Ignatius of Antioch alludes to Communion as the `medicine of immortality' which allows one to eternally abide with God. To believe, therefore, that one can contract sickness and AIDS from Holy Communion is blasphemy against the Holy Spirit. It is also to render everything that the Bible and the Church teaches about Communion meaningless."

As he spoke, he saw George near the back of the Church. Though only 47 years old, George looks 60. George was weak, abnormally thin, spoke with a rasp, and walked with a cane.

Before Sunday's Liturgy, Father Paul had discussed with George his pastoral concerns about the people's anxieties. Without asking, he proposed a solution, he would receive Communion last.

Father Paul introduced George to the congregation and announced that he would be receiving last.

At Communion time, several of the congregants assisted George to the front of the church. Then, the same individuals and several others lined up behind him.

About 10 people received Communion after George. Father Paul asked one why he did it. "Father, did you not tell us in your sermon that we had to be Good Samaritans. It would have been a very unloving and discriminatory act to allow George to go last."

George died several weeks later in New York City. The news was received with sadness.

George, thank you for coming to Jacksonville. God brought you to us to help us grow. May God remember you in his Kingdom.

(Adapted with permission from Father Paul Costopoulos, Jacksonville, Florida)

FREEDOM FOR COMPASSION: CHILDREN AND AIDS

Charlie the doll was pressed against the antique glass case. Jeff, a blue-eyed, blond-haired boy of 10, looked at him closely. "Someday Charlie will leave this cage," he pondered, "and someday he will be free."

A few visits later, Jeff devised a plan to buy Charlie. He began his task by seeking employment as a leaf raker, a car washer, and the best of panhandlers among friends. After a while his hope faded and his energy waned, but he did not despair. He had met adversity before, in fact, for most of his life. When Jeff was 4 years old, he had contracted AIDS.

The family of John Calvin Presbyterian Church met Jeff because other congregations had turned him away, telling his family that Jeff's illness was a punishment from God. Jeff planned his own memorial service, but five different congregations ignored him by making excuses that the songs he had chosen from the play, "Peter Pan," and the balloons he had requested would not be appropriate.

One Sunday morning as I was beginning my sermon, Jeff's mother wheeled him down the main aisle to a front pew. I wondered what would happen if this church rejected him, too? How would the other children treat him? Could this congregational family risk enough to love Jeff and his family in the same way in which God loved them? But my fears were relieved after church at the coffee fellowship. Parents introduced themselves to Jeff's mother and the children included Jeff within their circle of games. People earnestly gathered to accompany Jeff and his family on their special journey: members ran errands, provided transportation, and brought in food. This outpouring of help came at a crucial time: Jeff's mother had given up her own business to take care of Jeff, emotional pressures contributed to Jeff's parents' divorce, the family lost their home to bankruptcy court, and Jeff's brother and sister suffered from the prejudice of schoolmates and others.

A few weeks prior to Jeff's death, I bought Charlie the doll. As Jeff's fragile hands began to untie the shiny silver ribbon that secured the purple box, large tears began to trickle down his sunken cheeks. When he discovered what was inside, Jeff smiled and said, "Now he's free . . . and someday I will be, too."

Jeff's freedom arrived on March 2, 1988. Those of us who knew him have gained freedom as well. Jeff, and others, have introduced us to a new appreciation of life. Through them we have been reminded of how fragile we are and of our precious responsibility to live each moment fully. Together we have discovered the gift that no person, no circumstance, no condition—even the AIDS virus—can take from us. We have discovered God's gift to us in Jesus Christ.

John Calvin Presbyterian Church is now a better-educated congregation. Jeff helped to teach us the importance of risking and reaching out. Our church has adopted a resolution stating that we are committed to minister intentionally with people with AIDS and their families. We provide office space to the Tampa AIDS Network, an advocacy, support, and fund-raising group serving the Tampa Bay area. A number of members and I are part of a growing coalition of volunteers serving on task forces, care-giving programs, and support groups.

In the midst of our congregation's activity we are still keenly aware of the continuing apathy, ignorance, and prejudice permeating much of the religious community. Many underestimate the possibility of this disease intruding into their lives and communities. Much work remains to be done with few to accomplish it.

Jeff's memorial service was just as he had planned it. The sanctuary of the church was filled with the nurses and doctors who had worked with him, the many hospice volunteers who had given him solace, his buddies from the Tampa AIDS Network who had held his hand, the many other friends he had made on his journey. Hundreds of brightly colored helium balloons were released into the sky at the end of the service. We celebrated Jeff's life—and ours as well. Our celebration continues as we minister with others who are traveling this very difficult path. Our strength and hope are renewed with each encounter, for we have been given the freedom for compassion.

(Adapted from Rev. Jim Hedges, pastor of John Calvin Presbyterian Church, Tampa, Florida, in *Church and Society,* Vol. 79, No. 3(January/ February 1989). Reprinted with permission.)

Admiral James Watkins, Chairman of the 1988 Presidential Commission on the HIV Epidemic, reported that "33% to 50% of physicians in some of our major hospitals would not touch an AIDS patient with a ten-foot pole."

A friend of a dying AIDS patient who was in the hospital with pneumocystic pneumonia went to visit him. As he was leaving, his dying friend said, "Thank you for coming—thank you for touching me." He said, "I can't even imagine being at a point in my life that I would be so grateful for someone touching me, that I would have to say thank you."

It would appear that although biotechnology has provided methods of HIV detection, new drugs, and hope for a vaccine, human emotional responses have not changed much from those demonstrated during previous epidemics like the plague, cholera, influenza, and syphilis.

AIDS EDUCATION AND BEHAVIOR

> I said education was our "basic weapon." Actually it's our *only* weapon. We've got to educate everyone about the disease so that each person can take responsibility for seeing that it is spread no further.
>
> C. Everett Koop
> Former U.S. Surgeon General

BOX 14.4

THE WAY WE ARE

The young man worked alongside a 35-year-old woman helping to teach the disabled to function. She was very attractive with a wonderful sense of humor He watched her every movement - he was in love from a distance; she inspired him to new heights in his work and thoughts about his future. She understood his emotions so she was not surprised when, after work one evening, he offered dinner and a moonlight walk around the lake. During the walk, she could tell from the conversation that his young hormones were flowing - as were her own. In the awkwardness of saying goodnight she said, "I know you want me - I would like that very much." As his broad face glowed she said, "I must share something with you. I have been diagnosed with AIDS but there are no outward signs yet." The love that moments before surged through his body crashed down around him; he felt ill yet sympathetic - his urge for sex vanished. He could not bring himself to look at her as he said, "Please forgive me, I just can't." She nodded her understanding and explained it was either a blood transfusion in 1984 following an auto accident or death. "I made the choice for life and whatever comes with it." The young man cried as he walked home. He left the job the next morning.

The goals of educating people about HIV infection and AIDS are to promote social understanding and to prevent HIV transmission. To achieve these goals, accurate information must be provided that makes people aware of their risk status. People at minimum risk can continue their sexual lifestyles. People at high risk should determine their HIV status, alter behaviors, and practice safer sex.

This sounds so easy: Educate people and they will do the right thing. **Wrong.** Knowledge does not guarantee sufficient motivation to change sexual behavior or mitigate the biological urge to have sex. Education has not stopped teenage pregnancy, nor has the threat of lung cancer stopped people from smoking.

Perhaps the reason education is not as effective as it could be is because the public receives its education by daily doses from the mass media. With so much going on in the world, people have become more or less dependent on the media for information essential to their well being. Gordon Nary (1990) said, "The public wants to know what's right or wrong in five three-second images or 25 words or less. It wants simple problems with simple solutions. It wants *Star Wars* with good and evil absolutely defined. The media often responds to these demands."

Mathew Lefkowitz (1990) says that the word AIDS has been infused with an irrational fear that has nothing to do with the illness. He states that the word AIDS has been politicized in such a way that it can and has been used as a weapon. Lefkowitz relates the parallel between today's use of the word AIDS with Eugene Ionosco's classic absurdist play *The Lesson.* In the play, a professor stabs a girl to death with the word *knife*—not with a knife but with the *word knife.* It appears that today the word *AIDS* is being used to stab those whom we fear; namely the HIV-infected. How long will it take the educational process to work? *The virus is not as much our enemy as ourselves.*

Public AIDS Education Programs

The 1988 Presidential Commission on the Human Immunodeficiency Virus Epidemic stated

> No citizen of our nation is exempt from the need to be educated about the HIV epidemic. The real challenge lies in matching the right educational approach with the right people. During the last year, there has been a great deal of debate over the content of HIV/AIDS education. The Commission is concerned that, in the promotion of the personal, moral and political values of those from both ends of the political spectrum, the consistent distribution of clear, factual information about HIV transmission has suffered. HIV/AIDS education programs, for example, should not encourage promiscuous sexual activity; however, they need to be explicit in nature so that there is no confusion about how to avoid acquiring or transmitting the virus. The Commission firmly believes that it is possible to develop educational materials and programs that clearly convey an explicit message without promoting high-risk behaviors.

West Coast health officials told this same Presidential Commission that the censorship of sexually explicit materials is hampering the fight against AIDS. Many of those who testified before the Commission expressed frustration about the barriers posed by government bureaucracy. Several representatives of AIDS organizations told commissioners of the difficulties they have experienced in trying to produce effective educational materials and programs. They said that state officials prohibit the use of certain language when they fund educational programs. It is sometimes necessary, however, to use slang or sexually explicit language in order for readers to understand the material. As an example, they cited women who had given birth but claimed they had never had "vaginal intercourse." They did not know what *vaginal* meant, but they did know what *cunt* meant. Educational material must use colloquial or recognizable language to be effective.

Over the years many millions of dollars have been spent by federal and state health departments to inform the public about cardiovascular risks, health risks associated with sexually transmitted diseases (STDs), smoking and lung cancer, chewing tobacco and oral cancer, drug addiction, alcohol consumption, and seat belt use to name just a few. In some cases these campaigns were eventually supported by specific state and federal legislation. Tobacco advertisements were outlawed on TV and drivers in some states who are not buckled up must pay a fine. But even with laws to support these educational programs, the majority of adults have failed to change established behavior patterns. In the larger cities, educators must combat the fear that AIDS is a government conspiracy to eliminate society's "undesirables"—minorities, drug addicts, and homosexuals. They must overcome cultural and religious barriers that prevent people from using condoms to protect themselves.

Another problem is that educational programs are not preventing individuals from acquiring one or more STDs, using drugs, drinking to excess, driving drunk, failing to use seat belts or motorcycle helmets, and smoking. It might also be added that there have always been educational programs against crime, but in 1989–1990 more new jails were built in the United States than ever before. And this expanding jail-building program continues! In short, educational programs on TV, radio, in newspapers, and in the popular press have achieved only limited success in changing peoples' behavior.

It is not that education is unimportant; it is essential for those who will use it! But that is the catch. Although education must be available for those who will use it, too few, relatively speaking, are using the available education for their maximum benefit. In general, people, especially young adults, *do not do what they know.* They sometimes do what they see, but most often do what they feel. In short, knowledge in itself may be necessary but it is insufficient for behavioral change. A variety of studies have failed to show a consistent link between knowledge and preventive behaviors (Fisher, 1992; Phillips, 1993)

Costs Related to Prevention— The assertion that spending more money on educational programs will ensure disease prevention for the masses, as the examples given above suggest, may not be the case. In particular, peoples' behaviors regarding the prevention of HIV infection do not appear to be changing sig- nificantly despite the many millions of dollars being used to produce, distribute, and promote HIV/AIDS education. The major educational thrust is directed at how not to become HIV-infected. Most of this information is being given out to people from age 13 and up.

The problem with AIDS education is that communicating the information is relatively easy but changing behavior, particularly addictive and/or pleasurable behavior, is quite difficult. Most cigarette abusers know that smoking causes lung cancer and would like to quit or have tried to quit. Likewise, many alcoholics have tried to quit. But both cigarettes and alcohol are pleasurable to those who use them. The mass media have provided near saturation coverage of key AIDS issues and it is very unlikely that significant numbers of future HIV infections in the United States will occur in individuals who did not know the virus was transmitted through sexual contact and IV drug use. Yet new infections and AIDS cases continue to increase.

POINT OF VIEW 14.1

THE RED RIBBON

We were sitting in a small Italian restaurant. I had just come back to town from a presentation on AIDS. The jacket I wore still had the red ribbon on the lapel. As we enjoyed our meal I noticed a woman at the next table who appeared to be glaring at me and making statements to her companion. At one point her voice became loud enough for us to hear her say, "I am sick and tired of those people trying to push the lifestyle of homosexuals down our throats" as she was looking right at me. She then said, "That red ribbon is a sign of a sick person trying to make all of us sick too. That ribbon and all that it stands for ruins my day." With that she and her companion left the restaurant.

That outburst left my family and me embarrassed and confused. My children deserved an explanation. I don't think I have even explained the idea of the red ribbon to anyone before. Like so many things we observe in life, after a while they become understood by each in his or her own way. This woman expressed her way rather forcefully. To my children I said that the ribbon is a symbol to call attention to a social problem that needs a solution. I went on to say, "Do you recall the song 'Tie A Yellow Ribbon Round the Old Oak Tree' in 1973 and what that meant? And, do you recall the ribbons tied around trees, on car antennas, mailboxes and so on while our 56 service men were held captives in Iran in 1980 and again for out captives in the 1991 Persian Gulf War? Remember the first lady Nancy Reagan's campaign using red ribbons for 'Just say no to drugs' and more recently the pink ribbons for women against breast cancer and most recently the purple ribbons for stoppng violence in our schools? These are all symbolic gestures to show support for those enduring suffering and pain. All of the ribbons then and now serve to connect people emotionally, to help unite people in a common cause, to help people feel less isolated in a crisis."

I explained to my children that the problem with the red ribbon now is similar to what occurred over the long time period our soldiers were in captivity—people begin to wear the ribbon as an accessory.

Evidence accumulated between 1983 and 1987 indicates that homosexual and bisexual males modified their sexual behavior and this resulted in a drop in AIDS cases among them. There is also evidence that some IDUs have begun wearing condoms. But recent evidence suggests that some of these people are being drawn back to their former practice of unprotected sex and needle sharing. The disease is showing signs of a resurgence in the gay community as health workers struggle to get their message to a new generation and to older gays who seem to have lost the motivation to protect themselves.

In 1982, there were 18 new HIV infections for every 100 uninfected gay men in San Francisco. That rate dropped to 1 per 100 in 1987 but rose to 2 per 100 in 1993. For gay men younger than 25, it is 4 per 100.

Although humans are capable of dramatic behavioral changes, it is not known what really initiates the change or how to speed up the process.

BOX 14.5

ANECDOTE: FATHER AND SON EXCHANGE SEX INFORMATION

"Son, I think it's time we had a talk about sex." "O.K., Dad, what do you want to know?"

Public School AIDS Education

Some information relevant to AIDS education can be learned from educational programs that have been designed to reduce pregnancy and the spread of STDs among teenagers. However, data from a variety of high school sex education classes offered across the country indicate that teenagers are learning the essential facts but they are not practicing what they learn. **They do not do what they know.**

Risky sexual behavior is widespread among teenagers and has resulted in high rates of STDs. Over 25% of the 12 million STD cases

BOX 14.6

HIV-RELATED BELIEFS, KNOWLEDGE, AND BEHAVIOR AMONG HIGH SCHOOL STUDENTS

"Education concerning AIDS must start at the lowest grade possible as part of any health and hygiene program. The appearance of AIDS should bring together diverse groups of parents and educators with opposing views on the inclusion of sex education in the curricula. There is now no doubt that we need sex education in schools and that it must include information on heterosexual and homosexual relationships. The threat of AIDS should be sufficient to permit a sex education curriculum with heavy emphasis on prevention of AIDS and other sexualy transmitted diseases."

Up to 500,000, of those infected with HIV in the United States are **under** the age of 25, making HIV/AIDS a major concern for young adults. About 20%, or one in five people, who have AIDS are in their twenties. A large proportion of these individuals become infected during adolescence. It is clearly time to place a special emphasis on teenagers and AIDS.

Reported data suggest that HIV-related beliefs, knowledge, and behaviors among the students surveyed in 32 states and 10 cities in 1990 were generally similar in 1994. Many students incorrectly thought that HIV infection could be acquired from giving blood, using public toilets, having a blood test, and from mosquito or other insect bites. Most students knew intercourse and injection drug use could result in HIV infection.

State Mandated Policy on HIV/AIDS Education

Elementary and secondary school students in Nevada need written permission from their parents to participate in the state-mandated HIV and AIDS education program. In Minnesota, state law requires schools to target high-risk adolescents for education programs. But in California, where the incidence of AIDS is second highest in the country, an AIDS education law has not been passed.

These three policies represent the broad spectrum of approaches states have been taking toward HIV and AIDS education through 1993. By the end of 1993, at least 32 states had mandated some form of HIV/AIDS education in their school systems. Twenty-eight of these states determined that such education must be given during regularly scheduled classes in health, family life, or sex education. Only Washington state mandates that HIV/AIDS is to be presented specifically as part of a required course on sexually transmitted disease. Seven states do not, by law, specify the context in which HIV and AIDS education is to be presented (Voelker, 1989). Without a statewide policy, school districts may devise their own HIV/AIDS curricula. Because of a lack of national policy, students are receiving different HIV/AIDS educations. For example, even though 20 states require discusssion of HIV/AIDS prevention and 18 states stipulate that sexual abstinence be stressed, only three require discussion of condom use and only two require a discussion of homosexuality. Seven states require giving information on the risks of IV drug use and sharing needles.

Fourteen of the 32 states have requirements for training or for the credentialing of instructors who will teach HIV/AIDS programs. While some require unspecified training for the "appropriate" staff, others require teachers to have completed specialized in-service training. Nine states require some in-service training for school employees' the requirements vary from specialized health education training to attending annual AIDS awareness programs. In 1990, the CDC gave an average of $250,000 to each state to develop HIV and AIDS education programs, but only seven education departments received funds from their state budgets.

per year occur among teenagers. One teenager is infected with an STD every 30 seconds in the United States. One in six teens has been infected with an STD. Over 50% of sexually active teenagers (11 million) report having had two or more sexual partners; and fewer than half say they used a condom the first time they had intercourse (Kirby, 1988). A National Research Council panel (1989) stated that 75% of all female teenagers had sexual experience and that 15% had four or more partners.

Teenage Perceptions About AIDS and HIV Infection in the United States— A recent survey run by People magazine indicated that 96% of high school students and 99% of college students knew that HIV is spreading through the heterosexual population; but the majority of these students stated that they continued to practice unsafe sex. Combined data from surveys performed in 1988-1989 indicate that among sexually active teenagers, only 25% used a condom. Peter Jennings stated in a February, 1991, AIDS Update TV program that 26% of American teenagers practice anal intercourse. Data such as these have prompted a number of medical and research people to express concern for the next generation. If HIV becomes widespread among today's teenagers, there is a real danger of losing tomorrow's adults. Available data suggest that teenagers have not appreciably changed their sexual behaviors in response to HIV/AIDS information presented in their schools or from other sources (Kegeles et al., 1988).

Teenagers at high risk include some 200,000 who become prostitutes each year and others who become IDUs. About 1% of high school seniors have used heroin and many from junior high on up have tried cocaine (Kirby, 1988). A large number of children from age 10 up consume alcohol. Is it possible that too much hope is being placed on education to prevent the spread of HIV? Through mid-1995, teenagers made up about 0.5% of 476,500 AIDS cases, or about 2,383 cases. Teenagers must be convinced that they are vulnerable to HIV infection and death. Until then, it only happens to someone else. Jonathan Mann, past director of the World Health Organization estimates that worldwide, 1993, there were between 1 and 2 million HIV-infected teenagers.

Teenagers, like adults, must be convinced of their risk of infection but not with scare tactics. Behavior modification as a result of a scare is short lived. However the information is given, it must be internalized if it is to be of long-term benefit.

College Students— Everyone must know and act on the fact that a wrong decision about having sexual intercourse can take away the future. For example, a young college student had a 3-year nonsexual friendship with a local bartender. She was bright, well educated, and acutely aware of AIDS. After drinks one evening, as their friendship progressed towards sexual intercourse, she asked him if he was "straight" (a true heterosexual) and he said yes. But he was a bisexual! It was a single sexual encounter. She graduated and left town. She found out that the bartender died of AIDS 3 years later. She did not think much of it until she was diagnosed with AIDS 5 years after their affair. This young, talented, bright, and personable girl lost her future. This brings home the point that it is difficult to change something as complex as personal sexual behavior regardless of knowledge. It also brings up at least one other important point in personal relationships: telling the truth.

During the 1988 Psychological Association Convention, the following facts were presented with respect to telling the truth or lying in order to have sex. The data come from a survey of 482 sexually experienced southern California college students:

1. 35% of the men and 10% of the women said they had lied in order to have sex.
2. 47% of the men and 60% of the women reported they had been told a lie in order to have sex.
3. 20% of the men and 4% of the women said they would say they had a negative HIV test in order to have sex.
4. 42% of the men and 33% of the women said they would never admit a one-time sexual affair to their long-term partner.

Adult Perceptions About HIV Infection and AIDS in the United States— R.J. Blendon and colleague (1988) summarized the results of telephone surveys and personal interviews with a large number of adults. They provide an insight into adult knowledge and emotions regarding transmission of the AIDS virus. The data may also serve as a potential indicator for discrimination against HIV-infected people. Of the adults surveyed:

General Public—

1. Over 50% felt that the AIDS pandemic has lead to increased homophobia (fear of homosexuals) and discrimination.
2. 10% actively avoided social contact with homosexuals.
3. 20% said AIDS was punishment against immoral homosexual behavior and that the punishment was deserved.
4. 29% said HIV-infected people should wear a tattoo or other means of identification to warn the public.
5. 30% supported the idea of quarantine for HIV-infected and AIDS patients.
6. 40% believed that HIV-infected school employees should be fired.
7. 33% said they would keep their child out of school if a student there were HIV-infected or had AIDS.

The Workplace— AIDS can have a variety of impacts in the workplace. The obvious one, of course, is on the individual employee who is diagnosed with HIV. The probability of sickness and death obviously affects the individual and his or her ability to continue to contribute to the organization's activities and goals.

Employees fear AIDS can create a widespread loss of teamwork and productivity, and create an environment that is inhumane and insensitive toward the infected employee.

As the incidence of HIV and AIDS increases, the impact on organizations will obviously increase as well. While there are important logical and moral reasons for ensuring that infected people are not discriminated against, there are also practical reasons for addressing the employee HIV/AIDS problem.

An educated work force, aware of the facts regarding diagnosis, testing, treatment, and transmission of HIV, can have a positive impact on the overall health of all employees. People are more inclined to openly acknowledge their HIV status and to seek treatment when assured of a supportive workplace environment. This increases productivity.

The results of a survey of people in the workplace by Blendon and Donelan (1988) revealed that:

1. 25% believed HIV was transmitted by coughing, spitting and sneezing.
2. 20% believed HIV infection could occur from a drinking fountain or toilet seat.
3. 10% believed touching an HIV-infected or AIDS patient was dangerous.
4. 25% refused to work with an HIV-infected or AIDS person.
5. 25% believed employers should be able to fire people who were HIV-infected or had AIDS.

Whether additional public education will change these attitudes over time is unknown. The Surgeon General's brochure, "Understanding AIDS" (Figure 14-3), was sent to 107,000,000 homes in 1988 at a cost of 22 million dollars. Fifty-one percent of those who received the pamphlet did not read it because they did not remember getting it or they chose to ignore it (Eickhoff, 1989).

A recent Georgia Tech survey found that workers who received educational brochures or pamphlets about the disease were more likely to have negative feelings toward HIV-infected co-workers than employees who received no information. The results suggest companies should be more concerned about the kind of messages workers receive. By focusing only on practices that can transmit the disease, many educational materials neglect to deal with the social, emotional, and humanitarian aspects of the problem. Edu-cation may be the key, but we need to look closely at what kind of education that should be.

THE CHARACTER OF SOCIETY

Rumors of Destruction

Today, friends are asked on street corners, at social gatherings, or over telephones: "Did you hear that he/she has AIDS?" Or: "Do you believe that he/she might be infected? You never know with the life they lead!" Some of the famous people *rumored* to have HIV/AIDS are Madonna, Elizabeth Taylor, Burt Reynolds, Richard Pryor, and Joe Penny from the TV show *Jake and the Fatman.*

Rumors ruin lives. People suddenly subtly lose services; the lawn boy quits, no reason

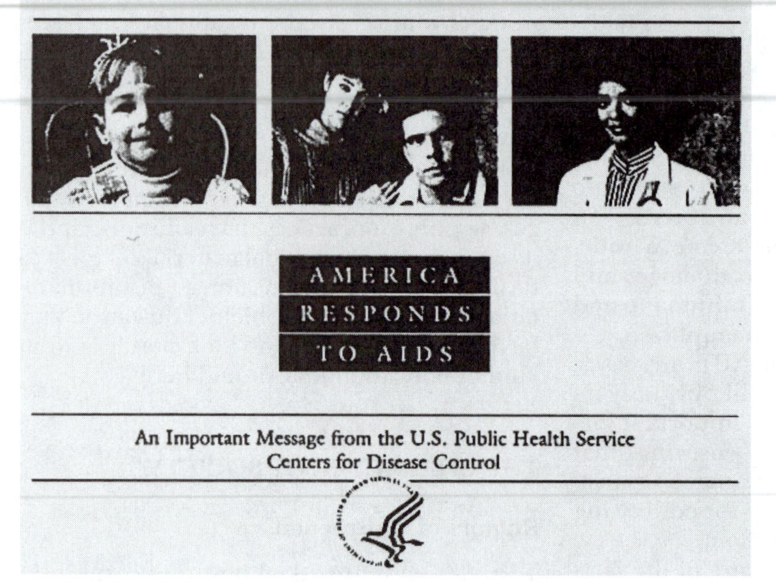

FIGURE 14-3 Understanding AIDS. This public health pamphlet contains eight pages of HIV/AIDS information. It was sent to 107million homes in the United States in 1988. Fifty-one percent of those who received the pamphlet did not read it!

given. Quietly job applications are turned down or car and homeowner insurance policies are canceled, and so on. In one case, after rumors of HIV infection spread in a small town, a man, if he was served in local bars at all, received his drinks in plastic cups. A health club refunded his membership dues. His apartment manager asked him to leave and when his toilet backed up the maintenance man came in wearing a hat over a World War II gas mask, deep water fishing boots, raincoat, and rubber gloves. In frustration, he had an HIV test. The results were negative and he gave copies of the test to every "joint" in town, his

POINT OF VIEW 14.2

THE RIGHT TO PRIVACY

Arthur Ashe died of AIDS in February of 1993; he was *forced* to go public about having AIDS. Did that affect his life? Yes. He had to alter a lifestyle he was trying to live with his family. He could no longer live a normal day with his family.

The immediate defense from the press, which forced Arthur Ashe to go public, is that it serves the public interest to identify prominent people with AIDS. The news media says that it increases awareness—and therefore, theoretically, action—to fight back against AIDS. *Do you agree?*

Organizations can write and broadcast about HIV/AIDS any time, about anybody they want to. *Is this morally right?*

Some defenders of the news media say that a public figure cannot have it both ways—cannot deliberately keep himself in the limelight with sports-equipment endorsements, and so forth, and then turn around and say, "I want to be a private person." But what is public and what is private?

As Ellen Hume asks, "Is there no moment of a public figure's life that is not open to prurient exposure? Does being a political officeholder or, as in Ashe's case, a sports champion, mean that the public owns all of your life, including your life in the bedroom, the doctor's office, the church confessional or the psychiatrist's couch?" *What is your reply to her?*

Ms. Hume asks, "Should journalists end their scrutiny of public figures?" She thinks not. But she says, "Not every revelation serves the public interest. No American president and few athletes, astronauts, journalists or other heroes could have survived this Spanish Inquisition. Isn't it time for the press to develop a more sophisticated sense of priorities and ethics to go along with its extraordinary new power?" *What is your reply?*

physician, dentist, theater manager, grocery store manager... He felt this approach was better than running. **Do you agree?**

In another case in Brantly County, Georgia, population 11,077, the 22-year-old mother of a 2-year-old son was the subject of a rumor that she was HIV-infected. The rumor also stated that she had had intercourse with 200 men in the past year. To convince the townspeople, she took the HIV test and was not HIV-infected. This young woman had to circulate the results of her blood test around town, but it was still not enough to stop the rumor. A newspaper in nearby Waycross quoted an unnamed source saying that this woman was HIV-positive. The rumor goes on!

There was the case of a compassionate person who opened a home for helping AIDS patients. Rumor quickly spread that the entire neighborhood was in danger, especially after the mail carrier refused to deliver mail and was ordered to wear rubber gloves and return to the post office for disinfection! To help the neighborhood understand AIDS and stop unfounded fears, a seminar was held at the AIDS home, but no one would enter the house.

A young person with AIDS reluctantly returned home—it meant revealing that he was gay to his family—and to the community. He said to his parents, "I have good news and bad. The bad is that I'm gay. The good is I have AIDS. I won't be around long enough to interfere with anyone." Once the word got out a catering service refused to do the annual family Christmas party They could not hire a practical nurse. Family and friends who used to drop in stayed away. People whispered that the son had gay cancer . . . that it was lethal . . . that it could be caught from dishes, linens, a handshake and breathing in the same air he breathed out.

In Athens, Alabama, the headline of the town's newspaper read, "Athens doctor: 'I don't have AIDS.'" This doctor, a prominent pediatrician in this town for 18 years, had to produce a public defense to dispel the gossip that he had AIDS. Because in a small town everybody knows everybody, the rumor spread with lightning speed to the town hospital, grocery store, hair salon, school, newspaper, and so on. The doctor offered a $2000 reward for any information about who began the rumor. To date no one has collected the money, but the townspeople have gathered to support him.

Mathilde Krim of the American Foundation of AIDS Research said, "From the beginning, the people with AIDS have been a disposable group—gays, blacks and drug users. People don't care about them. They'd rather they wouldn't be here anyway." When

BOX 14.7

ORPHANED CHILDREN DUE TO AIDS AND HIV INFECTION

An increasing number of HIV-infected children are being left in hospitals because their HIV-infected mothers and fathers are unable to care for them and no one else wants them. The hospital becomes their home. James Hegarty and colleagues (1988) reported that for 37 children at Harlem Hospital Center, one third of the total in-patient days and over 20% of the cost was for social rather than medical services. By the end of 1994, there were an estimated 24,000 AIDS-related orphan children in the state of New York.

As HIV continues to spread across the nation and HIV-infected women continue to become pregnant, the question is: What will happen to their HIV-infected babies? For one young woman who passed the AIDS virus to her baby 2 years ago, the decision has been made. The baby has AIDS and is in foster care. The mother is very ill. The courts are now deciding whether her six other children should also be put in foster care.

David Michaels and Carol Levine (1994) indicate that by the end of 1995, an estimated 24,600 children, 21,000 adolescents, and 35,100 young adults in the United States will have been orphaned by the HIV/AIDS epidemic. An estimated 13% of children and 9% of adolescents whose mothers died in 1991 lost their mothers to AIDS. More youths now lose their mothers to AIDS than to motor vehicle injuries. Unless the course of the epidemic changes drastically, by the year 2000, the cumulative number of U.S. children, teens, and young adults left motherless due to AIDS will exceed 144,000. The great majority of these children, uninfected by the virus—will begin to affect already burdened social services in major American cities. Things will get immediately worse in such places, where children already spend years going from foster home to foster home and caseworkers are overwhelmed by long lists of families needing everything from housing to medical care. Using the same projections, as many as 98,000 young people 18 and older will become motherless and in some cases be called upon to care for younger family members.

Orphans are often referred to as the **silent legacy** of AIDS. It is expected that about a third of the children orphaned will be from New York City, which has the nation's largest number of AIDS cases. Other cities expected to be hit hard are Miami, Los Angeles, Washington, Newark, and San Juan, Puerto Rico. Most of these orphans will be the children of poor black or Hispanic women whose families are already dealing with stresses like drug addiction, inadequate housing, and health care. Relatives who might in other circumstances be called upon to care for the children often shun them because of the stigma attached to AIDS.

ADOPTION ADVERTISEMENTS FOR PARENTS WITH AIDS

"AIDS. Kids. If you have both, maybe it's time to take a closer look at adoption. Call 1–800–NCFA" (National Council For Adoption). This is the shortest of the public service announcements that began in January of 1995.

The areas targeted by the ads are those with the highest incidence of AIDS cases. The ads have prompted hundreds of calls from people wanting to adopt.

The number of U. S. children orphaned by AIDS is estimated at around 35,000. By the year 2000 health officials say there will be between 70,000 and 145,000 AIDS orphans.

For additional information on pediatric HIV/AIDS research and community help, write The Pediatric AIDS Foundation, 2407 Wilshire Blvd., Suite 613, Dept. P, Santa Monica, CA 90403.

the National Gay Rights Advocates asked the nation's 1,000 biggest companies whether employee medical plans covered AIDS-related expenses, one anonymous answer read, "Just enough to defray the cost of the bullet." However, HIV has spread to infect most other groups of society and attitudes are slowly changing.

Good News, Bad News, and Late News

Good News— Good news is thinking and believing you're HIV-infected and you're not. There must be a reason to think you're infected, so not being infected is, as some would say, a new lease on life. All too often that feeling is soon forgotten and many people continue lifestyles that place them at risk for infection.

Bad News— Bad news is thinking you're HIV-infected and you are. It is difficult to predict what a person sees, hears, or does after being told he or she is HIV-positive. For example, some have contemplated suicide, some have committed suicide, others have become completely fatalistic and proceeded to live a reckless and careless lifestyle that endangered others. Some have said it's like death before you're dead.

You are never prepared to hear the bad news regardless of how sure you are that you're infected. For example, one man who had suffered from night sweats, fevers, weight loss, and other classic symptoms just knew he was infected. Yet when told of the positive test results he said "I got so angry, I ripped a shower out of the wall." Being told you are infected is totally devastating, said another infected person. "You feel that everyone is looking at you, everyone can tell you're dirty." Another person said, "The fact that I'm HIV-positive completely dominates my life. There is not a waking hour that I do not think about it. I feel like a leper. I live between hope and despair." Still another said, "I did not leave the house for two days after being told I was HIV-positive. The initial shock was that I was contaminated—unhealthy, soiled, unclean. I carried this burden in isolation for over two years. After all, I had met people who had AIDS but never a person who said—I'm HIV-infected."

The bad news is not confined to those hearing they are HIV-infected; it touches everyone they know—lovers, family, friends, and employers. Nothing remains the same. The more symptomatic one becomes, the greater the social and human loss. One symptomatic mother said, "Whenever I tell my four-year-old I am going to the doctor, he screams because he knows I could be gone for weeks." I try to put him in another room playing with his sister when they come for me." This woman has died. Relatives care for her children.

Late News— Late news is remaining **asymptomatic** after infection. Asymptomatic can be defined as when no clinically recognizable symptoms appear that would indicate HIV infection. During this time period, the virus can be transmitted to sexual partners. By the time either antibodies and/or clinical symptoms appear, the news is too late for those who might have been spared infection had their sexual partner tested positive or demonstrated clinical symptoms early on.

When People Pretend to Be HIV-Positive or to Have AIDS

Donald Craven (1994) reported that a growing number of people may pretend to have AIDS either because of emotional disorders or because they want to gain access to free housing, medical care, and disability income. In one case, seven patients with self-reported HIV infection were treated for an average of 9.2 months in a clinical AIDS program before their sero-negative status was discovered at the hospital (in general, hospitals in the United States do not require a written copy of the HIV test results proving that someone is HIV-positive). Craven noted that "because patients with AIDS often have preferred access to drug treatment, prescription drugs, social security disability insurance, housing and comprehensive medical care, the rate of malingering may increase and reach extremes."

Another doctor who treats many AIDS patients said that he and his colleagues have seen many patients who repeatedly come to their offices fearing that they have AIDS, even though multiple tests have shown that they do not.

An Oklahoma physician has written about the AIDS Munchausen's syndrome—an emotional disorder in which people pretend to have the disease simply to get attention from doctors. Confidentiality requirements makes AIDS a "perfect" illness for people suffering from Munchausen syndrome, because the laws shield them from being discovered.

Physicians' Public Duty: A Historical Perspective of Professional Obligation

Physicians enjoy a virtual monopoly on medical care, social status, and generous financial remuneration. Thus the medical profession is uniquely entrusted with the knowledge to care for those with HIV disease/AIDS or any other contagious disease and has a clear responsibility to do so, absent compelling considerations to the contrary. A fair and reasonable share of medical risk just naturally goes with the professional territory.

Robert Fulton and Greg Owen (1988) stated that throughout history, plagues and pestilences have challenged humankind. In his book, *Plagues and People,* William McNeill (1976) cited the many death-dealing epidemics in Europe. He wrote that one advantage the West had over the East in the face of deadly epidemics was that caring for the sick was a recognized duty among Christians. The effect of a prolonged epidemic more often than not strengthened the Church when other social institutions were discredited for not providing needed services. McNeill further observed that the teachings of Christianity made life meaningful, even in the immediate face of death: Not only would survivors find spiritual consolation in the vision of heavenly reunion with their dead relatives or friends, but God's hand was also seen in the work of the life-risking caregivers.

The United States has also had its share of plagues and epidemics; one of the most notable was the outbreak of yellow fever in Philadelphia in 1793. Thousands of citizens of the capital city perished. William Powell (1965), in his book *Bring Out Your Dead,* describes Philadelphia at the time of the yellow fever plague: the dying were abandoned, the dead left unburied, orphaned children and the elderly wandered the streets in search of food and shelter. Nearly all who could fled the city, including the President, leaving the victims of the fever to their fate. Among those who remained, however, were Benjamin Rush, M.D., the mayor, a handful of medical colleagues and their assistants, and a number of clergy. With the help of a small group of laborers and craftsmen, they undertook the enormous tasks of maintaining law and order, providing medical care, food and shelter to the sick and helpless, as well as gathering up and burying the dead.

Dr. Rush and the others remained at their posts because of their overriding sense of professional obligation along with a conviction inspired by the precept of the New Testament "Blessed are the merciful, for they shall obtain mercy" (Matthew 5:9).

But this vision, shared by Christians for centuries, along with a sense of professional commitment, may not be sufficient to persuade contemporary health care workers to stay at their posts.

The baby boom generation, well-educated and self-oriented, has learned to blame AIDS on groups whom society defines as deviant: homosexuals, prostitutes, and drug abusers. There is a significant probability, therefore, that today's young health care practitioner may turn away from HIV/AIDS patients despite the fact that a 1981 Gallup Poll of the religious beliefs and practices of 14 countries showed that the United States leads the world not only in church membership but also in charitable services.

According to an article in the November 13, 1987, issue of *The Wall Street Journal,* Arthur Caplan, a director for the Center of Biomedical Ethics at the University of Minnesota in Minneapolis, believes that doctors and nurses who refuse to treat AIDS patients do so out of disapproval. "They know how to deal with violent patients and infectious diseases like hepatitis." So why not treat someone with AIDS? "It's more than fear. They're making a value . . . judgment about AIDS victims. They're saying they won't treat people (they find) disgusting." Others refuse to place their lives at risk for someone who became HIV-infected through immoral behavior. C. Everett Koop said the refusal by some medical personnel to treat AIDS patients "threatens the very fabric of health care in this country." *Do you agree?*

Medical Moral Issues

HIV/AIDS represents a new era in medicine, one in which physicians are faced with complex moral issues. When the American Medical Association (AMA) issued a statement to the effect that it is unethical to refuse to treat HIV/AIDS patients, that statement reflected a deep concern in the medical community about the possibility of their becoming infected by treating patients with HIV/AIDS.

The AMA statement for an ethical call to arms is unprecedented in this century. It is the result of a spreading fear that HIV/AIDS is too contagious to tolerate in spite of the knowledge that the virus is not transmitted via casual contact. *Emotions,* not education, are in control of those whose fears exceed reality. But these emotions are real and they are having an impact on the medical community.

There is an ongoing dilemma concerning the rights of the physician and other health care workers to practice medicine in a safe environment as opposed to the rights of HIV-infected and AIDS patients to receive care and medical support. Although the risk of HIV transmission through medical occupational exposure appears to be quite low, the fact that it is possible at all, coupled with the uniformly fatal prognosis associated with AIDS, suggests that physicians, nurses, and other health care workers have legitimate concerns about risk to their health.

In a recent report by C.E. Lewis and colleagues (1992), almost half of the primary care physicians in the Los Angeles area have refused to treat HIV-infected patients or plan not to accept them as regular patients.

In a more recent survey of American doctors in residency training, 39% said that a surgeon or other specialist had refused to treat a patient with AIDS in the resident's care. In Canada, only 13% reported a specialist had refused to treat a patient with AIDS; in France, only 8% said a specialist had rejected care.

Further, 23% of American doctors would not care for AIDS patients if they had a choice as compared with 14% of Canadian physicians and 4% of French doctors.

The survey results may be a disturbing indicator of how American physicians view their work and a reflection of cultural and political attitudes here that view with veiled hostility those with AIDS.

To combat that fear, medical schools are now providing their students with disability insurance that covers AIDS. Hospitals have adopted policies that require physicians to treat AIDS patients or face dismissal.

AIDS Influencing Medical Students' Choices

Nathan Link and colleagues (1988) surveyed 250 first, second, and third year interns in two medical and two pediatric residency programs. Twenty-five percent said they would not continue to care for AIDS patients if given a choice. These data represent a significant degree of fear of contracting AIDS from patients.

A 1989 survey of 120 students in their second and third year of medical school (66% male; 91% had no experience with AIDS patients) revealed the following:

1. 75% worried that they might contract AIDS if they had to work with AIDS patients.
2. 25% felt that AIDS patients should be quarantined.
3. 25% said they would be afraid to care for AIDS patients.
4. 15% said they were morally offended by AIDS patients.
5. 33% said they would avoid caring for AIDS patients.
6. 50% said hospital personnel should not be required to care for AIDS patients.
7. 27% said they had considered changing their careers because they might be required to care for AIDS patients.

In another study, a survey on the attitudes of 1,045 internal medicine staff physicians revealed: (1) 63% said that they did not intend to treat people with HIV; (2) 17% had no objection to caring for HIV/AIDS patients; (3) about 66% stated that they would withhold lifesaving measures from a patient if they felt there was a 1-in-100 chance that they themselves might become infected. Such attitudes can be found in virtually all medical specialties (Driscoll, 1990).

Collectively, these data suggest that medical students and practicing physicians are deciding, on some level, whether they want to continue on in medicine. This decision has important ramifications for everyone. It would be interesting to know how many students decide against entering medical school because of the HIV/AIDS pandemic.

HIV-Infected Physicians

The fact that medical students and residents fear contracting HIV infection and AIDS can be tied to the reality that by mid-1991, 720 physicians were reported to the CDC as having

BOX 14.8

PHYSICIAN SHORTAGE—WHO SUFFERS?

A 1991 survey of physicians throughout the United States revealed that there is only one primary care physician for every 2,857 residents in rural areas compared to 1 for every 614 residents nationally. And there are 111 rural counties in 22 states with no physician at all. Texas has 18 counties without a physician. Rural America needs at least 35,000 more general practitioners.

Senator Max Bacus (Dem., Montana) said that in his state, eight counties have *no* physicians and 18 counties have no one qualified to deliver babies. He said, "There currently are 50 vacancies for family practice doctors in Montana. Thirty of our 56 counties are designated 'health-professional shortage areas.' In Montana, where we have no medical school, we have an additional disadvantage in that young doctors do not spend their learning years or their residencies anywhere in our state." Montana is only one of many states that face physician shortages in smaller cities, towns, and outlying areas. If HIV-infected physicians, whose numbers continue to climb, are denied the right to practice, the physician shortage will become worse. If physicians who are HBV-infected (carry the hepatitis B virus) or are infected with other serious sexually transmitted diseases are included among the HIV-infected, a very serious physician shortage would occur not only in the rural areas, but also in the larger cities.

Discussion Questions: At what point or for what reason should physicians and other health care workers be denied the right to practice?

Can these physicians still save lives even though their own may be forfeited?

AIDS. This number is probably underreported by 20% to 50%. At least 5,000 physicians were HIV-infected by 1990 (Breo, 1990). The question residents and medical students are asking is: How did so many become infected?

Along with the recognition of infected physicians come many disturbing questions on whether they should be permitted to continue their medical practice. In 1987, a Gallup Poll (as reported in January 1989 in *The Wall Street Journal*) asked that very question, and 57% of the general public said **not under any circumstances.**

Medical experts say the public should not be worried about patients contracting the virus during a routine physical examination or through casual contact with an infected doctor or hospital worker.

But the public does worry about what might happen during surgery and procedures involving contact with mucous membranes (Table 14-1). For example, some medical experts fear that if an infected surgeon is accidently cut in the operating room, the surgeon's blood could cause an infection. Because of the controversial dentist-to-patient HIV transmission that occurred in Florida, the CDC has convened its advisors to help revise CDC guidelines for infection control. A major question under review is whether any HIV/AIDS professional who performs invasive procedures should be allowed to continue. Restriction of HIV-infected surgeons and dentists would greatly curtail or even destroy their practices. It was suggested by one consultant to the CDC that any restriction would lead to mandatory screening of all health care workers. At the moment, the CDC says that the question of whether an infected physician or dentist should be allowed to perform invasive procedures (those in which bleeding may occur) can only be answered on a case-by-case basis.

Risk Protection of the Patient: Political Dimensions— The American Medical Association's position is that HIV/AIDS doctors "should

TABLE 14-1 Poll on Revelation of HIV Status

A. Should the following health care workers who are HIV-infected be forbidden to practice?

	Yes	No
Surgeons	63%	28%
All physicians	51%	42%
Dentists	60%	33%
All health care workers	49%	43%

B. Should patients be required to inform their physicians, dentists and other health care workers whether they are HIV-infected?

Yes	No
97%	2%

(Source: Newsweek, July 1, 1991)

POINT OF INFORMATION 14.1

HIV TRANSMITTED BY AUSTRALIAN SURGEON

A breakdown in infection control procedures is being blamed for the transmission of HIV to five patients of an Australian surgeon. It's believed the virus was transmitted from one patient to four others during minor skin surgery on a single day in November, 1989. Health officials say one patient, a gay man, is believed to have been the infection source. The CDC calls the case the first known patient-to-patient transmissions of HIV in a health care setting (*American Medical News*.. 1994 37:2.) Similar to the more recent dentist-Bergalis case, the source of HIV, will most likely, never be documented to everyone's satisfaction.

consult colleagues as to which activities the physician can pursue without creating a risk to patients."

There must be a rational relationship between the degree of risk, the morbidity and mortality of the disease, and the consequences of policies and procedures implemented to reduce the risk. Invasive surgery involves many risks. There is an overriding ethical obligation to reduce these risks in ways that do not create more harm than good. The justification of policies to prevent life-threatening illnesses with a risk factor of 1 in 10,000 is significantly greater than those with a risk factor of one in 100,000. More lives can be saved by innovative approaches to preventing the kind of injuries that have accounted for 75% of all cases of occupationally related HIV infection than by preventing HIV-infected health care workers from performing invasive surgery.

The risk of HIV infection by an HIV-infected surgeon is only one-tenth the chance of being killed by lightning, one-fourth the chance of being killed by a bee, and half the chance of being hit by a falling aircraft. The 1 in 100,000 risk of transmission from an infected surgeon equals the probability of death we face bicycling 2 miles each way to school for 1 month, or commuting 15 miles round-trip by car for a year.

Similarly, our chance of dying from anesthesia during an operation is roughly 10 times our chance of being infected by a surgeon known to be infected with HIV. A mother who approves a penicillin injection for her toddler with pharyngitis accepts a 1 in 100,000 risk of death from anaphylactic shock. In one study, the most successful coronary artery bypass graft surgeon surveyed had a 1.9% mortality rate, while the least successful had a 9.2% mortality rate. Patients selecting the least successful surgeon thus face 7,300 times the extra risk of death posed by an HIV-infected surgeon. The risk to a person undergoing invasive surgery by a surgeon of *unknown* HIV status is about 1 in 20 million of becoming HIV-infected (Daniels, 1992). The CDC estimates the risk to a patient by an HIV-infected surgeon to be between 1 in 42,000 and 1 in 420,000 (Lo et al., 1992).

Patients' Right to Know if Their Physician Has HIV/AIDS— In a 1987 Gallup Poll, 86% of those polled felt that they had the right to know if a health care worker treating them was HIV-infected. Many lawyers also take this position. The courts appear to be moving toward an interpretation of the doctrine of informed patient consent as "what a reasonable patient would want to know," rather than "what a reasonable physician would disclose." Because it is so difficult for surgeons to avoid occasionally cutting themselves during surgery, it has been suggested that the best solution is not to have HIV-infected surgeons perform surgery at all.

Public anxiety on HIV/AIDS and medical care is becoming increasingly tinged with hysteria. A national Gallup Poll undertaken for *Newsweek* (June 20, 1991) asked a representative sample of 618 adults, "Which of the following kinds of health care workers should be required to tell patients if they are infected with the AIDS virus?"

The answers were: surgeons 95%; all physicians 94%; dentists 94%; all health care workers 90%.

Clearly, people do not differentiate between doctors who perform invasive procedures and those who do not. However, the patient could ask what the probability is of a single dentist (Acer) infecting six of his patients (Bergalis, Web, and four others). Extremely low, **yet it did happen!** The lowest of probabilities and best of guidelines and precautions do not stop the fire of fear. It must also be mentioned that the same *Newsweek* poll found that 97% of those interviewed felt that HIV-infected patients should tell their health care workers that they are infected (Table 14-1B).

There is one important aspect related to this poll that needs to be addressed. That is, many of the people interviewed stated that if they knew their surgeon was HIV-infected, they would "get another surgeon." This *switching dilemma* would have the majority of the population needing surgery standing in line for the uninfected surgeons. Services provided by the reduced number of surgeons, it could be claimed, at some point, result in increased costs and diminished quality.

Physician–Patient Relationships

In most states, physicians may *not test* a patient for HIV antibodies without written permission from the patient. Physicians can run tests for any other infectious diseases without written permission.

Do you think this is fair and equal medical practice?

Because the majority of HIV-infected patients are asymptomatic, there is no way of telling **who is** or **is not** infected. Therefore, for the protection of health care workers, everyone must be treated as though they were HIV-infected.

BOX 14.9

MY FIRST AIDS EXPERIENCE

"A man was waiting for his mother in my office while she consulted me about a back problem," reports a family practitioner in a Gulf state city. "He had a grand mal seizure, bit his tongue and bled quite a bit. I put a tape-wrapped tongue depressor into his mouth to keep him from further injuring his tongue and then just supported him until the seizure was over. Later the physician who had been caring for him at a hospital clinic called to ask that I confirm the seizure, adding, "By the way, this man has AIDS." I never gave a thought to AIDS in this situation," continues the family practitioner. "It was my first experience in dealing with an AIDS patient" (Polder et al., 1989).

HIV is the silent medical threat of the 1980s and 1990s. Whenever blood is drawn, a wound is examined, a dressing is changed, or anything that involves blood, needles, or surgery is done, there is an unspoken fear that HIV might be present. The patient sees this preventive attitude of physicians and other health care workers by the new look of the 1980s and 1990s: wraparound smocks, gloved hands, and masks. The patient wonders whether his or her physician is an HIV carrier and the physician assumes that the patient may be a carrier. A recent Associated Press article presented some examples of how the AIDS pandemic has changed doctor–patient relationships:

1. In many operating rooms, doctors and nurses wear wraparound glasses in case of blood splashes.
2. In many emergency rooms, health care workers cover themselves with caps, goggles, masks, gowns, gloves, shoe covers, and blood-proof aprons.
3. Infection control specialists must spend time convincing hospital workers it is safe to enter an HIV/AIDS patient's room to perform normal duties ranging from picking up dinner trays to fixing the plumbing.
4. At some hospitals, all emergency room trash, no matter how innocuous, is treated as hazardous waste.
5. Many doctors and nurses routinely pull on gloves whenever they give an injection or draw blood.
6. Mouth-to-mouth resuscitation is simply not done at many hospitals. Instead a mask and valve device is used to avoid direct contact with the patient's mouth.
7. A surgeon at San Francisco General Hospital takes the AIDS drug zidovudine whenever he operates on people he thinks are infected.
8. Physicians are increasing life insurance policies to provide for their families in case they become HIV-infected.

The health care professionals' fear of getting AIDS will persist as long as there is a risk that HIV can be transmitted in the workplace. The goal is not to eradicate that fear, but to prevent it from compromising the quality of patient care and from threatening the health

BOX 14.10

THE PHYSICIAN'S RIGHT TO KNOW IF THE PATIENT IS HIV/AIDS INFECTED

PRO:

Recently there have been calls for attention to the rights of health care providers to know when they are being exposed to HIV-infected patients (Hagen et al., 1988; Fournier et al., 1989; Rhame et al., 1989).

(*A letter from a practicing nurse to the editor of a large southeastern newspaper*)

"Perhaps the physician's letter was a bit too harsh in the opening sentence when he stated that he was 'sick and tired of AIDS patients and their rights."

However, I don't think this doctor is hysterical or ignorant. I can only speculate on his feelings, but I assume that he is like other health care professionals who want to help, but think they also have rights to protect themselves.

We all use or are instructed to use universal precautions. These precautions can easily be violated when a patient with alcohol or drug withdrawal bites someone or a needle goes through a gloved hand.

I have been spat on, bitten, clawed and urinated on, among other things, in my years of nursing. It is not glamorous, but, at least, I knew if the patient had hepatitis or tuberculosis. Why shouldn't I know if he has AIDS?

We can't work as a team if we don't know what we're dealing with. When someone develops a sudden increase in temperature, we don't have to go through mounds of red tape to do cultures to determine the cause of illness. When the patient goes to the doctor with a symptom, he expects the doctor to make a diagnosis. What's the physician supposed to do if he suspects AIDS but can't confirm it because the patient has rights?

This disease should be treated like any other, beginning with a diagnosis, followed by treatment, concern and confidentiality among the patients and health care professionals.

Eventually, these people will realize that when they stop fighting us we will have the same genuine compassion for them that we have for all patients".

Behind physicians' anxiety about HIV/AIDS is anger about being obligated to take risks in an atmosphere of uncertainty. They feel that AIDS is an infectious disease that is not being treated like one. And according to law, HIV/AIDS is *not* an infectious disease, it is considered a disability. (See Chapter 16 for legal definition.) Most physicians feel it is absurd that they do not have the right to find out whether or not a patient is HIV-infected. The recommendation that doctors treat every patient as if he or she had HIV/AIDS is unrealistic in the hospital setting, especially in hospital emergency rooms. Currently, there is great pressure from the health care community to obtain legislation for health care workers' *right to know* patient HIV status.

CON:

There is another side to this conflict of rights, the side that says universal patient testing will not be useful. J.D. Gostin, executive director of the American Society of Law and Medicine says that there are no data to indicate that physicians would reduce their risk of exposure if they knew the HIV status of their patients (Mandelbaum-Schmid, 1990). Gostin believes that patients have a moral obligation, although not a legal one, to be retested after a health care professional is exposed to their blood. "It's true that a few patients may not consent," he concedes, "but the overwhelming majority will. One can't develop a policy of testing everyone in the country because of a hypothetical case where a doctor might be stuck, the patient won't disclose, and zidovudine might be effective. That is too speculative a basis for taking away people's rights.

THE COMPROMISE:

Sanford F. Kuvin, M.D. (Vice Chairman, Board of Trustees, National Foundation for Infectious Diseases, Washington) is of the opinion "all health care professionals involved in invasive procedures should have themselves tested for HIV and make their status known to their patients. Similarly, patients who will be undergoing invasive procedures should be tested and make their status known to those treating them."

THE QUESTION:

Are federal and state governments overstressing the need for privacy at the expense of prevention?

BOX 14.11

THE SECRET

In 1992, a 40-year-old gay family practice doctor had to decide on whether to tell his patients he had HIV disease. If the doctor tells his patients he has the virus, he will lose his business. At least that has been the case for the doctors, dentists, nurses, pharmacists, and surgical technicians who have come forward so far. If he lost his profession he could face the last years of his life not only grappling with a devastating and expensive illness, but also be deprived of income, health insurance, and the solace of employment. If he concealed his infection and continued to work, his infection could be revealed and his practice destroyed anyway, through lawsuits. That was the experience of one doctor who publicly announced he had AIDS in 1990, *after* another doctor reported him to the state board of medical examiners. This doctor was subsequently sued by 24 former patients for malpractice and personal injury. In another case, a Johns Hopkins University surgeon died of AIDS disease in 1990, since then, two patients have filed suit against his estate, claiming damages because they were so horrified to find they had been operated on by a doctor with the virus and because they now face the prospect of repeated HIV tests. About 50 more of this doctor's patients are contemplating similar actions. However, the charges against him were dismissed because the claimants couldn't show any actual damages. In addition, some hospitals and institutions have dismissed all medical or health care workers who were HIV-positive.

In a survey by the Medical Expertise Retention Program, a San Francisco-based program that helps infected health workers sort out their options, 67% of HIV-positive doctors said they have avoided, or plan to avoid, seeking treatment or submitting insurance claims because they fear their **secret** will be told.

Before this doctor died, he decided that "there were no good solutions." Left to his own conscience and reasoning, the doctor came to the conclusion that his doubts were based on emotion, not science—just like the fears of his patients. Technically, he decided, there was no way he could give the virus to a patient. "If there was the slightest possibility I could give it to them it would be their right to know I'm HIV-positive," he says. "But there is no conceivable way. So it is absolutely not their business. My patients like me, love me, depend on me. But if they find out I have HIV, they're going to leave me. How many are going to stay? Three out of ten? Why should they take the chance? Why should they be crusaders? They won't." (Adapted from Japenga, 1992)

QUESTION: Should the patient have the choice as to whether they wish to become a crusader? Compare your immediate response to the responses of physicians who read "The Secret".

RESPONSE from physicians who read this story, "The Secret":

1. "Thank you for your story 'The Secret." I, too, am a physician who learned of my HIV in fection one year ago. I have experienced many of the same feelings as the doctor you profiled in the article.

For the past year, I have lived much of my life "in secret. I am afraid to tell even my closest friends for fear of divulging my status to the hospital and medical school for which I now work. I have had to worry about who I might meet at a support group, about whether I might run into my patients at community meetings about HIV/AIDS, and about losing my job and health insurance if my employer finds out.

Just as other infected people, I have fought guilt, shame, fear, anger, and hopelessness. However, as a physician at an inner-city hospital, I am also responsible for a large number of patients with HIV/AIDS. Although I enjoy my work and feel fulfilled, it has been very difficult for me to care for people who are at a later stage of the same disease that I have, and watch as they decline mentally and physically.

Perhaps someday we may not have to keep this important part of our lives such a secret.

NAME WITHHELD

2. "My situation as a physician with HIV infection is complicated by the fact that I am a surgeon". I went through virtually the exact decision process as the doctor profiled in `The Secret' but I arrived at a different conclusion, and have been devastated by the results.

I told my chief of service, in confidence, of my diagnosis. Within two days, my privileges were suspended, and the hospital sued to get permission to disclose my condition to all patients I had treated while at the hospital, to the press, and to any other hospital I applied to. The court granted the request. My practice evaporated, and the hospital has made certain that my efforts to build an alternative non-operative practice would fail.

The doctor in `The Secret' made the right decision: Since he's not a danger to his patients, he should say nothing, and get on with his life.

The irony is that all this can be prevented: This 'crisis' is driven not by medical fact or necessity, but by the hospital industry's fear of being sued."

NAME WITHHELD

3. Bravo for publishing 'The Secret.' I am an HIV-positive operating room nurse, and I know this story all too well. I did what I thought was the moral and ethical thing to do: I disclosed my status to my supervisor. From that point on, all confidentiality went out the window. I discovered that confidentiality is only rhetoric.

After review by the hospital's 'expert review panel'—which did not include a peer or anyone else from the department of surgery—my practice was restricted. I could no longer work as a scrub nurse. No one ever noticed that I was the **only** one in my operating room who followed impeccable infection control and universal precautions.

Yes, doctor keep your mouth shut, and practice impeccable infection control. The review panel I dealt with provided no counseling, no follow-up, and even less support. To quote from one survey of high-risk and HIV-positive hospital workers like myself, 'Let us not forget that HIV-positive health care providers have saved and continue to save thousands of lives every year.'"

NAME WITHHELD

professional's own well-being (Gerbert et al., 1988).

In early 1990, Lorraine Day quit her post as chairperson of the Orthopedics Department at San Francisco General Hospital and abandoned her surgical practice because of her fear of exposure to HIV. "I have two children to think about and operating was too dangerous. If I was a skydiver, people would say I was an irresponsible mother, but to me, surgery now, it was just as risky."

Dr. Day said during a TV interview, "Our risk is one in 200 per single (needle) stick with AIDS blood and it can be the first one—it doesn't take 200. And I ask you, if you came to work every day and flipped the light switch on in your office and only one out of 200 times you were electrocuted would you consider that low-risk?"

While Dr. Day has been called a scaremonger, many surgeons in private conversations call her a "hero" for raising the risk issue.

Physicians with AIDS

According to Mandelbaum-Schmid (1990), one overriding issue facing physicians who become HIV-infected is that there is no support system to compensate them once they become too sick to work. For example, a 32-year-old gastroenterologist, claimed she was infected with HIV in 1983 when she accidently pricked herself with a needle that an intern had used to draw blood from an AIDS patient. She was working at the time at Brooklyn's Kings County Hospital.

She tested HIV-positive in 1985. On subsequent consultations with physicians at the National Institute of Health (NIH), she was told that she was a healthy carrier of the virus who could become ill. She continued training at Kings County, completing a residency in internal medicine and a fellowship in gastroenterology.

She became symptomatic in 1987. A year later, she filed a 175 million dollar lawsuit charging that the hospital's negligence had caused her illness. At the time of the trial, her life expectancy was estimated at less than a year. Following a stormy 2-month trial that challenged the integrity of all the physicians and expert witnesses who testified, she reportedly settled for just under 2 million dollars.

Another pressing issue pointed out by Mandelbaum-Schmid is that HIV-infected doctors are not protected against discrimination.

The experience of an otolaryngologist who died of AIDS in June, 1989, at the age of 46, set an unwelcome precedent. Before his illness, he had a thriving practice in Princeton, New Jersey. He believed he was infected in 1984 after being splashed in the face with blood while performing an emergency tracheotomy. He became ill with an undifferentiated pneumonia in 1987. Physicians performed a bronchoscopy and gave him an HIV test without telling him.

Word of his positive HIV test soon spread through the hospital and soon after into his community. By the time he was released from the hospital, his telephone lines were jammed with calls from hysterical patients. He eventually lost about half his practice. When he tried to schedule operating room time, the hospital's president convened an emergency meeting of trustees. They made the unprecedented decision that he may operate but only with the informed consent of his patients.

He filed a lawsuit based on breach of ethics and doctor–patient confidentiality—his diagnosis had been leaked by the hospital laboratory—and violation of antidiscrimination laws. In April, 1991, New Jersey Superior Court Judge Philip S. Carchman ruled that the Medical Center of Princeton, after learning the doctor had AIDS, made a "reasoned and informed response" in barring him from performing surgery without informed consent of his patients.

The last example of the plight of a physician with AIDS involves a physician at Johns Hopkins Medical Center. He contracted an HIV infection from a patient in 1983 while working as a resident in the bone marrow transplantation unit, he had an accident with the blood of a young leukemia patient who had been transfused many times The accident was followed 3 weeks later by an acute febrile illness with cough, sore throat, rash, and lymphadenopathy. After this, he was in good health for the next 3 years. He completed his residency and became a chief resident and a fellow in cardiology. He married, and had a daughter. In November of 1986, unexplained weight loss led him to be HIV tested. He tested positive for HIV.

The hospital's reaction was unexpected. He had to sue the institution and some members of the faculty in an effort to defend his reputation and obtain appropriate benefits. After endless months of legal battle, Johns Hopkins proposed a settlement 3 weeks before the trial date.

He said, "By actions like this, medical institutions send an awful message to the health care worker: we ask you to be in the front lines, but if something happens to you, we will not stand behind you, you will be abandoned, and you will be deprived of the privilege of practicing medicine" (Aoun, 1990). He died of AIDS in February of 1992, 9 years after becoming infected with HIV.

SUMMARY

In 1981, AIDS was announced as a new disease affecting the homosexual population. Many religious people believed this was a sign that homosexuality should be punished. The few facts available at that time gave rise to a great deal of fantasy and fear. Affected people were either innocent victims or they deserved the disease. Contracting AIDS labeled a person as less than desirable, a homosexual or one who practiced deviant forms of sexual behavior. But even the so-called innocent victims, the children, the hemophiliacs, and the recipients of blood transfusions were not spared social ostracism. If you had AIDS, you were twice the victim—first of the virus and second of the social behavior.

Children were barred from attending school, adults from their jobs, and both from adequate medical care. For example, there are still relatively few dentists who will treat AIDS patients and a significant number of surgeons refuse to operate on AIDS patients. Fourteen years have passed, but many misconceptions about HIV/AIDS linger on.

Fear is being casually transmitted rather than the virus. A significant number of people, after 12 years of broad scale education, still believe that the AIDS virus can be casually transmitted from toilet seats, drinking glasses, and even by donating blood.

The fallout from the fear of the AIDS pandemic has been a major change in sexual language in TV advertisements, magazines, and radio. Condoms once spoken about only in hushed tones in conversations and kept under the counter in most drug stores, are now spoken of everywhere as a means of safer sex. AIDS, perhaps more than any other disease, has demonstrated that ignorance leads to fear and knowledge can lead to compassion.

To achieve understanding and compassion, people must be educated as to their HIV risk status and how they can keep it low. Many hundreds of millions of dollars have been spent to inform the public of the kinds of behavior that either place them at risk or reduce their risk for HIV infection. The problem is that although people are getting the information, too many refuse to act on it. Former Surgeon General C. Everett Koop's office mailed 107 million copies of the brochure "Understanding AIDS" to households in the United States. Fifty-one percent of those who received it said they never read it. But even among those who read the brochure, are those who refuse to change their sexual behavior. Old habits are difficult to break.

To date, the hard evidence shows that only the homosexual population has significantly modified their sexual behavior as evidenced by the drop in the number of new cases of AIDS among them from 1988 through 1994.

A major problem looming on the horizon is the prospect of HIV being spread in the teenage population. Large numbers of teens use drugs and alcohol, have multiple sex partners, and believe they are invulnerable to infection.

One of the greatest tragedies of the AIDS pandemic is orphaned children. They are left in hospitals because (1) their parents have died of AIDS or cannot care for them, or (2) no one wants them.

The AMA stated in 1988 that physicians may not refuse to care for patients with AIDS because of actual risk or fear of contracting the disease. Some physicians get around this through referral to other physicians who will treat AIDS patients. There is one area of medicine that takes issue at having to treat AIDS patients. That area is surgery. Because it is difficult not to accidently get cut during surgery, surgeons have been the leading advocates for HIV testing of all surgical patients so they will know their risks before performing surgery.

On the other hand, patients feel they have a right to know if their physician, especially a surgeon, is HIV-infected. Surveys indicate that most people would not want to be treated by an HIV-infected physician.

REVIEW QUESTIONS

(Answers to the Review Questions are on page 483.)

1. Name three major sources of information that contributed to the early panic and hysteria about the spread of AIDS.
2. Give three examples of unfounded public fears to AIDS infection.
3. Fear of the casual transmission of AIDS parallels what other earlier STD epidemic?
4. What evidence is there that it is difficult to get people to change their behavior even though they know it is harmful to their well being?
5. What is the major thrust of AIDS education in the United States?
6. If education is the key to preventing HIV infection and new cases of AIDS; and most people interviewed say they have been 'educated,' why is it not working?
7. Why are today's teenagers in danger of contracting and spreading HIV?
8. Where do most of the orphaned AIDS children come from? Why are they called AIDS orphans?
9. Yes or No: Do physicians have a right to refuse to treat AIDS patients? Support your answer.
10. Do patients have a right to know if their physician is HIV-infected or has AIDS?
11. What is the primary means of offsetting the bias toward people with AIDS in the workplace?

REFERENCES

American Medical Association News. (1991). Ruling fuels debate over HIV-infected doctors. May:1,41–43.

Aoun, Hacib. (1990). A handful helped us. *Medical Doctor,* 34:31–32.

BLENDON, R.J., et al. (1988). Discrimination against people with AIDS: The public's perspective. *N. Engl. J. Med.,* 319:1022–1026.

BREO, DENNIS L. (1990). The slippery slope—handling HIV-infected health care workers. *JAMA,* 264:1464–1466.

CRAVEN, DONALD, et al. (1994). Factitious HIV Infection. *Ann. Intern. Med.,* 121:763–766.

DANIELS, NORMAN. (1992). HIV-infected professionals, patient rights and the 'switching dilemma'. *JAMA,* 267:1368–1371.

DRISCOLL, CHARLES E. (1990). AIDS: Issues for every woman and her physician. *Female Patient,* 15:11–12.

EICKHOFF, THEODORE C. (1989). Public perceptions about AIDS and HIV infection. *Infect. Dis. News,* 2:6.

FISHER, J.D., et al. (1992). Changing AIDS risk behavior. *Psychol. Bull.,* 111:455–474.

FOURNIER, A.M., et al. (1989). Preoperative screening for HIV infection. *Arch. Surg.,* 124: 1038–1040.

FULTON, ROBERT, et al. (1988). AIDS: Seventh rank absolute. In *AIDS: Principles, Practices and Politics.,* Inge B. Corliss, et al., eds. Bristol, PA: Hemisphere.

GERBERT, BARBARA, et al. (1988). Why fear persists: Health care professionals and AIDS. *JAMA,* 260:3481–3483.

HAGEN, M.D., et al. (1988). Routine preoperative screening for HIV: Does the risk to the surgeon outweigh the risk to the patient? *JAMA,* 259:1357–1359.

HEGARTY, JAMES D., et al. (1988). The medical care costs of HIV-infected children in Harlem. *JAMA,* 260:1901–1909.

HEREK, GREGORY M., et al. (1993). Public reaction to AIDS in the United States: A second decade of stigma. *Am. J. Public Health,* 83:574–577.

JAPENGA, ANN. (1992). The secret. *Health,* 6:43–52.

KEGELES, S.M., et al. (1988). Sexually active adolescents and condoms: Changes over one year in knowledge, attitudes and use. *Am. J. Public Health,* 78:460–461.

KIRBY, D. (1988). The effectiveness of educational programs to help prevent school-age youth from contracting AIDS: A review of relevant research. United States Congress.

LEFKOWITZ, MATHEW. (1990). A health care system in crisis: The possible restriction against HIV-infected health care workers. *PAACNOTES,* 2:175–176.

LEWIS, C.E., et al. (1992). Primary care physicians' refusal to care for patients infected with HIV. *West. J. Med.,* 156:36–38.

LINK, R. NATHAN et al. (1988). Concerns of medical and pediatric house officers about acquiring AIDS from their patients. *Am. J. Public Health,* 78:455–459.

LO, BERNARD et al. (1992). Health care workers infected with HIV. *JAMA,* 267:1100–1105.

MANDELBAUM-SCHMID, JUDITH. (1990). AIDS and MDs. *Medical Doctor,* 34:33–40.

MCNEILL, WILLIAM H. (1976). *Plagues and People,* Garden City: Anchor Press.

MICHAELS, DAVID, et al. (1992). Estimates of the number of youth orphaned by AIDS in the United States. *JAMA,* 268:3456–3461.

Morbidity and Mortality Weekly Report. (1990). HIV-related knowledge and behavior among high shool students—Selected U.S. cities, 1989. 39:385–396.

NARY, GORDON. (1990). An editorial. *PAACNOTES,* 2:170.

PHILLIPS, KATHRYN A. (1993). Subjective knowledge of AIDS and Use of HIV testing. *Am. J. Public Health,* 83:1460–1462.

POLDER, JACQUELYN A., et al. (1989). AIDS precautions for your office. *Patient Care,* 23:161–171.

POWELL, JOHN H. (1965). *Bring Out Your Dead.* New York: Time-Life Inc.

RHAME, FRANK S., et al. (1989). The case for wider use of testing for HIV infection. *N. Engl. J. Med.,* 320:1242–1254.

ROWE, MONA, et al. (1987). *A Public Health Challenge: State Issues, Policies and Programs, Volume 2.* Intergrovernmental Health Policy Project, George Washington University.

VOELKER, REBECCA. (1989). No uniform policy among states on HIV/AIDS education. *Am. Med. News,* Sept.:3,28–29.

CHAPTER

15

The Economics of HIV/AIDS

Chapter Concepts

- There is an AIDS industry.
- The medical cost of treating AIDS patients is in the billions of dollars.
- The direct or true costs for HIV disease and AIDS.
- The indirect costs for HIV disease and AIDS.
- The costs for AIDS research, education, and prevention.
- Public backlash to the high cost of the AIDS industry.
- Hospital space available for AIDS patients.
- Thirty-seven million people in the United States do not have health care insurance.
- Commercial health care insurers are leery of writing policies for HIV-infected people.
- Commercial life insurance carriers want to test for HIV infection before writing a policy.
- Funeral directors charge higher rates for burying the AIDS-related dead.

HIV disease and AIDS are producing a global economic challenge. Yet data on actual expenditures for services rendered to HIV/AIDS patients and for research and education are limited. However, it can be estimated that the economic impact of this disease will become as serious as the pandemic itself. The bulk of the expense is registered in the relatively affluent industrialized nations. Estimates of medical care costs for HIV/AIDS patients vary widely. Meanwhile, indirect costs (loss of productivity) dwarf the medical costs because it is the young and middle-aged who most often die.

NATIONAL HEALTH CARE SPENDING: 1993–1995

Health care spending in the United States was about $910 billion in 1993. This figure represents about $3,540 for every man, woman, and child. It costs about $75 billion a year just to treat the infectious diseases. And this item is increasing by $3 billion to $6 billion a year (Perkin, 1993). In 1994, costs exceeded $1 trillion. For 1995, health care spending will exceed $1 trillion, 100 billion. This exceeds any other country's spending on health care, either per capita or as a percentage of gross national product.

Former Health and Human Services secretary Louis Sullivan said in 1991 that health care costs were growing at an unsustainable rate and that something had to be done (Packer, 1991).

In 1993, Americans spent about $2.5 billion a day on medical care. That is twice what they spent 7 years ago. For the federal government, medical care has become the fastest growing item in the budget, increasing at more than 8% annually at a time when inflation is about 4%. Health care spending is expected to rise by 12% to 15% annually over the next 5 years (Weissenstein, 1993). For corporate America, health care has become a crippling expense. General Motors paid out $3.2 billion in 1990—more than it spent on steel—to provide medical coverage for 1.9 million employees, dependents, and retirees. Unchecked, the cost of medical care will more than double in the next 10 years to $2 trillion, crowding out spending for other needs.

Medicaid

Medicaid is a form of combined federal and state financing of health care for the **disadvantaged**. As increasing numbers of people infected with HIV exhaust their private insurance, lose their insurance, or become reliant on Medicaid, the problem of financing their health care becomes a pressing public policy issue. There is no really clear picture of the kinds of health insurance coverage found among the different socioeconomic groups represented by people with HIV disease/AIDS, because most studies have been narrowly focused.

POINT OF INFORMATION 15.1

BEHAVIORS ARE EXPENSIVE

Drug and alcohol abuse, smoking, failure to use seatbelts, unsafe sex, and sharing contaminated needles are all behaviors that account for more than one fourth of the billions of dollars that Americans spend on health care each year. It is estimated that a total of $188 billion of the dollars spent on health care in this country is attributable to unhealthy lifestyles (Health Insurance Association of America, 1994).

Obstacles to Medicaid Funding

An obstacle to medical care for persons with HIV disease and AIDS who qualify for Medicaid are the low reimbursement rates. Stunning examples of Medicaid physician compensation rates far below those by private insurance or Medicare were presented during a recent commission hearing. For example, a new patient intermediate office visit in New York City is compensated by Blue Cross at $78, by Medicare at $80, and by Medicaid at $7. One witness indicated that physicians in New York with large AIDS practices were reluctant to refer Medicaid patients for specialty consultations because of low levels of reimbursement—levels so low that several physicians said that the few dollars at stake per office visit were not worth the time and paperwork to bill the Medicaid program. Overall, however, Medicaid pays for the health care of at least 40% of all adult/adolescents with AIDS and 90% of all pediatric AIDS cases (Washington Outlook, 1993). Twenty-nine percent of AIDS patients are **uninsured** and those with private health insurance often have limited benefits or high out-of-pocket costs (Levi, 1994). While it is clear that some type of health reform will occur in 1995/1996, how well this reform plan will address the medical problems of people with HIV disease and AIDS is presently unknown.

Medicare

This $110 billion program which started out in 1965 with a budget of $5 billion was designed to provide medical care for those 65 and older and some people in exceptional medical categories. But the program gives the same benefits to those who are well-off as to the poor. Although the elderly do pay some of the costs, nearly 90% of Medicare funds come from income taxes. As a result, the burden falls partly on working people who often have no health insurance of their own.

The burden on younger Americans continues to increase as the population ages, bringing with it the responsibility of caring for millions of elderly with expensive medical needs. There are now about seven Americans under the age of 65 for every person over, compared with 11 to one in 1960. One of those seven is unemployed and two are children. That leaves about four workers to support each elderly American. And one of them does not even have his or her own health insurance (Castro, 1991).

THE HEALTH CARE INDUSTRY

As a disease increases in incidence, it demands greater expenditures for research, testing, education, and setting up a network of health care services to meet the needs of patients. In other words, a disease over time gives rise to its own medical industry. There are health care industries that focus on the brain (psychiatric disorders), cardiovascular disease (heart), and bone and eye diseases. The largest health care industries are those that deal with cancer and contagious diseases. ***Now there is the AIDS industry.***

Financing the AIDS Industry

Federal—In 1990, the United States Congress did something quite rare: it allocated money specifically for the treatment of one disease—HIV/AIDS.

In some ways the increased commitment of federal and state government to cancer research and treatment in the early 1970s is similar to what has happened in the war on AIDS in the 1980s. In both decades, there was a major funding surge to stimulate research, therapy, and prevention. A major difference, however, is that dollars for cancer came more slowly over a longer time period that began well before the 1970s. With AIDS, federal funding began in 1981 (Figure 15-1) and has increased at an unprecedented rate.

During the 12 years from 1982 to 1994, federal spending on AIDS-related projects increased from $8 million in 1982 to $6.2 billion in 1994. It is estimated to reach $8 billion for 1995. Figure 15-2 demonstrates the 1994 allocation of federal dollars for AIDS and non-AIDS programs within just three of the federal agencies allocating AIDS dollars; the Center for Disease Control and Prevention (CDC), the National Institute of Allergy and Infectious Disease (NIAID), and the National Institute on Drug Abuse (NIDA).

In 1989, the federal government spent $1.3 billion, or about 33% of total dollars spent, on AIDS-related projects. The other 67%, or $3.9 billion, came from the private sectors. In 1990, $2 billion was allocated by the federal government for AIDS projects. In 1992, the federal government spent $4.5 billion, in 1993 $4.9 billion, in 1994 $6.2 billion (Figure 15-1). In addition, the private sector also spent about $4 billion a year for 1992, 1993, and 1994. By the end of 1994, the federal government spent over 28 billion dollars for HIV/AIDS-related work. The cost of treating Americans with HIV disease/AIDS in 1995 is estimated to be over $15 billion. It is interesting to note that through 1994, only two states, Wyoming and West Virginia, provided no state funding for HIV/AIDS programs. Both states rely 100% on federal government funding for all HIV/AIDS programs.

The $4.9 billion in 1993 represented about 2% of the $238 billion federal health care budget. To place health care and AIDS expenditures in perspective, in 1989 the federal government allocated $159 billion to "bail out" the savings and loan industry over the next 10 years; however, along the way through 1994, an additional $7 billion was added. It is estimated that $500 billion will be needed over the next 40 years. In 1989, the Department of Energy estimated it would take $128 billion to clean up nuclear weapons plants. But in 1994, it was estimated that it will take 30 years and over $300 billion. In 1995, it was estimated that the cost to clean up nuclear waste dumps across the United States would be $1,000 billion (*Nature*, 1995). The government spends about $300 billion annually on its military machine.

BOX 15.1

AIDS INDUSTRY SPIN-OFFS

1. Selling of "AIDS-Free" Certificates

In Jacksonville, Florida, an entrepreneur promoted a service that would have allowed patients to know the names of doctors and dentists who have tested AIDS-free. Many medical community leaders thought the service would promote hysteria.

The president of Jacksonville-based National Free of AIDS Identification Service said he was going to recruit doctors, dentists, and other health care professionals for HIV testing (1991). His plan was that for those who paid the $189 fee and who tested HIV negative, they would be issued "Free of AIDS" certificates.

Prospective patients will be able to call the service's 24-hour information line and, for a $2 fee, get a list of doctors and dentists who have received the certificate.

List the major problems involved with this enterprise: biological (e.g., how might this list promote/prevent HIV transmission?) and the moral-social aspects. **Is the idea based on good biology**?

2. Clothier's Exploitation of the HIV/AIDS Pandemic

An apparel maker shrugged off complaints of exploitation and said it was having no problem finding U.S. magazines for a new advertisement that shows a person dying of AIDS and his grieving family.

The trendy fashion concern is pinning its United Colors logo on previously published news photographs including one that shows an AIDS patient on his deathbed being comforted by his family. The advertisement appeared in issues of *Vogue, Vanity Fair, Interview, Details, Elle, Mademoiselle, Us,* and *Spin* magazines.

3. Investors Promised Profits from AIDS Patient Insurance Policies

Investors around the country are invited to buy the life insurance policies of AIDS patients—and the sooner the patient dies, the better for the investor, who then collects the insurance.

Newspaper, wire, and staff reports that one company is giving would-be investors a patient list to help them pick people who will die soon. The list predicts how many months each patient is supposed to live, based on the health of their immune system, and lists the amount of insurance they have.

In a nutshell, the companies line up investors to buy the insurance policies of the dying, typically at a 33% discount from face value, and pay the premiums until the insured dies. Then the investor collects the money. The promotion is as follows: A non-HIV/AIDS person takes out, for example, a $100,000 policy. He or she is later diagnosed with AIDS. An investor may be able to buy that person's policy for, say, $65,000, most of which is used to pay for the person's medical expenses. After death, the investor, who became the beneficiary of the policy, collects the $100,000 for a net profit of $35,000. AIDS persons and potential investors are urged to contact their state insurance commissioners office to be certain that this activity is legal.

4. A few companies have begun to sell AIDS-related products of questionable taste.

For example, one AIDS promotional kit reads: "RED RIBBONS ARE NOT ENOUGH!" And then it proceeds with an attempt to sell name tags or dog tags—"polished silverstone, military-style dog tags, inscribed with 'ALWAYS REMEMBER,'" and the name of a lost loved one. Cost $25. It continues, "Red ribbons offer **no monetary donations to the fight against AIDS**. With a *Remembrance Tag,* you can remember the one you love while contributing to the defeat of the virus."

A second promotional package, for $25, describes a Director's Handbook that teaches one how to make a memorial videotape of oneself. It provides questions that "you don't want to forget to answer." It provides a format for telling your personal history. It also says, "Be remembered as *you* want to be remembered."

A third company offers a video package for mothers. "Leave a message for your children." (Cost not given)

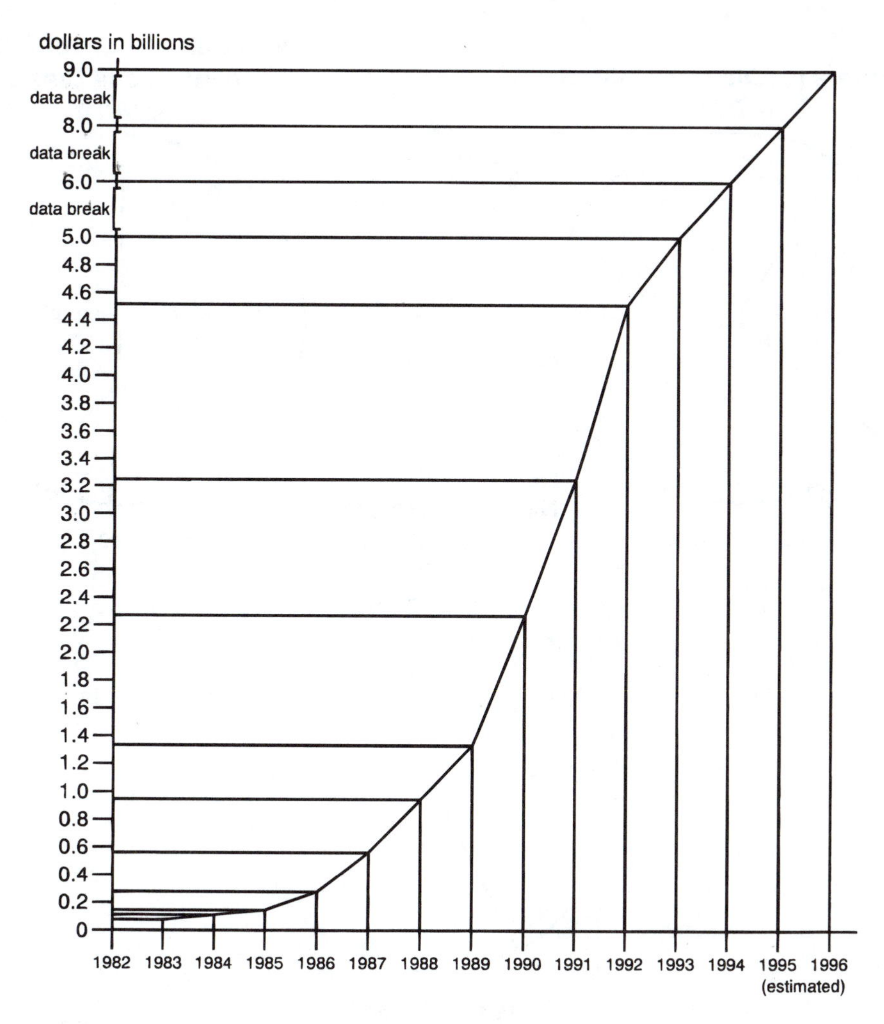

FIGURE 15-1 Federal Government AIDS Expenditures Projected to the Year 1998. Note the sharp rise in monies spent on AIDS-related projects by the Public Health Services between 1986 and 1996 (projected). Federal expenditures were $1.3 billion in 1989, $4.5 billion in 1992, $4.9 billion in 1993, $6.2 billion in 1994, and will be about $8 billion in 1995 and $9 billion in 1996.

Costs Related to Care—Right now, there is one HIV-related death about every 12 minutes in the United States (estimated 270,000 to 300,000 deaths through December 31, 1995). These data raise questions as to whether more money invested in AIDS research will slow the death rate and whether the money already spent was spent effectively. Timothy Murphy (1991) wrote that all the money spent so far on the HIV epidemic has not insured adequate medical care for all people with HIV-related conditions. This is especially true for the homeless. Neither have the dollars spent on HIV research produced a cure. Treatments with nucleoside analogs (ZDV, ddI, ddC, d4T, and 3TC) have proved ineffective for long-term care and there are still many unresolved questions about their short-term use. (See Chapter 7 for a discussion on the effectiveness of nucleoside analogs and other drug treatments.)

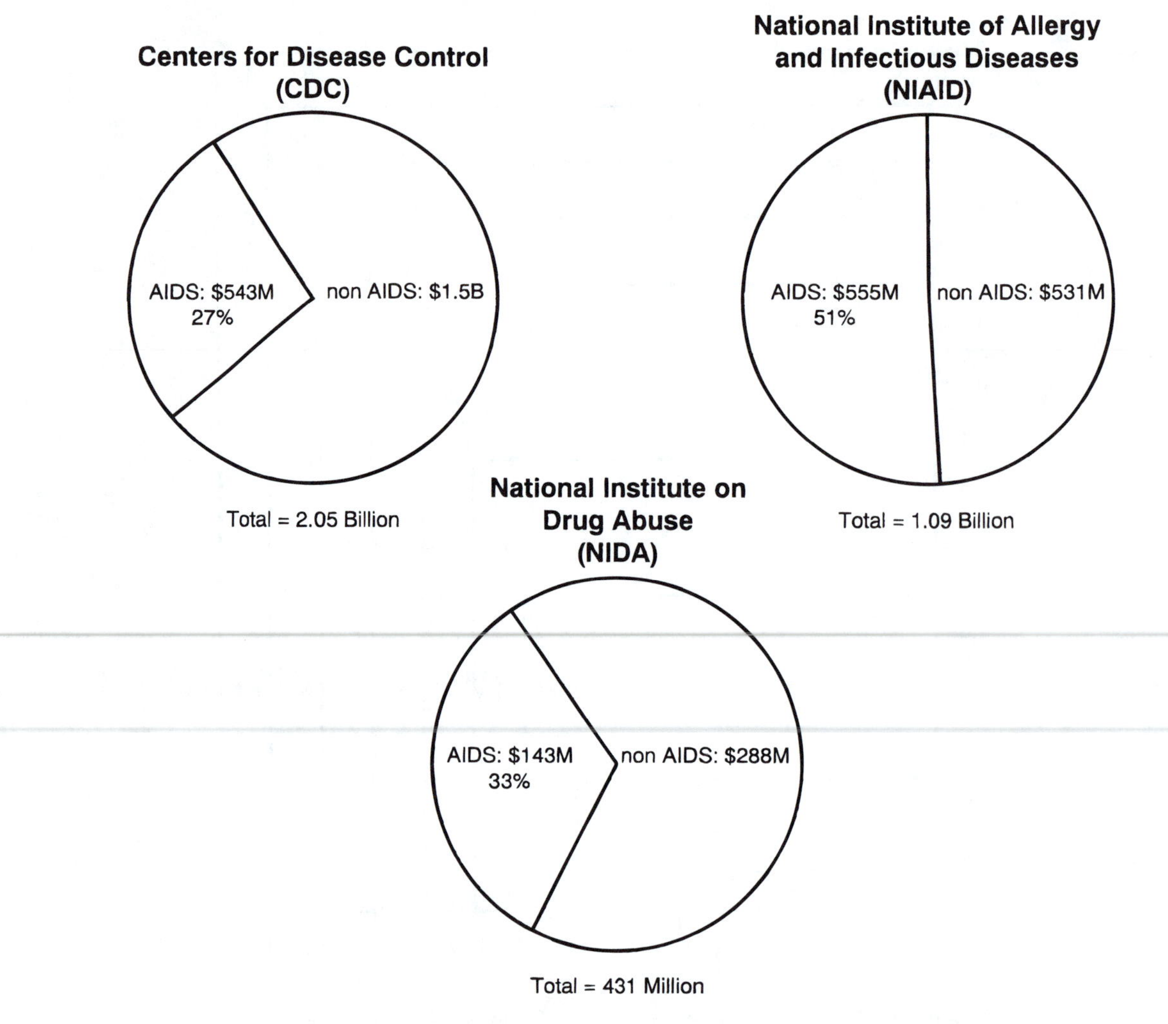

FIGURE 15-2 Three Major Federal Health Agency Budgets for 1994. The CDC, NIAID, and NIDA are three of the largest AIDS dollar consumers within the National Institutes of Health.

AIDS Expenditures Compared to Other Major Diseases

Federal spending for AIDS research, educational programs, counselor training, testing, and prevention programs has been compared with federal spending for other diseases (Table 15-1). There is a discrepancy between the federal dollars spent on certain diseases and the number of deaths they cause. In 1989, AIDS projects received $1.3 billion and there were about 19,000 AIDS-related deaths. In 1992, with 31,000 plus deaths, HIV/AIDS received $1.26 billion. In 1993, with 33,787 deaths, HIV/AIDS received $4.9 billion. In 1993, cancer caused about 526,000 deaths (about 1,500 people/day) and received $1.9 billion. During the same year, there were 1,170,000 new cases of cancer in the United States; 183,000 were new cases of breast cancer and there were over 46,000 breast cancer-associated deaths. One in seven to nine women will get breast cancer. Heart disease, which caused some 950,000 deaths in 1993 (43% of all deaths in that year),

BOX 15.2

THE COST FOR TREATING HEMOPHILIA—UNITED STATES

Before the blood supply in the United States became contaminated with HIV, the cost per unit of **blood factor VIII** was about 12 cents. The new technologies that are needed to establish and maintain a safe supply of factor VIII drove the price so high that it is jeopardizing the lives of patients. While some hemophiliacs are covered by private health insurance, many are not. Those who must depend on Medicaid and other state-supported programs are often forced to limit family income to maintain their eligibility, and it is not unheard of for husbands and wives to divorce in order to meet the requirements for this kind of financial aid.

In 1992, the television program "60 Minutes" interviewed people who had children with hemophilia. The cost of treatment was staggering—it may run as high as $200,000/year/child.

In order to stop a bleeding episode, hemophiliacs need an injection of a blood clotting factor (factor VIII). Clotting factor is isolated out of the blood of donors, concentrated, and sold. A batch of clotting factor may be separated out from the donated blood of 20,000 or more people. It is estimated that up to 50% of the 20,000 individuals affected by inherited bleeding disorders who used blood component therapy prior to 1985 are infected with HIV. In 1989, AIDS replaced hemorrhage, central nervous system (CNS) bleeding, and liver disease as the leading cause of death among hemophiliacs.

The reporter interviewed one family that had a 13-year-old son who was hemophilic. His condition was discovered at age 3, at a time prior to recognizing that much of the blood supply in the United States was contaminated with HIV. Somewhere along the way, he was injected with HIV-contaminated clotting factor. He now has AIDS.

The parents of this young man said that their expenses for HIV/AIDS therapy were between $45,000 and $50,000 a year. But that was small compared to the cost of the clotting factor. In April of 1992, just 1 month, his bill for clotting factor came to $24,000. One vial of clotting factor, enough for one infusion, cost $1000. Their son, in one episode, used 2 vials/day for 10 days. This family has been trying to pay bills like this for the past 5 years. Friends help with food and mortgage payments, but they owe too much to pay the 20 to 30 medical bills coming in each month. Because of their financial burden, the parents have considered divorce. This would allow their son to receive free medical benefits under Medicaid, and Social Security benefits.

The reporter interviewed a second family with a similar story: cost of clotting factor, $200,000/year and about $50,000 for AIDS treatment. In this case the husband and wife divorced so the son could receive the medical benefits.

TABLE 15-1 Federal Monies Spent on Five Major Diseases

Diseases	Millions of Dollars	Deaths[a] in 1993
Cancer	1,900	526,000
AIDS	4,900	36,787
Heart disease	900	950,000
Diabetes	287	200,000
Stroke, hypertension	186	150,000

1994 Federal expenditure figures are for research, education, and prevention programs and may underestimate actual amounts.

[a]Deaths in the United States (Source: Monthly Statistics Report, U.S. Dept. Health and Human Services, CDC. April, 1994; A. Cancer J. Clinic, 1993, 43:7–26)

received less than $1 billion. Some 2 million Americans require insulin injections for type I diabetes and perhaps as many as 10 to 12 million have type II diabetes (diet controlled). Diabetes, a severe progressive disorder, received $287 million, or about 5.8% of the AIDS budget in 1993. It is estimated that 200,000 people will die because of diabetes complications. Hypertension, which affects millions of Americans and is involved in about 100,000 to 200,000 deaths per year received $186 million. Overall, between 1981 and the end of 1993, while 212,000 people died of AIDS, 7.5 million died of heart disease and 4.5 million died of cancer.

In 1990, AIDS projects received $2.2 billion from the federal government. In 1993, $4.9 billion was allocated. To place these data in perspective, in 1993, the federal government paid farmers over $7 billion *not* to grow crops (production subsidies), and lost over $3 billion on defaulted student loans. Star Wars research in 1992 cost $4.2 billion.

Justification for AIDS Expenditures—William Winkenwerder and colleagues (1989) pointed out that if federal dollars for HIV/AIDS projects continue to increase at current rates, it will become difficult to justify the expenditures. They point out that over 63 million Americans have cardiovascular diseases and about 30% of the population will eventually have some type of cancer. Smoking, a preventable health risk, is associated with an estimated 400,000 deaths annually. Alcohol abuse is linked to premature death, accidents, crime, and lost productivity, with an associated cost estimated at over $150 billion a year.

Winkenwerder and colleagues also point out that spending more money on AIDS does not necessarily mean progress or a cure, and may, in fact, be wasted. In the 1970s the Nixon administration spent between $30 million and $50 million on cancer research on the assumption that a cure could be found if enough money was available to support basic research. But many years and billions of dollars later, a cure for cancer still eludes our best scientific efforts. But the cause of AIDS and means of its prevention are known. With many diseases such as hypertension, diabetes, heart disease, stroke, and cancer, cause and prevention are complex and not as easily defined. The questions now being asked by legislators are: How much money is enough for HIV/AIDS projects? What about all the other diseases that have to be funded?

BOX 15.3

HIV/AIDS FEDERAL FUNDING BEING MISDIRECTED?

According to an October 1992 report in the *Washington Post,* the National Institutes of Health is diverting millions of dollars away from research on adults with AIDS and toward children with HIV/AIDS.

As a result, pediatric AIDS now consumes nearly 40% of the federal budget for testing new AIDS drugs, despite the fact that only 1.3% of over 472,000 AIDS patients are children. Of 30 million children under the age of 5 in the United States, only 0.15% have AIDS. Of children ages 1 to 14, 42% of deaths result from accidents, 10% from cancer, 9% from congenital anomalies, 6% from homicide, 4% from heart disease, and so on. AIDS comes in ninth. NIH spending on new AIDS drugs for children is now 34 times higher per patient than for adults; and to fund the increases, medical centers treating adults have seen sharp cuts in their budgets.

The shift in resources represents the new political clout of the pediatric HIV/AIDS lobby and Congress, far greater funding for research to benefit children rather than for drug users and gay men who make up the bulk of the AIDS population.

In your opinion, is this turn of events morally correct? Economically correct? Politically correct?

AIDS: Direct Costs of HIV Disease

In 1991, the Department of Health and Human Services' Agency for Health Care Policy and Research determined that between 1991 and 1994, the costs of treating all people with HIV disease will increase 21% each year. In 1995 between $15 billion and $20 billion will be spent on people with HIV disease/AIDS).

Lifetime Costs for Treating People with HIV Disease/AIDS

Fred Hellinger's (1993) study on the lifetime costs of treating a person with HIV disease/AIDS assumes that an individual is identified and treated for HIV immediately following infection. The study presents data from a large multistate survey that collected data directly from persons with HIV from March, 1991 through August, 1992. Table 15-2 presents hospitalizations, costs of those hospitalizations, and the total cost of care during **all** stages of HIV disease. Data in Table 15-2 indicate that the mean survival time of a person diagnosed with AIDS in 1993 is 25 months. Multiplying this figure by the average monthly

POINT OF VIEW 15.1

EACH DISEASE DESERVES AN INDEPENDENT LEVEL OF FUNDING

The tragedy of cancer and other diseases cannot be denied. But should the distribution of funds be based on the number of people dying from a disease? It would appear that this type of judgment may be short-sighted because the cause of each disease must be taken into account. AIDS is caused by a transmissible virus: **It can be spread geometrically**! There is a real chance to prevent HIV infection. Can we say that about most other diseases whose cause is vague and not associated with a microorganism? The point is that **each disease** needs funding sufficient to service the needs of that particular disease spectrum. Money for one disease should not be taken from a pool of money needed to combat another disease. Funding for disease prevention should be taken out of the political arena; there should be no "pet" diseases sponsored by a single physician or group of politicians. People must resist the divisive effort to pit one disease group against another and to compare one disease against the other, simply because such comparisons are so often dealing with "apples and oranges." Instead, people fighting against all those life-threatening illnesses must band together and seek more money for use against all diseases. The monetary obligation to each disease should be determined by those who research and treat it.

cost of $2,764 indicates the lifetime cost after AIDS diagnosis until death in 1993 will be $69,100. Lifetime cost from HIV infection until death is estimated to be $119,274.

Direct medical costs per person for the State of Florida can be seen in Table 15-3. In San Bernadino County, California, it is estimated that 7,800 HIV-infected people cost $796 million for treatment until death. That cost is $102,051 per person (Kurata et al., 1993).

Hellinger (1993) estimated the average medical costs for an HIV-infected person with a T4 cell count of less than 200/μL to be about $990/month. The medical costs for an HIV-positive person with a T4 cell count greater than 200/μL but less than 500/μL was estimated to be $430/month. And for an HIV-positive person with a T4 cell count of 500/μL or higher, $282/month (Table 15-4). The lifetime costs of treating a person with HIV may be calculated by multiplying the average monthly cost of care in each of the four stages by the corresponding mean occupancy time (i.e., the average number of months an infected person spends in a given stage before proceeding to the next stage) and summing the four products (Table 15-2).

Worldwide Costs

According to the World Health Organization (WHO), through 1994, $50 billion has been lost due to lost productivity, lost markets, and

TABLE 15-2 HIV Disease, Stage, and Lifetime Treatment Cost (In 1992 dollars)

	Mean Occupancy Time (mo.)	Cost per Month ($)	Total Cost of Care During Time in Disease Stage ($)
Disease stage			
HIV-positive without AIDS ($T4$ cell count $\geq 0.50 \times 10^9/L$)	67.3	282 (216–348)	18,978 (14,537–23,420)[a]
HIV-positive without AIDS ($T4$ cell count ≥ 0.20 and $<0.50 \times 10^9/L$)	44.0	430 (353–507)	18,920 (15,532–22,308)
HIV-positive without AIDS ($T4$ cell count $<0.20 \times 10^9/L$)	12.4	990 (842–1138)	12,276 (10,441–14,111)
With AIDS	25	2764 (2610–2918)	69,100 (65,250–72,950)
Total lifetime cost of care	148.7	802	119,274 (105,760–132,789)

[a]Numbers in parentheses are 95% confidence intervals.
(Source: Hellinger, 1993)

TABLE 15-3 Current and Projected Costs for AIDS Patient Care—State of Florida

Year	Total Number Patients	Living[a] AIDS Patients	Direct Personal $ Cost / Patient	Total Direct Personal Cost In $ Millions
1988	6,205	4,715	44,114 (9.38)	208
1989	11,016	7,931	48,039 (6.04)	381
1990	14,875	8,925	52,074 (3.9)	465
1991	20,407	11,631	56,468 (2.5)	657
1992	26,098	10,962	62,500 (5.7)	685
1993	35,697	15,355	119,000 (7.8)	1,827
1994[b]	42,049	18,082	119,000 (6.6)	2,152

Total numbers of patients reported in the Florida health care system funded by state and federal programs. Actual number of AIDS patients in state of Florida is higher but difficult to estimate.

[a]Number of live AIDS patients at any time during the year, cost per patient, and total amount each year to be spent on persons with AIDS for direct medical care, 1988–1994.

[b]Estimates for 1994 based on first quarter report of 1,588 AIDS cases. Death rates for 1992–1994 at 57%.

retraining of people for jobs held by those who have HIV disease or have died of AIDS. The WHO projects that by the year 2000, the economic costs of HIV/AIDS could reach 1.4% of the world's gross national product—equal to the value of the economy of Australia.

AIDS: Indirect Costs or the Human Capital Approach

The human capital approach to the cost of AIDS takes into account the usual life cycle patterns of the labor market and potential earnings. Indirect cost is lost productivity due to premature death. Most people dying from AIDS are in the 20- to 45-year-old age bracket. The expected lifetime earnings of a 29-year-old male are $727,000. If he dies at age 29, society loses $727,000 worth of productivity.

Indirect costs are about five times higher per person than direct costs. For example, in 1986 direct costs for AIDS patients were $600 million, while the indirect cost of lost economic productivity was about $3 billion. Projections of direct costs for 1991 are about $11 billion and indirect costs are projected at $55 billion. While the direct costs of AIDS are about equal to those of cancer and heart disease, the indirect costs are much higher because AIDS is primarily a disease of the young and middle-aged. Heart attacks and strokes, in particular, are associated with older people with less economic potential. The future earnings of a 67-year-old male are estimated at $30,000 (Caldwell et al., 1988).

Nonpersonal Costs of AIDS

In 1986, the federal government spent $234 million on public education about AIDS; in 1987 it spent $494 million; and in 1988, $931 million. In addition, between 1986 and 1988, the federal government spent over $210 million on testing military personnel for HIV. In 1989, $2.2 billion in federal funds were spent on HIV/AIDS research, education, and prevention. The 1992 federal budget for these three programs was projected to be $4.3 billion. Estimates of nonpersonal costs are about

TABLE 15-4 Estimated Monthly Cost ($) of Treating a Person with HIV by Disease Stage

Service Component ($)	Persons with AIDS	HIV-Positive without AIDS (T4 Cell Count <0.20 × 10⁹/L)	HIV-Positive without AIDS T4 Cell Count ≥0.20 × 10⁹/L and <0.50 × 10⁹/L	HIV-Positive without AIDS (T4 Cell Count ≥0.50 × 10⁹/L)
Inpatient	1,890 (68)	456 (46)	119 (28)	54 (19)
Outpatient visits	380 (14)	344 (35)	191 (44)	151 (54)
Home health	174 (6)	80 (8)	21 (5)	10 (4)
Drug costs	265 (10)	110 (11)	99 (23)	67 (24)
Long-term care	55 (2)	0	0	0
Total	2,764	990	430	282

Charges in 1992 dollars. Percentage of total charges shown in parentheses. HIV, human immunodeficiency virus; AIDS, acquired immunodeficiency syndrome. Percentages may not total 100 due to rounding.

(Source: Hellinger, 1993)

BOX 15.4

PUBLIC BACKLASH TO AIDS

Because of TV, plays, magazine articles, newspapers, radio talk shows, pamphlets in physicians' offices, and courses in schools and universities, the public is feeling AIDS anxiety. Yet the general public does not feel it is in danger. Perhaps because they have been told repeatedly that the majority of people affected are homosexuals, bisexuals, IDUs, and prostitutes. Many people might think "I'm not one of them. I just want to be left alone. The problems they have could be prevented if they wanted to."

PLACING THE BLAME

The AIDS pandemic has provided individuals with a platform from which they can blame someone else for a disease. During the 14th century, Jews were burned at the stake for causing the plague. In the 19th century, cholera was called God's wrath on the poor and immoral. In the 20th century, polio in America was believed to be caused by Italian immigrants. Now it is AIDS, and some evangelists and politicians say it is God's condemnation of the homosexuals, injection drug users, and prostitutes. California Senator Jim Neilson said in 1989 that AIDS may be God's way of visiting a plague upon mankind (Silverman, 1990).

Former U.S. Surgeon General C. Everett Koop said he feared the American public may turn against AIDS patients as their numbers increase and the taxpayer has to pick up the tab for their health care.

> Such a public response would be tragic, but it is not unexpected among health professionals. Retribution may come about in the 1990s as Americans grow to resent the cost of caring for AIDS patients, estimated at over $5 billion a year, and as health workers burn out from the pressures of watching young people die. There is a public mood of retribution as evidenced by the spread of no-smoking areas aimed at smokers, as well as the crackdown against drunk drivers, against teenage pregnancies, wife beaters and drug addicts.

For whatever reasons, fund raisers say that almost none of the largest foundations in the United States have given a cent to fight AIDS. William Freeman, director of Institutional Affairs for the National AIDS Network, said that because 44% of AIDS patients are minorities, he fears that within the next 3 years AIDS will be considered just another disease of the poor.

An example of how individuals perceive the HIV/AIDS epidemic can be found in a letter to a newspaper columnist.

> In a recent column you said 47,000 people died of AIDS since the early '80s. You didn't say how many people died of cancer during the same period.
>
> When I saw that quilt commemorating AID victims on Ted Koppel's *Nightline* I was infuriated. My brother had just died of cancer. He was 44, didn't smoke, didn't drink and lived for his wife and three kids. According to the American Cancer Society, a half-million people like him will die this year. But federal funding for cancer research is being cut back because there isn't enough money to go around.
>
> I realize that AIDS is a terrible disease. But homosexuals who are monogamous do not get AIDS. I am also aware that some babies are born with AIDS and that a bad blood transfusion can result in AIDS. I am not talking about these people, I am talking about homosexuals who are promiscuous.
>
> I realize that people who have AIDS, from whatever source, are gravely ill and need our compassion and our sympathy, but skip the quilt. Just remember that AIDS is avoidable. Most cancer is not.

As the economic and medical impact continues to increase, resentment may grow in proportion. The burden of dealing with the AIDS pandemic is moving from the federal government onto city, state, and voluntary agencies, placing the issues of how much to spend and on what directly in the hands of the voters.

Aran Ron and David Rogers reported that

> The majority of new AIDS diagnoses are in injection drug users, their sexual partners, and infants born to these couples. More than 80% of these patients are black or Hispanic and almost all are poor. These groups, along with homosexual AIDS patients and substance abusers who don't have AIDS, are already placing great demand on limited hospital resources. It is becoming more difficult to arrange admission for patients with acute illnesses requiring hospitalization. There are anecdotal reports of patients who wait days in emergency departments before a hospital bed becomes available, and elective admissions are also becoming more difficult to arrange. If care for persons with AIDS is perceived as interfering with the health care of others, bitter conflicts between those with and without AIDS and acts of discrimination that may fall along racial lines seem likely. (Ron et al., 1988)

one third of the direct costs for any given year. For 1991, the research budget was in excess of $1.2 billion; for blood screening $930 million; and for education, $233 million.

Hospital Care for AIDS Patients

Projections on the number of cases into the 1990s indicate that the current number of HIV/AIDS cases will at least double. (This projection was made prior to the 1993 CDC definition for AIDS, which increased the total number of AIDS over 1992 by 111%.) Will there be a sufficient number of hospital beds available for these people? Hospital treatment remains the primary and frequently the only source of care for AIDS patients (Andrulis et al., 1987).

In 1987, the National Public Health and Hospital Institute conducted a national survey of 623 acute care hospitals to obtain information relating to inpatient and outpatient AIDS care. Two hundred seventy-six (44%) reported treating people with AIDS; the average stay was 16.8 days. Average cost and revenue per day were $681 and $545, respectively; a loss of $135 per day. The cost per year was $17,910. Estimated cost for AIDS inpatient care during 1987 was $486 million; Medicaid represented the primary payer. But Medicaid is available only to indigent patients. As a result, AIDS patients and even those who are HIV-infected must spend themselves into poverty (with assets of less than $2,000) in order to qualify for Medicaid. In 1989, one in five HIV-infected individuals had **no** insurance. As the disease progresses, they become indigent and have to rely on already overburdened public hospitals.

In 1987, the National Public Health and Hospital Institute in Washington, D.C., surveyed 276 hospitals that treated AIDS patients. The results showed that 10% of the hospitals treated 58% of all AIDS patients receiving treatment. Of these 28 hospitals, 10, including six public hospitals, cared for 32% of all AIDS patients. By the end of 1992, AIDS patients in New York City occupied about one in every four public hospital beds. In San Francisco, AIDS patients occupied about one in every five public hospital beds. It is believed that the same scenario will eventually be seen in all metropolitan public hospitals across the nation.

The Crowding-Out Phenomenon—In 1987, 72% of AIDS patients were treated in public hospitals; 26% in private hospitals and 2% in veteran's hospitals. Larry Gage, President of the National Hospital Association, said that there is a crowding-out phenomenon. AIDS patients are beginning to crowd out other indigent patients, and in some cases even insured patients who do not have the same urgent need of medical care. AIDS is changing the nature and mission of some hospitals.

Even the teaching hospitals in the United States are feeling the AIDS caseload crunch. Information from the Fifth International Conference on AIDS indicates that AIDS is having a negative impact on teaching hospitals. A survey reported at the conference indicated that:

1. Only 13% of teaching hospitals are reimbursed for counseling AIDS patients.
2. Infectious disease specialists may have to give short shrift to other problems, as they are now spending more than a third of their time in the hospital on AIDS-related cases.
3. Twenty percent of respondents from 88 hospitals reported medical school and house staff recruitment problems. These were more likely to be in high-incidence institutions.
4. Nineteen percent of the respondents reported that hospital personnel had quit because of AIDS-related fears and frustrations.
5. Twenty percent reported that physicians had refused to care for AIDS patients.
6. In 61% of the teaching institutions, employees had demanded that patients be tested for HIV.

THE INSURANCE INDUSTRY AND AIDS

Insurance is, by definition, a spreading of the risk, and AIDS most affects the age group that had previously been the healthiest and therefore the least likely to use health benefits. Because the cost of treating an AIDS patient is high (and group health and life insurance premiums are based in part on a group's loss-claims experience with its insurance carrier and also on actuarial tables, which forecast the probable cost of medical treatment for an age group), insurance costs have risen (and continue to rise) even for those companies in which no employee has contracted AIDS or a related illness. However, the cost for treating an individual with AIDS is actually less in many cases than treating an employee for cancer.

Fifty-nine percent of health care in America is financed primarily through private insurance and uninsured people who pay their own expenses. Forty-one percent is financed through public sector programs at the federal, state, and local levels. The problem of providing care for people with HIV infection and AIDS has financially strained the health care system.

Barriers to health care for HIV/AIDS patients include: (1) refusal by private insurers to underwrite individual policies for people who test positive for HIV; (2) loss of employment-related group health insurance; (3) variable coverage and eligibility policies of state Medicaid programs; (4) reimbursement by private insurance and public programs at levels that do not encourage use of services and facilities commensurate with need; and (5) lack of coordination between health care and social service systems. There is the additional problem of over 37 million uninsured individuals who do not qualify for public health care (Table 15.4) (Friedman, 1991). It should be mentioned that although this number, 37 million, has been used repeatedly in all types of forums, Katherine Swartz (1994) argues that the number is very misleading. Her statistics describe the dynamics of people moving in and out of particular insurance situations. Swartz writes that a large proportion of the uninsured pick up insurance within relatively short periods, but a significant number of people are uninsured for very long periods of time. For many people (at least 21 million in 1993), being without health insurance is not a temporary or transitory phase in their lives.

Over the course of a year, many more than 37 million Americans will be uninsured for 1 to 11 months, but not during the single month that the Census Bureau counts the uninsured. That 1-month survey is the basis for the point-in-time figure of 37 million. In fact, the number of Americans who are uninsured during a given year is closer to 58 million—about one quarter of the nonelderly population is uninsured.

About 36% of this total are uninsured for the entire year, some 21 million Americans. Thus, when the point-in-time estimate of 37 million is used, it represents 16 million people who will be uninsured for less than a year and 21 million long-term uninsured.

In 1988, of 31 million adolescents between ages 10 and 18, one in seven had no health insurance. In 1994, one in three had no health insurance (*Hastings Center Report*, 1991 updated). Between the ages of 18 and 44, 25% lacked health insurance (Diaz et al., 1994).

For the medically disenfranchised, there is no access to a system of care. For those who have no doctor, no clinic, no means of payment, access to health care services is most often through the emergency room door of one of the few hospitals the community that treats people with HIV infection and AIDS. Five percent of the nation's hospitals treat 50% of the people with AIDS.

As new therapies are developed, the gaps in the system may present even greater problems. In addition to the direct cost of therapy, prolonging life may result in additional costs. If new therapies are effective for asymptomatic HIV-infected people, who may outnumber other clinic patients by 20 or 50 to one, the financial implications will be profound. Moreover, as HIV/AIDS patients live longer, many may become eligible for Medicare, having outlived the 24-month waiting period following determination of disability. As patients live longer, many more will also outlive insurance coverage (*Public Health Reports*, 1988).

Is Insurance Obtainable and/or Affordable?

Industry trade groups estimate that health insurance claims and death benefits paid in AIDS-related cases totaled $1.6 billion in 1994, for a total of $7 billion since 1990.

Life insurance companies typically require individuals to take a blood test before writing a policy for a large amount of money. Insurance officials say they deny coverage to people who test positive for HIV because the odds are that those people will get AIDS and die, absorbing large claims or benefits after paying only a small amount in premiums. The insurance companies feel that if they continued paying those high claims, they would not be able to continue coverage for other customers and remain financially sound.

The American Council of Life Insurance and the Health Insurance Association of America conducted a survey of 325 insurance companies. All of these companies said they would refuse coverage to someone who had tested HIV-positive.

As a response to this, 14 states have set up a pool of money to help care for the uninsurable. Other states are considering such pools. California, the District of Columbia, and Maine have passed controversial bills concerning AIDS and insurance companies. These bills **prohibit** companies from requiring anyone to take the HIV antibody test or inquiring if they have had such a test. They also restrict the companies from basing rates or other aspects of coverage on whether a person has had such a test.

The latest trend among companies is an attempt to control, rather than avoid, the cost of AIDS care. In the earlier stages of illness, AIDS patients do not usually require acute care. Less expensive home or hospice care is an alternative to hospitalization. Insurance companies that do not normally cover this sort of care are beginning to investigate such alternatives.

As reported, over 37 million people in the United States are without health insurance (Wenneker et al., 1990). These people are not all poor and unemployed. Some make respectable wages but have simply been priced out of the private insurance market, and their employers refuse to cover them in a group plan because the cost of group insurance is skyrocketing. Some individuals are not insurable because they have certain illnesses such as cancer or diabetes.

Between 1980 and 1983, health insurance premiums increased 50%, while the average income went up only 17%. The rates are leveling off somewhat, but are still beyond the reach of many millions of Americans (Table 15-5).

Profile of the Uninsured

The General Accounting Office recently drew a profile of the uninsured population. Nearly three quarters are employed, but most work at part-time jobs where insurance is not part of the package (Table 15-5). The growth of employment in retail and construction has contributed to the number of uninsured workers because those industries traditionally are less likely to offer coverage.

Risk Classification for the Insured

From the insurance industry's point of view, the issue is one of risk classification. Life insurers have always used medical information to try to predict how long customers are likely to live. In a process known as underwriting, a company groups people with similar risk—based on factors such as age, current health status, family medical history, occupation, and lifestyle—and charges each member of a group the same rate, which is proportional to the amount of risk the company assumes in insuring them. In this way, the industry attempts to keep healthier individuals from subsidizing people with greater risks.

Depending on a physical examination and answers to specific questions asked by a physician, an individual may be able to obtain a policy by paying a higher than normal premium or by accepting a policy that contains a waiver (insured but not for a certain condition).

TABLE 15-5 The Uninsured: By Race and Employment Status

Race	Percentage of Uninsured People (1993)
White	11.7
Black	20.2
Hispanic	26.5
Employment status[a]	
Full-time[b]	62.0
Part-time	23.2
Unemployed	14.8

[a]Employment status for primary wage earner (head of household).

[b]Part-time includes those who worked full-time for only part of the year.

(Source: *The New York Times*, April 28, 1991, p. 28; updated)

BOX 15.5

THE RIGHT TO HEALTH INSURANCE?

A physician shared his concern over patients' rights this way: "You have the right to remain silent or to request that I not record any part of your medical history."

If abusive practices by insurance companies do not cease, this medical equivalent of a Miranda criminal rights statement could become necessary so physicians could warn their patients that what they say could be used against them—often unfairly.

To obtain private health insurance, the health consumer has no choice but to sign his or her name, allowing insurance companies to obtain medical records from any physician or health provider.

In the past, this would consist of a brief summary form completed by the physician. Now increasingly, insurance companies photocopy every page of the patients' medical records, opening their most intimate, nonmedically pertinent secrets to scrutiny.

It is not uncommon for insurance companies to turn down single men who happen to be waiters, decorators, or hairdressers for fear that some might be gay and more prone to AIDS. Even married men have been scrubbed because an unreliable test for AIDS falsely tagged them as HIV-positive. In 1991, the 5th U.S. Circuit Court of Appeals in New Orleans ruled that employers who provide *self-insured health plans* for their workers have the right to substantially reduce medical benefits to those with AIDS-related illnesses. The ruling stems from a case where a Houston company cut its plan for $1 million in lifetime health coverage to $5,000—but only for workers with AIDS. This is the first federal appeals court ruling of its kind to become law in Louisiana, Texas, and Mississippi, unless overturned by the U.S. Supreme Court. In November, 1992, the United States Supreme Court refused to hear an appeal of the 5th Circuit Court ruling. This decision may be used to reduce insurance coverage for many other illnesses. However, similar reduction in coverage for other such cases has now been ruled discriminatory under the Americans with Disabilities Act. (See ADA rulings in Chapter 16.)

There are, however, a number of health problems for which individuals are denied an insurance policy (Table 15-6). Diagnosed HIV infection and AIDS are both reasons for health care and death benefit insurance policy denial. In fact, the insurance industry is still reacting to a study done in late 1987 indicating that a 35-year-old man who is infected with HIV is 51 times more likely to die prematurely than a healthy male of the same age. Insurance applicants who are more than five or six times as likely to die prematurely are usually too expensive to underwrite. For example, a 35-year-old male with coronary heart disease would be five times as likely as a healthy applicant to die a premature death.

TABLE 15-6 Some Commercial Health Insurers: Classification of Risks

Higher Premium	Exclusion Waiver	Denial
Allergies	Cataract	AIDS
Asthma	Gallstones	Ulcerative colitis
Back strain	Fibroid tumor (uterus)	Cirrhosis of liver
Hypertension (controlled)	Hernia (hiatal/inguinal)	Diabetes mellitus
Arthritis	Migraine headaches	Leukemia
Gout	Pelvic inflammatory disease	Schizophrenia
Glaucoma	Chronic otitis disorders	Hypertension (uncontrolled)
Obesity	Spine/back disorders	Emphysema
Psychoneurosis (mild)	Hemorrhoids	Stroke
Kidney stones	Knee impairment	Obesity (severe)
Emphysema (mild–moderate)	Asthma	Angina (severe)
Alcoholism/drug abuse	Allergies	Coronary artery disease
Heart murmur	Varicose veins	Epilepsy
Peptic ulcer	Sinusitis, chronic or severe	Lupus
Colitis	Fractures	Alcoholism/drug abuse

Commercial Health Insurers

In 1988, Jill Eden and colleagues reported the results of a survey on AIDS and health insurance for the Office of Technological Assessment (OTA). The survey was sent to 88 commercial insurers, to 15 of 77 available Blue Cross/Blue Shield (BC/BS) plans, and to the 50 largest local and national Health Maintenance Organizations (HMOs). Sixty-one commercial insurers, all 15 BC/BS, and 39 of the HMOs responded to the survey. Several questions from that survey are presented along with the respondents' answers:

Question: Do health insurers attempt to identify applicants exposed to HIV?

Answer: Forty-one commercial insurers currently test applicants for HIV infection—10 are planning to test. If the applicant tests positive for HIV, he or she will be denied insurance.

Question: How do insurers screen applicants for HIV exposure?

Answer: Not all health insurers concerned with the applicant's HIV status demand HIV testing. Those that do not test rely on a review of the applicant's medical history questionnaire and the attending physician's statement (APS) to assess the risk of HIV exposure. Thirty-four of the 41 commercial health insurers have AIDS-related questions on the medical history form. The AIDS-associated questions vary with the insurance company. Some companies ask about AIDS-related signs and symptoms; some ask whether the applicant has ever been HIV tested and what test he or she has had (Table 15-7).

Through 1993, the states of California, Connecticut, Florida, Hawaii, Maine, and Washington, D.C. prohibited HIV testing as a condition for life and health insurability. Similar HIV testing bans for insurance applicants in New York, Wisconsin, and Massachusetts have been invalidated. Although California does not allow HIV testing, it does allow a T cell count to determine if the individual has a properly functioning immune system. Insurers and gay rights activist groups nationwide are escalating their fight over AIDS issues, with testing foremost in the struggle. The insurers say that if they are not allowed to test, then other policyholders will have to subsidize the costs. Gay activists say that those who most need access to health insurance are least able to get it.

Another effort by gay activist groups is to ban the limiting of AIDS-related coverage. By 1988, 19 states had already prohibited the practice.

Insurers say that if HIV testing is prohibited, they may experience **adverse selection**. As insurance companies raise their premiums, low-risk individuals will stop buying insurance. But individuals at high risk of developing AIDS will continue to want full coverage, and the percentage of AIDS patients among those insured will rise. As a result, insurance companies will again raise their premiums and more low-risk individuals will drop their coverage. Finally, only those individuals with the highest risk of developing AIDS will want to buy insurance at rates they may not be able to afford.

Testing is already affecting low-risk insurance applicants. A long-married Florida resident with two children had a chance to save $300 a year by switching life insurance carriers if he took the AIDS test the insurer now requires for policies of $250,000 or more. Rather than risk a false-positive result that would go on his record, he remained with the old insurer.

Question: Which applicants are to be tested?

Answer: Of the 61 insurers responding to the sur-

TABLE 15-7 Commercial Insurers, BC/BS Plans, and HMOs Screening for Exposure to HIV

Method(s) Used to Identify AIDS Exposure	Commercial Insurers[a] (*n* = 50)		BC/BS Plans[a] (n = 11)		HMOs[a] (n = 9)	
	Number	Percent	Number	Percent	Number	Percent
Question on application	44	88	11	100	9	100
Attending physician statement	42	84	9	82	6	67
T cell subset study	17	34	0	—	0	—

BC/BS, Blue Cross/Blue Shield; HMOs, health maintenance organizations (25% of medically insured Americans have BC/BS plans; BC/BS offers 69 different medical plans across the United States).

[a]Data included only those insurers or plans that screen or intend to screen for AIDS exposure.

(Adapted from Office of Technology Assessment, Eden et al., 1988; updated 1994)

vey, 31 routinely tested applicants. Seven of the 31 companies tested every applicant, 14 of 31 tested those who admitted to a lifestyle that placed them *at high risk* (high risk was defined differently by each company). Ten companies tested applicants depending on criteria such as residence, medical history, homosexuality, job, and amount of the policy. Three insurers stated that all applicants living in high HIV prevalence areas such as large cities in New York, California, and Florida were tested. Some insurance companies stated that they did not insure IDUs or hemophiliacs.

Question: What are the future plans of the 61 responding insurance companies to offset the financial impact of AIDS?

Answer: Only one insurer, an HMO, plans to withdraw from the marketplace. Thirty-four percent of the commercial insurers and 40% of BC/BS insurers plan to reduce individual and small group health markets (use more restrictive underwriting guidelines). Thirty-three percent of commercial insurers plan to expand HIV or other types of testing for applicants. Nine companies will add questions on AIDS to their medical history forms. Seven BC/BS companies plan to exclude HIV/AIDS and other STDs from individual health coverage. One commercial insurer plans to establish a 2-year waiting period for AIDS before the policy takes effect. And two commercial insurers plan to limit the dollar value for AIDS claims.

In summary, private insurance covers a large part of the medical cost of AIDS patients. AIDS patients without private insurance coverage must pay for treatment themselves. After they have spent nearly all their assets and are indigent, they become eligible for Medicaid coverage in most but not all states. Also, income and asset limits for Medicaid vary among states. The federal government pays 50% to 77% of Medicaid costs, depending on per capita state income, with the state governments, and in some instances, local governments paying the remainder.

Commercial Life Insurers

Life insurance companies say they need to be allowed to test for HIV because people who know they are HIV-infected can pool resources and take out large policies. In 1986, $20 billion worth of individual policies and $15 billion worth of group policies were written for HIV-infected people. If left unchecked, increased premium payouts for AIDS deaths could bankrupt many insurers. The gay community argues that to test for insurance purposes would breach individual confidentiality. The insurers argue that they have a right to protect their financial stability. They say that they are allowed to withhold insurance for certain health problems (Table 15-6), to increase premiums for people who practice destructive

BOX 15.6

NEW YORK'S NEW INSURANCE LAW—1992

In July of 1992, the New York State Legislature passed the Community Rating Bill. This law is a major victory for all people with HIV disease, AIDS, and chronic illnesses. It widely expanded the opportunity of buying insurance, and helps people hang on to coverage they already have.

"Rating" is insurance-speak for the way the insurance company sets the cost of the premium.

"Community Rating" means that the insurance company spreads the cost of claims across the community. All claims from all policyholders are added up and the average of the cost of providing coverage at the end of the year becomes the new premium. No one is penalized for being in poorer health or punished for using their health insurance by getting a huge increase at the end of the year.

When this law took effect on April 1, 1993, people were allowed to change jobs without fear of losing their coverage or having an additional "preexisting condition waiting period" imposed. In short, if you have the money for the policy, commercial insurers, through an **open enrollment**, must sell it to you. This means you can go *shopping*! Maybe you'd like a policy with better prescription coverage, or more home health care, a higher lifetime maximum, or a lower deductible. This is not to say that a perfect "dream" policy is out there, or that it is within your price range, but it means that people of New York State won't have to worry about being rejected because of their age, sex, health status, sexual orientation, etc.

lifestyles such as smoking or alcoholism, and to stipulate exclusion waivers. Why should it be different for HIV-infected or people with AIDS?

Finally, insurance companies are suspected of denying coverage to people who live in certain neighborhoods, in same-gender households, or who work in certain professions. Sometimes insurers cancel policies or refuse to pay on grounds of preexisting conditions, fraud, or the experimental nature of treatment.

There may be laws in your state which prohibit insurance companies from asking certain questions, requiring an HIV/AIDS test, denying coverage, or engaging in other discrimination. Federal law also prohibits certain practices.

If you have an insurance-related problem, you probably will need legal help if your state insurance department cannot provide it.

Insurance Breakthrough: Collection of Benefits Before Death

Insurance experts estimate that one in five deaths will be due to AIDS by the year 2000. The cost of these AIDS-related deaths to life insurance companies may reach $50 billion to $100 billion. In mid-1989, in a move praised by gay rights activists and members of the medical and health care communities, the Canadian branch of Prudential Life Insurance started a program in which victims of acquired immune deficiency syndrome can get benefits from their life insurance policies before they die. The program allows patients access to 40% to 70% of their death benefits to pay for health care. It is hoped that other insurers will follow this practice.

A Right to Treatment

Some hospitals, nursing homes, and doctors may deny treatment to persons living with AIDS (PLWA) or provide less or inferior care than they provide to other patients. Health care discrimination against PLWAs may be fought under a number of federal and state laws. The following are some examples. They are not intended to give legal advice. It is important that you contact your state department or health or county welfare program to determine if you are eligible for benefits or protection under these laws. If you encounter difficulties in obtaining the protection described or you think you have legal problems, you should consult your local AIDS organization, ACLU-legal services, or bar association. Assistance may also be obtained from:

NATIONAL HEALTH LAW PROGRAM
2025 M Street, N.W.
Suite 400
Washington, D.C. 20036
(202) 887-5310

Section 504 of the Rehabilitation Act—Prohibits discrimination against the handicapped, in certain situations, by hospitals, nursing facilities, and state agencies which receive federal funds. AIDS has been determined to be a handicap for these purposes. Other recipients of federal funds may be covered under this act.

Hill-Burton Act—Hospitals and nursing homes which receive federal funds to build and operate their facilities may be challenged for discrimination in certain circumstances.

Anti-Dumping Laws—New federal law and some state laws require hospitals to examine, treat, and stabilize people in need of emergency care before discharge or transfer to other facilities.

State Anti-Discrimination, Privacy, or Civil Rights Laws—Many states have new or existing laws which prohibit discrimination against the handicapped, invasion of privacy, and violation of civil rights.

Funeral Expenses

Funeral directors in some cities will not knowingly handle AIDS deceased. Others are charging $300 to $1,000 extra for handling the bodies. The directors explain that they often must hire outside embalmers and other additional personnel to prepare the bodies. They also point out that after working on the bod-

BOX 15.7

VIATICALS: INCOME FROM THE SALE OF LIFE INSURANCE POLICIES

In 1989, insurance companies began to purchase life insurance policies from the terminally ill to allow them to collect benefits before they die. This new industry offered cash (a "viatical settlement") help to a person in danger of death, in return for being named the irrevocable beneficiary of a life insurance policy. Viatical settlements offer people with HIV disease disposable income that would otherwise accrue to their beneficiaries.

Viatical companies or private investors typically purchase life insurance policies at 60% to 80% of face value; this payment increases if life expectancy is shorter. Companies generally acquire policies valued at $50,000 to $500,000 and are reluctant to buy a policy if minor children or other dependents are reliant on the policyholder for financial support.

To meet the requirement of a viatical settlement, terminally ill people must release their medical records for review to the viatical company, which will use these records to estimate life expectancy. Group life insurance coverage can be viaticated only after it has been converted to an individual policy, but some group policies preclude viatication. The entire viatication process can take 3 to 4 months.

Viatical settlements are considered taxable income. Receiving a viatical settlement also disqualifies recipients from any means-based entitlements such as Medicaid or Supplemental Security Income (Peterson, 1992).

ONE VIATICAL SURVIVOR ENJOYS JACKPOT

To those who bet $100,000 on his quick death, one AIDS person became a viatical nightmare.

For the last 2 years, he has defied the laws of AIDS, surviving with a T4 cell count of less than 200.

Thanks to his viatication, in which investors paid him a portion of his life insurance money for the rights to the policy's proceeds, he has a lot of money.

For premium payments totaling $857 a year, he wound up with $100,000 in cash from a viatical investor. He said, "You go through this guilt thing at first. But you know they are making money off your death."

In 1990, he began negotiating with three viaticals, receiving offers of $75,000, $85,000, and $100,000 before selling his $150,000 policy to the top bidder.

Immediately, he went on a spending binge: two new cars, home redecoration, and college tuition for his siblings.

"Since I sold my policy, I haven't thought about AIDS. What more can you ask for than that you forget about your disease?"

The settlement led to other fortuitous events. He had never gone near the stock market. But his settlement put him in a gambling mood. He plunked down $30,000 on assorted stocks, betting on their 1-day rise. A year later, he had $300,000.

"Most people that I know are living longer and are happier," he said. "That is the bottom line: Happiness creates longevity."

He is getting ready to viaticate his second policy. It has a face value of $500,000. He says he will probably get $350,000.

ies, they must disinfect their labs and throw away gloves and other items that may be contaminated.

SUMMARY

AIDS is an expensive illness. The average cost of treatment per patient from diagnosis to death is about $69,000. Because many health care services are required to treat this pandemic, there has evolved an AIDS industry. For 1994/1995, it was estimated that about $15 billion was spent on the care of people with HIV disease/AIDS; and the cost is expected to continue to rise throughout the 1990s. In terms of number of deaths from a given disease and the federal dollars spent on it, AIDS is receiving a disproportionately large sum. For example, in

1994, $6.2 billion in federal funds was allocated to AIDS projects.

The fact that so many federal dollars are being used in AIDS programs, seemingly at the expense of other projects, and that the majority of affected people are homosexuals, bisexuals, and injection drug users, has spawned a public backlash. There is an increasing number of low-risk Americans who resent the expenditure of vast sums of money on these people when so many others need those same federal dollars. The situation may worsen as more hospital beds are occupied by AIDS patients and non-AIDS patients experience shortages. This is particularly true for public hospitals that already have a high caseload of indigent patients. In 1987, 72% of all AIDS patients were being treated in public hospitals. As the number of AIDS patients increases in the 1990s, fewer and fewer hospital resources will be available for non-AIDS patients. In addition, there may be a physician and nurse burnout—they may simply get tired of treating AIDS patients.

The high cost of AIDS therapy and hospitalization is now being met by individual insurance, group insurance, Medicaid, and Medicare. But insurance companies are looking for ways to deny policies to people who might be HIV-infected. Applicants are asked to fill out forms that ask specific questions about their lifestyles and whether they have ever been HIV-tested. Insurers believe they have a right to stay solvent. They feel they owe it to those who are insurable. Some insurers have, since the AIDS pandemic started, raised their life insurance premiums because they will have to pay claims on many people who were HIV-infected prior to obtaining a policy. Life insurance companies estimate that the cost of AIDS-related deaths may reach $50 billion by the year 2000. In that year, they project that one in every five deaths will be due to AIDS. Even funeral directors have added extra charges for embalming.

REVIEW QUESTIONS

(Answers to the Review Questions are on page 483.)

1. What is the average cost of medical care for an AIDS patient in the United States? Is that significantly higher than for patients who die of cancer, chronic heart disease, or diabetes?

2. What are indirect costs with regard to AIDS; and do they amount to more than direct costs?

3. With respect to AIDS, what is the irony of the health insurance industry?

4. What is the major concern of life insurance companies?

5. Who is responsible for your not becoming HIV-positive?

REFERENCES

ANDRULIS, DENNIS, et al. (1987). Provision and financing of medical care for AIDS patients in US public and private teaching hospitals. *JAMA*, 258:1343–1347.

BAUM, RUDY M. (1992). Progress fitful on understanding AIDS, developing therapies. *Chem. Eng. News*, 70:26–31.

CALDWELL, JACQUES R., et al. (1988). Economic stresses of AIDS: Lessons for the United States and Florida. *Florida M.A.*, 75:449–452.

CASTRO, JANICE. (1991). Condition critical. *Time*, 138:34–42.

DIAZ, THERESA, et al. (1994). Health insurance coverage among persons with AIDS: Results from a multistate surveillance project. *Am. J. Public Health*, 84:1015–1018.

EDEN, JILL, et al. (1988). AIDS and health insurance: An OTA Survey. *OTA, United States Congress*, 20510–8025.

FRIEDMAN, EMILY. (1991). The uninsured: From dilemma to crisis. *JAMA*, 265:2491–2496.

Hastings Center Report. (1991). A generation at risk. 21:3.

Health Insurance Association of America (1994). Source book of health insurance data 1993. Washington D.C.

HELLINGER, FRED J. (1993). The lifetime cost of treating a person with HIV. *JAMA*, 270:474–478.

Intergovernmental AIDS Report. (1989). Non-medical funds for HIV patient care. George Washington Univ., 2:1–18.

KURATA, JOHN, et al. (1993). Seroprevalence of HIV among family practice outpatients. *J. Am. Board Fam. Pract.*, 6:347–352.

LEVI, JEFFREY. (1994). The AIDS agenda and reform. *FOCUS*, 9:4–6.

MURPHY, TIMOTHY F. (1991). No time for AIDS back lash. *Hastings Center Report*, 21:7–11.

Nature. (1995). Task force turns on sponsor (DoE). 373:457–458.

PACKER, JUDY. (1991). 1990 Health tab—666.2 billion. *Modern Health Care,* 21:3.

PERKIN, JUDY. (1993). Facing the health policy challenge of HIV infection. *Natl. Forum,* LXXIII:45–47.

PETERSON, D. (1992). Viatical settlements: Living benefits for the insured, terminally ill patient. *The Bulletin (New York City Association of Life Underwriters),* April 1–4.

Public Health Reports. (1988). Report of the work group on patient care/health care needs. 103:80–87.

RON, ARAN, et al. (1988). New York City's health care crisis: AIDS, the poor, and limited resources. *JAMA,* 260:1453.

SILVERMAN, MARVYN F. (1990). The social and political impact of the AIDS epidemic. *AIDS Patient Care,* 3:3–6.

SWARTZ, KATHERINE. (1994). Dynamics of people without health insurance. *JAMA,* 271:64–66.

Washington Outlook. (1993). AIDS tab to grow. *Hospitals,* 67:8.

WEISSENSTEIN, ERIC. (1993). Health spending hits $838 billion in 1992. *Modern Healthcare,* 23:2–3.

WENNEKER, MARK B., et al. (1990). The association of payer with utilization of cardiac procedures in Massachusetts. *JAMA,* 264:1255–1260.

WINKENWERDER, WILLIAM, et al. (1989). Federal spending for illness caused by the human immunodeficiency virus. *N. Engl. J. Med.,* 320:1588–1603.

CHAPTER

16

Legal Aspects of HIV/AIDS: A Review of Legislation and Court Decisions in the United States

CHAPTER CONCEPTS

- First HIV/AIDS legislation
- How a bill moves in the House or Senate
- AIDS litigation: The social impact of AIDS
- Discrimination on the basis of handicap
- American Disabilities Act of 1990
- Legal rights and duties in the AIDS pandemic
- Infected persons duties: Criminal law, civil law
- Uninfected persons' rights to protection
- Legal aspects of HIV/AIDS and health care workers
- HIV transmission during an invasive procedure
- HIV transmission from physician to patient and vice versa
- HIV infected physicians and the practice of invasive procedures

The information in this chapter is general in nature and not intended as legal advice. Always seek legal counsel with regard to specific questions and situations in your state.

Many articles have been published in the United States on the legal aspects of the HIV/AIDS epidemic. A few of these articles are presented with permission.

INTRODUCTION

The history of the HIV/AIDS pandemic is one of remarkable scientific achievement. A search of the literature does not reveal a single life-threatening disease where so much has been learned in so short a time. AIDS was clinically described in June, 1981, its epidemiology was known by 1983, the course of the disease was reported by early 1984, a blood test for antibodies to the virus was commercially available by June 1985 and in late 1986, zidovudine was being used to treat people with AIDS.

However, 15 years into this modern day plague, there is still no cure for those who are HIV-infected or have AIDS. Nor is there a clinical means of preventing the spread of infection. A vaccine is probably years away. In the meantime, it is estimated that 40,000 to 80,000 Americans became HIV-infected in each year of the 1990s. And the number of new HIV infections is expected to increase as the pool of HIV-infected people becomes larger. The majority of these people do not know they are HIV-infected. There are over 1 million HIV-infected people in the United States and the number is growing. In addition, by mid-1995 there were about 230,000 people living with AIDS in the United States.

A QUESTION OF RESPONSIBILITY

HIV/AIDS investigators say that the vast majority of HIV/AIDS cases could have been prevented. HIV infection is caused by a virus that in most cases is sexually transmitted, transmitted via blood or blood products, or transmitted by HIV-contaminated needles during injection drug use. Therein lie many of the legal and ethical problems that must be confronted. Bernard Dickens (1988) and others raise questions such as: Because people behave in a manner that causes their infection, should they be compelled to be tested and test results be made known to protect others? Should everyone be HIV tested? What about surgical patients? If they refuse, does a surgeon have the right to refuse to perform surgery? What are the obligations to prevent health care workers from being HIV-infected or from infecting their patients? What of confidentiality—who is responsible for it? Should confidentiality be preserved at any cost? Who may inform a spouse that his or her sexual partner is HIV-infected? Is it the responsibility of society to pay the medical costs of those who have been educated about HIV/AIDS and become infected anyway? Who is responsible for HIV-infected children? Who pays the medical bills? What if the child gets the virus from a blood transfusion? Who is liable—the blood bank, the hospital, the doctor who ordered the trans- fusion? And who pays—the insurance company or the taxpayer?

Questions such as these have spawned more HIV/AIDS-related lawsuits than have been associated with any other disease. But many of the court decisions appear to be based on fear and stereotype rather than fact. For example, jurors have been influenced to rule in favor of the prosecution in cases against HIV-infected people who bit or spit on someone. These jury decisions occurred even though there has never been a documented case that showed either of these acts to be a means of transmitting HIV. Brian McCormick (1992) cites a case where the jurors were shown evidence labeled *"DO NOT TOUCH—AIDS EVIDENCE."* An appeals court refused to overturn a guilty verdict, ruling that the display was not discriminatory and did not prejudice the jury.

David Schulman (1988) in his article "Remembering Who We Are: AIDS and Law in a Time of Madness" wrote that

> Fear and ignorance divide people. They pit infected against uninfected, threatening once again the web of relationships which enable us to understand each other as people. Law is rarely thought of as a healing social force, yet in the AIDS epidemic it can remind us of our highest ideals concerning ourselves, how we wish to treat others and would wish to be treated.

This chapter presents an overview of some major areas of legal concern in which the HIV/AIDS epidemic in the United States is having an impact. Where appropriate, legal concerns in foreign countries are presented.

FIRST HIV/AIDS LEGISLATION: SWEDEN

Sweden was the first country to introduce legislation on AIDS. Passed on March 8, 1983, regulations made mandatory the reporting of confirmed and suspected AIDS cases to the National Bacteriological Laboratory. Sweden also adopted the first legislation dealing with protection against HIV transmission in the health care environment. In March 1985, Sweden's National Board of Occupational Safety and Health issued general recommendations concerning protection against AIDS in the

BOX 16.1

LEGAL HIV/AIDS VIGNETTES—UNITED STATES

Portland, OR—An AIDS-infected man under court order to abstain from sex for five years has been charged with attempted murder for previously having unprotected sex with a 17-year-old teenager. The man was sentenced, in December of 1992, to 9.4 years in prison.

Pensacola, FL—An HIV-positive parolee who allegedly raped his former girlfriend and injected her with his blood because he wanted her to know what it was like to be HIV-infected, killed himself. He had a history of crime and drug abuse. (1992)

Jacksonville, FL—A 30-year-old gay male faces charges of first-degree attempted murder and sexual battery after he was accused by a former lover of infecting him with the virus that causes AIDS. He is being held in lieu of $1 million bail. In a second case, same city, a 22-year-old man was arrested and charged with attempted second-degree murder and knowingly engaging in heterosexual intercourse while infected with HIV. He has been sentenced to 4.5 years in jail and to serve 13 years of probation during which time he must do 1,950 hours of community service. In a third case (January 1994), same city, a 42-year-old male was charged with attempted murder for engaging in unprotected heterosexual intercourse while knowing he was HIV-infected. To date 6 women who had sex with him after he became HIV-positive have been contacted. The man now has AIDS. (Case is pending)

Miami, FL—A former exotic dancer was ordered to pay her ex-husband $18 million for knowingly infecting him with the AIDS virus. The award was described by an attorney as the largest U.S. civil verdict of its kind. (1993)

Miami, FL—An HIV-positive 32-year-old male was sentenced to 5 consecutive life terms in prison for kidnapping, sodomizing, and trying to kill three boys in 1991. It is the first case in the country of a rapist with HIV being convicted of attempted murder. Ending 1994 the boys remain HIV-negative.

Miami, FL—For 2 years, a Miami woman thought she was dying of AIDS. She would not let her children hug her. Friends would not visit. Family members refused to speak with her.

She gave legal custody of her three teenage children to her mother — who would wash her daughter's dirty dishes with bleach.

Finally, she returned to her hometown in Georgia, where her attorney said she planned to kill herself when the disease made her seriously ill.

But she never became seriously ill, because she was not HIV-infected!

A Circuit Court jury in September of 1994 ordered the state Department of Health and Rehabilitative Services to pay the Miami woman $390,000 for her pain and suffering after the agency misread her HIV test. The physician who perscribed anti-HIV medication was required to pay $250,000.

Philadelphia, PA—In October, 1992, he was working for a top Philadelphia law firm, billing clients $150 an hour to handle complex commercial litigation and antitrust suits, just 3years out of law school.

By early 1993, the attorney identified in court papers as Scott Doe Esq. had learned he was HIV-positive. He stated that his employer told him to find a new job within a year.

A bad situation grew worse when his employer learned Doe planned to sue for disability discrimination. An office administrator promised Doe "could kiss his legal career goodbye," Doe asserts, and he had to stand by as his belongings were packed. Doe said the firm's senior partner demanded his keys to the building and watched until he left. Doe sued for discrimination under the Americans With Disabilities Act and a similar Pennsylvania law. The federal law prohibits employers from discriminating against *people* with disabilities, including HIV disease and AIDS.

This case has haunting similarities to the fictional movie, "Philadelphia," in which a new law partner is drummed out of this prestigious frim after a colleague notices a tell-tale sign of AIDS. This case was settled out of court, in Scott Does' favor, on October 31, 1994, for 1 million dollars plus costs.

Oakland, CA—A man convicted of having unprotected sex with a 22-year-old woman in order to give her AIDS was sentenced to three years in prison. (1991)

Boston, MA— Wendy Doe (a pseudonym used in court papers) is a nurse struggling with AIDS. But she is also involved in a fight of another sort against the Lahey Clinic of Burlington, MA where she worked for six years in the 1980s.

The clinic is contesting her claim for workers' compensation benefits based on her belief that she contracted AIDS while working for the clinic, and denies she was routinely exposed to blood.

Ms. Doe's lawyer says the clinic is lying about her exposure, and has filed a lawsuit in Middlesex Superior Court accusing the health care institution of behavior that "shocks the conscience and violates the law."

Rarely sick throughout her life, Ms. Doe's first symptoms appeared in 1986. But they were not diagnosed as AIDS until 1990, four years and nine doctors later, she says. The test results came three weeks before her wedding. (Case pending, 1993)

Muskegon, MI—A woman quarantined by Michigan officials after having unprotected sex without telling her partners she's infected with the virus that causes AIDS, agreed to stay home for a month. No charges were filed against the woman, 31, who has an IQ of 72 and lives in an adult foster home. The case will be reviewed monthly.

Boston, MA—The U.S. government refused to appeal a $3.8 million judgment awarded to an HIV-infected marine whose wife and son died of AIDS after she received HIV-tainted blood at a Navy hospital.

The ruling ended a five-year court battle for the Marine, who is hospitalized and sought the money for his 8-year-old daughter.

The Marine charged in his lawsuit that doctors at the Long Beach, CA, Naval Hospital botched his wife's pregnancy in 1981 by failing to give her a cesarean section. She was two weeks late delivering the baby and required a blood transfusion. The blood was infected with HIV.

The infant was stillborn. The couple had another son, who died of AIDS at age 13 months. His wife died of AIDS in 1987.

The U.S. District Court Judge ruled in 1991 that if a cesarean section had been performed in time, a transfusion would not have been necessary.

Denver, CO—Jurors, who didn't know a woman had died the day before, ordered a blood bank to pay her $6.6 million for providing a transfusion tainted with the virus that causes AIDS. Her husband was awarded $1.5 million for loss of companionship.

The woman had contracted AIDS from a 1983 transfusion that came from United Blood Services of Albuquerque, NM. She died in a hospital as her attorney presented closing arguments in her case. (Case is on appeal, 1992)

Portland, OR—The American Red Cross settled out of court on a $10 million lawsuit. A man claimed he received HIV in blood supplied by the Red Cross. (1993)

San Diego, CA—A woman who became HIV-positive after being injected with a syringe that had been used on an AIDS patient in a hospital mix-up two years ago has settled her lawsuit against the hospital for $1 million—receiving $600,000 at the time of the settlement and $2,300 a month for life. (1991)

San Francisco, CA—The California Supreme Court has let stand a ruling that says convicted prostitutes and their customers must submit to HIV tests. The court declined to review a state appeals court ruling upholding the constitutionality of a 1988 law. A San Francisco public defender challenged the law on behalf of 11 prostitutes, who claimed it unfairly singled them out and subjected them to privacy violations. A state appeals court upheld the law earlier this year (1990), saying that the prostitutes' constitutional rights were outweighed by the danger to society of spreading HIV through multiple sex partners.

Charleston, WV—The state Supreme Court upheld a $1.9 million award to a security guard who sued a hospital after being bitten by a person infected with the virus that causes AIDS. (1991)

Jacksonville, FL—In 1991, a Jacksonville man who is HIV-infected was awarded $59,000 by a jury that found he was turned away from a homeless shelter because of his disease.

His lawsuit was the first major test of a 1988 Florida law that forbids discrimination against people who have AIDS or the virus that causes AIDS.

Orlando, FL—In December 1992, a 21-year-old woman with AIDS was arrested for the attempted murder of her 2-year-old daughter via multiple bites. The woman said she bit the child to infect her to prevent her grandmother from caring for her. The girl is now in the custody of state health officials.

Texas—In July of 1992, a mid-level appeals court *affirmed* the conviction and 99-year or life, whichever is longer, sentence of a man who has AIDS and spit on a prison guard. The man was charged with attempted murder. Ruth Harlow, staff attorney for ACLU AIDS Project said, "his sentence is to die in prison for the crime of spitting." During the trial, Texas prosecutors relied on the testimony of two "expert" witnesses to win a conviction. One witness has made a career of testifying against litigants who are gay or who are associated with AIDS. During the trial, he (erroneously) testified that not only could AIDS be transmitted by spitting, but he also said that it could be transmitted by mosquitoes and through the air. The Texas Court of Appeals has been petitioned to reverse the lower court decision. (Outcome pending).

Martin, TN—In 1991, when her fiance collapsed from a heart attack, a woman rushed desperately to a stranger and pleaded for help. She didn't say the dying man had AIDS. Because the woman knew the man had AIDS, she faced felony charges for not warning rescuers. The officer who administered mouth-to-mouth resuscitation fears he was infected. The woman, an unemployed nursing assistant, was jailed for five days. She was freed on $2,500 bond. A county grand jury later found her innocent of intentional wrongdoing.

Wilmington, DE—In 1988, the states Attorney General ordered one of the state's largest pediatric institutions to recind a controversial policy of not treating AIDS patients.

The order targeted a 90-bed pediatric hospital. The Attorney General stated that the hospital's policy violated the state's public accommodation policy.

New York City, NY—In February of 1994, a data supervisor at the New York City Health Department was charged with changing the computerized result of an AIDS test from positive to negative.

The supervisor knew the person whose test result he had changed.

The data supervisor's lawyer said: "He was trying to do a good deed. It was a matter of trying to protect the confidentiality of a patient or a testee." (Trial is pending.)

Albany, NY—In July of 1992, Court of Claims judge ordered the state to pay $5.4 million to a nurse and her husband. She became HIV-infected after being stuck with a needle used on an HIV-infected prisoner who became uncontrollable. She sued the state for $10 million, claiming that the guards should have helped control the inmate. The state claimed the guards were under no legal obligation to help. The state attorney said the state was liable and willing to pay $3 million but would appeal the remaining $2.4 million as excessive. (Outcome pending).

Bridgeport, CT—A mistrial was declared in the case of a man who beat his girlfriend to death with a hammer. The judge learned during the trial that the man demonstrated AIDS dementia. A competency examination was ordered. (Case pending, 1993)

Salt Lake City, UT—Two women with AIDS have filed suit in July 1993 to overturn a Utah law that bars those with the disease from marrying. Utah is unique in having such a law. The women are requesting immediate action on their suit. They feared that their families could lose financial benefits if they died before the law was revoked because their marriages could be ruled invalid. (Case pending)

In 1992, 1993, and 1994, a number of insurance companies in the United States attempted to reduce coverage after a person became HIV-infected or was diagnosed with AIDS. One case is cited herein—it aptly represents at least 50 such cases that have already been litigated.

Chicago, IL—Ruling for the first time that a dentist's office is a public accommodation and is therefore subject to the Ilinois Human Rights Act, the Chief Judge of the State of Illinois Human Rights Commission decided that a Chicago dentist broke the law in 1987 by refusing to continue treatment of a long-time patient solely because the patient disclosed that he was HIV-positive. In the October, 1994 ruling, Chief Administrative Law Judge concluded that the plaintiff is handicapped due to his HIV status (a precedent in Illinois law) under the Americans With Disabilities Act. Under the Act, a dental office is a place of public accommodation and the dentist, acted in a discriminatory fashion. The Judge awarded the patient $8,048, primarily for the emotional damages suffered due to discriminatory treatment.

St. Paul, MN (1993)—The health plan of local 110 of the International Brotherhood of Electrical Workers in St. Paul and the electrical contractors' association agreed to lift a $50,000 ceiling on payments for AIDS-related diseases. The health plan provided insurance up to $500,000 for other catastrophic conditions.

Settling charges that it had discriminated against members with AIDS, the union welfare fund also agreed to pay $100,000 to the estate of a 36-year-old construction worker who died in November 1992. This was the first large award in a case involving an AIDS-related denial of health insurance under the Americans with Disabilities Act.

These vignettes cover selected episodes that were written up in the newspapers in 13 states. Note that although the events vary, they are all concerned with who is or was responsible for HIV transmission. There are countless incidents and legal cases of HIV/AIDS-related events in the United States. Most likely there are countless similar legal cases occurring in other countries.

By the end of 1994, there were over 250 arrests made against persons who deliberately attempted to use their HIV infection as a weapon (to harm) against others. Numerous charges have also been filed against workers' unions and insurance companies for discrimination against persons with HIV diseases.

POINT OF INFORMATION 16.1

DNA AND AMINO ACID SEQUENCING OF HIV REVERSE TRANSCRIPTASE CONVICTS RAPIST: STOCKHOLM DISTRICT COURT

The male, a Swedish injection drug user, was HIV-positive. The woman he raped tested HIV-positive several weeks after the rape. Much of the trial evidence that led to his conviction was based on direct DNA sequence analysis of their HIVs. His and her viruses were "highly DNA homologous." Further, amino acid analysis of both individuals' HIV-produced reverse transcriptase were identical at 6 positions. Control samples taken from injection drug users and gay males in the same geographical region showed no more than 2 of the 6 amino acids to be similar.

This is believed to be the first case ever where DNA and amino acid sequencing of HIV was used to help in a conviction (Albert et al., 1993).

Over 25 states now have laws on the books making it a misdemeanor or felony for an HIV-positive person to spread HIV through methods ranging from sexual contact to the exposure of blood. Such laws in Louisiana carry a maximum punishment of a $5,000 fine and 10 years in prison.

course of the care and administration of patients along with highly detailed measures to be taken in work entailing a risk of infection with HIV.

As of September 1988, approximately 70 countries had introduced some form of legislation concerning AIDS and HIV infection, a significant number of which addressed specific issues concerning health care workers (HCWs). The following countries, among others, have addressed hospitals or HCWs in their legislation: Australia (New South Wales), Austria, Belgium, Brazil, Canada (Alberta), Chile, China, Dominican Republic, Greece, Guatemala, Indonesia, Luxembourg, Malta, Norway, Panama, Peru, Rwanda, South Africa, Spain, Sweden, Switzerland, and Turkey (Fluss et al., 1989).

LEGAL FRAMEWORK

The Congress of the United States has demonstrated its concern about the HIV/ AIDS epidemic by approving the expenditure of billions of dollars for educational programs, research, and medical care. But most of the legislative activity surrounding the issue of HIV/AIDS has been at the state level. Since 1987, state legislators have enacted over 200 bills addressing HIV/AIDS-related issues such as testing, blood bank screening, confidentiality, housing, insurance, prisons, informed consent, counseling, and medication programs (Rothstein, 1989).

Lawrence O. Gostin, J.D. (Juris Doctorate) has written a series of papers discussing legislative and regulatory policies regarding HIV/AIDS in the United States (Figure 16-1).

In his report "Public Health Strategies for Confronting AIDS," Gostin (1989a) presents evidence that, although state legislatures have responded well to health care and research, they have also been susceptible to attitudes that the primary modes of HIV transmission are immoral, even criminal. He says that both federal and state statutes, by placing special

Figure 16-1 Photograph of Lawrence O. Gostin, J. D.

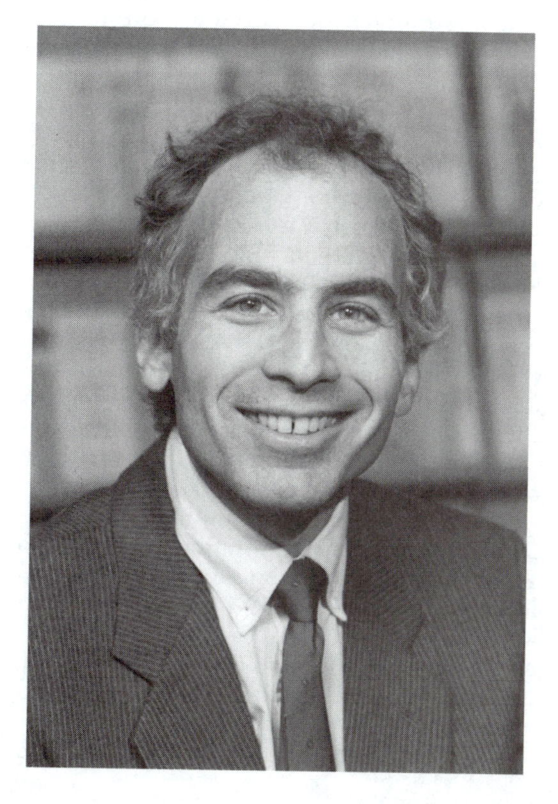

emphasis on warning against extramarital intercourse and drug use, choose to ignore that these behaviors have historically persisted. He writes that there is political pressure on legislators to use the coercive powers of the state to deal with the HIV/AIDS epidemic. And legislation for compulsory HIV screening, quarantine, and criminalization for behavior that spreads HIV has proceeded in some states without evidence that it would be effective.

In a follow-up 1989 article "The Politics of AIDS: Compulsory State Powers, Public Health and Civil Liberties," Gostin (1989b) reviews the various risks involved in the transmission of HIV and concludes that the risk of transmission from biting, spitting, or splattering blood is negligible. The risk of sexual transmission is much greater. Mr. Gostin is opposed to coercive or compulsory public health measures because they are likely to be ineffective and violate human rights. He reviews various suggestions such as isolation of the infected in AIDS care facilities, modified isolation based on behavior, and criminalization of HIV transmission, all of which he thinks are inappropriate. He urges focused education, testing, counseling, and treatment for drug dependency.

In 1990, Gostin examined public policy on AIDS. His exceptional two-part article reviews AIDS-related litigation and Human Rights Commission decisions in the United States since 1981 (Gostin, 1990a).

Gostin reports in his "AIDS Litigation Project, Part I," that sharp differences in perception of public health, ethics, and civil liberties have created the largest body of legal cases attributable to a single disease in the history of American jurisprudence. He reviews the areas of law that encompass 469 cases (cited in the bibliography), and of over 1,000 cases decided or pending, and notes that they show conflicts of values that will likely require legislative and policy resolution. But he also shows that there has been significant progress in addressing HIV/AIDS in school and the workplace. The courts have affirmed that a child with HIV/AIDS has a right to public education, and in most cases this has meant attendance in his or her usual classroom. Similarly, the right of employees with HIV/AIDS to remain on the job has been repeatedly upheld. In both areas, reasonable accommodations are made for the affected individual.

Most of the cases Gostin cites have escaped the attention of the public health community. They contain important information for everyone—health workers, blood bankers, policymakers, attorneys, legislators, and perhaps most of all, people with HIV/AIDS and people at risk.

In presenting legal and policy controversies in light of public health imperatives, Gostin's articles are significant for their potential to prevent enactment of unfounded HIV/AIDS legislation and to promote freedom from discrimination.

In Part I of the review Gostin also examines court and Human Rights Commission decisions since the start of the AIDS epidemic in 14 subject areas. These include AIDS education, testing, criminal law, state regulation of bathhouses, private tort actions, confidentiality and AIDS in prison populations.

Perhaps the most valuable lessons in Part I may be found in examples of sound and unsound public health policies and their consequences. Reasonable policy based on scientific fact promotes the public health, as is demonstrated by laws that require the testing of blood products, semen, and donated organs. In most cases, these laws followed, rather than preceded, the standard of practice. Similarly, laws that require AIDS education clearly serve the best interests of the public.

Unscientific or irrational policy, on the other hand, may harm the public health. For example, restrictions on HIV/AIDS educational content inhibit the ability of organizations to produce accurate and effective programs; as a result, more people may become infected. Laws and policies that compromise confidentiality may jeopardize efforts to prevent infection and provide early intervention to those infected by discouraging them from seeking care (Sherer, 1990).

Gostin addresses the futility of measures to prevent immigration and free travel of people with HIV/AIDS. Such measures are discriminatory and have no convincing public health rationale (Duckett et al., 1989; Gilmore et al., 1989). The Immigration and Naturalization

BOX 16.2

HOW A BILL MOVES IN THE HOUSE OR SENATE

Here is how a bill generally moves after a Member of Congress introduces it into either the House or Senate:

The parliamentarian and leadership of whichever body receives the bill refers it to a committee where the chairperson and staff determine what subcommittee, if any, is to receive it. If a bill is going to die, it usually dies at the committee or subcommittee level.

The subcommittee provides the forum where the bill is likely to receive its most thorough consideration and witnesses may testify for and against it. Included among the witnesses, if the bill affects a Federal agency, will be officials of that agency. If a majority of the subcommittee approves, the bill goes back to the full committee where it again must be approved by majority vote before it goes to the House or Senate floor. House bills must have cleared the Rules Committee where debate time limits are often established. Amendments may have been offered by the subcommittee or full committee and, with certain exceptions, may again be offered on the floor.

If the House or Senate passes the bill it then is moved to the other chamber where it is referred to a committee. If a majority of the committee approves, it goes to the floor. Amendments generally may be offered in committee or on the floor. Approval on the floor means both the House and Senate have separately cleared the bill and conferees from each chamber then are selected to work out any necessary compromise of differences between the House and Senate on the bill and to write a conference report. Final passage comes when the House and Senate approve the conference report.

The bill is then sent to the White House for Presidential action. If the President signs, it becomes law. If he sends it back unsigned to the original chamber and notes his objections, the bill has been vetoed. For it now to become law, both House and Senate, by roll-call votes of two-thirds, must agree to override the veto.

Bills not considered in a 2-year Congress such as the 101st, do not automatically carry over for the next Congress but must be reintroduced. And most bills are not considered at all. For instance, over the past 18 years (nine Congresses), an average of more than 20,000 bills have been introduced in the house during each 2-year term. Only slightly more than 10% have even been reported from committees to the House floor. And, of the 20,000 introduced, the average number that became law per Congress is under 5%.

TIPS ON WRITING A MEMBER OF CONGRESS

Senators and Representatives pay attention to their mail. It is good politics. Responding to mail is crucial to reelection. A member knows your vote can be won or lost by his or her response. The most effective letter is a personal one, not a form letter. It should be concise, informed, and polite. Some specific tips:

1. Try to stick to one typewritten page. Two pages at most. Don't write on the back of a page. If writing longhand, write legibly.
2. In a short first paragraph, state your purpose. Stick with one subject or issue. Support your position with the rest of the letter.
3. If a bill is the subject, cite it by name and number.
4. Be factual and support your position with information about how legislation is likely to affect you and others. Avoid emotional or philosophical arguments.
5. If you believe the legislation is wrong and should be opposed, say so, indicate the likely adverse effects, and suggest a better approach.
6. Ask for the legislator's view but do not demand support. Remember, Senators and Representatives respond to a variety of views, and even if your position is not supported on one issue or bill, it may be the next time.
7. Be sure your name and return address are legible.
8. The suggested address style is:

The Honorable ____________________
United States Senate
Washington, DC 20510

Dear Senator ____________________

The Honorable ____________________
United States House of Representatives
Washington, DC 20515

Dear Representative ____________________

(*PWA Newsline,* 1991, People With AIDS Coalition, "Surviving and Thriving With AIDS: Collected Wisdom")

Service can authorize HIV antibody testing on visitors to the United States or, through the Justice Department, bar their entry. This regulation was issued by the Justice Department in 1988. It was temporarily lifted in 1990 to permit HIV/AIDS-infected people to attend the Sixth Inter- national Conference on AIDS. Because the law is still in effect, sponsors for the Eighth International Conference on AIDS (May 24–29, 1992) moved it from the United States to Amsterdam.

Health workers may take particular interest in the section on private tort actions that involve health professionals. One clear lesson from this section is the imperative for all health workers, physicians in particular, to learn as much as possible about HIV/AIDS. Physicians who order HIV antibody tests without patient consent or who misdiagnose or improperly treat HIV-related disease may put themselves at risk for liability.

In Gostin's "The AIDS Litigation Project, Part II : Discrimination" (1990b), he reports on the most controversial area of human rights. He points out that public health and medical organizations that have issued HIV/AIDS papers have unanimously condemned discrimination as unjust and detrimental to public health. Case identification (testing, reporting, and partner notification) is of growing importance as the benefits of early intervention become clearer. Gostin looks at the 149 cases of discrimination reported by municipal and federal agencies and reviews the major areas of discrimination litigation: education, employment, housing, insurance, and health care. The bibliography includes citations to the discrimination cases. Gostin's report should be read with care as it explains why HIV/AIDS patients are considered handicapped even though HIV infection leads to an infectious, contagious disease. That is, the mental picture that one holds of a handicapped person (person living with disabilities, PLWD) is usually different from the legal definition. Take a moment. Think of the words **handicap** and **disability.** Form a mental image of a disabled or handicapped person. In a compelling review of these cases, Gostin concludes that there has been a critical mass of discriminatory behavior that warrants government action in the form of comprehensive federal antidiscrimination legislation. These cases underscore the imperatives of confidentiality and full, written, informed consent prior to HIV antibody testing.

In order to better understand Gostin's review of HIV/AIDS discrimination cases, it should be understood that people with HIV/AIDS have been disabled by the disease. Because of the disability imposed on those who have HIV disease and AIDS, they are said to be handicapped. As such, they receive the civil protection of the federal statutes regarding discrimination against the handicapped.

You are encouraged to read the excellent review of *Discrimination on the Basis of Handicap,* BOX 13.3, for a better understanding of the key statutory language of the federal legislation on handicap, clarification of who is to be considered a handicapped or disabled person, and who qualifies for federal protection from discrimination under the New Americans with Disabilities Act of 1990.

The Americans with Disabilities Act of 1990

The Americans with Disabilities Act (ADA) addresses the concern that society has been inclined to segregate individuals with disabilities. The ADA is a mandate to eliminate discrimination against those with physical and mental disabilities in *all* aspects of their lives. An employer, program, or health care provider must evaluate each person's ability to perform a given task and make *reasonable* accommodations that would allow the disabled person to perform.

Nondiscrimination obligation can be found in Section 504 of the Vocational Re-habilitation Act passed in 1973. The ADA is modeled after Section 504 and, for the most part, the difference between Section 504 and the ADA is a change in terminology from "otherwise qualified handicapped individual" to "otherwise qualified individual with a disability."

Every court case decision on the HIV/ AIDS discrimination issue has found that HIV-positive individuals are protected as handicapped under Section 504. Section 504 and the ADA protect not only the people with actual impairments but also those with a past history of an impairment and those **perceived by others** as being impaired, despite the fact that the individual has no past or present impairment at all (Palma, 1992). To demonstrate the extent of coverage in Section 504 Palma cites a recent AIDS discrimination case against Beth Israel Hospital. A resident teaching M.D. of a hospital refused to perform surgery on an HIV-infected patient. The court held that because the hospital received Medicare and Medicaid funds for services rendered, the hospital was liable under Section 504. However, the court dismissed the claim against the physician because he could not receive federal funds as a resident teaching M.D. The ADA eliminates such exclusions.

Discrimination Laws Have Social Limits— Discrimination laws provide a legal foundation for the rights of people with HIV infection and AIDS, but this foundation is not really adequate to ensure that they receive the humane treatment to which everyone is entitled as a basic human right. The statutes provide limited remedies, and their administration frequently takes more time than people with HIV infection or AIDS can afford. This means that the ethical issues must take precedence if true justice is to be done.

First Federal ADA Case— The first federal case of HIV/AIDS discrimination since the implementation of the ADA was filed against Westchester County Medical Center, Valhalla, New York in April 1992. According to an opinion issued by Department of Health and Human Services administrative law judge, Westchester did discriminate against a pharmacy job applicant, an HIV-infected pharmacist, under the Rehabilitation Act of 1973, and sanctioned the hospital from receiving Medicare and Medicaid payments until it "complies" with the act. The pharmacist was awarded $30,000 and the job without restrictions.

In defense, the hospital states that the pharmacist stated on his application that he had no infectious conditions. But the hospital learned—because the applicant was being treated at the facility—that he was HIV-positive. Following a policy the hospital has had in place for years barring employees with infectious diseases from preparing intravenous solutions, the hospital offered him a position with the provision that he could not prepare IVs. The applicant took action against the hospital through state and federal agencies, charging that he was discriminated against based on his HIV status.

The *Westchester* case illustrates the challenges that confront hospitals in dealing with HIV-positive health care workers, and the difficulties they face in trying to balance the protection of patients with the rights of workers. A spokesman contends that the hospital acted reasonably and fairly. "It's ridiculous to take what has always been a fundamental right of hospitals in this country and carelessly cast it aside based on someone's handicapped status." The spokesman also said that the hospital is one of 12 AIDS management centers in New York and acts as a clearinghouse for all AIDS activity in the surrounding counties. He adds that the center has a full-service dental clinic for HIV-positive patients, one of the few in the nation. "We know how difficult it is to cope with this disease. We know some of the social stigmas attached to it; we know how it is transmitted. Further, the applicant was offered a job with the same rate of pay and opportunities for advancement that anyone else in the pharmacy would have (Lumsdon, 1992).

On January 11, 1993, Westchester County Medical Center agreed to hire the HIV-infected pharmacist without restriction. Failure to comply would have cost the hospital $107 million in Medicaid and Medicare reimbursement.

What is your inital reaction to this situation? If you were the presiding hospital officer, how might you decide — Was the applicant discriminated against? Would you have employed him because of federal/state pressures? Why?

The ADA as Civil Rights Legislation— The ADA is the most sweeping piece of civil rights legislation since 1964. The goal is to remove barriers to employment, shopping, travel, and entertainment for the nation's 43 million disabled people.

The guidelines cover more than 5 million public facilities. Companies have begun making changes to their premises. They must do so as long as the changes can be done without excessive expense. The act is estimated to cost business as much as $2 billion.

ADA Highlights, First Phase, which began on January 26, 1992 include the following:

- Public accommodations may not discriminate on the basis of disability.
- Physical barriers in existing facilities must be removed if possible. If not, other methods of providing services must be offered. Alterations to existing facilities must be accessible.
- Public transit systems must provide comparable paratransit, such as vans, to people who cannot use a fixed-route bus service. New busses and rail vehicles must be accessible.

ADA Access Time Line—

- **January 26, 1992:** Organizations must take steps to assure that people with disabilities have access to existing public areas so long as such accommodations will not pose an unreasonable hardship. New buildings and renovations undertaken after this date must meet more stringent guidelines. Physicians may be sued for refusal to treat patients solely because of disability.
- **July 26, 1992:** Employers with 25 or more people on the payroll must make sure that persons with disabilities are not discriminated against in any employment practice. It takes effect July 26, 1994, for companies with 15 or more employees; those with fewer than 15 are exempt.
- **July 26, 1993:** Requires that states provide unrestricted telephone service for individuals who use telecommunications devices for the deaf.
- **July 26, 1995:** Providers of commuter rail transportation must have at least one passenger car per train readily accessible to individuals with disabilities.

The ADA will eventually apply to *all* employers with 15 or more employees. It will impact nearly every local government. For large cities, the impact began in January 1992; for smaller towns, 1994. ADA will underscore the rights of the HIV-infected worker by utilizing the same criteria for coverage that is currently used in Section 504 of the 1973 Vocational Rehabilitation Act. But ADA goes beyond existing legislation and strengthens the rights of HIV-infected employees in several ways. First, it is the specific intent of Congress to include HIV/AIDS as a handicap covered by ADA. Second, the legislation provides concrete examples of reasonable accommodation. Third, with the exception of drug testing, ADA will also prohibit employers from using preemployment medical examinations as a screening device. Employers will still be able to impose job-related physical examinations, but only after they have extended job offers to applicants. Moreover, HIV-infected people will benefit from the heightened stature of ADA in that its implementation and monitoring will now fall under the auspices of the Equal Employment Opportunity Commission (Slack, 1991). Key statutory language of ADA 1990 can be found in BOX 13.3.

Legal Rights and Obligations

In an attempt to place legal rights and obligations during this HIV/AIDS epidemic in perspective, Bernard M. Dickens provides us with some legal insight in his report "Legal Rights and Duties in the AIDS Epidemic" (1988) (BOX 13.4). In this report Dickens reviews the rights of infected individuals with regard to testing, treatment, and confidentiality; and looks at discrimination in access to health care, employment, housing, education, and insurance. He outlines the obligation that an infected person has to prevent transmission of the virus, including liability for contaminated blood. The author also considers the rights of the uninfected to protection, the rights and duties of health pro- fessionals and health authorities, and international legal developments outside the United States.

Confidentiality Laws

The word *confidential*, according to Webster's dictionary, means *private or secret, to entrust* (*information*) *with confidence*. In medicine this means that a patient's records, including name, address, phone number, medical history, and so on must be kept confidential. This means that the results of an HIV test may not be released

BOX 16.3

"DISCRIMINATION ON THE BASIS OF HANDICAP"

I. FEDERAL STATUTES REGARDING HANDICAPPED DISCRIMINATION

Congress has enacted two federal laws designed to eliminate discrimination on the basis of handicap. These two laws are known as the Rehabilitation Act of 1973 and the Americans with Disabilities Act of 1990. As its name indicates, the Rehabilitation Act of 1973 has been in effect for almost 20 years. The Americans with Disabilities Act of 1990 did not become effective until July 26, 1992. Those provisions of each Act which are of particular interest to colleges and universities are set out below.

A. The Rehabilitation Act of 1973

Section 504 of The Rehabilitation Act of 1973, 29 U.S.C. Sec. 794, was designed to eliminate discrimination on the basis of handicap in any program or activity receiving financial assistance from the federal government. Because most colleges and universities receive some form of financial assistance from the federal government—whether in the form of grants, loans, or contracts—most colleges and universities have been subject to the provisions of the Rehabilitation Act of 1973.

1. The Key Statutory Language

The key language of Section 504 reads as follows:

> No otherwise qualified individual with handicaps . . shall, solely by reason of her or his handicap, be excluded from the participation in, be denied the benefits of, or be subjected to discrimination under any program or activity receiving Federal financial assistance. . .

Section 504, thus, protects otherwise qualified handicapped persons from discrimination based on their handicapped status.

2. Who Is an "Individual with Handicaps"

An individual with handicaps is any person who has a physical or mental impairment which substantially limits one or more of the person's major life activities. Any person who has a record of having such a physical or mental impairment or who merely is regarded as having such an impairment is also protected by the statute as a handicapped person. 29 U.S.C. Sec. 706(8).

a. What Is a "Physical or Mental Impairment"?

A physical impairment is any physical condition or disorder which affects a major system of the body. The term "physical impairment" includes orthopedic, visual, speech, and hearing impairments, cerebral palsy, epilepsy, muscular dystrophy, multiple sclerosis, cancer, heart disease, and diabetes. A mental impairment includes disorders such as mental retardation, emotional or mental illness, and specific learning disabilities. 45 C.F.R. Sec. 104.3

b. What Is Meant by "Substantially Limits"?

A determination as to whether a person is "substantially limited" by his or her handicapping condition depends upon the nature and severity of the condition. Courts, for example, have held that fear of heights and left-handedness do not qualify persons as "handicapped" because such conditions do not substantially limit major life activities.

c. What Is a "Major Life Activity"?

A major life activity means a function such as caring for one's self, performing manual tasks, walking, seeing, hearing, speaking, breathing, learning, and working. 45 C.F.R. Sec. 104.3

d. Who Has a "Record" of Having an Impairment?

A person will be protected by Section 504 as a handicapped individual if the person has a history of, or has been formally classified as having, a physical or mental impairment which substantially limits one or more major life activities.

e. Who Is Merely "Regarded" as Having an Impairment?

A person will be protected by Section 504 as a handicapped individual **even if the person has no handicap** if the person is perceived and treated by others as a person with a physical or mental impairment which substantially limits one or more major life activities.

3. Who Is an "Otherwise Qualified" Individual with Handicaps?

A person is not entitled to protection under Section 504 just because the person has a handicap; the person also must be "otherwise qualified" to perform the essential requirements of the job or program in question in spite of the handicap. In the employment context, an otherwise qualified handicapped person is a person who, **with reasonable accommodation**, is able to perform the essential functions of the job in question. In the student context, an otherwise qualified handicapped person is a person who, in spite of his or her handicap, is able to meet the academic and technical standards for admission to and participation in his or her institution's educational programs. 45 C.F.R. Sec. 104.3

a. What Is "Reasonable Accommodation"

Reasonable accommodation is a concept that is central to handicap law. It essentially requires that institutions adopt a reasonable and flexible attitude toward handicapped applicants, employees, and students. Reasonable accommodation does *not* require that institutions undertake accommodations which fundamentally alter the nature of their academic programs, which lower or substantially modify their academic standards, which result in safety risks to the handicapped individual or others, or which impose undue administrative or financial burdens on the institution.

In the employment context, reasonable accommodation might entail making facilities readily accessible to and usable by handicapped employees, restructuring jobs to eliminate duties that are peripheral to the position in question but which eliminate handicapped persons, permitting part-time or modified work schedules, or purchasing specially modified equipment. In the student context, reasonable accommodation might entail modifying building access routes to permit entrance by wheelchair, permitting light course loads or additional time to complete exams, or providing readers, interpreters, or special tutors.

b. Court Decisions Interpreting the "Otherwise Qualified" Standard

(1) Tuberculosis-Infected Teacher

A federal court held that a schoolteacher with tuberculosis was "otherwise qualified" to remain on the job, since the court concluded that she posed no threat of transmitting tuberculosis to her students. *School Board of Nassau County v. Arline,* 692 F.Supp. 1286 (1988)

(2) HIV-Infected Teacher

A federal court held that an elementary schoolteacher with AIDS was "otherwise qualified" to remain on the job, since the court concluded that the teacher posed no threat of transmitting HIV to his students. *Chalk v. US District Court,* 840 F.2d 701 (9th Cir. 1988)

(3) Hearing-Impaired Nursing Student

The U.S. Supreme Court held that a hearing-impaired nursing student was *not* "otherwise qualified" to perform the essential aspects of a nursing program because of concerns about patient safety. With a hearing aid, the student could hear gross sounds occurring in the listening environment. However, to understand speech, she relied on lipreading. The student proposed that she be given individual faculty supervision when attending patients directly and that certain required courses be dispensed with altogether since it was unnecessary that she be trained to undertake all of the tasks a registered nurse is licensed to perform. The Supreme Court held that Section 504 does not require colleges and universities to make fundamental alterations in their academic programs or to lower or substantially modify their academic standards in order to accommodate a handicapped individual. *South-eastern Community College v. Davis,* 442 U.S. 397 (1979)

(4) Hand-Function Impaired PT Student

A Texas court held that a physical therapy student with deformed fingers was *not* "otherwise qualified" because he could not perform the manipulations required for graduation from the physical therapy program. *Samelson v. Texas Woman's University,* (not reported) (S.D. Tex. 1989)

4. Can an Institution Find Out if an Individual Has Handicaps?

a. Employment Context

As a general rule, the regulations do not permit an institution to make a preemployment inquiry as to whether an applicant for employment is handicapped or to conduct a preemployment medical examination. An employer may, however, describe the functions of an open position and ask if the applicant is able to perform those functions. For example, an employer may not ask if an applicant is visually impaired, but may ask if the applicant holds a current drivers' license—if a license is a necessary qualification for the position in question. In addition, an employer may condition an offer of employment on the results of a medical examination to be conducted after the offer is extended but before the first day of work, *if but only if*, (1) such an examination is administered to all entering employees, (2) the results are used in accordance with the laws on handicapped discrimination (which means that the results cannot be used to deny employment unless the revealed conditions indicate that the person is not "otherwise qualified") and (3) the results are treated on a confidential basis. 45 C.F.R. Sec. 104.14

b. Student Context

As a general rule, the regulations also do not permit an institution to make a preadmission inquiry as to whether a prospective student is an individual with handicaps. *After* admission, however, an institution may inquire on a confidential basis as to whether a newly admitted student has handicaps that may require accommodation. 45 C.F.R. Sec. 104.42

B. The Americans with Disabilities Act of 1990

The Americans with Disabilities Act of 1990, 42 U.S.C. Sec. 12101 et seq., extends the reach of federal protection for people who are disabled. Whereas the Rehabilitation Act of 1973 only applies to federal contractors and programs and activities receiving federal financial assistance, the Americans with Disabilities Act (popularly known as the ADA) will eventually apply to all private employers with 15 or more employees. Colleges and universities already in compliance with Section 504 of the Rehabilitation Act of 1973 will need be make sure that they will also be in compliance with the ADA.

1. The Key Statutory Language

The key language of the ADA is contained in Section 12112 which reads as follows:

> No covered entity shall discriminate against a qualified individual with a disability because of the disability of such individual in regard to job application procedures, the hiring, advancement, or discharge of employees, employee compensation, job training, and other terms, conditions, and privileges of employment.

Section 12132 similarly prohibits public entities from discriminating against qualified individuals with a disability. Section 12182 prohibits discrimination on the basis of disability in the full and equal enjoyment of places of public accommodation such as schools, hospitals, banks, and gas stations.

2. Who Is an Individual with a "Disability"?

The ADA's definition of an individual with a "disability" is almost identical to the Rehabilitation Act's definition of an "individual with handicaps." The term "disability" is used, however, instead of the term "handicap." An individual with a disability is an individual who has a physical or mental impairment that substantially limits one or more of the major life activities of the individual. An individual with a record of such an impairment and an individual merely regarded as having such an impairment are also considered to be individuals with a disability.

3. Who Is a "Qualified Individual with a Disability"?

Under the ADA, a "qualified individual with a disability" is an individual with a disability who, with or without reasonable accommodation, can perform the essential functions of the employment position that such individual holds or desires. "Reasonable accommodation" under the ADA is defined in substantially the same way that it is defined under the Rehabilitation Act.

4. Can an Institution Find Out if an Individual Has a Disability?

Under the ADA, an employer will not be permitted to use qualification standards, employment tests, or other selection criteria that screen out or tend to screen out an individual with a disability or a class of individuals with disabilities unless the standard, test, or other selection criteria is shown to be job-related for the position in question and consistent with business necessity. As a general rule, an employer will neither be permitted to make preemployment inquiries as to whether an applicant for employment has a disability or to conduct preemployment medical examinations. An employer may, however, describe the functions of an open position and ask if the applicant is able to perform those functions. In addition, an employer may condition an offer of employment on the results of a medical examination to be conducted after the offer is extended but before the first day of work, *if but only if,* (a) such an examination is administered to all entering employees in the same job category, (b) the results are treated on a confidential basis, and (c) the results are used only in a manner consistent with the provisions of the ADA. This means that an employer may withdraw an offer of employment on the basis of medical examination results only if the revealed conditions are job-related, consistent with business necessity, and no reasonable accommodation is possible. 42 U.S.C. Sec. 12112(c)

II. CONTAGIOUS DISEASES AND FEDERAL LAW

A. Specific Statutory Provisions

1. Individuals with a "Currently Contagious Disease"—The Rehabilitation Act of 1973

In 1986, the Rehabilitation Act was amended. The amended statute specifically provides that, in the employment context, the definition of an "individual with handicaps" does not include an individual who has a currently contagious disease and who, by reason of such disease or infection, would constitute **a direct threat to the health or safety of other individuals** or who, by reason of the currently contagious disease or infection, is unable to perform the duties of the job. 29 U.S.C. Sec. 706(8) (C). Thus, in circumstances where a person with a currently contagious disease poses a direct threat to others, the infected person will not be deemed to be "handicapped" within the meaning of the statute and will not be entitled to the Section 504's protection.

2. Individuals Who Pose a "Direct Threat"—The Americans with Disabilities Act

Under the ADA, an employer will be permitted to require that an individual not pose a direct threat to the health or safety of other individuals in the workplace. 42 U.S.C. Sec. 12113. The ADA defines "direct threat" to mean a "a significant risk to the health or safety of others that cannot be eliminated by reasonable accommoda- tion." 42 U.S.C. Sec. 12111. According to proposed regulations, in order to reject an applicant or employee on this basis, an employer must consider the (a) duration of the risk, (b) the nature and severity of the potential harm, and (c) the likelihood that the potential harm will occur. The employer's decisions in this regard must also be based on either valid medical analysis or on other objective evidence individualized for the particular individual and job. 56 Fed. Reg. 8578 (Feb. 28, 1991)

B. Application of the Law

1. Is AIDS or HIV Infection a Handicap/Disability?

a. AIDS

AIDS has been found to be a "handicap" under the Rehabilitation Act of 1973. In *Chalk v. U.S. District Court,* 840 F.2d 701 (9th Cir. 1988), a federal court of appeals ruled that AIDS was a handicap covered by the Rehabilitation Act and held that the dismissal of a elementary school teacher because he had AIDS violated the Act. There have also been a number of federal suits involving elementary school children with AIDS. In virtually all of these cases, the courts have deemed the children to be protected by the Rehabilitation Act and the federal Education for All Handicapped Children Act and have ultimately ordered school systems to permit such children to attend school in normal classroom settings. *See Thomas v. Atascadero Unified School District,* 662 F.Supp. 376 (C.D. Cal. 1987).

b. Asymptomatic HIV Infection

The analysis is more difficult as to whether HIV infection alone is a "handicap" or "disability." Many people who are infected by HIV appear to be healthy; they have no physical or mental symptoms which incapacitate them. Nonetheless, the Rehabilitation Act and the ADA protect not only individuals who are handicapped, but also individuals who are perceived to be handicapped. It is safe to assume that, in most cases, asymptomatic HIV infection—like AIDS—will be deemed a "handicap" or "disability" protected under federal law.

2. Is an Individual with HIV Infection or AIDS "Otherwise Qualified"

In order to fall within the protection of federal law, it is not enough to be an "individual with handicaps"; one must also be "otherwise qualified." The U.S. Supreme Court has stated that "**[a] person who poses a significant risk of communicating an infectious disease to others in the work place will not be otherwise qualified for his or her job if reasonable accommodation will not eliminate that risk.**" *School Board of Nassau County v. Arline,* 480 U.S. 273, 287 (1987). Thus, in evaluating whether an employee or student with HIV infection is "otherwise qualified," a two step analysis is required.

a. Significant Risk

First, an institution must decide if the employee or student poses a significant risk of communicating HIV to others. The U.S. Supreme Court has enumerated four factors that must be considered in determining whether a person poses a "significant risk" of transmitting a communicable disease to others. Those four factors are as follows:

(1) The nature of the risk (how the disease is transmitted);

(2) The duration of the risk (how long the carrier is infectious);

(3) The severity of the risk (the potential harm to the third parties); and

(4) The probability that the disease will be transmitted and will cause the varying degrees of harm.

In evaluating these factors, sound medical advise should be sought. It was important to the Court that decisions in this area be based on reasonable medical judgments.

b. Reasonable Accommodation.

Second, if there is a "significant risk" to others, an institution must determine if reasonable accommodation would eliminate that risk. According to the Supreme Court in *Arline,* an accommodation will not be deemed reasonable, if it either (1) poses undue financial and administrative burdens on an institution, or (2) requires a fundamental alteration in the nature of the institution's programs.

3. Can an Institution Find Out if an Employee or Student Is Infected with HIV or Has AIDS

a. Employment or Academic Setting.

Under the federal laws prohibiting discrimination on the basis of handicap or disability, an institution is to focus on an individual's ability to perform all of the essential requirements of the job in question or the academic program in question. Except in health care fields such as medicine, dentistry, and nursing where an individual's HIV infection might pose a significant risk to others, it is difficult to envision an employment or academic situation in which an individual's HIV status would be job- or school-related. Thus, as a general rule, school supervisors and administrators should avoid making inquiries as to an individual's HIV-infection status.

b. Student Health Setting.

The federal laws which prohibit discrimination on the basis of handicap do not in any way dictate how a physician should practice medicine. If, in the context of rendering good and complete medical care to students, a physician deems it necessary or appropriate to inquire about HIV infection, then that inquiry should be made. With limited exceptions, medical information obtained by a student health physician should be treated as confidential medical information and not shared with other college or university administrators.

III. STATE LAWS

In addition to the Rehabilitation Act of 1973 and the Americans with Disabilities Act, most states have state laws which prohibit discrimination on the basis of handicap or disability in employment settings.

A. Florida

Florida has a state statute which specifically prohibits discrimination on the basis of AIDS, ARC, and HIV. Paragraphs (2) and (3) of Section 760.50 of the Florida Statutes state as follows:

(2) Any person with or perceived as having acquired immune deficiency syndrome, acquired immune deficiency syndrome related complex, or human immunodeficiency virus shall have every protection made available to handicapped persons.

BOX 16.3 *(continued)*

(3)(a) No person may require an individual to take a human immunodeficiency virus-related test as a condition of hiring, promotion, or continued employment unless the absence of human immunodeficiency virus infection is a bona fide occupational qualification for the job in question.

B. Maryland

Maryland has a state statute which prohibits discrimination on the basis of handicap. Maryland Annotated Code, Art. 49B, Section 16(a) (1) provides as follows:

(a) It shall be an unlawful employment practice for an employer:

(1) To fail or refuse to hire or to discharge any individual, or otherwise to discriminate against any individual with respect to his compensation, terms, conditions, or privileges of employment, because of such individual's . . . physical or mental handicap unrelated in nature and extent so as to reasonably preclude the performance of the employment.

C. New York

New York has a state statute which prohibits discrimination because of disability. Section 296.1 of Article 15 of the New York Human Rights Law (Consolidated Laws Service) provides as follows:

It shall be an unlawful discriminatory practice:

(a) For an employer . . . , because of the . . . disability . . . of any individual, to refuse to hire or employ or to bar or to discharge from employment such individual or to discriminate against such individual in compensation or in terms, conditions or privileges of employment.

D. Pennsylvania

Pennsylvania has a state statute which prohibits discrimination of the basis of handicap. Section 955 of Chapter 17 of Title 43 of the Pennsylvania Statutes reads as follows:

It shall be an unlawful discriminatory practice, unless based upon a bona fide occupational qualification . . .

(a) For any employer because of the . . . non-job related handicap or disability of any individual to refuse to hire or employ, or to bar or to discharge from employment such individual, or to otherwise discriminate against such individual with respect to compensation, hire, tenure, terms, conditions or privileges of employment, if the individual is the best able and most competent to perform the services required.

Promoting Student Health '91 Legal Issues. Peter H. Ruger, Leslie Chambers Strohm, The Washington University, St. Louis, Missouri. Outline prepared for the New Jersey Collegiate Summer Institute for Health in Education held July 28–August 2, 1991.)

BOX 16.4

LEGAL RIGHTS AND DUTIES IN THE AIDS EPIDEMIC

Bernard M. Dickens

The impact of the acquired immunodeficiency syndrome (AIDS) on human interactions mediated by law has been felt at all levels of society. Early questions about legal protections against the spread of infection are now balanced by questions about the rights of those infected with the human immunodeficiency virus (HIV) and about confidentiality and nondiscrimination. The recognition of such AIDS patients as children infected prenatally or recipients of contaminated blood in transfusions has mitigated an early response within the general population that those infected were culpable and undeserving of legal rights (1, 2).

Governmental responses to the AIDS epidemic, at least in the United States, have in part been punitive, reinforced by a conviction that infection comes from outside and that only a few citizens bear responsibility for causing infection. New immigration laws have been proposed, on the view that national boundaries can be secured against invasion by the virus that causes the disease. An extension of attributing the spread of AIDS to restricted populations is seen in legislative proposals targeting prisoners and prostitutes for compulsory testing and control.

While initial legislative proposals often have been moralistic and largely irrelevant to pragmatic management of the problem, private individuals and organizations have invoked laws in practical pursuit of their perceived interests. Fears of infection in the workplace, educational system, hospital and health care system, and the home have led to resourceful invocations of the law. Conventional legislation against sodomy and illicit drug-taking has proved ineffectual and perhaps counterproductive in containing the spread of infection. In this overview of legal rights and duties in the AIDS epidemic I focus in minor part on laws newly enacted and predominantly on established legal principles that are invoked by motivated individuals and interest groups.

It is conventional jurisprudence that a legal right available to one person depends on a legal duty that binds others. Competing interests may each claim a different right and the other's correlative duty. Litigation requires courts of law to resolve conflicting claims, but in the absence of authoritative rulings mutually incompatible claims to rights are likely to be asserted. Thus, although in the following sections I discuss claimed rights, the identification of a right is often indeterminative of which right the courts of final authority would hold to prevail over others.

Infected Persons' Rights

Testing and treatment. Access to voluntary testing for exposure to HIV is not dependent on the status of the applicants as members of low-risk or high-risk populations. However, rights to testing and to treatment may be only theoretical where, under principles of private law, health professionals have no reciprocal duty to enter into contracts with prospective patients. Public hospital and health authorities are likely to accept a volunteer's right to be tested where this appears to be in the public interest, but might charge nonresidents of their areas the commercial cost of the testing service (3). Similarly, private sector agencies might recognize the right to be tested, but condition it on due payment.

Those who prove HIV-positive, and who even without testing are in high-risk populations, such as actively homosexual and bisexual men, drug-takers who have shared needles or syringes, and hemophiliacs and others who have used blood products [particularly before late 1985, when blood product screening in developed countries became relatively reliable (4, 5)], may claim a right to additional care. Counseling a person before testing, and before or after giving the test results, is considered essential by public health professionals, to give advice both on safer life-style options and on implications of a finding of seropositivity. The rates of clinical depression and suicide among persons testing positive or suspecting positivity reinforce the claim to due counseling (6).

The rights of AIDS patients to medical care apply to the conditions of disease they suffer because of their lack of immunity. These patients have the rights to appropriate care that is routinely available from public or private health insurance plans according to the prevailing local pattern of health service funding. Their right to coverage is in no way diminished when their disease is indirectly attributable to voluntary life-style factors.

No right to treatment of AIDS per se can be claimed while no treatment exists. Rights to unproven therapies are more contentious and revive controversies similar to those raised when laetrile was offered as treatment for cancer (7, 8). Personal autonomy and rights to the benefits of science that are not yet recognized by conservative health service and drug approval administrations may be invoked. A legal compromise may be that health authorities compelled to permit use of such treatments can decline to pay for them (7, 9).

Patients with AIDS may also demand the exemption of potential treatments from the regular process of drug approval, which usually requires premarketing trials extending over a longer time than the patients are likely to survive. Some would-be entrepreneurs have invoked legal defenses of the necessity to save life to found a right to supply unproven drugs to AIDS patients. Jurisprudentially, however, no such right may exist and claiming it may at most be only an excuse for illegal supply of a drug (10).

Confidentiality. Rights to confidentiality of test results are frequently compromised by legislation and judicially declared law concerning the duty and privilege of an individual to warn of anticipated peril. Public health legislation often compels reporting of otherwise confidential information of, for instance, contagious, infectious, or sexually transmitted diseases to designated authorities (11). Such authorities and their officers must protect data from improper release, but in some cases may undertake tracing of contacts in ways that identify patients. Claims of rights to confidentiality are reinforced by policy arguments that the possibility that seropositive results may be released improperly will deter members of high-risk populations from submitting to testing (12, 13).

At various points the law mandates and tolerates disclosures of sensitive and potentially harmful medical information. It is a matter of jurisprudence whether such disclosures constitute permissible breaches of confidentiality or limits beyond which the protected right to confidentiality does not extend. There is growing recognition that the physician–patient relation creates a legal obligation on the physician toward an identifiable third party who may be endangered by the patient. The Supreme Court of California has summarized the principle in the observation that: "The protective privilege ends where the public peril begins" (14). The protective duty owed to third parties may be discharged by warning them of the source and nature of danger or notifying public authorities that exercise the state's police powers, which include public health authorities.

All states require that specified "listed" or "notifiable" diseases be reported to public health departments. AIDS is uniformly notifiable, but AIDS-related complex (ARC) usually is not. A few states, including Arizona, South Carolina, and Wisconsin, expressly require reporting of positive HIV-antibody tests, but others such as Minnesota have more generally expressed provisions that require reporting of any "case," "condition," or "carrier state" relating to listed diseases, including AIDS (15). Reports of anonymous epidemiological monitoring may be unobjectionable, but if reports will disclose identities, they may deter people who fear they may be infected from approaching physicians or hospitals (13).

Where medical confidentiality is not limited by a duty of disclosure, courts may recognize a privilege of disclosure if exercised in good faith to protect another against perceived serious risk. Disclosure of only necessary information is protected, and publication must be confined to persons with a need to know for protection of the threatened vital interest (16). This protection of disclosure is part of the law's accommodation of necessity to act to preserve human life. Disclosure is based on a reasonable perception of danger—the privilege of disclosure covers the situation in which an individual is informed of positive HIV-antibody test results that prove to be false positives.

Nondiscrimination Laws

Because the rights to confidentiality of people who have been exposed to (or who are actually infected by) the virus are so compromised in law that their status may become known, they have to invoke related rights to nondiscrimination as disabled or handicapped persons (17). Private persons and bodies in some states are governed by antidiscrimination legislation only when government is involved, such as through financing of subsidizing a private enterprise. Patients affected by AIDS and ARC may establish their disabled status, but asymptomatic patients showing seropositivity have an unconfirmed status as disabled persons (18). They are not handicapped according to common law or statutory definitions (19) and face limitations primarily through restrictions of life-style they adopt and through others' responses to them.

Health care. Rights to nondiscrimination in health care are important particularly if hospitals and health care facilities test patients for HIV antibodies and health professionals are disposed to deny services to proven seropositive patients. Attending physicians, hospitals, and health facilities have duties not to abandon their existing patients, but when hospital or facility admission is refused and health professionals decline to enter into treating relationships (20), nondiscrimination rights become central to the affected persons' welfare. Legislation, notably in California, Wisconsin, and Michigan, prohibits health professionals from discriminating against persons having or suspected of having conditions associated with AIDS (21).

Employment. Retention and acquisition of employment may depend on rights of nondiscrimination (22). If AIDS, ARC, or seropositivity does not impair employment performance or place other employees or the employer's customers at risk, discrimination on grounds of health status is unjustifiable. Further, where impairment or risk of infection exists, a right may be claimed to alternative work deployment where there is neither impairment nor risk to others before dismissal is justifiable. City ordinances, notably in California, and legislation, most explicitly in Wisconsin, regulate employers' use of HIV-antibody tests (2, 23).

It appears that other employees' fears of working at close quarters with an infected person that lead to disruption in the workplace are not sufficient in themselves to justify the person's dismissal. As the U.S. Supreme Court has observed on prohibited discrimination: "Society's accumulated myths and fears about disability and disease are as handicapping as are the physical limitations that flow from actual impairment"

(24). Courts may occasionally be sympathetic to employers' extraordinary hardship because of customer or even co-workers preferences, but have not been sympathetic in race and sex discrimination suits. A restaurant owner known to employ an HIV-infected waiter or chef, for instance, might consider himself to have legitimate grounds for dismissal of that employee. Unusual hardship because of an employee's AIDS or ARC may be claimed to constitute a "just cause" for discharge under collective bargaining agreements, although seropositivity alone probably would not be justification (25).

Housing. Infected persons may have to consider their legal rights in order to keep or obtain housing. Zoning prohibitions against group homes for the infected raise legal issues of substantive and procedural rights to have planning legislation properly applied. More common, however, are invocations of rights against public and private landlords and participants in the housing market. Public housing is often subject to antidiscrimination laws, and these may also apply to private housing, but their application beyond racial, sexual, and marital-status distinctions is contentious unless the laws clearly prohibit handicap or disability discrimination (26).

Tenants who are infected or are in high-risk categories of infection have no better rights than other tenants to lease renewals or against eviction for breach of applicable clauses in tenancy agreements, and they benefit no more than others from tenant-security laws governing rental agreements. Clauses in tenancy agreements on eviction for misconduct or "good cause" may be applied, for instance, against criminal drug-users (27). Consumer protection laws now often reinforce tenants' rights to resist landlords, however, because leases and rental agreements are viewed less as property transactions than as landlords' service undertakings.

Consumer protection legislation may also work to the disadvantage of infected persons. The sale of accommodation formerly occupied by such persons was historically governed by the principle "let the buyer beware." Legislation or case law may have been developed, however, that requires disclosure of invisibly unsafe conditions in property and of material facts that significantly reduce its value (27). An HIV-infected occupant as such apparently leaves no risk in a home that jeopardizes its safety, but knowledge of the former occupancy may lower the resale value (27, 28).

Education. School-aged children with HIV infection and their parents who invoke rights and indeed obligations under compulsory school attendance laws may be resisted through argument based on public health laws on contagious and infectious diseases, through picketing, boycotts of schools by other parents and children, and worse. Rights of access to public education below school-leaving age are not necessarily certain, but are increasingly viewed as a matter of entitlement (29). Compulsory school attendance laws seem in principle to confer corresponding rights. Admission may depend, however, on immunization and hygiene tests that HIV-infected children fail. The U.S. Supreme Court has upheld laws conditioning public school attendance on vaccination (30), and similar laws requiring proven immunity from contagious disease have been approved at lower levels of courts as a valid exercise of police power even in the absence of emergency or threatened epidemic (31). Again, children's rights of school attendance, in the absence of an imminent danger of spread of disease, have been based on laws prohibiting discrimination on grounds of handicap (32), and establishment that seropositivity is a handicap.

More refined arguments may be made that the right to an education cannot be satisfied through public provision of isolated instruction (33), since an important component of education is socialization with peers. The right of peer contact may be unenforceable at one level in that other children may be directly and indirectly induced to ostracize an infected child, but the right may be asserted against a public school board rather than against other children. The claim will be for an opportunity of broadly defined classroom education, not for achievement of an educational outcome. If educational malpractice claims against school and education authorities gain recognition, however, failure to achieve standards of literacy and other skills in children may become actionable.

Insurance. The ability to obtain insurance protection has been a source of bitter controversy (34). Seropositive applicants have complained of discrimination when denied insurance coverage, and private insurance companies have complained of exploitation and abuse by AIDS patients. Health insurance is distinguishable from disability and life insurance, but all forms of insurance are subject to legal principles of fiduciary obligation. Because parties seeking insurance know their circumstances better than those offering coverage, they are required to redress the imbalance of power derived from knowledge by making full and frank disclosure of material information. Knowledge of HIV infection appears material, but problematic is whether knowledge of membership in a high-risk group must be disclosed. The law often imputes knowledge to those who should make relevant inquiries to obtain it. An insurance policy may be voided in legal principle for lack of an insured's due disclosure of what is, or should be, known.

Health insurance is particularly costly to provide to the population of AIDS patients, not only because of high treatment costs but also because sufferers tend to be young and have thus not paid premiums long enough to permit insurers to accumulate capital. Life insurance is similarly costly, and companies cite patients with full-blown AIDS taking out large policies at high premiums for the short time before they die, when their beneficiaries, who may have contributed to payment of premiums, recover the high sums insured. Insurance company problems are aggravated by their common practice of contracting to offer group insurance to classes of persons not dependent on individual health examination (35).

Those claiming rights of insurance say that it is discriminatory to require the population with AIDS to furnish the funds they cause to be spent, when other populations, such as alcoholics and elderly drivers, are not expected as a group to cover their costs. Distribution of costs over an undifferentiated population is said to be the function of insurance. Further, health insurance and disability insurance in the United States have remained largely privatized, unlike in most other developed countries, because government has been persuaded by the insurance industry that the industry can provide adequate coverage. Government regulation requires that companies do so comprehensively, without discriminating unduly against the sick and handicapped. Patients with AIDS cause large but limited health care expenditures, but companies are particularly apprehensive of uncontrollable costs of maintaining the health of seropositive insureds.

Rights of HIV-infected people to insurance depend significantly on government regulators of the insurance industry disallowing AIDS-based discrimination, such as by exclusions from coverage and prohibitive premiums (36). Regulation may prohibit or control questioning of applicants (37), but also may permit limits on coverage when health information is not given or applicants do not agree to testing. Conditions may also be set for testing, such as that it be medically indicated and not simply based on life-style.

Related areas. A sizable array of additional activities exists that may be subject to laws governing discrimination against AIDS patients or HIV-infected persons. Public sporting or recreational clubs may fear members inadvertently exchanging such body fluids as perspiration and saliva, which have not been shown to cause infection, and blood. Public ambulance and paramedical services seem to deny their purpose when they refuse assistance to persons who are sick due to AIDS, and these services and privately operated common carriers may be liable under antidiscrimination laws (21). Embalmers, funeral homes, and cemeteries may be reluctant to manage corpses of AIDS patients, but may violate rights of AIDS victims' families to proper and prompt disposal of relatives' remains (21).

A number of bills have been introduced in state legislatures to control the right of HIV-infected persons to marry (38). Drawing on conservative laws that made satisfactory testing for certain sexually transmitted diseases a condition of obtaining marriage licenses, some have urged that no marriage license be issued without a negative antibody test result (39). This condition appears constitutionally flawed (40), would have no effect on homosexual couples who cannot legally marry, and seems overreaching in attempting to enforce the moral duties couples contemplating marriage owe each other. Further, it is counterproductive to prevent informed couples, one or both of whom are infected, from marrying, since their sexual fidelity to each other is better encouraged than obstructed. This issue requires attention to be given to the legal duties of infected persons.

Infected Persons' Duties

Criminal law. HIV-infected persons are bound by criminal laws that govern offenses ranging from the most heinous classical crimes to relatively minor modern administrative infractions (41). Some jurisdictions, such as Florida and Idaho, have introduced a new crime of willfully or knowingly exposing another to the AIDS virus, but most jurisdictions seem able to rely on existing offenses of (attempted) homicide (42, 43) and, for instance, assault with a deadly weapon. The latter was successfully charged in Minnesota when an infected prisoner bit two prison guards (42, 44).

Those who know of their infection, but still have sexual relations without condoms, and infected drug-takers who share needles or syringes may be charged with attempted murder or assault with intent to kill, although if their intent to kill cannot be shown the charge will be dismissed or reduced. Manslaughter may be charged against those proved to have caused death when they knew or should have known of their liability to transmit the infection. Blood donation when it was possible that the donor was infected is difficult to charge. Such an offense might be prosecuted as manslaughter or negligent killing if death were to be caused, but would not otherwise be indictable if the purpose of donation was to have the blood tested and rejected, with notification to the donor if it tested positive for HIV antibodies.

Risking the transmission of AIDS may lead infected persons to be charged with related offenses. Prostitution-based crimes may be charged when paid sexual relations are involved, and even without commerce, sodomy may be charged in cases of both unprotected and protected homosexual sex (45). Drug offenses may similarly be pursued when they are the origin of risk of transmission (46). More specifically, offenses relating to the running of such enterprises as gay clubs and bathhouses may be charged, although these may shade into zoning or comparable regulatory infractions. Charges relating to sexually transmitted diseases may be pressed where the law penalizes infected persons' failure to report, to seek testing or treatment, or to remain celibate, but enforcement questions are then raised regarding infections such as AIDS that are transmissible both sexually and nonsexually.

Civil law. Noncriminal law seeks to deter harmful conduct not by imposing punishment, but by such means as ordering wrongdoers to pay compensation for the injuries they have caused (47, 48). The duty of care that the tort of negligence requires to be observed is often supplemented by statutes that require proper care of others. Civil actions arising from transmission of AIDS range from wrongful death claims for wrongfully causing a victim to die to so-called "wrongful birth" (49) or "wrongful life" (50) claims. The latter charge is brought by or on behalf of a child who contracted infection *in utero* (51). The essence of such a claim is that, where the infection was unavoidable, the child should not have been conceived or born. Lingering doctrines of parental immunity may protect mothers against suit, but render liable those other than their husbands whose wrong caused their infection or pregnancy. Few jurisdictions, in fact, recognize wrongful life actions, and, because liability to such action may lead to abortion, some jurisdictions have prohibited them (52).

Sexual transmission of HIV fits within the rather unclear framework of legal liability for spreading venereal disease and, for instance, herpes (53). The duty each person has to protect a sexual partner against a contagious disease (54) is defined by the policy of the law to require infected persons to exercise ordinary caution. Those who know or reasonably should know of their liability to have and therefore to transmit HIV are responsible to inform or otherwise protect sexual partners. In contrast, an asymptomatic sex partner not in a high-risk group may not be liable for failing to recognize presence or risk of infectivity.

A party seeking compensation is legally required to show that infection was caused by breach of duty by the party sued. The long incubation period of AIDS may obstruct the tracing of an alleged source and make it difficult to establish that party's wrongful nondisclosure or failure to follow prudent sexual behavior, or the plaintiff's seronegativity prior to the sexual encounter and low-risk conduct thereafter. Further, even when causation can be shown, a defense exists that the plaintiff voluntarily accepted the risk of infection. This defense is defined by the legal principle that requires persons voluntarily placing themselves at risk to protect themselves (54). Many claims for venereal infection and pregnancy, and defenses to paternity and child maintenance claims, have failed on grounds of the assumption of risk doctrine. Some courts compromise through recognizing a claim for spread of infection, but reducing recoverable compensation by finding that the claimant contributed to the injury (47).

Liability for battery is unlikely since consent is a full defense, and consent need be only to the sexual encounter in general rather than to an act of the specific nature and quality that occurred. Ignorance of a sexual partner's infection does not convert voluntary intercourse into rape in criminal law, and is equally unlikely to convert it into battery in civil law. A claim for fraudulent misrepresentation may succeed, however, if an infected person deliberately gives an assurance of noninfectivity that induces the sexual act (55). An assurance may be made by silence when a trust or fiduciary obligation of disclosure arises, as in marriage or other confidential relationship. Other tort claims may be for inflicting emotional damage or causing outrage by deliberately risking AIDS transmission, and for causing psychic injury through negligently spreading infection, although courts may find particularly the latter claim too speculative and open to abuse.

Liability for provision of contaminated blood products concerns both blood donors and intermediate processors such as hospitals and blood banks (56). They may bear liability to recipients, however, only when their actual negligence can be shown and not under legal principles that impose strict (no-fault) liability on producers of certain items (57). Product liability principles are inapplicable where supplying blood is considered to be a service rather than a commodity transaction, as it is in most states at least in clinical cases (as opposed to large volume blood sales). Blood product consumers' rights of informed decision-making on use of products entitles them to general information on the origin and safety processing of materials they propose to receive, although information may have to be given only on their request. They have no right, however, to identifying information about specific blood donors (58).

In addition to liabilities under general civil laws, infected persons may bear special liabilities, for instance, to involuntary detention on grounds of dangerousness or incompetency arising under mental health legislation. Dementias objectively discernible by psychological tests appear to occur in over 50% of AIDS patients (59), and other neurological conditions associated with different stages of disease development may bring affected persons within controls of mental health systems. Indications for engagement of mental health laws include general dangerousness, danger of spreading HIV infection, inability to maintain self-care and, for instance, microcephaly in children born with HIV infection.

Uninfected Persons' Rights to Protection

Persons not infected with HIV have numerous legal rights to protect their own welfare and that of others that their infection might endanger, such as their unborn children. Their rights correlate to others' duties, notably infected persons' obligations to exercise due care not to transmit HIV. Health professionals have special duties to screen and control agents of HIV transmission such as blood, to warn of known risks outside their control, and to advise on conduct and life-style that will reduce risk of infection. Observance of others' rights must be carefully judged, however, because persons' rights to be informed and counseled, when served by aggressive and directive counselors, may endanger their rights not to be unduly alarmed. The rise of the medical malpractice action for induction of cancer phobia (60) and of, for instance, clergy liability for negligent counseling causing or aggravating distress and suicidal tendencies (61), indicates a line between rights to be informed about AIDS and not to be harmed by misinformation. Uninfected persons may have to compromise their preferred conduct or life-style when they lack rights to receive the protective services or devices they want; prisoners may be unable to receive condoms, for instance (43, 62), and illicit drug-takers may have no claim to clean needles or syringes. Where legal rights to goods or services exist in principle, they may be unavailable to indigents (9) because while other persons or bodies have duties not to obstruct access to such goods or services, they have no duties to supply them without charge. Legal rights to self-provision of costly preventive services or treatments may alone be inadequate to ensure their availability.

Rights and Duties of Health Professionals and Authorities

Several jurisdictions have recently enacted laws of differing scope and terms that allow AIDS patients to be detained and isolated (15), but historic unrepealed laws are frequently found to contain isolation and quarantine powers (63). Particularly in developed countries, public health standards have so improved and epidemic disease has become so infrequent that it is easy to forget that legislation once led public officers to exercise the state's police powers with considerable invasiveness and coercion. Compulsory testing for venereal disease and the subjection of prostitutes to detention, quarantine, and internment are well within living memory: during World War I more than 30,000 prostitutes were incarcerated in federally supported institutions in the United States (64). Legislation accommodated both moral and public health panic, both of which are apparent in some responses to AIDS.

Some health authorities have proposed that they have legal powers of nonconsensual screening of high-risk populations for AIDS. The military initiated screening in 1985 and has tested over 3 million individuals (65), on the explanation that, in combat, the military constitutes its own supply of transfusable blood. Particularly targeted by other screening programs have been such legally accessible groups as immigrants and refugees, prisoners, convicted prostitutes, and known drug addicts. Several proposals invoke control measures traditionally used to contain airborne contagious diseases, and often reflect misunderstanding of the principal modes of AIDS transmission. Requests that public health authorities exercise existing or newly acquired legal rights of quarantine presume that this is a preferable means of disease containment. More specific proposals have been made to use legal powers, which include due-process protections, to isolate "incorrigible" or "recalcitrant" persons aware of their infection who continue to engage in high-risk conduct dangerous to others despite warnings given by health professionals (11).

Hospital staff make a case for a legal right of routine (that is, involuntary) screening of patients on admission because of the risk they present of exposing hospital personnel to their body fluids. Apart from inapplicability of such testing to emergency admissions, particularly trauma cases, results of testing may yield little useful information. False-positive results will lead to the same precautions as true-positive results, but true-negative results may indicate only that the incubation period of HIV infection has not been sufficient. Routine precautions that are available, and those that hospital authorities often legally require to be taken against hepatitis may achieve a high level of protection. The AIDS policy of the American Medical Association rejects mandatory testing of hospital patients (66).

Health care workers have stronger legal remedies against their employers than they have against AIDS patients to protect their own well-being. Under occupational safety and health laws, they are entitled to high standards of personal safety in their work environments (21). Hospitals and comparable facilities must train and equip their staff for safe practice and enforce legally mandated standards of protection. Availability and use of gloves and gowns are minimum conditions of safety; provision of such clothing and of sterile equipment protecting both patients and staff members is to be expected. New U.S. federal guidelines (20) to protect health care workers, reflecting earlier recommendations of the U.S. Public Health Service and the American Hospital Association, stress that all patients be viewed as potentially infected, and the Occupational Safety and Health Administration has power to penalize hospitals and other medical facilities that fail to observe prevailing safeguards to protect health care workers. Staff who suffer work-related infection may take legal action against their employers or present claims before workers' compensation boards.

Health care workers, including physicians and nurses, who feel inadequately protected against AIDS-infected patients may decide to withdraw from the workplace or decline to treat known AIDS patients or identified members of high-risk groups (20). They may be in breach of service contracts unless it can be shown that the employers were in breach of express, implied, or legislated provision on employee protection, or that withdrawal was for adequate cause. Whether refusal of professional services of AIDS-infected persons for instance, by hospital staff not bound by contracts, legally justified condemnation as misconduct by the disciplinary tribunal of licensing authority has not yet been litigated (67).

Authorities with legal responsibility for individual health protection of dependent or captive populations often aim to prevent sexual and drug-related conduct for reasons of morality, discipline, and policy, not simply to contain HIV infection. Prisons, adolescent correctional facilities, group homes, and, for instance, homes for retarded persons may accordingly be reluctant to offer instruction in safer sex practices and to make condoms available (62). Denying mentally incompetent persons means of self-protection in indulging their sexual instincts and leaving anyone exposed to risk in the sexually brutal or callous conditions that prevail in some prison and comparable facilities open authorities to legal liability to nonculpable victims of HIV infection that reasonable care could have prevented.

Public health authorities and public and private sanitation undertakings have legally enforceable duties to dispose of pathological and comparable wastes in a manner that protects both handlers and communities from risk of infection. Laws on public nuisance must be observed in waste storage and disposal, and waste collection must be under instructions and supervision that are protective of personnel. Legal duties must be observed under specific legislation contract law, negligence law, and occupiers' liability and land law or escape of dangerous materials brought onto or otherwise not naturally accumulated on premises.

International Legal Developments

International collaboration on the epidemiology, control, and searches for cures of AIDS, ARC, and HIV infection is gathering momentum, particularly through the instrumentality of the World Health Organization (WHO) (68). Legal and regulatory initiative are essentially national, however, with minor exceptions regarding international travel, where collaboration has occurred

BOX 16.4 *(continued)*

to reduce obstacles to transit (69). The Health Legislation Unit of WHO continues to amass an unrivaled collection of information on different countries' enacted and proposed laws specific and relevant to aspects of AIDS. Particularly through the Unit Director, information is promptly and systematically published in the WHO's quarterly journal *The International Digest of Health Legislation* and synthesized in various other publications (70).

Legal rights and duties outlined above reflect general approaches in jurisdictions of the United States and other countries of the common law tradition such as England, Canada, Australia, New Zealand, and many other members of the British Commonwealth. The prominence given to constitutional provisions in the United States is not common, however, in other jurisdictions. By 9 December 1987, 128 countries had reported at least one AIDS case (71) and have had to engage their legal systems at different levels in management of clinical and public health aspects of these cases. Legislative proposals elsewhere often parallel U.S. developments on, for instance, reporting requirements and control of high-risk populations and immigrants. Several countries, such as Sweden (but not the United Kingdom), have used regulatory changes to bring AIDS infection within existing legal frameworks governing sexually transmitted and contagious diseases.

Coercive legislation has been specially enacted in Austria (72) and in Bavaria [West Germany (73)] that controls prostitutes, and in the latter provides for compulsory testing of suspected persons, prisoners, and refugees. Infected persons are required to inform prospective partners in sexual and other contacts of their liability to transmit infection. Aliens may be denied residence permits and, if medical orders are disregarded, may be deported. In April 1987, Iraq went further and required compulsory testing of returning nationals (74). In August 1987, the Soviet Union adopted strong measures (75) for mandatory testing of selected Russian and foreign citizens and stateless residents, with liability to expulsion for non-Russian citizens who evade testing. Up to 5 years of incarceration may be imposed on those who knowingly expose others to risk of infection, and up to 8 years if infection is actually transmitted.

Countries in some regions of the world where AIDS is widespread, such as Central Africa, have been slow to invoke or implement laws. Much legislation in the early to mid-1980s in Europe and, for instance, Australia, was concerned with control of blood donations and screening of blood products, and may have contributed to success in reducing transmission of infection by this route. Other laws tend to reflect the conviction that the disease is primarily of alien origin and to adopt stereotypical views of the necessity to protect national boundaries against outsiders. Marginal domestic groups may also receive stereotyped attention. For instance, in June 1986, Guatemala introduced remarkably detailed AIDS regulations (76) to control women prostitutes; female employees in bars and cafes; dancers in bars, shows, nightclubs, and cabarets; and women working in men's saunas and massage parlors. The United States, in whose state legislatures 51 bills on AIDS were passed in 1986 (77) and 550 such bills were introduced in the first 8 months of 1987 (78), may be pioneering recognition, however, that AIDS has become a feature of the environment.

References and Notes— Original article contains the 78 references cited.

Update 1995—Twenty-two states now have laws making it a felony to have unprotected sex if you know you are HIV-positive.

without the patient's written consent or a court order. All states have laws on the books to protect medical and public health records from unauthorized disclosure. But some believe that these laws are inadequate and vulnerable to court orders for the release of confidential medical information on individuals' HIV status (Dickens, 1989). It is felt that new laws that apply directly to the confidentiality of HIV information should be passed to protect people from social bias. Such new laws were passed in a number of states in 1988 (e.g., California, Florida, Massachusetts, New York, and Vermont.) In Florida, the person to be tested, or the parents of a child to be tested, are given the following statement on confidentiality to read:

Confidentiality

You should be aware that there is some risk associated with letting others know about your test results. It is advised that you keep this information very private and inform only your physician/dentist. It is also advised that you inform your sexual or needle sharing contacts that they may have been exposed to the virus that causes AIDS and recommend that they be tested.

Parents of children taking the test should be aware that there may be some risk associated with letting others know about their child's test results. It is advised that parents keep this information very private and inform only their child's physician/dentist or foster home. In each of the above cases, using test results as grounds for discrimination in insurance or employment is prohibited in some states. How-ever, the burden of proof is on the persons discriminated against.

Every effort is made to insure the confidentiality of the test results. Any information that may identify you is kept in your medical records at the health department and available only to a limited number of people who have a "need-to-know." The "need-to-know" refers to **Allowable Disclosure** (see BOX 16.5). These people are your physician, nurse, or counselor. In some states, laws prohibit the release of HIV antibody test information without your written consent.

Many people want new laws that require the tracking and reporting of HIV carriers and their partners. It is doubtful that a single law can be so constructed that it will please everybody. In 1988, there was a fierce battle between opposing forces concerning the Dannemeyer-Gann AIDS Initiative, or Pro-position 102 on the California ballot. If this proposition had passed, it would have eliminated confidentiality for people taking the HIV test. Physicians would have had to report names and addresses of those who tested positive and those they reasonably believed to be infected. Failure to report a case would have meant a fine of $250. In addition, the infected would have been required to produce a list of sexual partners to public health officials or be charged with a misdemeanor.

The Confidentiality Dilemma

There appears at the moment to be no legal balance between a physician's obligation to his or her patients and the obligation to the public good. The physician is in a "Catch-22" position: There does not appear to be a clear moral or legal choice. The following cases help highlight the moral and legal morass confronting physicians in the United States.

Case 1— A physician said he knew that a heart bypass surgery patient was HIV-infected and advised the man against having sex for several weeks after surgery for the sake of his heart. Six months later, the man died of a heart attack. Six months after that, his wife developed AIDS. Was this physician *legally obligated* to make sure that both the patient and his wife knew of his HIV infection? The wife decided not to sue the physician. Note that the question emphasizes legal obligation. Physicians often fail to exercise their moral obligations when they conflict with the law; especially when lawyers and physicians are groping for mutual agreement on the legality of confidentiality with regard to HIV-infected patients.

Case 2— Key West, Florida (population 30,000) has one of the highest AIDS rates in the United States. Ninety-five percent of AIDS cases are in the homosexual population. It is estimated that one in four people in Key West is homosexual and one in two carries HIV (Breo, 1988).

The wife of the owner of Sloppy Joe's Saloon died of AIDS. After the memorial service for his wife, his pregnant girlfriend filed a suit wherein her attorney asked that the Monroe County Health Department. and the Florida Department. of Health and Rehabilitative Services (HRS) release the bar owner's medical records. The order was granted allowing her personal physician to view the medical file. The judge prohibited further disclosure of the records by either the pregnant woman or her physician.

The lawsuit provoked anger and unrest in Key West and caught private physicians and public health officials in the middle of the dilemma of how to balance the rights of individual patients against the rights of those whomay become infected.

The wife had told her physician that both she and her husband tested HIV-positive at out of state laboratories. They were both counseled extensively, in particular about the risk of transmitting the virus to others. After the lawsuit was filed, the counseling physician was outraged. He said "I knew that he had understood what I had told him because he told me, 'Well, Doc, this little bugger is a bastard of a virus and there's nothing we can do to beat it

BOX 16.5

ALLOWABLE DISCLOSURE

Allowable disclosure refers to the special circumstances which justify disclosure of a patient's HIV status without that patient's authorization. The impact of these disclosures may vary greatly. Extreme caution should be taken when making an allowable disclosure; professionals in all areas, health, education, police, and so forth, are advised to consult an attorney before doing so. Typically, the following exceptions to maintain confidentiality are recognized as allowable disclosures:

1. As necessary for health care personnel to proceed with appropriate treatment as determined by physicians
2. To conduct epidemiological research
3. To respond to potentially significant exposures of health care or public safety personnel to contaminated blood or body fluids. Thus exception is applied to discrete exposure incidents, evaluated through risk assessment on a case-by-case basis.
4. As required by law or regulation for reporting child abuse, sexually transmitted diseases, including HIV/AIDS, or cause of death
5. As required for the welfare of the patient, as in cases of attempted suicide or dementia
6. As required for the welfare of third parties. This is applicable in cases where third parties are faced with possible harm due to the conduct of a patient or the nature of his or her illness.
   a. There is presently no established *legal* duty for a health care provider to warn sexual or needle-sharing partners of HIV-infected patients, making **duty to warn** one of the most challenging HIV-related determinations for health care providers.
      i. There is no certainty about who must be warned or under what circumstances.
      ii. The more specific the knowledge of who and under what circumstances a third party is at risk, the more compelling the duty to warn that specific third party.
      iii. The legal case most often cited as precedent for disclosure in this type of situation is the *Tarasof* case. [*Tarasof v. Regents of the University of California,* 551 P.2d 334 (CA 1976)] (See BOX 13.6)
         (a) The majority legal opinion held that "the protective privilege ends where the public peril begins."
         (b) However, the justices did not state what should be done to adequately warn a potential victim or what constitutes "reasonable efforts to warn."
         (c) *Tarasof* may have more bearing on mental health practitioner decisions to warn third parties because they may be held to a somewhat different legal standard than physicians in many jurisdictions.
      iv. Physicians may be absolved of any potential duty to warn by making a statutorily required report to local health department.
      v. Legislation in some states focuses on "privilege to disclose" rather than on duty to warn.
         (a) Under these laws, partner notification is a routinely allowable disclosure and the provider is protected from civil or criminal liability when disclosure is made in good faith.
         (b) **It is important to review state laws affecting these situations.**
   b. Confidentiality may be breached in third party situations only when all of the following conditions have been met:
      i. It is known that the infected individual will not or cannot carry out the responsibility to warn others known to be at risk;
      ii. Reasonable efforts have failed to persuade the patient to give voluntary disclosure consent;
      iii. There is a high probability both that harm will occur if the confidential information is not disclosed, and that the disclosed information will in fact be used to prevent harm. This is most easily established in the instance of a patient's specific threat of imminent physical violence or harm against a specific person;
      iv. The harm that others at risk would suffer would be serious harm; *and,*
      v. Adequate precautions are taken to guarantee that only necessary information is disclosed (i.e., protecting the identity of the infected person).

BOX 16.6

THE HIPPOCRATIC OATH AND CONFIDENTIALITY

"Whatsoever I shall see or hear in the course of my profession, in my intercourse with men, if it is that which should not be broadcast about, I will never divulge it but consider it a holy secret."

The commitment of a physician to his or her patient has a historical basis. But the commitment of a physician to society is just as strong and historically precedented. The rate at which the AIDS virus is being transmitted worldwide has put the historical debate of confidentiality versus the public's right to know in a new perspective. Oliver Wendell Holmes wrote that when the public's right to know and an individual's right to privacy come into conflict, the public's right to know comes first.

Harold Schwartz (1988) reported on a 37-year-old bisexual married man whose lover had recently been diagnosed with AIDS. He was worried that he may have acquired the infection and wanted to be tested After appropriate counseling the test was arranged and he turned out to be HIV-positive. When asked how he planned to bring up this matter with his wife, he said that he had no intention of telling her. She knew nothing about his bisexuality and he would be humiliated and disgraced if she learned of it now. He promised that he would reduce the number of sexual contacts with his wife, but he could not eliminate them entirely or even rely on safer sex practices because his wife was trying to become pregnant. What should the physician have done?

Duty to Protect Whom?

When an HIV-infected person behaves in a manner that the physician knows will endanger others, the physician has both a professional and moral obligation to protect the patient's confidentiality and a duty to protect those who may be in danger.

Precedent for the legal obligation to protect those in jeopardy from someone who behaves in a reckless or dangerous manner is the case of *Tarasof v. Regents of the University of California*. A mentally disturbed psychiatric patient told his psychiatrist the name of a person he was going to kill. The person was not warned. The psychiatrist kept the information confidential and his patient committed murder. The *Tarasof* case is now interpreted with respect to HIV-infected people as the physician's duty to protect people from potential harm.

But individuals in general have an obligation not to harm others. This was made abundantly clear in the case of Marc Christian, age 35, after he initially won 21.7 million dollars from the estate of movie star Rock Hudson. Hudson died in 1985 of AIDS. The jury found that Hudson was guilty of outrageous conduct in concealing that he had AIDS from his homosexual lover. The jury ruled that Hudson conspired with secretary Mark Miller to keep secret the actor's disease to induce Christian to continue having high-risk sex with Hudson.

State Laws and Patients' Rights

Because of the conflict between a patient's right to confidentiality and the public's right to be warned, in 1988, 10 states passed laws authorizing physicians to inform spouses of HIV-infected individuals. The laws absolve the physician from civil or criminal liability so long as he or she informs the patient of the intent to contact the partner in advance of making the actual contact. Ten states established voluntary partner notification programs or programs under which infected individuals can ask public health officials to notify contacts. Thirty two states and the District of Columbia have passed antidiscrimination laws, 16 states have passed legislation restricting the use of blood tests by insurance companies, and 12 states have made it a felony to willfully or knowingly transmit or expose another individual to HIV.

As of April 1992, 37 states required that HIV infection in people who do not yet meet the criteria for CDC-defined AIDS be reported; these states account for 50% of all AIDS cases reported in the United States (Table 10-6). Twenty-two of the 37 states have enacted legislation or promulgated regulations that require reporting HIV-infected people by name to state or local health departments. These 22 states accounted for 16% of all reported AIDS cases. All 22 states require information to include the person's sex, age, and race/ethnicity; 19 states, require mode of transmission; six, clinical status; and three, CD4 T cell count. Sixteen of the 22 states that require reporting by name offer the option of anonymous HIV testing in some circumstances. Thus patient names are not always provided.

In 12 of the 37 states, *anonymous* individual reports of HIV infection must be provided to the state health department; these 12 states account for 22% of all reported AIDS cases. Eleven of the 12 states require reporting only sex and age; nine, only race/ethnicity; and six, mode of transmission. None of the 12 requires reports on clinical status or CD4 T cell count (*MMWR*, 1991).

A 1988 Florida law requires all testing sites to provide pre- and posttest counseling and stipulates that anyone offering posttest counseling must have special training that includes recognition of suicidal behavior.

California requires that people convicted of first-time prostitution must complete an AIDS education course. Washington and Florida require most health care providers to complete an educational course on HIV and AIDS as a condition of licensure. All states prohibit the sale or delivery of HIV self-testing kits. By the end of 1988, 32 states had laws requiring that health care workers, primarily emergency medical personnel and funeral directors, be notified if the patient or deceased was HIV-infected.

so we have to be careful.'" Should the husband and wife's treating physician have been permitted to warn those the carriers might have exposed? Should public health officials be empowered with emergency sanctions to override patient confidentiality? Are such powers needed?

Justice Abbott Goldberg (1989) carefully and precisely defines the legal issue of confidentiality, particularly concerning physician charting on AIDS patients. He states his position: "Physicians are liable if they fail to disclose that a patient has AIDS and this non-disclosure subsequently harms someone. The questions are not whether, but when, to whom, and for how much physicians may be liable for concealing the fact that a patient is infectious for AIDS." Thus the intentional breach of confidentiality is legally expected from physicians who care for patients with AIDS. This stems, Goldberg argues, from two sources: case law establishing that physicians ". . . [have] both the authority and the duty to violate a patient's confidence in order to protect those persons to whom the patient may communicate a disease" and from the professional view that physicians ". . . have a duty to keep accurate patient records on which they know other providers may rely."

From a legal standpoint, these points are hardly arguable (Murphy, 1989). Justice Goldberg is saying that confidentiality ends where public peril begins. The precedent for Justice Goldberg's interpretation of the current confidentiality laws may have come from the ruling by the California Supreme Court in the case of *Tarasof v. Regents of the University of California* (1976). In this case, the defendants argued that a legal obligation of confidentiality prevented warning a person who was known to be in danger of being attacked by a psychiatric patient. The Court observed, "We recognize the public interest in supporting effective treatment of mental illness and in

POINT OF INFORMATION 16.2

A PENALTY FOR VIOLATING PATIENT CONFIDENTIALITY

In 1988, an orthopedic surgeon settled out of court to end a suit for breach of patient confidentiality. The surgeon was charged with violating a provision of the California Health and Safety Code that prohibits disclosure of a patient's HIV status without the patient's written consent.

The surgeon stated that in late 1985, a few months after the confidentiality statute went into effect, a patient informed him that he was infected with HIV. The patient was scheduled for surgery and the surgeon was concerned about the possible risk of becoming infected.

The patient verbally agreed that his HIV status could be revealed to members of the surgical team to lessen their chances of becoming infected. The surgeon subsequently entered HIV status into the medical record.

The patient later sued the surgeon for breach of confidentiality under the new law. He asserted that by entering his HIV status in the medical record, the surgeon had violated his privacy and statutory rights.

The suit was ultimately settled, in part because of the patient's reluctance to pursue a public trial. This case illustrates the tug-of-war in the era of AIDS between the obligation to protect patient privacy and the need for physicians and other health professionals to share medical information about their patients.

protecting the rights of patients to privacy, and the consequent public importance of safeguarding the confidential character of psychotherapeutic communication. Against this interest, however, we must weigh the public interest in safety from violent assault."

In prioritizing confidentiality and safety, the Court concluded, "The public policy favoring protection of the confidential character of patient–psychotherapist communications must yield to the extent to which disclosure is essential to avert danger to others. The protective privilege ends where the public peril begins" (Dickens, 1989).

Under *Tarasof*, physicians are obligated to inform a third party when they have reason to believe that he or she may be endangered by the actions of a patient. Based on the *Tarasof* decision, physicians may assume that if a patient's sexual partners are in danger, they should be notified. There must, however, be a specific target involved. In addition, the physician may be obligated to notify others, including the employer if a patient is involved in an occupation where job responsibilities could put others at increased risk of infection (Hirsh, 1988).

LEGAL ASPECTS OF HIV/AIDS AND HEALTH CARE WORKERS

HIV/AIDS is preventable. Therefore people must be educated on how to prevent HIV infection. They need to be taught how to protect themselves. According to national polls, the United States is doing a reasonably good job in educating the general public about the virus, its transmission, and how to avoid it. However, because thousands of health care workers (HCWs) are known to be HIV-infected or to have AIDS, the public has raised questions concerning the possibility that their doctors, nurses, dentists, and other HCWs might be HIV-infected. They began to ask whether or not they had a right to know the HIV status of their health care professionals. At the same time, doctors, nurses, and other medical professionals, in fear for their own safety, began to raise questions about testing their patients prior to treatment, especially prior to invasive surgery. But it took the transmission of HIV from dentist David Acer of Stuart, Florida to his patient Kimberly Bergalis in 1987 and the publicity of that case to bring the concerns, fears, and liability of both patients and health care professionals to national debate.

Following numerous reports, much publicity and pressure from its members over the Bergalis case, the American Dental Association sent out the following 1991 news release:

> The recent case of possible HIV transmission from dentist to patient has raised some uncertainty about the risk of transmission from health care provider to patient. While there is evidence that this dental practice did not consistently adhere to all recommended guidelines for prevention of disease transmission, the precise mechanism of transmission in this case remains unknown. This uncertainly leads to the conclusion that the foremost concern of the dental profession must continue to be protection of the patient. Thus, until the uncertainty about transmission is resolved, the ADA believes that HIV-infected dentists should refrain from performing invasive procedures or should disclose their seropositive status.

In addition to the American Dental Association's news release of January 16, 1991, the American Medical Association issued a January 17, 1991 news release regarding its position on HIV-infected physicians. The statement says:

> The American Medical Association believes that physicians who are HIV-positive and who must restrict their normal professional activities have a right to continue their career in medicine in a capacity that poses no identifiable risk to their patients. The American Medical Association pledges its support and protection of these physicians and believes the profession and the public have a need and an obligation to ensure that they continue to be productive as long as they practice medicine safely and responsibly.

The positions of the CDC and the major medical/dental professional associations are constantly shifting. Since issuing its July 27, 1990 report, "Possible Transmission of Human Immunodeficiency Virus to a Patient During an Invasive Dental Procedure," the CDC has issued at least two updates on the

Florida situation (January 18, 1991 and June 14, 1991). On July 12, 1991, the Centers for Disease Control and Prevention published its recommendations for preventing HIV and hepatitis B virus (HBV) transmission to patients during exposure-prone invasive procedures.

HIV/AIDS: A DOUBLE-EDGED SWORD FOR THE PRACTICING PHYSICIAN AND OTHER HEALTH CARE WORKERS

Questions have been raised concerning the legal obligation of health care personnel to treat HIV/AIDS patients. In November 1987, the Council on Ethical and Judicial Affairs of the American Medical Association issued a statement saying that a physician may not ethically refuse to treat patients who are infected with the virus It called on physicians who are infected to act in such a manner that transmission of the virus to patients is not possible. Clearly this statement says that physicians may not refuse to treat HIV/AIDS patients if the physician is qualified to treat such patients. Physicians do have legal obligations to their patients, including those who have HIV/AIDS. Physicians who refuse to treat HIV/AIDS patients may be accused of violating the New Americans with Disabilities Act. This law specifies that a physician's office is a public accommodation and HIV infection, HIV disease, and AIDS are recognized as disabilities. Refusing to treat a disabled person would, in the opinion of most lawyers, be a violation.

HIV Transmission from Physician to Patient and Vice Versa

Communicability of HIV is an important liability issue for personnel involved in the care of HIV/AIDS patients. Those who come into contact with bodily fluids, blood, blood products, or who receive accidental needle pricks are at risk for infection, and they can also spread the virus to other patients Lawrence Gostin (1989a) wrote that physicians involved in medically invasive procedures have claimed the right to know whether their patients are HIV-infected. Yet that information is of limited value because: (1) the physician should be using **universal precautions** which dictate that all patients be treated as though they were HIV-infected (this may be true, but the author believes that no matter how careful a physician is, if he or she knew someone had HIV disease/AIDS, he or she would be more careful); and (2) physicians have a professional, if not legal, responsibility to treat infected patients.

Patients also claim the legal right to know if their physician is HIV-infected or has AIDS. If this information were available, especially to those who were to have invasive surgery, which includes intraabdominal, colon or rectal, thoracic, cardiac, orthopedic, gynecological, cesarean section, oral surgery, and so forth, many would opt for an HIV-free surgeon. Withholding seropositive information from a patient who then becomes HIV-infected may make the physician and the hospital liable for damages.

In November 1991, Texas became the first state to pass a bill that puts into law the CDC guidelines calling for health care workers with HIV to stop performing "exposure-prone procedures" unless they obtain consent from a peer review group and the patient. Failure to comply could result in disciplinary action by the State Board of Medical Examiners. It may also be used by attorneys to file charges of malpractice on behalf of a client who was not informed. The bill broadly defines an HIV exposure-prone procedure as one that poses a direct and significant risk. The procedures listed in the bill are:

- Any surgical entry into tissue, cavities, or organs
- Repair of major traumatic injuries in an operating or delivery room, emergency department, or outpatient setting
- Vaginal or cesarean delivery or other invasive obstetric procedure during which bleeding may occur
- Cardiac catheterization or angiography
- Cutting of oral or perioral tissues where bleeding may occur.

Although the Texas legislature passed the bill, physicians may have the final word on how the law is applied, since physicians will decide which invasive procedures are "exposure-prone."

POINT OF INFORMATION 16.3

A PATIENT'S RIGHT TO KNOW A SURGEON'S HIV STATUS

A recent example of a patient's right to know the HIV status of a physician performing an invasive medical procedure is cited in: *Application of The Hersey Medical Center,* Pennsylvania Superior Court, July 30, 1991. In this case Dr. "John Doe," an obstetrician/gynecologist, was cut by a member of the operating team. Although it was unlikely that Dr. Doe's blood was transferred to the patient, Dr. Doe voluntarily took the HIV test. He was HIV-positive. Dr. Doe notified the two hospitals in which he worked and took a leave of absence. The hospitals notified 447 patients who may have had invasive procedures by Dr. Doe. The hospitals further filed petitions with the court alleging that it was their duty to inform potentially exposed patients and a limited number of physicians who worked with Dr. Doe, who could in turn inform their patients. Dr. Doe responded to the petition by asserting his right to privacy and that a compelling need, as required under the Confidentiality of HIV-Related Information Act, did not exist.

The county court authorized disclosure of Dr. Doe's identity and HIV status to the obstetrics and gynecology attending and resident staffs; and to any physician authorized by a patient for whom Dr. Doe participated in a surgical procedure; and an anonymous description of the situation was ordered for the media and all patients identified on the hospital's list.

The appellate court upheld the lower courts order to disclose. The appellate court stated that a "compelling need" was met. On Dr. Doe's right to privacy the court held that his medical problem was not solely his. It became a public concern the moment he became involved in the invasive procedure. The court held that the public's right to be informed in these situations is compelling and far outweighs a practicing surgeon's right to keep information regarding his or her disease confidential (Landwirth, 1992).

Lawrence Gostin (1989a) does not argue for the physician's or the patient's right to be informed of HIV/AIDS status, rather he makes the case that the risks inherent in invasive medical procedures are sufficient for the medical profession to hold patient safety from HIV, hepatitis, and other pathological organisms in high regard.

Gostin writes that professional guidance is required to identify when and where the physician should withdraw from performing an invasive procedure. This is the position the AMA supports.

American Bar Association Legal Directory

A comprehensive listing of programs and organizations that provide free legal services to people with HIV/AIDS is available. The 368-page publication was compiled by the American Bar Association's AIDS Coordination Project.

The Directory of Legal Resources for People with AIDS and HIV is organized by state, and each listing includes name, address, telephone number, and a brief description of the project. It also has information on national and state organizations.

For information on the AIDS Coordina-tion Project or to obtain copies of *The Directory,* contact ABA AIDS Coordination Project, 1800 M Street N.W., Washington D.C., 20036, (202) 331-2248.

SUMMARY

This chapter is not an exhaustive treatment on HIV/AIDS and the law and ethics. Many excellent papers have not been included because of space limitations. Papers that are included were selected based on the advice of practicing attorneys, members of the medical profession, and colleagues.

HIV/AIDS law has had a mixed record across the United States. Many states have come to accept research that has shown the remarkable efficacy of well-targeted education and counseling. There has also been wide acceptance of the importance of confidentiality and guarantee of antidiscrimination. Ensuring the privacy and equal treatment of people with HIV/AIDS is essential to the success of epidemiological studies, testing, outreach programs, and treatment for injection drug users. Public health officials will not gain the confidence and cooperation of infected individuals if these individuals are not legally protected from stigma and irrational prejudice (Gostin, 1989a,b).

While legislatures have responded well to health service research, they have also been susceptible to the attitude that the primary modes of HIV transmission are immoral, even criminal. Federal and state statutes, by requiring special emphasis on abstinence from extramarital sex and drug use, ignore the fact that these behaviors have persisted unabated throughout history.

There is political pressure on legislators to use the coercive powers of the state to combat the epidemic. Legislation for compulsory screening, isolation, and criminalization has proceeded despite evidence that these measures are not efficacious and often contradict advice from the Public Health Service. The use of coercive powers, far from impeding the epidemic, may well fuel it (Gostin, 1989a,b).

REVIEW QUESTIONS

(Answers to the Review Questions are on page 483.)

1. What is the confidentiality dilemma in medicine?
2. With respect to the HIV testing confidentiality controversy, what do you think is more important: A person's right to privacy or the public's right to know?

For discussion:

1. A female physician specializing in emergency medicine at an urban hospital learns that she is HIV-positive. Should any of her patients be informed of her HIV status? If so, when? Before, during, or after treatment? Refer back to Chapter 14 for additional information on HIV-infected physicians—it may help you formulate an opinion.
2. A 13-year-old runaway female who has exchanged sex for drugs or money enters a drug and rehabilitation program. She reveals her recent lifestyle to a counselor. Should this counselor advise the agency that is providing food, clothing, and shelter to this girl about her lifestyle?

REFERENCES

ALBERT, J., et al. (1993). Forensic evidence by DNA sequencing, *Nature,* 361: 595–596.

BREO, DENNIS. (1988). Patient confidentiality: With AIDS where do you draw the line. *Am. Med. News,* 31:3–7.

DICKENS, BERNARD. (1988). Legal rights and duties in the AIDS epidemic. *Science,* 239:580–586.

DICKENS, BERNARD. (1989). Legal limits of AIDS confidentiality. *JAMA,* 259:3449–3451.

DUCKETT, MELVIN J. et al. (1989). AIDS related migration and travel policies and restrictions: A global survey. *AIDS,* 3:S231–S252.

FLUSS, SEV S., et al. (1989). AIDS, HIV, health care workers: Some international legislation perspectives. *Maryland Law Rev.,* 48:77–92.

GILMORE, NORBERT J., et al. (1989). International travel and AIDS. *AIDS,* 3:S225–S230.

GOLDBERG, ABBOTT. (1989). Physicians' notes can be deceptive—or revealing. *Consultant,* 29:69–72.

GOSTIN, LAWRENCE O. (1989a). Public health strategies for confronting AIDS. *JAMA,* 261:1621–1630.

GOSTIN, LAWRENCE O. (1989b). The politics of AIDS: Compulsory state powers, public health and civil liberties. *Ohio State Law J.,* 49:1017– 1058.

GOSTIN, LAWRENCE O. (1990a). The AIDS Litigation Project. A national review of Court and Human Rights Commission decisions. Part I: The social impact of AIDS. *JAMA,* 263: 1961–1970.

GOSTIN, LAWRENCE O. (1990b). The AIDS Litigation Project. Part II: Discrimination. *JAMA,* 263: 2086–2093.

HIRSH, HAROLD. (1988). Patient confidentiality: New legal risks emerge. *Phys. Manage.,* 28:37– 41.

LANDWIRTH, JULIUS. (1992). Courts look at disclosure of physician's HIV status. *Infect. Dis. News,* 5:13.

LUMSDON, KEVIN. (1992). HIV-positive health care workers pose legal, safety challenges for hospitals. *Hospitals,* 66:24–32.

MCCORMICK, BRIAN. (1992). HIV-related discrimination lawsuits on the rise. *Am. Med. News,* Feb. 3:9.

Morbidity and Mortality Weekly Report. (1991). Publicly funded HIV counseling and testing—United States, 1990. 40:666–675.

MURPHY, DALE P. (1989). Confidentiality and the AIDS patient: The true dilemma. *Consultant,* 29:3.

PALMA, LYNNE L. (1992). Americans with Disabilities Act (ADA): Take the first steps now. *AIDS Newslink: Mountain Plains Regional AIDS Education and Training Center,* 3:8–10.

ROTHSTEIN, MARK A. (1989). Medical screening: AIDS, rights, and health care costs. *Natl. Forum,* 99:7–10.

SCHULMAN, DAVID. (1988). Remembering Who We Are: AIDS and Law in a Time of Madness. *AIDS Public Policy J.*, 3:75–77.

SCHWARTZ, HAROLD I. (1988). AIDS: Confidentiality versus the duty to warn. *Med. Asp. of Human Sexuality*, 22:13.

SHERER, RENSLOW. (1990). AIDS policy into the 1990s. *JAMA*, 263:1972–1974.

SLACK, JAMES D. (1991). *AIDS and the Public Work Force.* Tuscaloosa: University of Alabama Press.

Tarasof v. Regents of the University of California. (1976).

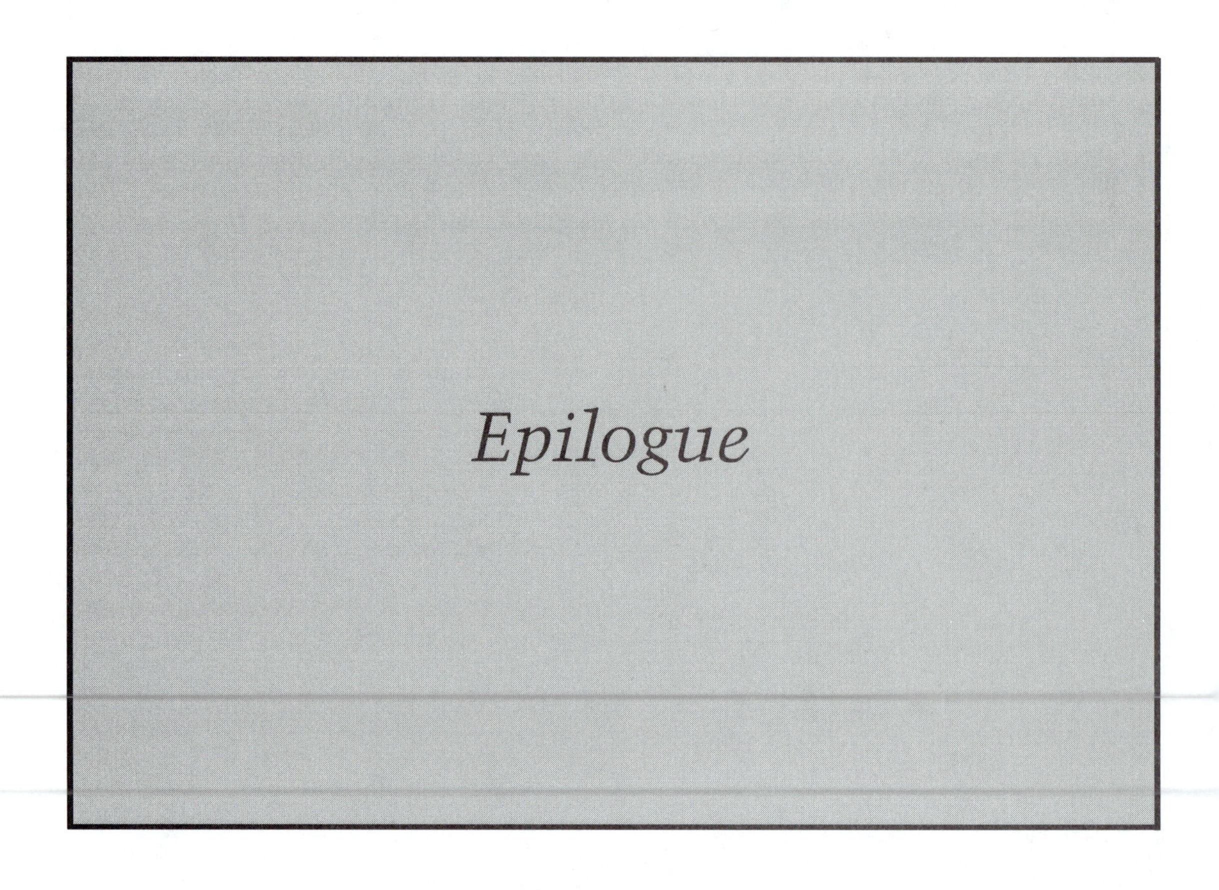

While the achievements of the global response to date should not be underestimated, neither should the challenge ahead. HIV disease/AIDS is a catastrophe in slow motion, and it is essential that the world community pace itself for the long haul. The task ahead calls for clear vision, renewed will, and greatly increased resources. But it also calls for greater determination to use the resources in the interest of everyone: HIV disease or AIDS must not be allowed to join the list of problems, like poverty and hunger, that those world has learned to live with because the powerful have lost interest, and the powerless have no choice.

In the United States, midway through 1995, or halfway through 15 years of the HIV/AIDS epidemic, we can reflect on the fact that we have learned a lot about this new disease but there is a long way to go. While it is easy to criticize, condemn, ridicule, and find mistakes in the way the HIV/AIDS pandemic has been handled, society should not lose sight of the outstanding scientific and social achievements made since HIV/AIDS was discovered.

Excellent progress has been made in understanding the biology of the virus, its transmission, therapy, and its relationship to the progression of AIDS. If the 1980s are to be remembered as the period of AIDS violence, hatred, and irrational fears, the 1990s will hopefully be remembered as the time of optimism. HIV disease has become a chronic treatable illness wherein the quality and duration of life are being extended. Promising antiviral treatments as well as vaccines for the prevention of HIV infection are in development. HIV/AIDS education will soon reach every grade school, high school, and workplace in the United States. Courts have affirmed the rights of HIV-infected/AIDS patients to a public education and to remain at their jobs.

Two areas of concern that have not improved are HIV/AIDS discrimination based on fear and obtaining insurance coverage. Moving through the 1990s, although legislation may help, these two problems may remain.

There is great hope that at some point during the 1990s, the diagnosis of HIV infection will *not* indicate the almost certain destruction of the immune system, the onset of AIDS, and death. It is hoped that before the 1990s are out, HIV will be just another controllable viral infection.

The divisiveness that has marked the 1980s has been too costly, the human toll too great. The way for us to get through this crisis is hand in hand.

Humans shall overcome HIV!

Answers to Review Questions

CHAPTER 1

1. Acquired Immune Deficiency Syndrome
2. No. AIDS is a syndrome. A syndrome is made up of a collection of signs and symptoms of one or more diseases. AIDS patients have a collection of opportunistic infections and cancers. Collectively they are mistakenly referred to as the AIDS disease.
3. In 1983 by Luc Montagnier
4. 1981
5. LAV
6. Five; 1982, 1983, 1985, 1987, and 1993
7. The ARC or AIDS Related Complex definition was a middle ground used before AIDS was better understood. It became meaningless after the 1985 expanded definition listed organisms and symptoms which indicated that two states existed: HIV infection and progression to AIDS.
8. It allows HIV-infected persons earlier access into federal and state medical and social programs.

CHAPTER 2

1. The unbroken transmission of infection from an infected person to an uninfected person.
2. The answer to both questions is unknown at this time.

CHAPTER 3

1. Because it contains RNA as its genetic message and a reverse transcriptase enzyme to make DNA from RNA

2. GAG-POL-ENV; at least seven
3. Because HIV has demonstrated an unusually high rate of genetic mutations; (1) the reverse transcriptase enzyme in HIV is highly error prone (makes transcription errors), and (2) a variety of HIV mutants have been found within a single HIV-infected individual.
4. The reverse transcriptase enzyme is highly error prone, making at least one, and in many cases more than one, deletion, addition, or substitution per round of proviral replication.

CHAPTER 4

1. T4 helper cells; because T4 cells are crucial for the production of antibodies, a depletion of T4 cells results in immunosuppression which results in OIs.
2. CD4 is a receptor protein (antigen) secreted by certain cells of the immune system, for example, monocytes, macrophages, and T4 helper cells. It becomes located on the exterior of the cellular membrane and happens to be a compatible receptor for the HIV to attach and infect the CD4-carrying cell.
3. The question of true latency after HIV infection has not been settled. Most HIV/AIDS investigators currently believe there is a latent period, a time of few if any clinical symptoms and low levels of HIV in the blood. Other scientists, currently the minority, believe there is no true latency. The virus hides out in the lymph nodes slowly reproducing, and slowly killing off the T4 cells. The virus is always present, increasing slowly in numbers over time.
4. True
5. False
6. True
7. False
8. False
9. True
10. False
11. True
12. True
13. True

CHAPTER 5

1. OI is caused by organisms that are normally within the body and held in check by an active immune system. When the immune system becomes suppressed, for whatever reason, these agents can multiply and produce disease.
2. *Pneumocystis carinii*; lungs, pneumonia
3. *Isospora belli*
4. *Mycobacterium avium intracellulare*
5. False. HIV has not been found in KS tissue. KS is believed to develop as a result of a suppressed immune system and not the virus *per se*.
6. Classic KS, as described by Moritz Kaposi; and KS associated with AIDS
7. False. KS normally affects gay males. It is highly unusual to find KS in hemophiliacs, intravenous drug users and female AIDS patients.
8. True
9. True

CHAPTER 6

1. The 6-stage Walter Reed System and the 4 group CDC system
2. About 30%; about 90%
3. AIDS dementia complex
4. Skin—Kaposi's sarcoma
   Eyes—CMV retinitis
   Mouth—thrush or hairy leukoplakia
   Lungs—pneumocystis pneumonia
   Intestines—diarrhea
5. True
6. False. The average time is 6 to 18 weeks.
7. False. HIV infection leads to HIV disease. AIDS is the result of a weakened immune system that allows opportunistic infections to occur.
8. False. The average length of time is about 10 years.

CHAPTER 7

1. Something that would *prevent* HIV infection
2. Zidovudine, dideoxyinosine and dideoxycytosine

3. In case of terminal illness. phase III may be omitted from the drug approval process.
4. To be corrected by instructor or sample student reading in class and discussion
5. HIVs that have mutated, and as a result are more resistant to zidovudine, will survive zidovudine therapy and multiply.
6. Soluble CD4 protein units
7. Because a new therapy is needed. To date, drug and immunomodulator therapies are inadequate to save lives or significantly relieve pain and suffering over the lifetime of an AIDS patient. If the structure of a gene product is revealed, drugs can be designed to block effectively its use by the virus.
8. From a scientific viewpoint anything is possible, but in this case not reasonable. Many healthy people on excellent diets have become infected. There is no knowledge as to what an HIV prevention diet could or should consist of. To date, no single viral infection has even been known to have been prevented or cured by a specific diet.

CHAPTER 8

1. False. The United States currently reports most of the world's AIDS cases.
2. Cases of AIDS-related death, according to the CDC definition, can be traced back to 1952 in the United States and to the mid-1950s in Africa. In addition, studies since 1902 indicate that non-African men have been diagnosed with an aggressive form of Kaposi's sarcoma, a criterion for AIDS in homosexual males.
3. HIV-1 and HIV-2 show a 40% to 50% genetic relationship to each other.
4. False. HIV-1 and HIV-2 are both transmitted via the same routes. HIV-2 is spreading globally in similar fashion to HIV-1.
5. True. All scientific and empirical evidence to date indicates that HIV is not casually transmitted.
6. Through sexual activities; exchange of certain body fluids—blood and blood products, semen and vaginal secretions; and from mother to fetus or newborn by breast milk.
7. False. There is not a single documented case of HIV infection caused by deep kissing. HIV has been found in the saliva of infected people in very low concentration, and saliva has been shown to have anti-HIV properties.
8. True; but this assertion has been proven to be untrue. Insects, in particular mosquitoes, have not been shown to transmit HIV successfully.
9. False. According to studies involving the sexual partners of injection drug users and hemophiliacs, HIV transmission from male to female is the more efficient route. This is believed to be due to a greater concentration of HIV found in semen than in vaginal fluid.
10. The answer may be True or False. There have been cases in which a single act of intercourse has resulted in HIV infection. However, the majority of surveys on the sexual partners of injection drug users and hemophiliacs indicate that the number of sexual encounters may increase the risk of HIV infection but does not guarantee infection. Sexual partners of infected people have remained HIV-free after years of unprotected penis–vagina intercourse.
11. The percentage of fetal risk varies widely in a number of hospital studies. At the moment, the risk as reported varies from less than 30% to over 50%. The figures most commonly used are 30% to 50%.
12. D, all of the above
13. True
14. True
15. True
16. True
17. True
18. False
19. True
20. True
21. False
22. True
23. False

CHAPTER 9

1. Latex condoms. They are known to stop the transmission of viruses. This may not be true for animal intestine condoms.

2. Water-based lubricants. Oil-based lubricants weaken the later rubber causing them to leak or break under stress.
3. Safer sex is having sexual intercourse with an *uninfected* partner while using a condom.
4. The answer may be True or False. There have been cases where a single act of intercourse resulted in HIV infection. However, the majority of surveys completed by sexual partners of injection drug users and hemophiliacs indicate that the number of sexual encounters may increase the risk of HIV infection but does not guarantee infection. Sexual partners of infected persons have remained HIV-free after years of unprotected penis-vagina intercourse.
5. No. IDUs exist between "fixes." They lose things, they may not care to pick up new equipment—they need the "fix" now, it may be easier to share. Circumstances vary considerably among the IDU. Just giving them free equipment is no assurance that they will use it.
6. Between 1 in 39,000 and 1 in 200,000.
7. Have several students read their answers for promoting class discussion. Compare their response to that given in the text (that they should be punished).
8. Because attenuated HIV may mutate to a virulent form causing an HIV infection; there is no absolute guarantee that 100% of HIV are inactivated.
9. Because at no time will a whole HIV be present in the vaccine. Only a specific subunit of the HIV will be present in pure form so the vaccine should be free of any contaminating proteins that might prove toxic to one or more persons receiving the vaccine.
10. It is a situation wherein HIV antibodies might predispose the host to become more easily HIV-infected. For whatever reason, it appears that the HIV antibody complex enters the cell more easily than HIV alone.
11. Because of the severe forms of social ostracism that occur when it is learned that someone is HIV-positive or belongs to a high-risk group (gay, injection drug user, bisexual).
12. Universal precautions are a list of rules and regulations provided by the CDC to help prevent HIV infection in health care workers.
13. False
14. False
15. True
16. True
17. True
18. False
19. False

CHAPTER 10

1. The CDC said for each AIDS case there are from 50 to 100 HIV-infected people in the population. They got the 1 to 1.5 million figure using the 50 HIV-infected/AIDS cases; 1986; they are believed to be within plus or minus 10%.
2. 96%; 85%
3. 72%; 10%
4. 77%
5. Because their social and sexual behaviors and medical needs place these people at a greater risk for HIV exposure than those not practicing these social and sexual behaviors or who do not need blood or blood products.
6. False. Studies show that the time for progression from HIV infection to AIDS is the same regardless of parameters.
7. 52%
8. 30% to 50%
9. 99%
10. Two per 1,000 students; more: The rate for military personnel is 1.4 per 1,000.
11. College students 2/1,000, general population 0.02/1,000; this means the rate of HIV infection on college campuses is about 10 times higher than in the general population.
12. One in 200 to 300
13. Needlestick injuries
14. 5.4%
15. Hepatitis B virus
16. Montana, North and South Dakota, and Wyoming. It probably implies that HIV infection in the heterosexual population in these states is lower than in other states. This would translate into fewer HIV-infected women and few, if any, pediatric cases.

17. GAO—300,000 to 485,000
CDC—270,000

18. Student's answer; text says no. People most often do not tell the truth—much depends on where, when, why, and who is doing the survey. There are just too many variables involved to believe sexual surveys.

19. 263,000

20. Over 92%

21. False

22. True

23. True

CHAPTER 11

1. 26 HIV infections per minute
2. Heterosexual
3. France and Italy in that order
4. The number of reported AIDS cases is doubling every 11 months.
5. IDUs—the frequency of new HIV infections appears to be leveling off in all other risk categories.
6. Mexico; Cuba; Soviet Union and Pakistan
7. Italy and Spain

CHAPTER 12

1. ELISA; enzyme linked immunosorbent assay
2. That the body will produce antibody against antigenic components of the HIV virus after infection occurs
3. No; a positive antibody result must be repeated in duplicate and if still positive, a confirmatory test is performed prior to telling people they are HIV-infected.
4. No; AIDS is medically diagnosed after certain signs and symptoms of specific diseases occur.
5. Western blot
6. Indirect immunofluorescent assay
7. By a color change in the reaction tube; the peroxidase enzyme oxidizes a clear chromogen into color formation. This occurs if the HIV antibody–antigen enzyme complex is present in the reaction tube.
8. False. Some newborns receive the HIV antibody passively during pregnancy. About 30% to 50% of HIV-positive newborns are truly HIV-positive; it is unknown whether all HIV-positive newborns go on to develop AIDS. Not all have been discovered and it has not been determined whether 100% of HIV-infected adults or babies will develop AIDS.
9. They are not 100% accurate.
10. Determining that positive and negative tests are truly positive and negative and not falsely positive or negative.
11. Using either too high or too low cutoff points in the spectrophotometer and the presence of cross-reacting antibodies
12. The percentage of false positives will increase as the prevalence of HIV-infected people in a population decreases.
13. It is a screening test value that represents the probability that a positive HIV test is truly positive; because screening tests are not 100% accurate.
14. Western blot
15. There is no standardized WB test interpretation. Different agencies use different WB results (reactive bands) to determine that the test sample is positive.
16. Because the PCR allows for the detection of proviral DNA in cells before the body produces detectable HIV antibody; PCR reactions can be used to determine if high-risk (or anybody) antibody-negative people are HIV-infected but not producing antibodies and whether newborns are truly HIV-positive or passively HIV-positive.
17. False. The FDA has not approved a single home-use HIV antibody test kit.
18. Between 6 and 18 weeks after HIV infection.
19. As early as 2 weeks after infection.
20. (1) Changes in their lifestyles that reduce stress on their immune systems may delay the onset of illness.

    (2) They can practice safer sex and hopefully not transmit the virus to others.

    (3) The earlier the detection, the earlier they can enter into preventive therapy.
21. Mandatory with confidentiality; voluntary with confidentiality, anonymous and blinded.

22. For anonymous testing no personal information is given; in blind tests, the name is deleted but the demographic data remain.
23. Because there are many example of breaches of confidence, which destroys trust and subjects people to social stigma.
24. False
25. True

CHAPTER 13

1. Education, counseling, and signing the test consent form
2. Directive and nondirective counseling
3. To give the test results and counsel the person based on the outcome of those results
4. Denial; anger, bargaining, depression, and acceptance
5. D
6. B
7. A
8. True
9. True
10. False

CHAPTER 14

1. Newspapers, TV, radio, magazines, etc.
2. Barring children from public schools, police wearing rubber gloves during arrests, not going to a restaurant because someone who works there has AIDS, firing AIDS employees, etc.
3. Syphilis
4. Use of tobacco products, alcohol, drugs; nonuse of seat belts and motorcycle helmets, etc.
5. The ways by which one can become HIV-infected and how not to become HIV-infected.
6. Because most of the new cases of HIV infection and AIDS occur in high-risk groups that will not or cannot change sexual and drug practices.
7. Because a larger percentage of teenagers are sexually active with more than one partner, use drugs, use alcohol, and think that they are invulnerable to infection and death.
8. Most orphaned AIDS children have mothers who are IDUs and are themselves HIV-infected. They are AIDS orphans because (1) their parents abandon them due to illness or death; and (2) these children are HIV-infected or demonstrate AIDS and therefore no one wants them.
9. According to the AMA, No. Physicians may not refuse to care for patients with AIDS because of actual risk or fear of contracting the disease.
10. The CDC and AMA feel that a patient's right to that information should be determined on a case-by-case basis where surgery will be performed. There is no legal requirement for physicians to tell their patients of their HIV status.
11. Worker information sessions that explain how the virus can and cannot be transmitted.

CHAPTER 15

1. About $69,000; No, the cost of health care for a number of chronic diseases comes to about $69,000.
2. Indirect costs are the costs of lost productivity due to premature death. They are about five times higher per patient than direct costs.
3. Those who need insurance most are not insurable.
4. If they were to underwrite all the HIV-infected people, it would bankrupt the system, leaving everyone else without insurance.
5. **YOU**

CHAPTER 16

1. There does not appear to be a legal balance between a physician's duties to his or her patients and duties to public health in general. The physician is in a "Catch-22" position.
2. Class discussion topic or student essay on why they take their position.
   (1) The late Justice Oliver Wendell Holmes said that the public's right to know comes first.
   (2) Justice Goldberg (1989) said that the public's right to know is first.
   (3) 72% of Americans oppose the confidentiality of HIV tests.

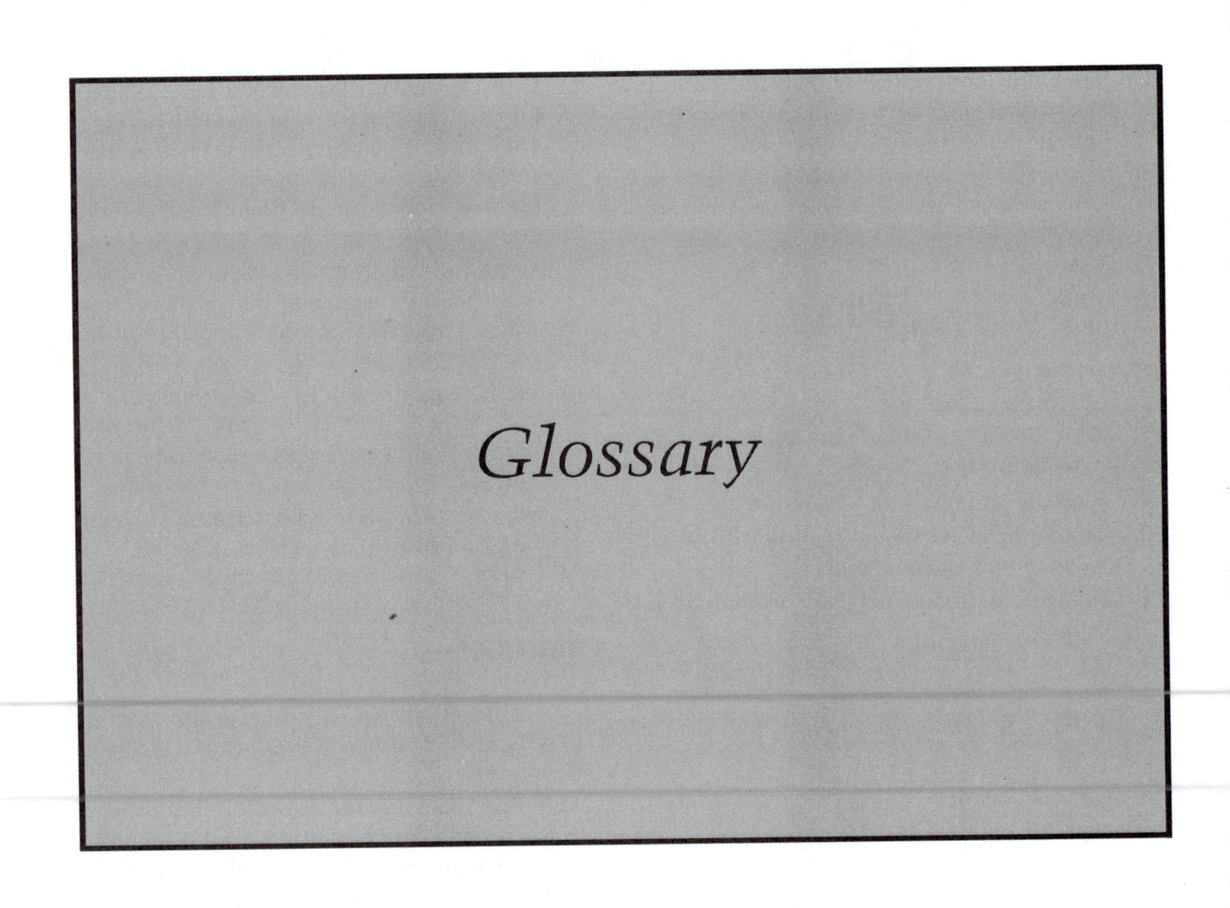

Glossary

Acronyms

AIDS acquired immunodeficiency syndrome

ARC AIDS-related complex.

ARV AIDS-related virus

AZT azathioprine (this is not zidovudine or azidothymidine)

CD4 reception site on a T4 cell to which HIV most often binds

CDC Centers for Disease Control and Prevention (part of PHS)

3CT lamivudine; nucleoside analog

CTS Counseling and Testing Services

DHHS Department of Health and Human Services

DNA deoxyribonucleic acid

d4T stavudine; nucleoside analog

ddC dideoxycytosine; nucleoside analog

ddI dideoxyinosine; nucleoside analog

FDA Food and Drug Administration (part of PHS)

HTLV-I human T cell lymphotropic virus, type I

HTLV-II human T cell lymphotropic virus, type II

HTLV-III human T cell lymphotropic virus, type III

IDAV immune deficiency-associated virus

IgG human immunoglobin G

LAV lymphadenopathy-associated virus

NCI National Cancer Institute (part of NIH)

NEI National Eye Institute (part of NIH)

NHLBI National Heart, Lung and Blood Institute (part of NIH)

NIAID National Institute of Allergy and Infectious Diseases (part of NIH)

NIDA National Institute on Drug Abuse (part of PHS)

NIDR National Institute of Dental Research (part of NIH)

NIH National Institutes of Health (part of PHS)

NIMH National Institute of Mental Health (part of PHS)

NINCDS National Institute of Neurological and Communicative Disorders and Stroke (part of NIH)

OTA Office of Technology Assessment (part of U.S. Congress)

PHS Public Health Service (part of DHHS)

RNA ribonucleic acid

ZDV zidovudine main drug in treating HIV/AIDS persons; nucleoside analog

Terms

Acquired immunodeficiency syndrome (AIDS): A life-threatening disease caused by a virus and characterized by the breakdown of the body's immune defenses. (See AIDS.)

Active immunity: Protection against a disease resulting from the production of antibodies in a host that has been exposed to a disease causing antigen.

Acute: Short-term with severe symptoms.

Acyclovir (Zovirax): Antiviral drug for herpes 1 and 2 and herpes zoster.

AIDS (acquired immunodeficiency syndrome): A disease believed to be caused by a retrovirus called HIV and characterized by a deficiency of the immune system. The primary defect in AIDS is an acquired, persistent, quantitative functional depression within the T4 subset of lymphocytes. This depression often leads to infections caused by opportunistic microorganisms in HIV-infected individuals. A rare type of cancer (Kaposi's sarcoma) usually seen in elderly men or in individuals who are severely immunocompromised may also occur. Other associated diseases are currently under investigation and will probably be included in the final definition of AIDS.

Allergic reaction: A reaction that results from extreme sensitivity to a drug or agent and is not dependent on the amount of drug given. These may be classified into two types, immediate and delayed, based on the time it takes for the reaction to occur.

Anemia: Low number of red blood cells.

Anorexia: Prolonged loss of appetite that leads to significant weight loss.

Antibiotic: A chemical substance capable of destroying bacteria and other microorganisms.

Antibody: A blood protein produced by mammals in response to a specific antigen.

Antigen: A large molecule, usually a protein or carbohydrate, which when introduced into the body stimulates the production of an antibody that will react specifically with that antigen.

Antigen-presenting cells: B cells, cells of the monocyte lineage (including macrophages and dentritic cells) and various other body cells that 'present' antigen in a form that T cells can recognize.

Antisense RNA: A strand of RNA that will complementary base pair with messenger RNA.

Antiserum: Serum portion of the blood that carries the antibodies.

Antiviral: Means against virus; drugs that destroy or weaken virus.

Arthritis: Inflammation of the joints and the surrounding tissues.

Arthropod: An insect-like animal.

Aspiration: The removal of fluids by suction.

Asymptomatic carrier: A host which is infected by an organism but does not demonstrate clinical signs or symptoms of the disease.

Asymptomatic seropositive: HIV-positive without signs or symptoms of HIV disease.

Ataxia: Inability to coordinate movement of muscles.

Atrophy: The wasting away or decrease in size and function of a body part.

Attenuated: Weakened.

Atypical: Irregular; not of typical character.

Autoimmunity: Antibodies made against self tissues.

Autoinoculation: A secondary infection originating from an infection site already present in the body.

Blymphocytes or B cells: Lymphocytes that produce antibodies. B lymphocytes proliferate under stimulation from factors released by T lymphocytes.

Bacterium: A microscopic organism composed of a single cell. Many but not all bacteria cause disease.

Blood count: A count of the number of red and white blood cells and platelets.

Bone marrow: Soft tissue located in the cavities of the bones. The bone marrow is the source of all blood cells.

Cancer: A large group of diseases characterized by uncontrolled growth and spread of abnormal cells.

Candida albicans: A fungus; the causative agent of vulvovaginal candidiasis or yeast infection.

Candidiasis: A fungal infection of the mucous membranes (commonly occurring in the mouth, where it is known as Thrush) characterized by whitish spots and/or a burning or painful sensation. It may also occur in the esophagus. It can also cause a red and itchy rash in moist areas, e.g., the vagina.

Capsid: The protein coat of a virus particle.

Carcinogen: Any substance that causes cancer.

Carcinoma: A form of skin cancer that occurs in tissues that cover or line body organs, e.g., intestines, lungs, breasts, uterus, etc.

Cardiovascular: Pertaining to the heart and blood vessels.

CD: Cluster differentiating type antigens found on T lymphocytes. Each CD is assigned a number: CD1, CD2, etc.

Cell-mediated immunity: The reaction to antigenic material by specific defensive cells (macrophages) rather than antibodies.

Cellular immunity: A collection of cell types that provide protection against various antigens.

Central nervous system (CNS): The brain and spinal cord.

Cerebral spinal fluid (CSF): The fluid which surrounds the brain and spinal cord.

Chain of infection: A series of infections that are directly or immediately connected to a particular source.

Chemotherapy: The use of chemicals that have a specific and toxic effect upon a disease-causing pathogen.

Chlamydia: A species of bacterium, the causative organism of *Lymphogranuloma venereum*, chlamydial urethritis and most cases of newborn conjunctivitis.

Chromosomes: Physical structures in the cell's nucleus that house the genes. Each human cell has 22 pairs of autosomes and two sex chromosomes.

Chronic: Having a long and relatively mild course.

Clinical manifestations: The signs of a disease as they pertain to or are observed in patients.

Cofactor: Factors or agents which are necessary or which increase the probability of the development of disease in the presence of the basic etiologic agent of that disease.

Communicable: Able to spread from one diseased person or animal to another, either directly or indirectly.

Condylomata acuminatum (venereal warts): Viral warts of the genital and anogenital area.

Congenital: Acquired by the newborn before or at the time of birth.

Core proteins: Proteins that make up the internal structure or core of a virus.

Cryptococcal meningitis: A fungal infection that affects the three membranes (meninges) surrounding the brain and spinal cord. Symptoms include severe headache, vertigo, nausea, anorexia, sight disorders and mental deterioration.

Cryptococcosis: A fungal infectious disease often found in the lungs of AIDS patients. It characteristically spreads to the meninges and may also spread to the kidneys and skin. It is due to the fungus *Cryptococcus neoformans.*

Cryptosporidiosis: An infection caused by a protozoan parasite found in the intestines of animals. Acquired in some people by direct contact with the infected animal, it lodges in the intestines and causes severe diarrhea. It may be transmitted from person to person. This infection seems to be occurring more frequently in immunosuppressed people and can lead to prolonged symptoms which do not respond to medication.

Cutaneous: Having to do with the skin.

Cytokines: Powerful chemical substances secreted by cells. Cytokines include lymphokines produced by lymphocytes and monokines produced by monocytes and macrophages.

Cytomegalovirus (CMV): One of a group of highly host-specific herpes viruses that affect humans and other animals. Generally produces mild flu-like symptoms but can be more severe. In the immunosuppressed, it may cause pneumonia.

Cytopathic: Pertaining to or characterized by abnormal changes in cells.

Cytotoxic: Poisonous to cells.

Cytotoxic T cells: A subset of T lymphocytes that carry the T8 marker and can kill body cells infected by viruses or transformed by cancer.

Dementia: Chronic mental deterioration sufficient to significantly impair social and/or occupational function. Usually patients have memory and abstract thinking loss. They may have impairment of more specific higher cortical functions. Frequently progressive and irreversible.

Dendritic cells: White blood cells found in the spleen and other lymphoid organs. Dendritic cells typically use threadlike tentacles to "hold" the antigen, which they present to T cells.

Dermatitis: Inflammation of the skin.

Diagnosis: The identification of a disease by its signs, symptoms and laboratory findings.

Didanosine: Also known as Videx; see ddI.

Direct transmission: A manner of transmitting disease organisms in which the agent moves immediately from the infected person to the susceptible person, as in person-to-person contact and in droplet contact.

Disease intervention specialist (DIS): A person who performs STD patient interviewing/counseling and field investigation.

Dissemination: Spread of disease throughout the body.

DNA (deoxyribonucleic acid): A linear polymer, made up of deoxyribonucleotide repeating units. It is the carrier of genetic information in living organisms and some viruses.

DNA viruses: Contain DNA as their genetic material.

Dysentery: Inflammation of the intestines, especially the colon, producing pain in the abdomen and diarrhea containing blood and mucus.

Efficacy: Effectiveness.

ELISA test: A blood test which indicates the presence of antibodies to a given antigen. Various ELISA tests are used to detect a variety of infections. The HIV ELISA test does not detect AIDS but only indicates if viral infection has occurred.

Endemic: Prevalent in or peculiar to community or group of people.

Enteric infections: Infections of the intestine.

Envelope proteins: Proteins that comprise the envelope or surface of a virus.

Enzyme: A catalytic protein that is produced by living cells and promotes the chemical processes of life without itself being altered or destroyed.

Epidemic: When the incidence of a disease surpasses the expected rate in any well-defined geographical area.

Epidemiologic studies: Studies concerned with the relationships of various factors determining the frequency and distribution of certain diseases.

Epidemiology: The study of the factors that impact on the spread of disease in an area.

Epitopes: Characteristic shapes of antigens found on an organism or virus.

Epstein-Barr virus (EBV): A virus that causes infectious mononucleosis. It is spread by saliva. EBV lies dormant in the lymph glands and has been associated with Burkitt's lymphoma, a cancer of the lymph tissue.

Etiologic agent: The organism which causes a disease.

Etiology: The study of the cause of disease.

Extracellular: Found outside the cell wall.

Exudate: To produce liquid in response to disease.

Factor VIII: A naturally occurring protein in plasma that aids in the coagulation of blood. A congenital deficiency of Factor VIII results in the bleeding disorder known as hemophilia A.

Factor VIII concentrate: A concentrated preparation of Factor VIII that is used in the treatment of individuals with hemophilia A.

Fallopian tube: A slender 4-inch-long tube extending from the ovary to the uterus. Eggs released during ovulation pass through this tube to reach the uterus.

False negative: Failure of a test to demonstrate the disease or condition when present.

False positive: A positive test result caused by a disease or condition other than the disease for which the test is designed.

Fellatio: Oral sex involving the penis.

Fomite: An inanimate object which transfers infectious organisms from one individual to another.

Fulminant: Severe.

Fungus: Member of a class of relatively primitive organisms. Fungi include mushrooms, yeasts, rusts, molds and smuts.

Gammaglobulin: The antibody component of the serum.

Ganciclovir (DHPG): An experimental antiviral drug used in the treatment of CMV retinitis.

Gene: The basic unit of heredity; an ordered sequence of nucleotides. A gene contains the information for the synthesis of one polypeptide chain (protein).

Gene expression: The production of RNA and cellular proteins.

Genital warts: Soft warts that grow in and around the entrance of the vagina and the anus and on the penis. They are transmitted by sexual contact and are caused by a human papilloma virus.

Genitourinary: Pertaining to the urinary and reproductive structures; sometimes called the GU tract or system.

Genome: The genetic endowment of an organism.

Giardiasis: Infection of the intestinal tract with *Giardia lamblia* (a protozoan) which may cause intermittent diarrhea of lengthy duration.

Globulin: That portion of serum which contains the antibodies.

Glycoproteins: Proteins with carbohydrate groups attached at specific locations.

Glycosylation: The attachment of a carbohydrate molecule to another molecule such as a protein.

Gonococcus: The specific etiologic agent of gonorrhea discovered by Neisser and named *Neisseria gonorrhoeae.*

Gonorrhea: A sexually transmitted disease, caused by the bacterium *Neisseria gonorrhoeae,* that is one of the most common infectious diseases in the world. Untreated gonorrhea may spread to other parts of the body and is a frequent cause of infertility.

Granulocytes: Phagocytic white blood cells filled with granules containing potent chemicals that allow the cells to digest microorganisms. Neutrophils, eosinophils, basophils and mast cells are examples of granulocytes.

Hemoglobin: The oxygen-carrying portion of red blood cells which gives them a red color.

Hemophilia: A hereditary bleeding disorder caused by a deficiency in the ability to synthesize one or more of the blood coagulation proteins, e.g., Factor VIII (hemophilia A) or Factor IX (hemophilia B).

Hepatitis: Inflammation of the liver; due to many causes including viruses, several of which are transmissible through blood transfusions and sexual activities.

Hepatosplenomegaly: Enlargement of the liver and spleen.

Herpes simplex virus I (HSV-I): A virus that results in cold sores or fever blisters, most often on the mouth or around the eyes. Like all herpes viruses, it may lie dormant for months or years in nerve tissues and flare up in times of stress, trauma, infection or immunosuppression. There is no cure for any of the herpes viruses.

Herpes simplex virus II (HSV-II): Causes painful sores on the genitals or anus. It is one of the most common sexually transmitted diseases in the United States.

Herpes varicella zoster virus (HVZ): The varicella virus causes chicken pox in children and may reappear in adulthood as herpes zoster. Herpes zoster, also called shingles, is characterized by small, painful blisters on the skin along nerve pathways.

High-risk behavior: A term used to describe certain activities that increase the risk of disease exposure.

High-risk groups: Those groups of people that show a behavioral risk for exposure to a disease or condition.

Histoplasmosis: A disease caused by a fungal infection that can affect all the organs of the body. Symptoms usually include fever, shortness of breath, cough, weight loss and physical exhaustion.

HIV (human immunodeficiency virus): A newly discovered retrovirus that is said to cause AIDS. The target organ of HIV is the T4 subset of T lymphocytes, which regulate the immune system.

HIV-positive: Presence of the human immunodeficiency virus in the body.

Homophobia: Negative bias towards or fear of individuals who are homosexual.

Human leukocyte antigens (HLA): Protein markers of self used in histocompatibility testing. Some HLA types also correlate with certain autoimmune diseases.

Humoral immunity: The production of antibodies for defense against infection or disease.

Hybridoma: A hybrid cell created by fusing a B lymphocyte with a long-lived neoplastic plasma cell, or a T lymphocyte with a lymphoma cell. A B-cell hybridoma secretes a single specific antibody.

Idiotypes: The unique and characteristic parts of an antibody's variable region, which can themselves serve as antigens.

Immunity: Resistance to a disease because of a functioning immune system.

Immune complex: A cluster of interlocking antigens and antibodies.

Immune response: The reaction of the immune system to foreign substances.

Immune status: The state of the body's natural defense to diseases. It is influenced by heredity, age, past illness history, diet and physical and mental health. It includes production of circulating and local antibodies and their mechanism of action.

Immunoassay: The use of antibodies to identify and quantify substances. Often the antibody is linked to a marker such as a fluorescent molecule, a radioactive molecule or an enzyme.

Immunocompetent: Capable of developing an immune response

Immunocompromised: Denotes an individual whose immune system is deficient in defending the body against infection and tumors.

Immunoglobulins: A family of large protein molecules, also known as antibodies.

Immunostimulant: Any agent that will trigger a body's defenses.

Immunosuppression: When the immune system is not working normally. This can be the result of illness or certain drugs (commonly those used to fight cancer).

Incidence: The total number of new cases of a disease in a given area within a specified time, usually 1 year.

Incubation period: The time between the actual entry of an infectious agent into the body and the onset of disease symptoms.

Indirect transmission: The transmission of a disease to a susceptible person by means of vectors or by airborne route.

Infection: Invasion of the body by viruses or other organisms.

Infectious disease: A disease which is caused by microorganisms or viruses living in or on the body as parasites.

Inflammatory response: Redness, warmth and swelling in response to infection; the result of increased blood flow and a gathering of immune cells and secretions.

Injection drug use: Use of drugs injected by needle into a vein or muscle tissue.

Innate immunity: Inborn or hereditary immunity.

Inoculation: The entry of an infectious organism or virus into the body.

Interferon: A class of glycoproteins important in immune function and thought to inhibit viral infection.

Interleukins: Chemical messengers that travel from leukocytes to other white blood cells. Some promote cell development, others promote rapid cell division.

Intracellular: Found within the cell wall.

In utero: In the uterus

In vitro: 'In glass' pertains to a biological reaction in an artificial medium.

In vivo: 'In the living' pertains to a biological reaction in a living organism.

IV: Intravenous.

Kaposi's sarcoma: A multifocal, spreading cancer of connective tissue, principally involving the skin; it usually begins on the toes or the feet as reddish blue or brownish soft nodules and tumors.

Keratin: A waterproofing protein in the skin.

Lamivudine: Also known as 3CT; see 3CT.

Langerhans cells: Dendritic cells in the skin that pick up antigen and transport it to lymph nodes.

Latency: A period when a virus or other organism is still in the body but in an inactive state.

Latent viral infection: The virion becomes part of the host cell's DNA.

Lentiviruses: Viruses that cause disease very slowly. HIV is believed to be this type of virus.

Lesion: Any abnormal change in tissue due to disease or injury.

Leukocyte: A white blood cell.

Leukopenia: A decrease in the white blood cell count.

Lymph: A transparent, slightly yellow fluid that carries lymphocytes, bathes the body tissues and drains into the lymphatic vessels.

Lymph nodes: Gland-like structures in the lymphatic system which help to prevent spread of infection.

Lymphadenopathy: Enlargement of the lymph nodes.

Lymphadenopathy syndrome (LAS): A condition characterized by persistent, generalized, enlarged lymph nodes, sometimes with signs of minor illness such as fever and weight loss, which apparently represents a milder reaction to HIV infection. LAS is also known as generalized lymphadenopathy syndrome.

Lymphatic system: A fluid system of vessels and glands which is important in controlling infections and limiting their spread.

Lymphocytes: Specialized white blood cells involved in the immune response.

Lymphoid organs: The organs of the immune system where lymphocytes develop and congregate. They include the bone marrow, thymus, lymph nodes, spleen and other clusters of lymphoid tissue.

Lymphokines: Chemical messengers produced by T and B lymphocytes. They have a variety of protective functions.

Lymphoma: Malignant growth of lymph nodes.

Lymphosarcoma: A general term applied to malignant neoplastic disorders of lymphoid tissue, not including Hodgkin's disease.

Lytic infection: When a virus infects the cell, the cell produces new viruses and breaks open (lyse) releasing the viruses.

Macrophage: A large and versatile immune cell that acts as a microbe-devouring phagocyte, an antigen-presenting cell and an important source of immune secretions.

Macule: A discolored spot or patch on the skin which is not raised or thickened.

Major histocompatibility complex (MHC): A group of genes that controls several aspects of the immune response. MHC genes code for self markers on all body cells.

Malaise: A general feeling of discomfort or fatigue.

Malignant tumor: A tumor made up of cancerous cells. The tumors grow and invade surrounding tissue, then the cells break away and grow elsewhere.

Messenger RNA (mRNA): RNA that serves as the template for protein synthesis; it carries the information from the DNA to the protein synthesizing complex to direct protein synthesis.

Microbes: Minute living organisms including bacteria, viruses, fungi and protozoa.

Microorganisms: Microscopic plants or animals.

Molecule: The smallest amount of a specific chemical substance that can exist alone. To break a molecule down into its constituent atoms is to change its character. A molecule of water, for instance, reverts to oxygen and hydrogen.

Monocyte: A large phagocytic white blood cell which, when it enters tissue, develops into a macrophage.

Monokines: Powerful chemical substances secreted by monocytes and macrophages. They help direct and regulate the immune response.

Morbidity: The proportion of people with a disease in a community.

Morphology: The study of the form and structure of organisms.

Mortality: The number of people who die as a result of a specific cause.

Mucous membrane: The lining of the canals and cavities of the body which communicate with external air, such as the intestinal tract, respiratory tract and the genitourinary tract.

Mucous patches: White, patchy growths, usually found in the mouth, that are symptoms of secondary syphilis and are highly infectious.

Mucus: A fluid secreted by membranes

Neisseria gonorrhoeae: The bacterium that causes gonorrhea.

Neonatal: Pertaining to the first 4 weeks of life.

Nodule: A small node which is solid and can be detected by touch.

Nosocomial: Hospital-acquired infection.

Nucleic acids: Large, naturally occurring molecules composed of chemical building blocks known as nucleotides. There are two kinds of nucleic acid, DNA and RNA.

Nucleotide of DNA: Made up of one of four nitrogen-containing bases (adenine, cytosine, guanine or thymine), a sugar and a phosphate molecule.

Oncogenic: Anything that may give rise to tumors, especially malignant ones.

Opportunistic disease: Disease caused by normally benign microorganisms or viruses that become pathogenic when the immune system is impaired.

p24 antigen: A protein fragment of HIV. The p24 antigen test measures this fragment. A positive test result suggests active HIV replication and may mean the individual has a chance of developing AIDS in the near future.

Parasite: A plant or animal that lives, grows and feeds on another living organism.

Pathogen: Any disease-producing microorganism or substance.

Pathogenic: Giving rise to disease or causing symptoms.

Pathology: The science of the essential nature of diseases, especially of the structural and functional changes in tissues and organs caused by disease.

Perianal glands: Glands located around the anus.

Perinatal: Occurring in the period during or just after birth.

Phagocytes: Large white blood cells that contribute to the immune defense by ingesting microbes or other cells and foreign particles.

PID (pelvic inflammatory disease): Inflammation of the female pelvic organs; often the result of gonococcal or chlamydial infection.

Plasma: The fluid portion of the blood which contains all the chemical constituents of whole blood except the cells.

Plasma cells: Derived from B cells, they produce antibodies.

Platelets: Small oval discs in blood that are necessary for blood to clot.

PLWA: Persons Living With AIDS.

Poppers: Slang term for the inhalant drug amyl nitrate.

Positive HIV test: A sample of blood that is reactive on an initial ELISA test, reactive on a second ELISA run of the same specimen and reactive on Western blot, if available.

***Pneumocystis carinii* pneumonia (PCP):** A rare type of pneumonia primarily found in infants and now common in patients with AIDS.

Prenatal: During pregnancy.

Prevalence: The total number of cases of a disease existing at any time in a given area.

Primary immune response: Production of antibodies about 7 to 10 days after an infection.

Prophylactic treatment: Medical treatment of patients exposed to a disease before the appearance of disease symptoms.

Protease (protienase): An HIV enzyme essential in processing HIV polyproteins into individual functional units.

Proteins: Organic compounds made up of amino acids. Proteins are one of the major constituents of plant and animal cells.

Protocol: Standardization of procedures so that results of treatment or experiments can be compared.

Protozoa: A group of one-celled animals, some of which cause human disease including malaria, sleeping sickness and diarrhea.

Provirus: The genome of an animal virus integrated into the chromosome of the host cell, and thereby replicated in all of the host's daughter cells.

Pruritis: Itching.

Receptors: Special molecules located on the surface membranes of cells that attract other molecules to attach to them.

Recombinant DNA techniques: Techniques that allow specific segments of DNA to be isolated and inserted into a bacterium or other host (e.g., yeast, mammalian cells) in a form that will allow the DNA segment to be replicated and expressed as the cellular host multiplies.

Rectum: The end part of the large intestine through which feces are excreted from the body.

Remission: The lessening of the severity of disease or the absence of symptoms over a period of time.

Retroviruses: Viruses that contain RNA and produce a DNA analog of their RNA using an enzyme known as reverse transcriptase.

Reverse transcriptase: An enzyme produced by retroviruses that allows them to produce a DNA analog of their RNA, which may then incorporate into the host cell.

Ribozyme: An RNA molecule with catalytic or enzyme-like function.

RNA (ribonucleic acid): Any of various nucleic acids that contain ribose and uracil as structural components and are associated with the control of cellular chemical activities.

RNA viruses: Contain RNA as their genetic material.

Salmonella: A bacterium that may cause diarrhea with cramps and sometimes fever.

Sarcoma: A form of cancer that occurs in connective tissue, muscle, bone and cartilage.

Secondary immune response: On repeat exposure to an antigen, there is an accelerated production of antibodies.

Sensitivity: The probability that a test will be positive when the infection is present.

Septicemia: A disease condition in which the infectious agent has spread throughout the lymphatic and blood systems causing a general body infection.

Seroconversion: The point at which an individual exposed to the AIDS virus becomes serologically positive.

Serologic test: Laboratory test made on serum.

Serum: The clear portion of any animal liquid separated from its more solid elements, especially the clear liquid which separates in the clotting of blood (blood serum).

Shigella: A bacterium that can cause dysentery.

Specificity: The probability that a test will be negative when the infection is not present.

Spirochete: A corkscrew-shaped bacterium; e.g., *Treponema pallidum.*

Spleen: A lymphoid organ in the abdominal cavity that is an important center for immune system activities.

Squamous: Scaly or plate-like; a type of cell.

Stavudine: Also known as Zerit; see d4T.

STD (sexually transmitted disease): Any disease which is transmitted primarily through sexual practices.

Subclinical infections: Infections with minimal or no apparent symptoms.

Subunit vaccine: A vaccine that uses only one component of an infectious agent rather than the whole to stimulate an immune response.

Suppressor T cells: A subset of T cells that carry the T8 marker and turn off antibody production and other immune responses.

Surveillance: The process of accumulating information about the incidence and prevalence of disease in an area.

Susceptible: Inability to resist an infection or disease.

Symptomatology: The combined symptoms of a disease.

Syndrome: A set of symptoms which occur together.

Systemic: Affecting the body as a whole.

T cell growth factor (TCGF, also known as interleukin-2): A glycoprotein that is released by T lymphocytes on stimulation by antigens and which functions as a T cell growth factor by inducing proliferation of activated T cells.

T Helper cells (also called T4 cells): A subset of T cells that carry the T4 marker and are essential for turning on antibody production, activating cytotoxic T cells and initiating many other immune responses.

T lymphocytes or T cells: Lymphocytes that mature in the thymus and which mediate cellular immune reactions. T lymphocytes also release factors that induce proliferation of T lymphocytes and B lymphocytes.

T8 cells: A subset of T cells that may kill virus-infected cells and suppress immune function when the infection is over.

Thrush: A disease characterized by the formation of whitish spots in the mouth. It is caused by the fungus *Candida albicans* during times of immunosuppression.

Thymus: A primary lymphoid organ high in the chest where T lymphocytes proliferate and mature.

Titer: Level or amount.

Tolerance: A state of nonresponsiveness to a particular antigen or group of antigens.

Toxic reaction: A harmful side effect from a drug; it is dose dependent, i.e., becomes more frequent and severe as the drug dose is increased. All drugs have toxic effects if given in a sufficiently large dose.

Toxoplasmosis: An infection with the protozoan *Taxoplasma gondii*, frequently causing focal encephalitis (inflammation of the brain). It may also involve the heart, lungs, adrenal glands, pancreas and testes.

Transcription: The synthesis of messenger RNA on a DNA template; the resulting RNA sequence is complementary to the DNA sequence. This is the first step in gene expression.

Translation: The process by which the genetic code contained in a nucleotide sequence of messenger RNA directs the synthesis of a specific order of amino acids to produce a protein.

Treponema pallidum: The bacterial spirochete that causes syphilis.

Tuberculosis: An infectious disease caused by the organism *Mycobacterium tuberculosis*. It most frequently infects the lungs; however, other organs also may be infected.

Tumor: A swelling or enlargement; an abnormal mass that can be malignant or benign. It has no useful body function.

Urethra: The tube conveying urine from the bladder out of the body.

Urethritis: Inflammation of the urethra.

Uterus: The womb; a pear-shaped, muscular organ which holds the fetus during pregnancy.

Vaccine: A preparation of dead organisms, attenuated live organisms, live virulent organisms, or parts of microorganisms that is administered to artificially increase immunity to a particular disease.

Vagina: The canal which leads from the external female genitalia to the cervix.

Vector: The means by which a disease is carried from one human to another.

Venereal warts: Viral *Condylomata acuminata* on or near the anus or genitals; see Genital warts.

Vesicle: A small blister on the skin.

Virulence: The ability on the part of an infectious agent to induce, incite or produce pathogenic changes in the host.

Virus: Any of a large group of submicroscopic agents capable of infecting plants, animals and bacteria; characterized by a total dependence on living cells for reproduction and by a lack of independent metabolism.

Vulva: The external parts of the female genitalia including the labia majora, labia minora, mons pubis, clitoris, perineum and vestibulum vagina.

Western Blot: A blood test used to detect antibodies to a given antigen. Compared to the ELISA test, the Western Blot is more specific and more expensive. It can be used to confirm the results of the ELISA test.

X-ray: Radiant energy of extremely short wavelength used to diagnose and treat cancer.

Zalcitabine: Also known as HIVID; see ddC.

Zidovudine: Also known as Retrovir; see ZDV.

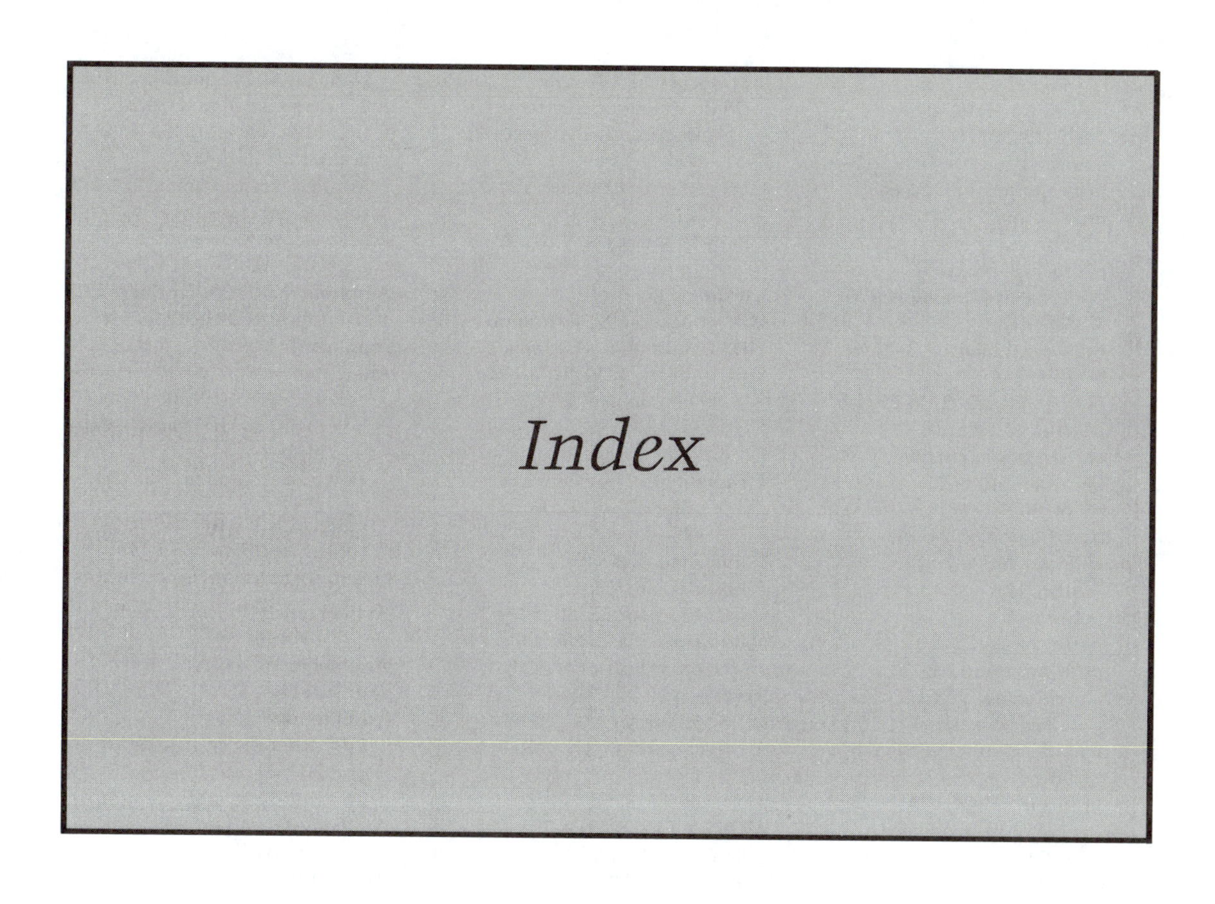

Index